Refining of Lignocellulosic Biomass to Bioenergy and Value-added Products

A Process Engineer's Perspective

Edited by

Mamilla Shyam Sunder and Sundergopal Sridhar

CRC Press
Taylor & Francis Group
Boca Raton London New York

CRC Press is an imprint of the
Taylor & Francis Group, an **informa** business

Designed cover image: © Shutterstock

First edition published 2026
by CRC Press
2385 NW Executive Center Drive, Suite 320, Boca Raton FL 33431

and by CRC Press
4 Park Square, Milton Park, Abingdon, Oxon, OX14 4RN

CRC Press is an imprint of Taylor & Francis Group, LLC

Library of Congress Cataloging-in-Publication Data
Names: Sunder, M. Shyam editor | Sridhar, Sundergopal editor
Title: Refining of lignocellulosic biomass to bioenergy and value-added products : a process engineer's perspective / edited by M. Shyam Sunder and Sundergopal Sridhar.
Description: First edition. | Boca Raton : CRC Press, 2026. | Includes bibliographical references.
Identifiers: LCCN 2025051051 (print) | LCCN 2025051052 (ebook) | ISBN 9781032355993 hardback | ISBN 9781032356006 paperback | ISBN 9781003327608 ebook
Subjects: LCSH: Lignocellulose—Biotechnology | Plant biomass | Biomass conversion | Biomass energy
Classification: LCC TP248.65.L54 R44 2026 (print) | LCC TP248.65.L54 (ebook)
LC record available at https://lccn.loc.gov/2025051051
LC ebook record available at https://lccn.loc.gov/2025051052

ISBN: 978-1-032-35599-3 (hbk)
ISBN: 978-1-032-35600-6 (pbk)
ISBN: 978-1-003-32760-8 (ebk)

DOI: 10.1201/9781003327608

Typeset in Times
by Apex CoVantage, LLC

Contents

About the Editors

Mamilla Shyam Sunder completed his M.Sc. in environmental sciences with distinction from Osmania University, Hyderabad, in 1998 and his Ph.D. in environmental sciences from Osmania University, Hyderabad, in 2012. He has been working as a technical officer in process development in the Chemical Engineering Division at the CSIR-IICT (Indian Institute of Chemical Technology), Hyderabad, for the past 30 years. He has contributed to the development of several technologies for chemical industries as a team member, besides contributing immensely to academic progress. Mamilla Shyam Sunder has published 16 research papers in reputed international journals, such as *Journal of Chemical and Engineering Data*, *Journal of Bioengineering and Bioprocessing*, *Sugar Technology*, and *Journal of Separation Technology*. He has two foreign patents, one book chapter, and ten papers presented in the proceedings of various symposia/conferences to his credit. He has trained more than 300 diploma, B.Tech./M.Tech., and M.Sc. students from various universities and institutes, including Birla Institute of Technology and Science (BITS)-Pilani, Indian Institute of Technology (IIT), National Institute of Technology (NIT), Osmania University-Hyderabad, and Jawaharlal Nehru Technological University (JNTU) for project work. He is a recipient of four prestigious awards: Two CSIR best performance awards and two technology awards for Hydrazine Hydrate and JCERDC projects.

Sundergopal Sridhar is a chemical engineer from the University College of Technology, Osmania University, Hyderabad. He has been working as a scientist in the area of membrane separation processes at the CSIR-IICT, Hyderabad, for the past 27 years, during which time he has developed several technologies for chemical and allied industries through gas separation, effluent treatment, and solvent recovery, besides completing 75 industrial and societal projects. He has also contributed immensely to rural welfare through water purification projects and academic development via extensive HRD and laboratory development in several schools and colleges. He has published 191 research papers in reputable international journals, such as Journal of Membrane Science and Macromolecules, which have been widely cited by peers, totaling more than 12,000 times in high-impact journals, with an h-index of 55. He has 20 foreign patents to his credit, as well as 54 book chapters and 200 papers presented at various symposia/conferences. Sundergopal Sridhar has trained 500 B.Tech./M.Tech and M.Sc. students from different universities and institutes for project work, apart from guiding six scholars in their Ph.D. program. He is a recipient of more than 75 prestigious science awards, including 35 national awards and 3 state awards, such as IIChE Amar Dye-Chem Award 2003; CSIR Young Scientist Award 2007; Engineer of the Year Award from the State Government of Andhra Pradesh in 2009; Scopus Young Scientist Award 2011; NASI-Reliance Industries Platinum

Jubilee Award 2013; VNMM Award from IIT-Roorkee 2015; CIPET national awards for 2016 and 2017; Nina Saxena Excellence in Technology Award from IIT-Kharagpur in 2017; HPCL NGIC Awards for 2019 and 2021; IIChE Jubilant Award; ASSOCHAM Award in 2023; FRSC in 2024; Outstanding Scientist Award from NFED, 2025; and Distinguished Scientist from NESA, New Delhi, in 2025.

Contributors

Mihir Acharya
Cavitation & Mechanochemistry Lab, Department of Chemical Engineering & Process Technology
CSIR-Indian Institute of Chemical Technology
Hyderabad, Telangana, India

Shashi Bhushan
Department of Pharmaceutical Sciences
North Dakota State University
Fargo, North Dakota

Sai Kishore Butti
Membrane Separations Laboratory, Chemical Engineering and Process Technology Division, CSIR-Indian Institute of Chemical Technology
Hyderabad, Telangana, India

Sajja Srinivas Chandrasekhar
Membrane Separations Laboratory, Chemical Engineering and Process Technology Division
CSIR-Indian Institute of Chemical Technology
Hyderabad, Telangana, India

Sugali Chandra Sekhar
Membrane Separations Laboratory, Chemical Engineering and Process Technology Division
CSIR-Indian Institute of Chemical Technology
Hyderabad, Telangana, India

Unnikrishnan Jayakrishnan
Cavitation & Mechanochemistry Lab
Department of Chemical Engineering & Process Technology
CSIR-Indian Institute of Chemical Technology
Hyderabad, India

Boya Jithendra Sai
Sai Department of Nanotechnology
JNTU College of Engineering
Ananthapuram, Anantapur, India

Madupathi Madhumala
Membrane Separations Laboratory, Chemical Engineering and Process Technology Division
CSIR-Indian Institute of Chemical Technology
Hyderabad, Telangana, India

Bishnupada Mandal
Department of Chemical Engineering
IIT Guwahati
Assam, India

Siddhartha Moulik
Membrane Separations Laboratory, Chemical Engineering and Process Technology Division
CSIR-Indian Institute of Chemical Technology
Hyderabad, Telangana, India

Nishnat Muley
Department of Chemical Engineering
Shri Guru Gobind Singh Ji Institute of Engineering and Technology
Nanded, India

Ganugula Naga Srinivas
Membrane Separations Laboratory, Chemical Engineering and Process Technology Division
CSIR-Indian Institute of Chemical Technology
Hyderabad, Telangana, India

Thangsei Nengneilhing Baite
Department of Chemical Engineering
IIT Guwahati
Assam, India

Manideep Pabba
Membrane Separations Laboratory, Chemical Engineering and Process Technology Division
CSIR-Indian Institute of Chemical Technology
Hyderabad, Telangana, India

Pratap Pullammanappallil
Department of Agricultural and Biological Engineering
Innovation Center of Yangtze River Delta
Zhejiang University
Jiashan, China

Mihir Kumar Purkait
Department of Chemical Engineering
IIT Guwahati
Assam, India

Prasansa Rai
Cavitation & Mechanochemistry Lab, Department of Chemical Engineering & Process Technology
CSIR-Indian Institute of Chemical Technology
Hyderabad, Telangana, India

Nivedita Sahu
Membrane Separations Laboratory, Chemical Engineering and Process Technology Division
CSIR-Indian Institute of Chemical Technology
Hyderabad, Telangana, India

Nazia Shaik
Membrane Separations Laboratory, Chemical Engineering and Process Technology Division
CSIR-Indian Institute of Chemical Technology
Hyderabad, Telangana, India

Shrisha Shailendra Raj
Membrane Separations Laboratory, Chemical Engineering and Process Technology Division, CSIR-Indian Institute of Chemical Technology
Hyderabad, Telangana, India

Debosmita Sharmmah
Cavitation & Mechanochemistry Lab, Department of Chemical Engineering & Process Technology
CSIR-Indian Institute of Chemical Technology
Hyderabad, Telangana, India

Mamilla Shree Veena
Department of Chemical Engineering
Anurag University
Ghatkesar, India

Mamilla Shyam Sunder
Membrane Separations Laboratory, Chemical Engineering and Process Technology Division

CSIR-Indian Institute of Chemical Technology
Hyderabad, Telangana, India

Rebba Sowmya
Department of Pharmaceutics
Vijaya Pharmacy College
Vijayawada, India

Sundergopal Sridhar
Membrane Separations Laboratory, Chemical Engineering and Process Technology Division
CSIR-Indian Institute of Chemical Technology
Hyderabad, Telangana, India

Spyros Svoronos
Department of Chemical and Biomolecular Engineering
University of Florida
Gainesville, Florida

Bukke Vani
Membrane Separations Laboratory, Chemical Engineering and Process Technology Division, CSIR-Indian Institute of Chemical Technology
Hyderabad, Telangana, India

Vikonoksh
Department of Chemical Engineering
IIT Guwahati
Assam, India

Na Wu
Department of Agricultural and Biological Engineering
Institute of Zhejiang University
Quzhou, China

Shunchang Yang
Department of Agricultural and Biological Engineering
Innovation Center of Yangtze River Delta
Zhejiang University
Jiashan, China

1 An Overview of Biomass

Shrisha Shailendra Raj, Mamilla Shyam Sunder, and Sundergopal Sridhar

1.1 INTRODUCTION

Biomass is a renewable lignocellulosic material derived from plants available globally in different varieties. Biomass is an organic plant material with heterogeneous and chemically complex renewable resources, which consist of leaves and stalks that do not go directly into food or consumer products. Biomass constantly undergoes complex physical and biochemical transformations to produce many value-added bioproducts. It is reported that 3×10^{10} tons would be generated annually through photosynthetic reactions by taller plants. The biomass cell consists of two major components: the cell and its cell wall. The plant cell wall has cell fractions that contain fats, organic acids, proteins, soluble ash, and carbohydrates. The cell wall contains a fraction of cellulose, hemicellulose, lignin, silica, and cutin. The cell wall fraction contains 60–80% of the total dry matter. The primary crop residues in India include paddy, wheat, cotton, mustard, sorghum, pulses, oilseeds, maize cobs, corn cobs, jute sticks, and sugarcane trash (Wyman, 2018; McKendry, 2002; Chen et al., 2022).

The plant cell wall is primarily composed of three major components: cellulose, hemicellulose, and lignin (Chen et al., 2022). Cellulose, the most abundant organic polymer found in nature, is made up of six-carbon sugar units. Hemicellulose, the second most prevalent constituent of biomass, mainly consists of five-carbon sugars such as xylose. The cellulose and hemicellulose components of lignocellulose are both carbohydrates. Lignin is the third-largest complex amorphous hydrocarbon molecule, comprising many chemical components, including phenols and benzene (Collinson, 2010). Different types of biomass are collected from other sources, as shown in Figure 1.1.

Many countries worldwide utilize lignocellulosic biomass to generate renewable energy, but most lack awareness and continue to rely on nonrenewable energy production. Using nonrenewable energy resources has many disadvantages, as they are limited in supply and may be exhausted quickly. In ancient times, many countries used biomass feedstocks such as cow dung cake, husk, and firewood for their livelihoods. The word "biomass," in general terms, refers to organic material

DOI: 10.1201/9781003327608-1

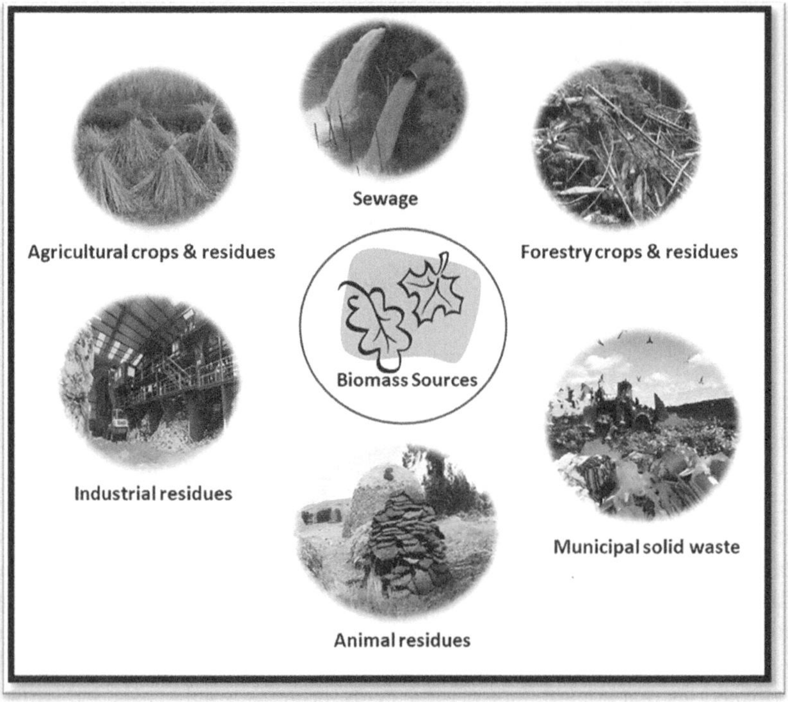

FIGURE 1.1 Different sources of biomass.

that stores sunlight's energy in chemical form, excluding oil, coal, and other fossilized remnants of organisms (Präger et al., 2019).

1.2 BACKGROUND ON TYPES OF BIOMASSES AND SOURCES

There is global concern about the depletion of petroleum-based fossil fuels and their combustion, driven by changes in the global climate and rising carbon emissions. The steady rise in oil prices, supported by convincing evidence, will have a substantial negative impact on economies, reducing economic growth. To address the financial impacts and reduce carbon emissions, many developed and developing countries worldwide need to consider alternatives to fossil fuels. Many challenges involve identifying the best option for sustainable, renewable bioenergy.

Due to increased oil prices and environmental concerns, the global production and use of biofuels have increased dramatically over the past two decades. Second-generation biofuels have generated much interest because they offer the potential to avoid direct conflict with food markets and to rely on feedstocks that could be produced on more marginal lands than prime croplands. The primary feedstock for biofuels and other bioproducts are leaves, stalks, and the residues of sugarcane, maize, and, to a lesser extent, wheat, rice, cotton, sweet sorghum, sugar beet, cassava, and oil crops like rapeseed, oil palm, Jatropha, and Pongamia. Second-generation biofuels are common in the developed world and developing countries. However, they need to embrace the technologies after a careful assessment of the availability of land that has potential for biomass production, besides efficient conversion technologies while adhering to the principles of sustainable biofuels development such as legality; planning and monitoring; greenhouse gasses; sustainability of natural resources (air, water, and land); human rights; food security; and technology innovations. Recent reports from the International Renewable Energy Agency (IRENA) estimate that by 2030, biomass could account for 60% of total biomass production (Makavana et al., 2018).

Developing cost-effective new technologies for biofuels from lignocellulose biomass is a priority for the world community. The following meet the future demand for fuels and other products: various agricultural residues like wheat straw, rice straw, corn stovers; agricultural processing by-products such as rice hulls and sugarcane bagasse; and energy crops such as gasses and tubers, which are abundantly available biomass materials as feedstock and considered to be low-cost, attractive carbohydrate sources for biofuel production. Although several process configurations for biofuel production from lignocellulose biomass have been studied and tested on a pilot scale, no mature technologies producing biofuels at cost-effective prices have been reported. The feedstock collection, material handling issues, pretreatment strategies, cellulose conversion costs, process engineering limitations, and water and energy requirements are predominant technological constraints (Jawaid et al., 2017).

The growing demand for biomass sources necessitates estimating the current availability and prospects of these sources to ensure a sustainable supply. A consortium of seven institutes from the European Union (EU) and six institutes from India took up a study and prepared an inventory of biomass resources in India and in the member states of the EU through a networking initiative sponsored by the Department of Biotechnology and the European Commission under its program (Kenney et al., 2013). The program includes an intensive consultation for the existing and new collection database systems. The information collected in the reports was compiled across biomass sectors such as agriculture, forestry, and biowaste. The results of the studies deliver an overview of the total biomass resources present. Storage and supply management, along with other logistics issues that are largely overlooked, can be considered the central area of study to be prioritized. The biomass databases generated in the inventory show that many countries worldwide, including India, are rich in agricultural biomass and municipal waste. However, due to government rules and regulations, many countries have substantial forest areas that cannot be considered available resources.

1.2.1 Agricultural Residue

Various plants grow seasonally worldwide, depending on climate and water conditions. Agricultural residue is plant material left in the field after harvest. They are grown over multiple seasons each year and vary by plant species, local climate, feedstock, and production technique. Agricultural residues are an important source of biomass that can provide substantial feedstock for the conversion into a wide range of value-added bioproducts. A large area of agricultural land is available in India and some other countries which produce massive agricultural residues, potentially as biomass feedstock for conversion into energy generation. Further, these agricultural residues are categorized into primary and secondary forms. The primary form is obtained in the field after harvesting a plant, and the secondary form is available during processing. Agricultural biomass residues are widely utilized in various applications, including cooking, boilers, and heating furnaces.

Agricultural biomass residues contain high levels of cellulose, hemicellulose, lignin, proteins, starch, and lipids, which constitute inexpensive feedstocks for the production of bioethanol and biodiesel without disrupting the world's food supply. The agricultural biomass residues, such as straws, stalks, bagasse, stems, husks, leaves, peel, shells, pulp, stubble, and cobs, are produced annually.

Straw is an important biomass-based residue. Straws produced after harvesting grains have a yearly production of 520 million tons. Straws are composed of internodes (60%), nodes (11%), leaves (20%), chaffs (12%), and rachis (7%). Among straws, wheat straw is abundantly available and consists of primary cellulose (28–39%), hemicellulose (23–24%), lignin (16–25%), and low levels of ash and protein. Wheat straw has shown potential as an effective biosorbent for treating wastewater contaminated with heavy metal ions. Researchers have investigated its use in a fixed-bed absorber systems for metal removal. Due to its low cost and widespread availability in modern agricultural practices, wheat straw is a suitable reinforcement and filler material for both structural and nonstructural composites (Ahorsu et al., 2018).

1.2.1.1 Bagasse: Sugarcane Bagasse, Sweet Sorghum Bagasse

In tropical regions worldwide, sugarcane is a significant crop across large areas of tropical and subtropical countries. Due to the rising global demand for sugar, sugarcane has become an increasingly attractive crop for farmers, driven by its high productivity and economic potential. The height and diameter of the commercial crop kinds cultivated in tropical areas under typical field conditions are 1.5–3.0 m and 1.8–5.0 cm, respectively. The surface of the sugarcane stalk may appear greenish, yellowish, or reddish and is covered with a thin layer of wax. The stalk comprises shorter segments with joints varying in length from 5 to 25 cm. Each joint contains two distinguishing components, the node and internodes, with the bottom joint being longer and broader than the higher joints. The root band, the bud, the growth ring, and the leaf are all related to the stalk through the stalk structure (Tan et al., 2021; Mahrous et al., 2011).

Bagasse is a fibrous residue containing short fibers obtained after crushing stalks. The composition of bagasse consists of 49.0% moisture, 48.7% fiber, and 2.3% solids. Bagasse is mainly used for burning, and 85% is burned. Bagasse also contains soil or soil deposits in the harvesting conditions. Bagasse contains insoluble materials, such as ash, and soluble materials, such as Brix. Sugarcane bagasse consists of 50% cellulose, 35% hemicelluloses, 15% lignin, and 5% other extractives. But it varies with sugarcane varieties, plant maturity, and soil properties. Brazil is the first country in the world to produce bagasse from sugarcane, which is dedicated to producing sugar and ethanol (Timunget al., 2016).

Sweet sorghum is a potential and essential millet crop, next in importance to rice. Sweet sorghum bagasse is utilized for second-generation biofuel (bioethanol). Sorghum is native to Australia, with some varieties extended to Africa, Asia, and Meso-America. The stem of sweet sorghum contains about 73% moisture, and the solids of carbohydrates are composed of sucrose, glucose, and fructose. Sweet sorghum stalks are used to produce value-added products (Zhu Z et al., 2021; Piskorz et al., 1998).

1.2.1.2 Stalks

Cotton stalks are left in the field, and they are a potential biomass source for the manufacture of value-added bioproducts. Lignocellulose biomass has become a driving force in developing alternative energy, especially for automobile fuels, one of the promising alternative biofuels for disposing of problematic lignocellulose stalk waste from agricultural residues, thereby lowering greenhouse gas emissions (Tatsiopoulos et al., 2003).

1.2.1.3 Cobs

Corn cobs are a cereal grain generally known as maize, which is derived from the Spanish word "maíz." Its height ranges from 2.5 to 7.0 m, and it is a facultative long-night plant with various colors: black, bluish-grey, red, white, and yellow. Corn cobs are the central cone of maize on which kernels grow. Young corn cobs, known as baby corn, can be eaten raw. As the plant matures, its kernels become edible as well (Shariff et al., 2016).

Corn cobs contain 40% cellulose, 42% hemicellulose, 9% lignin, 2% protein, and 2% ash. Corn cob residue has excellent potential as a renewable raw material for the conversion into value-added products and chemicals (Wang et al., 2018).

The following are the uses of corncobs: (1) fiber in fodder for remnant livestock (despite low nutritional value), (2) an industrial source of chemicals and biofuels, (3) for traditional preparation of sweet jelly, (4) in charcoal production, and (5) for household purposes.

1.2.1.4 Husk

Most of the world's population depends on paddy as a staple food, and the biomass residues generated by harvesting and processing include straws, husks, and bran. The husk is the most complex outer coat of the paddy. Rice husk is produced after the processing of paddy at the rice mill, which is used for combustion in the par-boiler or steam boiler in mills. The surplus paddy husk can be used to produce by-products (Pode, 2016).

The physical properties of the husk are crucial for transportation, storage, and related processes. At the same time, thermal characteristics provide specific information about energy production potential – burning crop residue results in

TABLE 1.1
Thermal and Physical Properties of Different Agricultural Residues

Properties	Cotton Stalks	Sugarcane Bagasse	Rice Straw	Rice Husk
Ash content (%)	6.93	3.28	15.20	18.60
Volatile matter (%)	76.07	86.15	64.43	70.70
Moisture content (%)	10.01	11.11	9.89	7.52
Porosity (%)	59.37	84.26	77.24	67.86
Bulk density (kg/m^3)	206.14	723.2	380.54	331.59
Angle of repose (degrees)	43.18	43.24	38.23	37.04

nutrient loss and pollution. Therefore, using agricultural waste as biofuel provides farmers with the best option for handling it. Every phase of calculating the fuel potential of agricultural leftovers uses thermal characteristics (Makavana et al., 2018). Table 1.1 gives the physical and thermal properties of several farm residues.

1.2.2 Forestry Residue

Forest-based biomass is gaining interest as a potential and renewable industrial energy source. Due to changes in climate and rising energy demand, renewable biomass from forests has become indispensable. Trunks, crowns, and branches of unwanted wood from forests, as well as waste products from the production and processing of timber, together constitute the lignocellulose biomass resource known as "forest residue." Forest biomass residue is essential for developing biofuels and other value-added products that replace fossil fuels. The evaluation of the forest area depends on the structure, topography, climate, and soil. The feedstock of forests as a pallet supply is increasing and expanding across larger areas, helping avoid the worst impacts of climate change. The tropical and temperate forests in developing and developed countries, through their supply, are driving industry growth, with increased production of heat and electricity over the past decades. However, the industrial utilization of wood as an energy source is a very complex process with environmental, social, and economic consequences. Recently, there has been concern about climate change, and many legislative measures have been taken to reconsider the role of forest biomass in a modern energy economy (Widjaya et al., 2018). The different types of forest biomass are given in Figure 1.2.

In developed and developing countries, wood is the primary resource for alternative energy derived from globally available harvested wood. Estimates suggest 55% is burned as fuel, and the remaining 45% is used as industrial raw material. Wood biomass consists of stems, branches, twigs, and so forth. Other sources of forest biomass include wood-processing units such as sawmills, plywood mills, and particleboard mills.

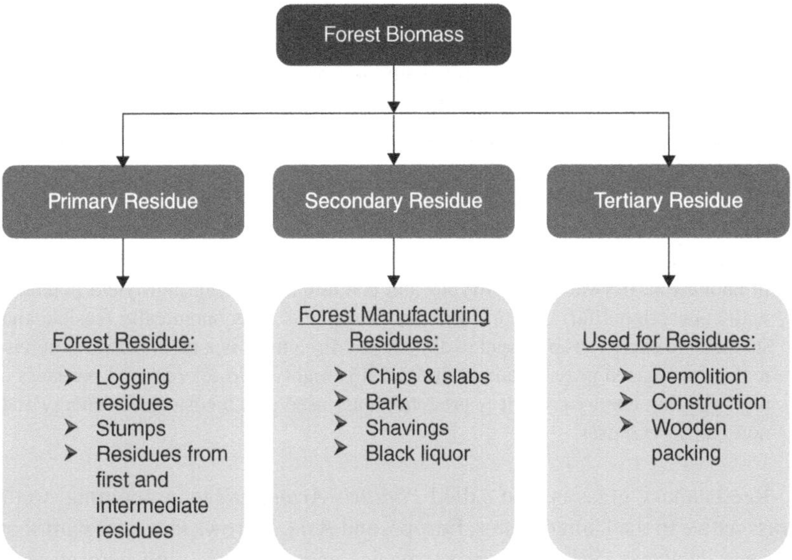

FIGURE 1.2 Various types of forest biomass.

1.2.3 Grasses

The evolution of grasses as an energy source took place in the 1800s. Grasses were widely used for heating fuel in many regions with little forest land. Today, the evolution of highly engineered, automated, and clean biomass burning is taking place. In the near future, the pelleting of grasses may be delivered in bulk via mechanical atomization and combusted for energy production. To substitute for depleting fossil fuels, such as wood, grasses can be used as a stored-energy source. This requires harvesting and processing crops into pellets using pelletizers commercially, after drying in the field. This approach reduces operational costs and makes the process more manageable. Grasses are abundant worldwide and widespread. They are an attractive lignocellulose feedstock for many value-added bioproducts. Grasses offer an innovative approach to biomass utilization, featuring lignin-polysaccharide linkages and elevated carbohydrate content, making them suitable for producing value-added products like bioethanol. Moreover, a deeper understanding of grass-based feedstocks contributes to advancements in *in planta* genetic engineering, enabling the design of synthetic genetic circuits for enhanced application in biorefineries and the production of other bioproducts (Abhijeet al., 2020).

Some researchers suggest that grass serves not only as a primary feed for ruminants such as cows and sheep but also as a promising source of biomass for future sustainable energy and material production. Further, grass can produce high-value protein-rich animal feed, gut health-promoting food, fibers, and biofuel. Perennial grasses have the greatest potential and promise as lignocellulosic biomass for conversion into various value-added products. Grasses grow repeatedly from their roots and do not require re-plantation each year. They also accumulate less fertilizer, energy, and water for production (Shinners et al., 2010). They also tolerate poor soil, flooding, and drought, reducing erosion. Some of the most valuable grass species with potential for conversion into value-added products include the following:

> switchgrass, also known as Panicum virgatum, is one of the best herbaceous (non-woody) energy crops, primarily found in the United States. It grows perennially in habitats across various soil types and conditions, offering high yield potential with conventional farming practices and serving as an economically feasible and sustainable energy crop (Vogel et al., 2002). Miscanthus is a natural hybrid perennial warm-season grass obtained in Asia. It is highly cold-tolerant and produces a high-yielding energy crop. It is predominantly used as a feedstock for energy and non-energy end uses.

Reed canary grass is also called *Phalaris Arundinacea*, a perennial wetland grass native to the United States, Europe, and Asia. It grows in winter with shorter seasons. However, it is an invasive species and competes with natural wetland species (Kukk et al., 2011).

Hemp, also called *Cannabis sativa*, grows worldwide as a fiber crop. It provides fiber for many uses such as animal bedding, paper, canvas, clothing, and rope. Hemp is also recognized for its high nutritional value, similar to that of hemp oil. It is used for food, cosmetics, paint, and as a fiber feedstock for biofuel (Zhao et al., 2020).

1.2.4 Nonwoody Biomass

With the increasing world population over the past few decades, energy demand has risen, leading to the depletion of fossil fuels and necessitating the search for alternative energy sources. Biomass and other biodegradable organic wastes, which are renewable sources, have attracted researchers for their high potential for conversion into biofuels. Abundant raw materials, such as algae, are among the most efficient and promising feedstock sources. As reported, the researchers conducted algal studies many years ago. Still, it has become necessary because the global economy requires energy for various uses such as lighting, mining, transportation, and everyday activities. Energy demand has been steadily increasing, driven by population growth, industrial development, and the rising use of modern amenities. Renewable energy sources can replace fossil fuels and provide greater access to fuel resources for both developing and developed nations. Several countries have developed many technologies, but no single strategy has combined them to substantially decrease our dependence on fossil fuels (Azeez, 2018).

In recent years, there has been growing interest in utilizing non-wood sources as raw materials for pulping and paper production. According to Wisur (1993), only 8% of the raw materials used in 1989 for pulp and paper manufacturing came from non-wood biomass. Currently, less than 10% of global pulp and paper production relies on non-wood sources. These include approximately 44% straw, 18% bagasse, 13% bamboo, 14% reeds, and 11% various other materials. Non-wood fibers produce pulps and papers with unique strengths and properties. Unlike wood, which requires long growth cycles, non-wood fibers can be harvested in a single year, making them a faster, more renewable resource. The fibers derived from plants other than wood are comparable to those of hardwoods. Their fibers have been found to be roughly 1 mm long, thin, and typically lignified (Azeez, 2018).

Algae are a diverse group of organisms and are abundant. This provides researchers with the opportunity to convert these strains into promising sources of biofuels and valuable bioproducts. The production of algae biomass requires only water, carbon dioxide, and other low-nutrient inputs in ponds and pools, making it economically feasible. Algae are a renewable biomass source and provide energy security as a sustainable resource for biofuel production. Algae can produce a high potential of 1,000–5,000 gallons of oil per acre. The major challenge in converting algae biomass feedstock for fuel production is a barrier that accounts for 80–90% of the final fuel cost. The alternative for algal-based valuable products, such as nutrients or pharmaceuticals, will be through the economic viability of the downstream process of the post-oil extraction residues, which consist of large quantities of protein, carbohydrates, and other nutrients that are an attractive source for use as animal feed and other valuable products (Vassilev and Vassileva, 2016).

Regarding their composition, algae are single-celled photosynthetic organisms that require sunlight to convert nutrients into bioactive components of their cell structure. The major bioactive components of algae are proteins, carbohydrates, lipids, and trace amounts of antioxidants and pigments. The cell constituents of various algae majorly acquire lipids, proteins, and carbohydrates (Kartik et al., 2021). Ecologically, filamentous algae and seaweed have different environmental requirements that vary by location and species. They are commonly found in photosynthetic plants, particularly in the microscopic cells of freshwater and marine environments, where they assimilate carbon.

1.2.5 Biomass from Other Sources

Biomass waste is abundantly available in both developing and developed countries and can be efficiently converted into biofuels through biochemical, biological, and thermochemical conversion processes. The following are the sources of biomass that are available for conversion into value-added biofuels and bioproducts economically:

Food industry waste: A significant amount is generated by hotels, restaurants, and community kitchens, including vegetable peelings and vegetable rejects, fruit rejects, and stale food from dishwashers, such as uneaten bread, vegetables, and rice. Food manufacturing units, such as confectioneries and other food processing industries, produce significant waste.

Wastewater and industrial waste: Wastewater generated by industry can cause severe water and soil pollution by discharging into water bodies, leading to health problems and affecting fish and other wildlife. It can serve as a biomass source that can be transformed into valuable bioproducts through a straightforward bioprocess.

Solid wastes: Solid wastes are obtained from fruit and vegetable scraps, pulp, nonstandard food, and fibers from extraction units and filter sludge industries. Usually, these wastes are disposed of in landfills, which can be used to generate biogas through a bioprocess.

Liquid waste: These are produced from meat-processing units, poultry and fish processing, fruits and vegetable cleaning and processing units, and distillery processing units. Wastewater from these industries contains organic compounds that can be fermented into biofuels.

Municipal solid waste: Municipal solid waste (MSW) is a significant source of biomass that can be obtained from households annually, in the order of millions of tons. It is dumped in a landfill, and methane and carbon dioxide can be produced by decomposition. Furthermore, this solid waste is converted into the most efficient biofuel through aerobic, anaerobic processes, or direct combustion (Klemetsrud et al., 2016). Municipal solid waste is generated by domestic, residential, commercial, industrial, and institutional activities. Urbanization, driven by high population density, increases municipal solid waste, a serious concern for local governments' proper waste management. MSW is rich in organic matter, particularly food and vegetable waste, which can be effectively converted into biofuels.

Due to its year-round availability, established infrastructure for collection and disposal, and potential for low cost, MSW is an appealing biofuel feedstock. As preprocessing is required to extract valuable fractions, enhance quality, and alter particle size, MSW has negative costs and is likely less costly than other herbaceous feedstocks. The use of organic components in MSW for biofuels has the potential to reduce greenhouse gas emissions and generate financial benefits, as landfills are the third-largest source of anthropogenic methane from the breakdown of organics in MSW. The situation of MSW in the United States was described by Klemetsrud et al. (2016). The typical mix of MSW produced in the United States is shown in Table 1.2. This indicates that various organic components – such as paper, paperboard, wood, yard waste, and certain plastics – can serve as excellent feedstocks for producing bio-based fuels and chemicals.

Sewage: It is the most important source of biomass that can be converted into energy. The sewage obtained can be collected and processed for biogas production using anaerobic digestion.

TABLE 1.2
National Average Municipal Solid Waste Composition in the United States

Material	Percentage Total MSW before Recycling (251 MT)	Percentage Total MSW after Recycling (164 MT)
Glass	4.6	5.1
Steel	6.7	6.8
Wood	6.3	8.2
Food	14.52	21.1
Paper and paperboard	27.4	14.8

Animal waste: Manure consisting of moisture, organic material, and ash, which can be dried into cakes for use as solid fuel. Animal waste can be converted into biogas, which typically contains 50–60% methane (CH_4) and 30–40% carbon dioxide (CO_2), along with small amounts of nitrogen and hydrogen sulfide. This biogas can be used for electricity generation and domestic purposes, such as cooking, by direct combustion (Zhu et al., 2015).

1.3 CONCLUSION

Biomass is a carbon-neutral energy source because the quantity of carbon dioxide formed during the entire combustion of biomass is equal to the amount removed from the atmosphere throughout the growth stage. Biomass is widely recognized as a renewable energy source and plays a crucial role in shaping future fuel supply trends. In boilers, biomass is an emerging energy source. Numerous aspects of biomass have been researched, including its conversion rates, compositions, assessment of its higher heating value, comparison to other fuels, combustion of biomass, co-firing of biomass and coal, effects of economic and social analysis of biomass, transportation of biomass, densification of biomass, issues with biomass, and prospects for biomass. Biomass from woody and nonwoody renewable resources, which are widely available globally, can be converted into biofuels and value-added products using inexpensive, eco-friendly processes.

Paper mills can employ non-wood biomass to mitigate the environmental hazards caused by ecosystem imbalance resulting from deforestation. Non-wood biomasses, such as crop residues and annual crops, are suitable for manufacturing high-quality pulp and paper due to their favorable properties. They share qualities with those discovered in paper forests. Compared to wood resources, non-wood biomasses are widely available. Non-wood biomass, including crop residues and annual plants, is well suited for producing high-quality pulp and paper due to its desirable characteristics and affordability. For simple manufacturing, effective pulping and bleaching procedures must be developed. Most non-wood fibers exhibit morphological and chemical characteristics comparable to those of wood fibers. As a result, they are practical and helpful in producing pulp with the necessary properties and for specialist papers. Fibers with higher lignin content are more difficult to pulp, resulting in lower-yielding pulps.

On the other hand, biomass presents certain drawbacks, such as high moisture content (ranging from 4% to 60%) and significant investment costs. These challenges have contributed to the slower global adoption of biomass applications.

REFERENCES

Abhijeet P, Swagathnath G, Rangabhashiyam S, Asok Rajkumar M, Balasubramanian P. Prediction of pyrolytic product composition and yield for various grass biomass feedstock. *Biomass Conversion and Biorefinery*. 2020 Sep;10:663–74.

Ahorsu R, Medina F, Constantí M. Significance and challenges of biomass as a suitable feedstock for bioenergy and biochemical production: A review. *Energies*. 2018 Dec 1;11(12):3366.

Azeez MA. Pulping of non-woody biomass. *Pulp and Paper Processing*. 2018 Nov 5:55–86.

Chen D, Cen K, Zhuang X, Gan Z, Zhou J, Zhang Y, Zhang H. Insight into biomass pyrolysis mechanism based on cellulose, hemicellulose, and lignin: Evolution of volatiles and kinetics, elucidation of reaction pathways, and characterization of gas, biochar and bio-oil. *Combustion and Flame*. 2022 Aug 1;242:112–42.

Collinson SR, Thielemans W. The catalytic oxidation of biomass to new materials focusing on starch, cellulose, and lignin. *Coordination Chemistry Reviews*. 2010 Aug 1;254(15–16):1854–70.

Jawaid M, Paridah MT, Saba N. Introduction to biomass and its composites. In *Lignocellulosic Fiber and Biomass-Based Composite Materials* (pp. 1–11). Woodhead Publishing, 2017 Jan 1.

Kartik A, Akhil D, Lakshmi D, Gopinath KP, Arun J, Sivaramakrishnan R, Pugazhendhi A. A critical review on production of biopolymers from algae biomass and their applications. *Bioresource Technology*. 2021 Jun 1;329:124868.

Kenney KL, Smith WA, Gresham GL, Westover TL. Understanding biomass feedstock variability. *Biofuels*. 2013 Jan 1;4(1):111–27.

Klemetsrud B, Ukaew S, Thompson VS, Thompson DN, Klinger J, Li L, Eatherton D, Puengprasert P, Shonnard D. Characterization of products from fast micropyrolysis of municipal solid waste biomass. *ACS Sustainable Chemistry & Engineering*. 2016 Oct 3;4(10):5415–23.

Kukk L, Roostalu H, Suuster E, Rossner H, Shanskiy M, Astover A. Reed canary grass biomass yield and energy use efficiency in Northern European pedoclimatic conditions. *Biomass and Bioenergy*. 2011 Oct 15;35(10):4407–16.

Mahrous AA, El-Shafie MH, Abdel-Khalek TM. Performance of growing lambs fed fungus treated sugarcane bagasse. *Egyptian Journal of Sheep and Goats Sciences*. 2011 Apr 1;6(1):1–10.

Makavana JM, Agravat VV, Balas PR, Makwana PJ, Vyas VG. Engineering properties of various agricultural residue. *International Journal of Current Microbiology and Applied Science*. 2018;7(6):2362–7.

McKendry P. Energy production from biomass (part 1): Overview of biomass. *Bioresource Technology*. 2002 May 1;83(1):37–46.

Piskorz J, Majerski P, Radlein D, Scott DS, Bridgwater AV. Fast pyrolysis of sweet sorghum and sweet sorghum bagasse. *Journal of Analytical and Applied Pyrolysis*. 1998 Jun 1;46(1):15–29.

Pode R. Potential applications of rice husk ash waste from rice husk biomass power plant. *Renewable and Sustainable Energy Reviews*. 2016 Jan 1;53:1468–85.

Präger F, Paczkowski S, Sailer G, Derkyi NS, Pelz S. Biomass sources for a sustainable energy supply in Ghana – A case study for Sunyani. *Renewable and Sustainable Energy Reviews*. 2019 Jun 1;107:413–24.

Shariff A, Mohamad Aziz NS, Ismail NI, Abdullah N. Corn cob as a potential feedstock for slow pyrolysis of biomass. *Journal of Physical Science*. 2016 Jul 1;27(2).

Shinners KJ, Boettcher GC, Muck RE, Weimer PJ, Casler MD. Harvest and storage of two perennial grasses as biomass feedstock. *Transactions of the ASABE*. 2010;53(2):359–70.

Tan J, Li Y, Tan X, Wu H, Li H, Yang S. Advances in pretreatment of straw biomass for sugar production. *Frontiers in Chemistry*. 2021 Jun 7;9:696030.

Tatsiopoulos IP, Tolis AJ. Economic aspects of the cotton-stalk biomass logistics and comparison of supply chain methods. *Biomass and Bioenergy*. 2003 Mar 1;24(3):199–214.

Timung R, Naik Deshavath N, Goud VV, Dasu VV. Effect of subsequent dilute acid and enzymatic hydrolysis on reducing sugar production from sugarcane bagasse and spent citronella biomass. *Journal of Energy*. 2016 Jan 1;2016.

Vassilev SV, Vassileva CG. Composition, properties and challenges of algae biomass for biofuel application: An overview. *Fuel*. 2016 Oct 1;181:1–33.

Vogel KP, Brejda JJ, Walters DT, Buxton DR. Switchgrass biomass production in the Midwest USA: Harvest and nitrogen management. *Agronomy Journal*. 2002 May;94(3):413–20.

Wang Z, Smith AT, Wang W, Sun L. Versatile nanostructures from rice husk biomass for energy applications. *Angewandte Chemie International Edition*. 2018 Oct 15;57(42):13722–34.

Widjaya ER, Chen G, Bowtell L, Hills C. Gasification of non-woody biomass: A literature review. *Renewable and Sustainable Energy Reviews*. 2018 Jun 1;89:184–93.

Wisur H, Sjöberg L-A, Ahlgren P. Selecting a potential Swedish fibre crop: Fibres and fines in different crops as an indication of their usefulness in pulp and paper production. Industrial. *Crops and Products*. 1993;2(1):39–45.

Wyman CE. Ethanol production from lignocellulosic biomass: Overview. *Handbook on Bioethanol*. 2018 May 2:1–8.

Zhao J, Xu Y, Wang W, Griffin J, Roozeboom K, Wang D. Bioconversion of industrial hemp biomass for bioethanol production: A review. *Fuel*. 2020 Dec 1;281:118725.

Zhu G, Zhu X, Xiao Z, Zhou R, Feng N, Niu Y. A review of amino acids extraction from animal waste biomass and reducing sugars extraction from plant waste biomass by a clean method. *Biomass Conversion and Biorefinery*. 2015 Sep;5:309–20.

Zhu Z, Liu Y, Yang X, McQueen-Mason SJ, Gomez LD, Macquarrie, DJ. Comparative evaluation of microwave-assisted acid, alkaline and inorganic salt pretreatments of sugarcane bagasse for sugar recovery. *Biomass Conversion and Biorefinery*. 2021;11:2681–2693.

2 Biomass Today and Tomorrow

Shrisha Shailendra Raj, Sundergopal Sridhar, and Mamilla Shyam Sunder

2.1 INTRODUCTION

Modern bioenergy, which is environmentally friendly, is often regarded as a potential replacement for fossil fuels to lessen humanity's reliance on them (Saidur et al., 2011). The industry is expanding more quickly than others, and 2050 emissions are expected to quadruple. India's rapid economic development is driving a significant increase in the number of vehicles on the road and in motorized mobility, thereby increasing air pollution and greenhouse gas (GHG) emissions from the transportation sector. The Southeast Asian nations, particularly Indonesia, the Philippines, Thailand, and Vietnam, must begin investing quickly in renewable energy generation to address the effects of climate change (Tursi, 2019; Abbasi and Abbasi, 2010). Humanity's primary source of bioenergy, which makes up around 12.2% of world energy consumption, is biomass. In recent years, renewable biomass energy has emerged as an alternative to fossil fuels, which are nonrenewable and deplete quickly. Biomass is available in many countries as indigenous energy sources, including animal waste, agricultural residues, municipal solid waste (MSW), wood residues, fuel wood, oil-rich algae, and market waste, which can generate employment and income for local people. Biomass is also sourced from traditional plantations, home gardens, forest plantations, and other nonwoody grasses, which can produce biofuels and value-added products (Johnson et al., 1995). In developed and developing countries, wood biomass is the primary energy resource, primarily for household fuels and, in developing countries, for industrial energy consumption.

Wood biomass consists of stems, branches, and twigs and is used in saw-milling, particleboard, and plywood manufacturing. Perennial plantation crops such as rubber, coconut, oil palm, cinnamon, tea, cocoa, coffee, and palmyra palm produce large amounts of wood residues that can be converted into valuable products. Agriculture is an essential economic resource in many developing countries and generates large quantities of residues annually, totaling about 140 billion tons. Renewable agricultural biomass materials, such as rice straw, maize stalks, tobacco stalks, and sugarcane bagasse, are generated during the processing of agricultural residues and products. Large amounts of agricultural residues are used as domestic fuels and dumped or burnt openly in the field, a practice referred

DOI: 10.1201/9781003327608-2

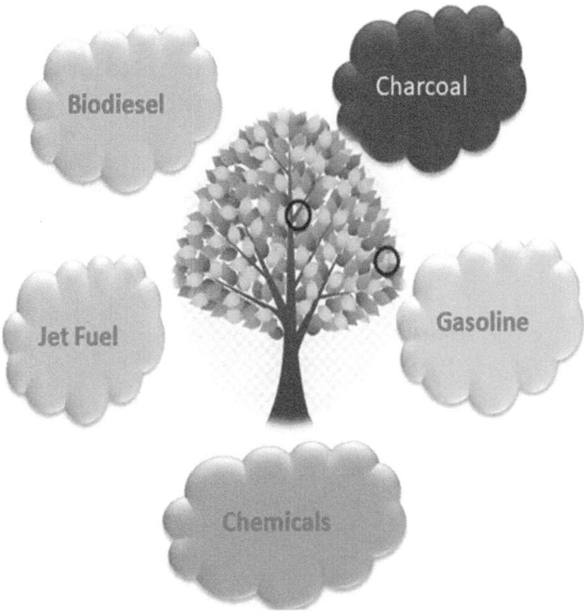

FIGURE 2.1 Various applications of woody biomass.

to as waste-farming biomass (Danish and Ahmad, 2018;Pan et al., 2013). The various uses of woody biomass are shown in Figure 2.1.

2.2 DISTRIBUTION OF BIOMASS RESOURCES ACROSS THE GLOBE

Global biomass demand is expected to double between 2005 and 2050. Due to its rapid economic expansion and extensive industrialization, China has experienced an unparalleled enhancement in energy demand. As the second-largest energy user and owner of the second-largest electrical sector in the world, China has today greatly influenced global energy demand. The primary reason for its rapid development is the use of biomass waste as a renewable source (Wise et al., 2015; Roni et al., 2017). International primary energy consumption over recent years is shown in Figure 2.2.

The major global issue in recent years is coal-fired power. Coal is not only the most prominent source of electricity worldwide, but it is also the primary source of carbon dioxide (CO_2). So, by substituting some of the coal used in co-firing with biomass, CO_2 emissions can be reduced. Co-firing reduces waste and the environmental crisis associated with its dumping because it can reduce the potential ecological impacts associated with burning fossil fuels. Biomass co-firing can play a significant role in achieving this new energy objective. Woody biomass

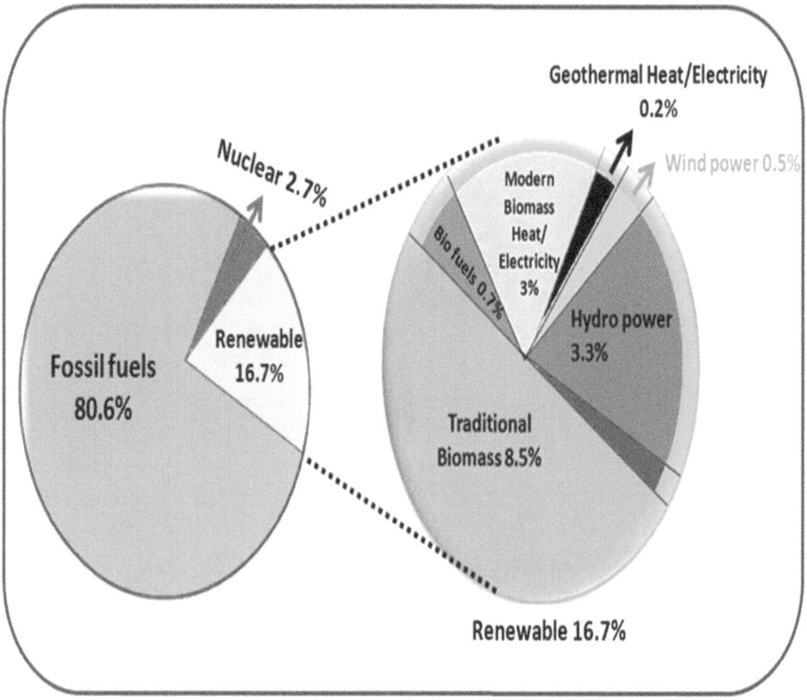

FIGURE 2.2 Global primary energy consumption in recent years.

contains no sulfur, so adding it to coal will help reduce emissions of harmful gases into the environment. Biomass co-firing, however, is not applied in most countries because it is a new concept. A significant part of biomass co-firing plants is sited in European countries such as Germany, Denmark, the UK, and Finland (Baxter, 2005;Vassilev et al., 2015). A review of biomass co-firing across different countries is presented in Table 2.1.

Overall global advantage: The benefits of employing multiple biomass sources primarily focus on overall system cost reduction. As biomass intake throughout the year might be more consistent, the amount of storage space needed could be smaller, enabling essential savings in the storage stage. Additionally, smoother resource needs at the biomass supply chain, including labor and equipment, might significantly reduce costs.

Global limitations: The challenges and constraints this technique poses are largely to blame for the scant research on the multi-biomass approach to date. When multiple biomass streams are involved, logistics can get rather complicated. It is necessary to thoroughly investigate organizational elements, differences in storage, availability, and backup fuel, particularly during wintry weather.

The capacity of the existing energy conversion technology to utilize a fuel mix comprising many biomass types with varied fuel properties, or a fuel whose characteristics change with the season, is one of the primary technical hurdles of

TABLE 2.1
Review of Biomass Co-Firing in Different Nations

Countries	Primary Feedstocks	Biomass Utilization Target	Greenhouse Gas Emission Target	Co-Firing Methods	Average Co-Firing Mixing Rates	Future Outlook
Germany	Straw, sewage sludge, organic residue, waste wood	35% renewable energy share by 2020.	Cut off 65% GHG emission levels by 2030 (compared to 1990 levels)	Direct	5–20%	Germany has begun converting organic waste into biomass in place of specialized energy crops.
Brazil	Rice straw	45% share of renewables in the energy mix by 2030.	The reduction rate in 2024 is 1.5%, and it is expected to be 65% by 2030.	N/A	Expected 30% share of biomass on heat basis	Co-firing is still in its infancy.
The UK	Wood pellets, miscanthus, short rotation coppice, olive/palm residues	15% renewable share by 2020	30% decrease from 1990 emissions by 2030; decrease by 6.2% by 2025; 80% decrease from 1990 emissions by 2050	Direct	3% by heat input	To continue operating and secure subsidies, coal-fired plants might transition to specialized biomass.
The United States of America	Wood pellets, wood chips, railroad ties, and wood wastes	Increase non-hydro renewables generation to 20% of total electricity by 2030;	Reduce net GHG emissions by 17% below 2005 levels by 2020. 2.5% increase in emissions in 2025 and 50–52% by 2030.	Direct	Typically around 5% on an energy basis	According to J.P. Morgan, biomass is expected to account for 6.4% of the targeted 15% of RES by 2020.
The Netherlands	Palm kernel shells, imported wood pellets, waste wood, and cocoa shells	30% biomass substitution of fossil fuels (through time)	43% decrease from 1990 emissions by 2025 and a 90% reduction by 2040.	Direct, indirect	5–34% biomass	It is less economically viable due to reduced subsidies, limited financing, and expensive imports.
Denmark	Straw, wood pellets, wood chips, and waste wood	30% renewable energy in total consumption by 2020, 100% renewable energy supply by 2050	20% reduction in GHG emissions in 2020 compared to 2005. 50–54% reduction by 2025 and expected to be 70% by 2030.	Direct, Indirect	5–100% biomass (100% for parallel boiler)	Co-fired plants may fully transfer to biomass plants shortly. International import costs will still be a problem.
Japan	Wood pellets	N/A	3.8% decrease from 2005 levels by 2020 and 2.5% decline by 2025; about 80% deduction from 1990 emissions by 2050	Direct	3% by mass	47 new coal-fired facilities are under construction, planned, or being assessed for their environmental impact.

the multi-biomass approach. There isn't a perfect answer to this problem. While specific energy conversion systems are susceptible to even small fluctuations in fuel properties, others tolerate variability in fuel characteristics. It is recognized that systems are available that can handle concurrent use of different biomass types with varying fuel characteristics or contamination levels. Additionally, multiple families of biomass types share many of the same traits and features as fuel. The equipment used to handle and treat the various biomass sources is another challenge brought on by the multi-biomass strategy. Most biomass types may be transformed into multiple forms, each needing unique loading, handling, unloading, fuel feeding equipment, and transport. All prospective biomass sources must be handled so that a single type of handling and feeding equipment can be used, or so that only minor, simple, and readily achievable adjustments and customizations are necessary. Otherwise, the benefit of employing different types of biomass to reduce equipment capital costs may be lost. As a result, the multi-biomass strategy requires that the biomass types under consideration have a similar form to allow the use of the same equipment for all of them (Wartha, 1997; Karsch et al., 1983; Ravindranath and Balachandra, 2009).

2.3 AVAILABILITY OF BIOMASS RESOURCES IN INDIA

With continuous GDP growth of more than 8% over the past few years, India is quickly becoming one of the world's fastest-growing nations, which is anticipated to continue. Given that energy is the primary force behind this expansion, maintaining this rate of increase depends critically on its availability. In another 25 years, the official forecasts indicate that energy consumption will have increased by more than three to four times from its current levels. Numerous academics have thoroughly examined the historical development of bioenergy generation in India, including analyses of energy efficiency, decentralized biomass gasification systems, the potential for global warming mitigation, and sustainability. In India, various biomass resources are easily accessible in multiple forms. They are grasses, vegetables, fruits, aquatic plants, and woody plants (Hiloidhari et al., 2014). In India, biodiesel is manufactured by algae and Jatropha. In recent years, power generation applications have mainly relied on various available feedstocks for conversion to biofuels. The conversion of biomass involves two chief process technologies: thermochemical and biochemical. Etherification (mechanical extraction) is the next technology for converting biomass to energy. Thermal conversion includes pyrolysis, combustion, liquefaction, and biomass gasification (Cardoen et al., 2015). With industrial and high economic growth, energy demand in India is also rising, and the country is rapidly developing to meet its energy requirements. In India, mostly nonrenewable energy resources are widely used due to a lack of awareness. Exploring clean, renewable energy sources that can provide reliable, grid-quality power is necessary. In India, biomass has been used for centuries in the form of cake, husk, and cow-dung fuel. Biomass resources available in India, such as grasses, woody plants, vegetables, Jatropha, aquatic plants, and nonwoody algae, are used to produce biofuels. The other biomass sources are energy plantations, crop residues, and domestic or industrial waste (Rai and Proctor, 1986; Tripathi et al., 1998).

2.3.1 Agricultural Feedstock

India has relied on the agricultural sector and rapidly developing agricultural areas for many decades for livelihoods, as most of the population lives in rural areas (i.e., 70% of the overall population). There are millions of villages in India, and even today, many villages still lack electricity. Therefore, there is a plan to electrify the towns using renewable energy sources. Governments in India and other countries have taken alternative steps to utilize agricultural residues for bioenergy. The new renewable energy ministry provides cogeneration and gasification through sustainability and subsidies for biomass. Governments in India and other countries have focused on deploying biomass-based energy (Jain et al., 2018). Biomass from wheat, rice, maize, cotton, pulses (gram and tur), sugarcane, and oilseed (groundnut, mustard, and castor) crops in different states of India is used for biofuel production.

Because of their potential impact and environmental friendliness, biofuels promise an ideal energy solution. Further, biomass resources play a vital role in enhancing the rural economy and generating employment, contributing to overall socio-economic development in the country. The cultivation of biomass at the grassroots level is significant; it is essential to focus on the development of advanced technologies for biofuel production and their applications. India has also recognized the importance of effective biomass utilization to realize the potential of biofuels as excellent technologies and business opportunities. In this context, it became imperative to review and assess the prioritized availability of potential biomass from the Indian perspective. The Technology Information, Forecasting and Assessment Council (TIFAC), India, has surveyed and studied current generation levels, the availability of surplus biomass from selected agro- and forest-residues, and their consumption patterns nationwide. Following up, the National Institute for Interdisciplinary Science and Technology (NIIST), Trivandrum, India, set up a center for biofuels to undertake cutting-edge research on bio-refinery-related technologies (Kumar et al., 2015).

Abundant residues are produced in India due to the availability of vast agricultural land. These residues constitute a potentially available biomass feedstock for energy generation. These biomass residues are obtained from agricultural crop processing after harvesting. While those formed during processing are referred to as processing-based residues, the field-based residues are those formed at the time of yield. The field-based biomass residues are used for animal feed and fertilizers, but can be better utilized for energy applications by processing them.

2.3.2 Source-Wise Classification of Potential Biomass Energy in Indian States

Sustainable biomass resources have been receiving attention worldwide due to the depletion of nonrenewable fossil fuels, which harms the environment

TABLE 2.2
Survey and Data Collection of Some Biomass Residues with the Quality Available in India

Crop	Residues	Biomass Potential (kt/yr)
Paddy	Straw, husk, stalks	169,965.1
Wheat	Stalks, panicle	112,034
Cotton	Stalk, husk, bollshell	52,936
Maize	Stalks, cobs	26,957.7
Jowar	Cobs, stalks, husk	24,207.8
Bajra	Stalks, cobs, husk	15,831
Groundnut	Shell, stalks	15,120.4
Banana	Residue	11,936.5
Coconut	Fronds, husk, pith, shell	10,463.6
Mustard	Stalks, husk	8,657.1

(Murali et al., 2008; Katiyar et al., 2020). Based on the data collection and survey, biomass residues and the quality accessible in India are listed in Table 2.2.

In Indian villages, biomass is abundant because a large population relies heavily on agriculture and cattle. Crops utilized for biomass power include sugarcane, pulses, rubber, grains, and so forth. These crops' various characteristics, such as moisture content, carbon content, and ash content, make them a potential source of biomass. These elements are essential for converting dry and wet biomass into usable energy. Recent research has demonstrated that crops with high yield potential have higher dry-matter yields. Kadam, bamboo, *Melia dubia, and Julie flora are prominent biomass sources used for energy plantations* (Sadi et al., 2021). Table 2.3 shows the zone-wise distribution of available agro-feedstock.

Meisam Sadi et al. (2021) explained the scale-up of biomass-based building cooling system with an innovative design. In this work, an off-grid biomass-based building cooling system was developed, given that India is one of the most populous, hot, and carbon-intensive countries and that its economic and thermal conditions are characteristic. The most advantageous scenario was chosen by comparing three specially designed biomass-firing heaters with varying costs and efficiencies and the two cooling system configurations most useful for the project's goals. The four most frequently used biomass types in India are wood chips, Prosopis, sugarcane bagasse, and rice husk. To investigate the presentation of every situation, MATLAB programming was used to break down hourly, monthly, and yearly financial and natural indicators. These records are the CO_2 emission file, LCOC, and COP. The effect of each biomass cost variance on the FPS was assessed (Sadi et al., 2019;Chaitanya et al., 2018).

TABLE 2.3
Zone-Wise Distribution of Available Feedstock in India

Obtainable Agro-Feedstock	Indian Region	States	Estimated Cost Range of feedstock (Rs/t)
Mustard stalk straw, rice husk, straw and wheat husk, cane trashes, and juliflora	North	Himachal Pradesh, Punjab, Haryana, Uttaranchal, Uttar Pradesh	1,550–3,000
Wood chips, rice husk, and sugarcane	North-east	Jharkhand, West Bengal	1,100–2,600
Stalks of mustard, juliflora, maize, *dhaniya*, cotton, *tuvar*, soybean, and sesame	North-west	Rajasthan, Gujarat	1,300–2,500
Juliflora, rice husk, groundnut and coconut shell, Bengal gram, cane trash, maize stalk, and channa stem	South	Andhra Pradesh, Karnataka, Tamil Nadu, Kerala	1,200–2,500
Cotton stalk, soy and mustards, maize stalks, rice husk, chili, juliflora, and bamboo	Central and south-west	Madhya Pradesh, Maharashtra	1,500–2,800
Rice husk, cotton stalk, sawdust, and Julie flora	Central and south-east	Orissa, Chhattisgarh	1,100–2,600

2.4 CONCLUSION

India has significant potential for biomass as a cheap, environmentally friendly fuel. The necessary knowledge and infrastructure already exist for most biomass energy technologies. Only the required funding must be set aside to advance these technologies and create a strategy for wide-scale adoption. The future of biomass energy hinges on offering trustworthy energy services at reasonable prices. This will only occur in India if biomass energy providers can compete fairly on the market. At the central and state levels, there is an urgent need for a well-organized, centralized, cogent, and consistent biofuel policy. Programs for bioenergy need incentives. Thus, this is a must. Partnerships between the public and business sectors should be supported in the development of biomass energy technologies. For India's bioenergy journey to succeed, a long-term vision is also needed. Traditional plantations, wild forests, forest plantations, backyard gardens, other usable agricultural areas, animal wastes, oil-rich algae, and the organic portions of municipal and industrial wastes are all biomass sources. Another abundant biomass resource available in both developing and developed countries is municipal and industrial waste, which can be used to produce biofuels, chemicals, and value-added products. The expanding bioeconomy industry attempts to increase recycling and safe disposal rates, decrease waste production, and promote waste that cannot be avoided as a resource. In addition to its numerous advantages, biomass as an energy source has several drawbacks. Biomass cannot compete economically with fossil fuels like other renewable energy sources. A significant portion of the loss in India's agricultural biomass is due to post-harvest losses.

REFERENCES

Abbasi T, Abbasi SA. Biomass energy and the environmental impacts associated with its production and utilization. *Renewable and Sustainable Energy Reviews*. 2010 Apr 1;14(3):919–37.

Baxter L. Biomass-coal co-combustion: Opportunity for affordable renewable energy. *Fuel*. 2005 Jul 1;84(10):1295–302.

Cardoen D, Joshi P, Diels L, Sarma PM, Pant D. Agriculture biomass in India: Part 1. Estimation and characterization. *Resources, Conservation, and Recycling*. 2015 Sep 1;102:39–48.

Chaitanya B, Bahadur V, Thakur AD, Raj R. Biomass-gasification-based atmospheric water harvesting in India. *Energy*. 2018 Dec 15;165:610–21.

Danish M, Ahmad T. A review on utilization of wood biomass as a sustainable precursor for activated carbon production and application. *Renewable and Sustainable Energy Reviews*. 2018 May 1;87:1–21.

Hiloidhari M, Das D, Baruah DC. Bioenergy potential from crop residue biomass in India. *Renewable and Sustainable Energy Reviews*. 2014 Apr 1;32:504–12.

Jain N, Sehgal VK, Singh S, Kaushik N. *Estimation of surplus crop residue in India for biofuel production*. Technology Information, Forecasting and Assessment Council (TIFAC), New Delhi; 2018.

Johnson JM, Coleman MD, Gesch R, Jaradat A, Mitchell R, Reicosky D, Wilhelm WW. Biomass-bioenergy crops in the United States: A changing paradigm. *Americas Journal of Plant Science and Biotechnology*. 2007 Jan 1;1(1):1–28.

Karsch T, Stahl U, Esser K. Ethanol production by Zymomonas and Saccharomyces, advantages and disadvantages. *European Journal of Applied Microbiology and Biotechnology*. 1983 Nov;18:387–91.

Katiyar P, Srivastava SK, Kushwaha D. Bioethanol extraction and its production from agricultural residues for sustainable development. *Waste to Energy: Prospects and Applications*. 2020:143–63.

Kumar A, Kumar N, Baredar P, Shukla A. A review on biomass energy resources, potential, conversion, and policy in India. *Renewable and Sustainable Energy Reviews*. 2015 May 1;45:530–9.

Murali S, Shrivastava R, Saxena M. Quantification of agricultural residues for energy generation – a case study. *J Inst Public Health Eng*. 2008;3:27.

Pan Y, Birdsey RA, Phillips OL, Jackson RB. The structure, distribution, and biomass of the world's forests. *Annual Review of Ecology, Evolution, and Systematics*. 2013 Nov 23;44:593–622.

Rai SN, Proctor J. Ecological studies on four rainforests in Karnataka, India: I. Environment, structure, floristics and biomass. *The Journal of Ecology*. 1986 Jun 1:439–54.

Ravindranath NH, Balachandra P. Sustainable bioenergy for India: Technical, economic and policy analysis. *Energy*. 2009 Aug 1;34(8):1003–13.

Ravindranath NH, Hall DO. *Biomass, energy, and environment: A developing country perspective from India*. Oxford University Press; 1995.

Roni MS, Chowdhury S, Mamun S, Marufuzzaman M, Lein W, Johnson S. Biomass co-firing technology with policies, challenges, and opportunities: A global review. *Renewable and Sustainable Energy Reviews*. 2017 Oct 1;78:1089–101.

Sadi M, Arabkoohsar A. Modelling and analysis of a hybrid solar concentrating-waste incineration power plant. *Journal of Cleaner Production*. 2019 Apr 10;216:570–84.

Sadi M, Chakravarty KH, Behzadi A, Arabkoohsar A. Techno-economic-environmental investigation of various biomass types and innovative biomass-firing technologies for cost-effective cooling in India. *Energy*. 2021 Mar 15;219:119561.

Saidur R, Abdelaziz EA, Demirbas A, Hossain MS, Mekhilef S. A review on biomass as a fuel for boilers. *Renewable and Sustainable Energy Reviews*. 2011 Jun 1;15(5):2262–89.

Tripathi AK, Iyer PV, Kandpal TC, Singh KK. Assessment of availability and costs of some agricultural residues used as feedstocks for biomass gasification and briquetting in India. *Energy Conversion and Management*. 1998 Oct 1;39(15):1611–18.

Tursi A. A review on biomass: Importance, chemistry, classification, and conversion. *Biofuel Research Journal*. 2019 Apr 1;6(2):962.

Vassilev SV, Vassileva CG, Vassilev VS. Advantages and disadvantages of composition and properties of biomass in comparison with coal: An overview. *Fuel*. 2015 Oct 15;158:330–50.

Wartha C. Advantages and disadvantages of biomass fuels on a fundamental combustion basis in fluidized beds. In *Fuel and energy abstracts*. Elsevier BV (Vol. 6, No. 38, p. 409); 1997.

Wise M, Hodson EL, Mignone BK, Clarke L, Waldhoff S, Luckow P. An approach to computing marginal land use change carbon intensities for bioenergy in policy applications. *Energy Economics*. 2015 Jul 1;50:337–47.

3 Resources of Biomass, Storage, and Supply Chain

Shrisha Shailendra Raj, Sai Kishore Butti, Mamilla Shyam Sunder, and Sundergopal Sridhar

3.1 INTRODUCTION

Biomass is a stable biological material derived from animals and plants. Biomass was the primary energy source until the 1850s. It is a vital fuel for cooking and heating in many countries, particularly in developing countries. Many countries are promoting the use of biomass fuels in transportation and power generation to reduce carbon dioxide emissions from fossil fuels. Bioenergy is a crucial factor in mitigating climate change, providing more energy than any other renewable energy source. Bioenergy innovation must effectively meet national and international emission reductions across all primary energy sources, including heating and cooling, electricity, and transportation (Adekoya et al., 2023; Balat and Ayar, 2005). In 2015, the world's biomass produced 48 exajoules (EJ) of energy.
In contrast, global total energy production in the same year was approximately 560 EJ. However, there is still considerable untapped potential. The IEA expects the bioenergy supply to reach 160 EJ by 2050 (Adekoya et al., 2023).

This is both an opportunity and a challenge. Biomass chain stakeholders must work hard to increase biomass use to 3.5 times the current levels. The transition to energy technologies and the management of forests and plants have received significant attention, as they are essential to increasing bioenergy potential and ensuring employment security. However, logistics decisions are as crucial as the design and coordination of the entire supply chain to improve delivery and reduce overall cost. Therefore, the supply chain's general theory must realize its potential by developing efficient, economical, and effective sustainable bioenergy products (Ramanauske et al., 2023; Scarlat et al., 2015). There are many plans for bioenergy supply chains. Compared to other renewable sources, bioenergy is more flexible, as it can be stored at various points along the supply chain, giving manufacturers greater control over production schedules and the opportunity to balance energy sources such as wind and solar. The primary focus of this chapter is on the supply chains of biomass from forestry, agriculture, and the cultivation of certain crops. More details on bioenergy and the

DOI: 10.1201/9781003327608-3

associated supply chain for MSW can be found in the WBA report on energy-to-waste recovery (Manzano-Agugliaro et al., 2013). While there are many ways to convert biomass into fuel, some methods are commonly used in supply chain planning. This section describes the purchasing, refining, storage, transportation, and processing of fuel before it reaches the end of the energy transition (Xiong et al., 2023).

The many advantages of using biomass include the following. Emissions of greenhouse gases can be decreased by using biomass energy. Burning biomass emits carbon dioxide, just as burning fossil fuels does. However, the carbon dioxide released by fossil fuels is a "new" greenhouse gas that photosynthesis has trapped for millions of years. In contrast, depending on the energy required for growing, collecting, and processing the oil, the carbon dioxide emitted by biomass is typically influenced by the carbon dioxide it absorbs during natural growth (Ba et al., 2016; Yu et al., 2009). It is ideal for growing biomass on land that has been previously cleared, such as unused cropland, because research has shown that deforestation for biomass results in carbon losses that take years to offset. Thanks to new technologies, agricultural products such as rice straw and corn stalks, leaves, and bark will also be utilized (Deshmukh et al., 2023). Algae, fast-growing trees, and grass are just a few energy crops that require dedicated cultivation and can take a long time to mature. These ingredients can be grown sustainably in areas that cannot support the cultivation of heavy food crops. Fossil fuels, including oil, coal, and natural gas, are now the world's leading energy source. However, energy resources are expected to run out within the next 40–50 years (Deshmukh et al., 2023; Geronimo et al., 2022; Manzano-Agugliaro et al., 2013).

Additionally, the world is striving to reduce carbon emissions by 80% and utilize renewable sources such as solar, wind, and biomass. It seeks to switch to more environmentally friendly renewable energy sources (RES). Further, these sources of renewable energy are less likely to cause environmental hazards such as global warming, precipitation, and urban smog. One of the oldest forms of energy, biomass has unique properties. Biomass waste worldwide makes it very important to discuss all biomass in bioenergy production. The availability of biomass determines the technology used to convert it into bioenergy.

3.1.1 Biomass Sources

Biomass consists of solar energy produced by photosynthesis (Figure 3.1). This energy can be converted into various forms of electricity by combining thermal energy directly or through multiple processes, which are used for business and transportation, continuously converting it into other fuels. Biomass supports farming and agriculture. Primary biomass feedstocks used for energy include municipal waste, wood mill waste, and paper mill products. Soybean oil and corn kernels (used to produce ethanol and biodiesel, respectively) are currently the two most widely used biomass fuel feedstocks (Ghosh, 2016).

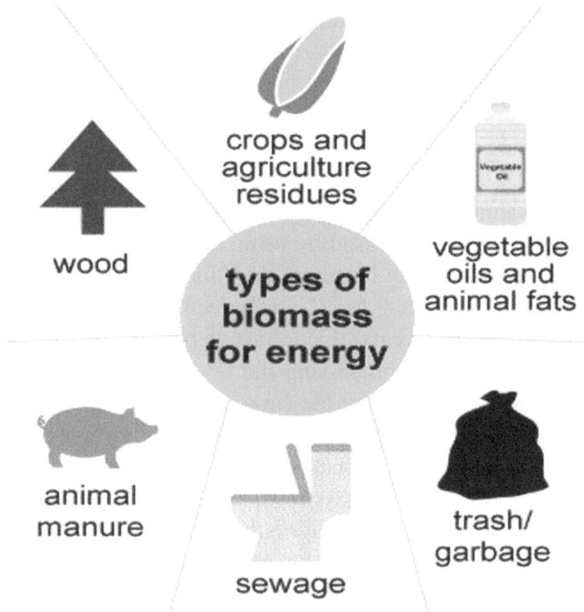

FIGURE 3.1 Types of biomass produced from different sources available for conversion into value-added products (Olatoyan et al., 2023).

Thanks to new technologies, agricultural products such as corn cobs and rice straw, especially the stems, leaves, and bark, will soon be utilized. In the long run, only a few energy crops are suitable for planting and use, including algae, fast-growing trees, and grasses. These can be grown in the sustainable areas that cannot support heavy food crops. "Feedstock" generally refers to sources of biomass that can be used directly as fuel or converted into other energy products. Crops, crop waste, forest leftovers, rare herbs, energy crops, algae, solid waste, and various waste materials, including municipal solid waste and food waste, are examples of biomass feedstocks (Schmidt et al., 2010; Sunde et al., 2011).

The sources of biomass energy are as follows:

- Miscanthus, bamboo, twig grass, kochia, long fescue, wheatgrass, and sweet sorghum are a few of these. Short-term crops are grown and harvested five to eight years after sowing.
- Waste products from agricultural production, such as soybeans, corn, woody plants, sugarcane, algae, switchgrass, and waste from food processing units, are mainly used to make biofuels.
- Paper, wool, cotton, and food wastes are all examples of biological solids that are found in municipal waste.
- Human and animal wastes are used to create biogas and sustainable natural gas.

Nonfood products that are grown marginally, especially for biomass production, are referred to as cash crops. Herbaceous and woody plants form the two main groups of these plants. Perennial plants with more than two years of lifespan are harvested each year when vigorous crops reach the fertile stage. Miscanthus, bamboo, long fescue, kochia, twig grass, wheatgrass, and sweet sorghum are a few of these. Fast-growing trees harvested some years after planting are considered short-term crops.

In addition to sycamores, silver maples, Eastern poplars, walnuts, frankincense, hybrid willows, and poplars are included. Many of these plants can increase agricultural output, provide animal shelter and support annual crops, improve soil and water quality, and generate revenue in various ways.

Agricultural crop residues on lands currently in use offer various options to maximize agricultural resources without obstructing day-to-day food processing, fiber, feed, and other forest products. In a developed country like the United States, there are many types of agricultural crop waste, including stalks and leaves. Examples include wheat, oats, barley, and rice straws. Maize stover (stalks, leaves, husks, and cobs) is another. Selling these wastes to a neighboring biorefinery allows farmers to earn extra money.

The two primary forest biomass feedstocks are whole-tree biomass, specifically harvested for its biomass content, and forest leftovers from timber extraction. After logging, dead, sick, malformed, and other unsaleable trees are frequently left in the forest. This woody waste can be gathered for bioenergy generation while still leaving enough to support habitat and maintain essential hydrological and nutrient processes. There are options for using surplus biomass on the millions of acres of forested land. Overharvesting of woody biomass can reduce the risk of fire and pest infestations and support forest regeneration, productivity, vitality, and resilience. This biomass can be gathered for conversion into bioenergy without impairing the health and stability of the forest's biological structure and function.

Various highly productive species of macroalgae (seaweed), microalgae, and cyanobacteria (formerly known as "blue-green algae") are referred to as "algal feedstocks" for bioenergy. Lipids, proteins, and carbohydrates are fundamental components of biomass produced by many organisms through photosynthesis and nutrient uptake. These materials can be transformed into various biofuels and other valuable products. Algae can grow in fresh, salty, or brackish surface water, groundwater, or ocean water, depending on the strain available. They can also thrive as a secondary source of water forms, such as other agricultural, industrial, municipal, and aquaculture waste, as well as oil and gas drilling activities. They can also grow in water that is used once and discarded, such as that from agriculture, industry, municipalities, and aquaculture.

Mixed business and home garbage is an example of solid waste from municipalities, which includes plastics, paper and paperboard, rubber, textiles, leather, yard trimmings, and food waste. Municipal solid waste presents an opportunity to reduce home and commercial waste, diverting sizable amounts from landfills to bioenergy refineries. Wood-processing leftovers, waste streams, and by-products have high potential. For instance, when wood is processed to obtain various products, sawdust, bark, branches, leaves, or needles are produced. The leftovers can then be used to make bioproducts such as biofuels. As they are already gathered for further processing, these leftovers can serve as useful and affordable biomass sources for electricity generation. Food waste from residential, commercial, and institutional sources is especially problematic because it is currently dumped in landfills. Moreover, the organic-rich solids, which include organic wastes from industrial operations, treated sewage sludge from municipal operations, and various wastes (wet waste), are examples of damp waste feedstocks. Rural economies can generate more revenue and alleviate disposal challenges by converting these "waste streams" into energy.

The three different biomass resources are primary, secondary, and tertiary. Plantation includes trees, herbaceous grasses, and grain biomass. Secondary sources refer to crops or main crops harvested for grain, not for energy generation; however, their by-products, such as husks, shells, straw, and stalks, are used for bioenergy production. Similarly, woody biomass, the main crop such as wood used as planks or in paper production, is not used for energy generation. Still, its logging bioproducts are used for energy production. Tertiary sources of available biomass include end-of-life materials such as discarded wood products.

3.1.2 Biomass Supply Chain

Biomass and bioenergy are essential resources for electricity generation, and they require the right technology to convert biomass into commercial, valuable products. Additionally, managing the preparation and use of biomass products ensures the effective management, storage, and supply chain of plants and their associated nutrients. Supply chain management also encompasses the demand and performance management of various types of biomass. In terms of management, situational analysis is crucial in developing solutions to address primary and secondary sources of biomass and waste products for conversion into biofuels and value-added products (Jazinaninejad et al., 2022; Loy et al., 2023).

Lignocellulosic biomass for sugar production is available as agricultural residues. Chains of slag, corncob, straw, wood biomass, and forest residue are essential for developing and customizing technologies for converting waste into biofuels and other value-added products.

Additionally, trials are currently underway to process municipal waste and other biomass, including algae, into precursors. Only when the unique characteristics of the production process (such as technology, weather, and topography) and the end application result in the generation of environmental, economic, and social benefits from bioenergy is the optimization of the supply chain's operation conceivable (Makepa et al., 2023; Mottaghi et al., 2022). Figure 3.2 shows a graphical representation of the waste biomass supply chain.

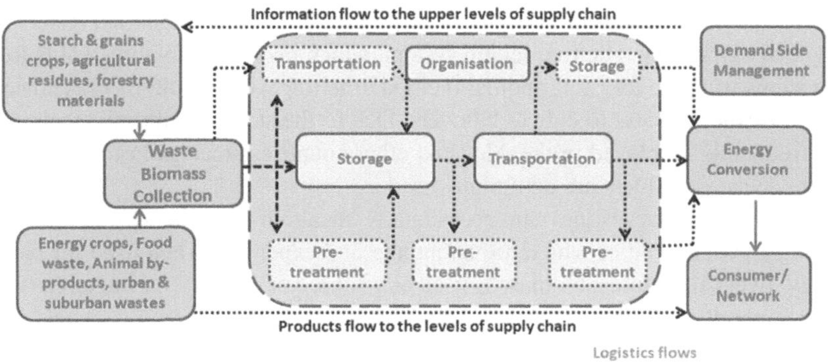

FIGURE 3.2 A typical waste biomass supply chain.

3.1.2.1 Harvesting and Transportation

Depending on the type of feedstock, environmental factors in the area, and the intended use, biomass harvesting and collection vary substantially. Some of these activities include large-scale agricultural harvesting systems, manual gathering of firewood for traditional biomass use in impoverished nations, and cutting-edge methods for collecting and harvesting lumber and forest leftovers. The collection of biomass from various sources and the intended uses of the initial feedstock impact how it enters the feedstock-to-energy supply chain. For example, specific forests or plantations are planted specifically for energy crops. At the same time, other feedstock is gathered from sawmills, conventional forest industry waste, or harvesting waste that cannot be utilized in the wood sector. Leftover foliage and small branches, often left on the site after wood harvesting, are collected for biomass fuel in slash harvesting.

Additionally, residues are produced when specific trees are cut to make room for other trees to expand in diameter. The thinning procedure can also be applied to plantations where most trees are grown for electricity. Chipping is possible along the road or at terminals, either at intermediate storage locations or upon arrival at the plant that converts gasoline or electricity. Tree-falling methods, cut-to-length systems, and tree-length systems comprise the two main types of tree-falling systems and associated equipment. Trees are directly treated after being felled in cut-to-length systems in the forest (Xiong et al., 2023).

They are typically felled and immediately cut into logs 2–4 m long, with branches and crowns removed. These leftovers are in the forest, dispersed across the harvested region, or gathered in unkempt mounds. As a result, gathering slash for energy needs is a distinct phase in the process that incurs extra expenditures. Usually, the slash is left in the forest to dry naturally for a while before being collected. When fuel is required, collection may be preferred to storing large volumes in plant or port storage facilities. Mobile chippers can chop the cut along the roadside, or more often for bigger plants, at or near the plant. The cut-to-length technique is widely used in northern Europe, and forwarders and harvesters are typical machinery. The tree-length system, which involves removing whole trees or stems from the forest, is another method of felling. As a result, there is no need for a further process to collect leftovers. Due to the steep terrain, this technique is frequently employed in the Alps and other countries, such as France and Germany, where skidders are commonly used.

Traditional harvesting can occasionally result in significant pollution and energy losses, both of which are damaging and expensive when used for bioenergy. Every time forest biomass is used as a source of energy, traditional harvesting methods must be adjusted to ensure that the biomass obtained is of very high quality for energy use without negatively impacting the biomass supply chain. Medium-sized to small-scale, partially forest-owner-based harvesting and collection of biomass for heating is another method, considerably distinct from mechanized large-scale systems. Typically, the wood is cut and gathered for individual use in wood boilers and stoves or for sale. These woods are responsibly maintained, and most of the time, a mechanized handheld saw is used for harvesting. The manual collection of biomass for home heating and cooking, which involves cutting trees with axes and other tools, is the final type of harvesting and gathering common in underdeveloped nations. The WBA brief on efficient biomass cookstoves describes this conventional biomass usage.

Residues from crops, unlike biomass from forests and agricultural wastes, are typically harvested in easily accessible locations using procedures similar to those for traditional farm goods, which are often highly mechanized. However, harvesting generally must be completed within a short timeframe and is highly dependent on the weather. Various harvesting equipment for agricultural waste, as well as the biomass produced by the selected harvesting method and feedstock, is displayed. Balers are machines that collect agricultural waste, which is often packaged in bales. Grain is harvested first, leaving other plant materials in the field if it is the primary product of the harvest. After that, a device known as a windrower collects these in rows. The leftovers are then compressed into bales using a baler. Depending on the baler being used, bales can be square, rectangular, or circular and come in various sizes. Square bales are typically denser and easier to handle and carry, even though round bales are generally less expensive to produce. Additionally, bales of certain energy crops are regularly gathered. Simultaneously, windrowing and cutting are to be done if the biomass has a low moisture content; it may not need to be dried on the field before baling; instead, the baling can be completed as part of an integrated process (Nandi et al., 2023; Nunes et al., 2020; Ooi et al., 2022).

- **Forage harvesters**
  Another option for collecting entire materials for use as forage harvesters is to gather standing plants and place them onto trucks using this method. The feedstock is frequently sized down throughout the process, potentially eliminating later stages such as grinding. However, this approach prevents natural field drying.

- **Mobile pelletizers**
  Mobile pelletizers are a less common harvesting option than harvesters. They can function as palletizers, allowing the plants to be pulled by trucks or tractors, or as mobile transport around the field while filled with bales, saving money by avoiding the need to transport the bales to the pellet plant. Alternatively, they can serve as moving pelletizers, eliminating the need for conventional harvesting equipment.

3.1.2.2 Cost Factors in Harvesting and Transportation of Woody Biomass

The availability of biomass resources determines which technologies can be used to convert it into biofuels. Each technology type and choice depend on the number of generic supply chains and the availability of biomass. Obtaining a clean and eco-friendly technology that is cost-effective also differs from harvesting and transportation, as well as screening from the field to the production unit, and thereafter processing whole biomass materials collected into an effective technological process of biofuels at the productive unit until end use (Mutascu, 2023; Ramanauske et al., 2023). A constructive system for evaluating bioenergy production should be adopted, encompassing components of various biomass resources, supply systems, and transportation, as well as enhancing conversion technologies and energy services (Han and Murphy, 2012). The cost of harvesting and refining biomass is a key issue that must be addressed. Supply chain and operations management play a role in selecting the most appropriate technology for converting biomass into biofuels.

Harvest systems for herbaceous feedstocks include combines, rakes, forage harvesters, choppers, and windrowers, while those for woody feedstocks may include skidders, feller-bunchers, and chipper harvesters. Variations occur depending on growing seasons, crop conditions, and environmental factors. The harvested biomass is collected at a centralized location with equipment such as loaders, roadsides, skidders, and cable systems. The processed biomass conventional harvest and collection employ a multi-step system that involves cutting the feedstock and another process to stabilize it, thereby increasing dry matter loss in storage. Biomass storage aims to preserve the valuable qualities of feedstocks until they are utilized in a conversion process and prevent degradation of beneficial components such as sugars. The conventional feedstock system for herbaceous and lignocellulosic biomass shifts the burden of making the resource usable to the producer.

Utilizing logging waste and unsaleable wood for energy involves significant transportation costs. The low bulk density, high moisture content, and lack of homogeneity of the biomass material are the primary reasons for its high energy prices. The costs for transporting various biomasses and converting them into products are fixed per distance traveled, regardless of the distance traveled. Because biomass has a higher density than traditional fossil fuels, transportation costs are undoubtedly significant. Therefore, improving the efficiency of woody biomass during transportation ought to significantly lower overall production costs. In addition to the financial savings, there will likely be fewer adverse environmental effects. Chip vans are typically used to transport woody biomass in supply chains, as they are the most economical method for moving this material. The primary duty is transporting woody goods from saw mills or harvesting sites to pulp and heating plants or export harbors. Planning for the transportation of woody biomass is complicated by the demands of the supply system, including locations, material varieties, vehicle and trailer designs, and the periods involved (Yu et al., 2009).

Transport planners usually organize and send fleets of woody biomass trucks based on their knowledge and experience of the local area. Transport planners cannot efficiently plan transportation routes for small truck fleets without scheduling technologies. However, expanding fleet numbers and supply and demand points often create inefficient, disorganized truck schedules, resulting in long working hours for each truck and protracted wait times at loading and unloading locations. These inefficiencies increase transportation costs and reduce overall output. Many efficient truck scheduling and dispatching technologies have reportedly led to significant reductions in costs and fleet size, thereby increasing transportation logistics efficiency. Using ASICAM, a heuristics-based model created for the Chilean log transport industry, truck fleet size, working hours, and operational costs were all reduced by 31%, 13%, and 13%, respectively. To lower total transportation costs and fleet size while adhering to constraints, quick, precise procedures are essential to provide the planner with thorough routes. These problems have been solved using various algorithms. These answer the truck route scheduling problem using integer linear programming (ILP). However, as computing time quickly grows with problem size, these ILP techniques frequently fail in large-scale situations.

3.1.2.3 Screening of Biomass Supply

Screening is one of the processes in biomass conversion technology and is most commonly used for various biomass feedstocks that are size-reduced by chipping. The obtained ground material is then used for energy conversion. The distribution of particle sizes of feedstocks is one of the essential characteristics that directly affect efficient utilization and handling. Biomass feedstocks, including agricultural residues, forest residues, and other sources, offer opportunities to produce bioenergy and bio-based products. Increasing fuel costs make renewable biomass energy an appealing alternative to nonrenewable fossil fuels. Biomass feedstock size characteristics and specification requirements, such as moisture content and particle size, are essential for biomass conversion technologies (BCTs). Oversized biomass material leads to bridging and inefficient handling, while materials under 3 mm in length reduce air circulation in storage, compromising decay rate and durability. Table 3.1 shows the desired specification for BCTs. Various new technologies are utilized to achieve feedstock specifications for BCTs, and commonly used machinery for biomass size reduction includes chippers and grinders. Chippers are homogeneous in terms of the shape and size of the ground material.

The screening technologies improve product quality by ensuring that the feedstock meets the size requirement for emerging BCTs. Three different sizes of screeners were tested, categorized as under, acceptable, and oversized, and were weighed and independently screened to measure productivity. The biomass materials were divided into two heaps for the star and deck screen machines. The screened materials were collected throughout the screening process to assess the size distribution and moisture content for each size class, categorized as under, acceptable, and large. To analyze the accuracy of biomass size distribution, the screen machine for the samples was studied in a laboratory using an oscillating sieve shaker. Different sieves, numbered six, seven, and eight, are used in the shakes, which are categorized as under, acceptable, and oversized biomass materials. The feedstock material was screened using screening machines, and the definition of sizes under, receive, and oversized should be refined further.

Based on FAO data, Table 3.1 provides an estimate of the total biomass used globally in Europe and the European Union, which includes food crops, fodder, agricultural residues, wood, industrial crops, animal products, and aquatic biomass. The data, however, do not include some of the waste created, such as food-related and other biogenic waste. According to the data, nearly 15 billion tons of biomass were used globally in 2011, many billion tons of biomass were used globally as food and feed, and for processing to produce sugar, starch, vegetable oils, and other items used in the food industry and for materials, and 2.1

TABLE 3.1
Biomass Supply Worldwide

Biomass	World [Million Tons]
Aquatic biomass	181
Meat and animal products	1,153
Wood	2,389
Fiber crops	35
Stimulants and spices	28
Vegetables	1,082
Starchy roots	796
Pulses	68
Tree nuts	15
Sugar crops	2,093
Cereals	2,318
Forest and agricultural biomass	13,434
Stimulants and spices	28
Crops	8,686
Meat and animal products	1,153

billion tons were used for energy. As a result, various semipermeable membranes can be found in the biomass (Zahraee et al., 2020).

3.2 STORAGE AND HANDLING

Most of the time, biomass and biofuels must be stored for shorter or longer periods before being used to generate electricity or heat, depending on the stage of the supply chain. While the forest business operates year-round, in some areas, the demand for heat and power fluctuates significantly by season (S. Zhang et al., 2023). As crop harvesting seasons are sometimes brief, storage methods are crucial for ensuring a consistent supply of biomass that can always meet demand. The primary challenge is frequently placing the solid fuel and feedstock dry, shielding them from rain and groundwater. There are many different storage alternatives, including above- or below-ground buildings designed for a specific location and application, adapted units such as silos and shipping containers, and prefabricated buildings tailored for a particular fuel, such as pellets (J. Zhang et al., 2023).

- **Storage size**
  The storage facility's size is crucial for optimization. A larger storage facility is often recommended, as purchasing larger quantities simultaneously can result in a lower unit price. Additionally, it offers greater scheduling flexibility for deliveries and serves as a backup if a delivery is delayed.
- **Ventilation**
  In addition to avoiding condensation and mold, both of which pose serious health risks if inhaled, it's crucial to ensure adequate ventilation when considering dry biomass to facilitate further drying and reduce decomposition, which can result in energy loss. Furthermore, it's essential to have adequate ventilation to stop high temperatures from becoming a fire threat. Carbon monoxide production is another risk that may be avoided with sufficient ventilation. Due to the hazardous gas produced when biomass is stored in environments with insufficient oxygen, stringent safety norms and regulations now exist.
- **Drainage**
  Additionally, drainage must be included to allow for cleaning of the space if necessary and to prevent water from inadvertently entering the storage area. For below-ground systems, which are often more expensive to construct than above-ground alternatives, ensuring adequate ventilation and drainage can be more challenging. However, the advantage of below-ground systems is that they facilitate easier distribution from tipper-type vehicles and require less space above ground.
- **Wet biomass**
  Just as traditional liquid fossil fuels are transported via pipelines, wet biomass, such as animal slurries and liquid biofuels, is stored in tanks.

Considering how long biomass can be stored without losing quality is crucial, as liquid biofuels can degrade over time, leading to biological deterioration and reduced energy content.

3.3 CONCLUSION

The supply of biomass, the screening process, which involves size reduction through chipping and grinding of feedstock materials used for energy conversion into economical, eco-friendly value-added products, and the control of biomass supply chain resources determine the efficient and effective flows, storage, and consumption of plant-origin materials.

REFERENCES

Adekoya, O.B., Akinbayo, S.B., Ishola, O.A., Al-Faryan, M.A.S., 2023. Are all the U.S. biomass energy sources green? *Energy Policy* 179, 113614. https://doi.org/10.1016/j.enpol.2023.113614

Ba, B.H., Prins, C., Prodhon, C., 2016. Models for optimization and performance evaluation of biomass supply chains: An Operations Research perspective. *Renew. Energy* 87, 977–989. https://doi.org/10.1016/j.renene.2015.07.045

Balat, M., Ayar, G., 2005. Biomass energy in the world, use of biomass and potential trends. *Energy Sources* 27, 931–940. https://doi.org/10.1080/00908310490449045

Deshmukh, S.M., Shekh, M.I., Samal, K., Geed, S.R., Ganguly, A., 2023. Utilization of biomass for energy conservation in agricultural usage. *Bioresour. Technol. Reports* 22, 101480. https://doi.org/10.1016/j.biteb.2023.101480

Geronimo, C., Vergara, S.E., Chamberlin, C., Fingerman, K., 2022. Overlooked emissions: Influence of environmental variables on greenhouse gas generation from woody biomass storage. *Fuel* 319, 123839. https://doi.org/10.1016/j.fuel.2022.123839

Ghosh, S.K., 2016. Biomass & bio-waste supply chain sustainability for bioenergy and biofuel production. *Procedia Environ. Sci.* 31, 31–39. https://doi.org/10.1016/j.proenv.2016.02.005

Han, S.-K., Murphy, G.E., 2012. Solving a woody biomass truck scheduling problem for a transport company in Western Oregon, USA. *Biomass and Bioenergy* 44, 47–55. https://doi.org/10.1016/j.biombioe.2012.04.015

Jazinaninejad, M., Nematollahi, M., Shamsi Zamenjani, A., Tajbakhsh, A., 2022. Sustainable operations, managerial decisions, and quantitative analytics of biomass supply chains: A systematic literature review. *J. Clean. Prod.* 374, 133889. https://doi.org/10.1016/j.jclepro.2022.133889

Loy, A.C.M., Kong, K.G.H., Lim, J.Y., How, B.S., 2023. Frontier of digitalization in Biomass-to-X supply chain: Opportunity or threats? *J. Bioresour. Bioprod.* 8, 101–107. https://doi.org/10.1016/j.jobab.2023.03.001

Makepa, D.C., Chihobo, C.H., Ruziwa, W.R., Musademba, D., 2023. A systematic review of the techno-economic assessment and biomass supply chain uncertainties of biofuels production from fast pyrolysis of lignocellulosic biomass. *Fuel Commun.* 14, 100086. https://doi.org/10.1016/j.jfueco.2023.100086

Manzano-Agugliaro, F., Alcayde, A., Montoya, F.G., Zapata-Sierra, A., Gil, C., 2013. Scientific production of renewable energies worldwide: An overview. *Renew. Sustain. Energy Rev.* 18, 134–143. https://doi.org/10.1016/j.rser.2012.10.020

Mottaghi, M., Bairamzadeh, S., Pishvaee, M.S., 2022. A taxonomic review and analysis on biomass supply chain design and planning: New trends, methodologies and applications. *Ind. Crops Prod.* 180, 114747. https://doi.org/10.1016/j.indcrop.2022.114747

Mutascu, M., 2023. Is biomass energy really sustainable in the United States? *Renew. Sustain. Energy Rev.* 181, 113325. https://doi.org/10.1016/j.rser.2023.113325

Nandi, S., Gonela, V., Awudu, I., 2023. A resource-based and institutional theory-driven model of large-scale biomass-based bioethanol supply chains: An emerging economy policy perspective. *Biomass and Bioenergy* 174, 106813. https://doi.org/10.1016/j.biombioe.2023.106813

Nunes, L.J.R., Causer, T.P., Ciolkosz, D., 2020. Biomass for energy: A review on supply chain management models. *Renew. Sustain. Energy Rev.* 120, 109658. https://doi.org/10.1016/j.rser.2019.109658

Olatoyan, O.J., Kareem, M.A., Adebanjo, A.U., Olawale, S.O.A., Alao, K.T., 2023. Potential use of biomass ash as a sustainable alternative for fly ash in concrete production: A review. *Hybrid Adv.* 4, 100076.

Ooi, W.J., How, B.S., Ng, D.K.S., Yin Ng, L., Andiappan, V., 2022. Analysing the impact of stakeholder relationships in the optimisation of biomass supply chains. *Comput. Chem. Eng.* 168, 108035. https://doi.org/10.1016/j.compchemeng.2022.108035

Ramanauske, N., Balezentis, T., Streimikiene, D., 2023. Biomass use and its implications for bioeconomy development: A resource efficiency perspective for the European countries. *Technol. Forecast. Soc. Change* 193, 122628. https://doi.org/10.1016/j.techfore.2023.122628

Scarlat, N., Dallemand, J.-F., Monforti-Ferrario, F., Nita, V., 2015. The role of biomass and bioenergy in a future bioeconomy: Policies and facts. *Environ. Dev.* 15, 3–34. https://doi.org/10.1016/j.envdev.2015.03.006

Schmidt, J., Leduc, S., Dotzauer, E., Kindermann, G., Schmid, E., 2010. Cost-effective CO_2 emission reduction through heat, power, and biofuel production from woody biomass: A spatially explicit comparison of conversion technologies. *Appl. Energy* 87, 2128–2141. https://doi.org/10.1016/j.apenergy.2009.11.007

Sunde, K., Brekke, A., Solberg, B., 2011. Environmental impacts and costs of woody Biomass-to-Liquid (BTL) production and use – A review. *For. Policy Econ.* 13, 591–602. https://doi.org/10.1016/j.forpol.2011.05.008

Xiong, J., Zhang, S., Ke, L., Wu, Q., Zhang, Q., Cui, X., Dai, A., Xu, C., Cobb, K., Liu, Y., Ruan, R., Wang, Y., 2023. Research progress on the pyrolysis of nitrogen-containing biomass for fuel, material, and chemical production. *Sci. Total Environ.* 872, 162214. https://doi.org/10.1016/j.scitotenv.2023.162214

Yu, Y., Bartle, J., Li, C.-Z., Wu, H., 2009. Mallee biomass as a key bioenergy source in Western Australia: Importance of biomass supply chain. *Energy & Fuels* 23, 3290–3299. https://doi.org/10.1021/ef900103g

Zahraee, S.M., Shiwakoti, N., Stasinopoulos, P., 2020. Biomass supply chain environmental and socio-economic analysis: 40-year comprehensive review of methods, decision issues, sustainability challenges, and the way forward. *Biomass and Bioenergy* 142, 105777. https://doi.org/10.1016/j.biombioe.2020.105777

Zhang, J., Wei, J., Guo, C., Tang, Q., Guo, H., 2023. The spatial distribution characteristics of the biomass residual potential in China. *J. Environ. Manage.* 338, 117777. https://doi.org/10.1016/j.jenvman.2023.117777

Zhang, S., Zou, K., Li, B., Shim, H., Huang, Y., 2023. Key considerations on the industrial application of lignocellulosic biomass pyrolysis toward carbon neutrality. *Engineering*. https://doi.org/10.1016/j.eng.2023.02.015

4 Development of High Biomass Varieties for Value-Added Products

Shrisha Shailendra Raj, Nazia Shaik, Ganugula Naga Srinivas, Mamilla Shyam Sunder, and Sundergopal Sridhar

4.1 INTRODUCTION

A research study on the agro-morphological characterization of chosen accessions of pearl millet has been undertaken to encourage the use of global genetic resources for agricultural biomass. Twenty-two thousand eight hundred eighty-eight accessions of the genus *Pennisetum* from 51 nations make up the pearl millet reference collection, with 13,185 from Africa (Upadhyaya et al., 2007). Locating trait-specific genetic material for crop development requires genetic resources and their characterization for agronomic evaluation, and breeding populations are crucial to ensuring long-term selection advantages.

In the United States and certain other countries or areas, maize-derived sugars are fermented to produce bioethanol, a first-generation biofuel (Reddy and Elanchezhian, 2008). Bioethanol is produced daily for industrial and human use due to intense competition from this feedstock (Jia et al., 2013). The "food versus fuel" argument is usually framed alongside ethical concerns (Chakravorty et al., 2009; Rosegrant and Msangi, 2014). Depending on the inputs required, such as fertilizer, water, and agrochemicals, the environmental benefits of producing these feedstocks might be modest (Fargione et al., 2008). Due to a lack of raw materials and the expansion of the relevant sector, alternative or additional feedstocks for biofuel production became essential (Shen et al., 2011). The best scenario would be for these basic materials to be produced on low-productivity land with little input from crops that aren't currently widely used for food or feed. In addition to bio-based financial systems, crops provide a new application for producing the cells to create feedstocks with unique qualities, either from newly developed crops or from current crops that have been appropriately optimized for bio-based product applications. Biomass such as sweet sorghum is an outstanding renewable energy source with many innovative features (Rooney, 2007; Vermerris et al., 2007). Sweet sorghum is a nonfood feedstock that is notably available to meet the high demand for industrial biofuel and demonstrates the following features.

DOI: 10.1201/9781003327608-4

Initial research indicates that it contains a wealth of liquid and solid sugars and bioactive components, making it possible to create a range of beneficial atomic particles (Dar et al., 2018; Tian et al., 2009). First, the species produces biomass that can exceed 60 tons per hectare and seeds that range from 2,250 to 6,000 kg per hectare, providing a high-quality feedstock for subsequent industrial applications. Second, it uses less nitrogen fertilizer and is more water-efficient than maize (Zea mays L.), resulting in lower input costs (Maw et al., 2019). Third, it may be cultivated everywhere because of its extensive drought tolerance and resilience to saltwater pH fluctuations. Notably, compared to the outcome on a nonsaline site, a 25% reduction in biomass building occurred when cultivated in border and salinized soils (Tang et al., 2018). Specifically, China has over 49 million hectares of low-lying areas suitable for extensive sweet sorghum production, yielding 13.57 million tons of grain and providing sustainable methods for effectively using dry-farming agricultural assets (Jiang et al., 2019; Appiah-Nkansah et al., 2019).

Sweet sorghum is a new-generation crop with a highly effective pigment structure and is highly effective at utilizing soil nutrients to produce bioenergy. It also is a climate-resistant crop that matures earlier on hot, long days. The crop, also known as a crop of the four Fs, can produce high-quality biomass and has a stalk that contains juice rich in sugar, much like sugarcane. It is referred to as "the camel among crops" for its drought endurance and as a "high-energy crop" for its high photosynthetic rate. This crop requires lower water volume, around 8,000 m^3/ha. The development of germplasm is necessary to achieve high biomass and sugar yields for production across various agro-climatic conditions, and this is only achievable by leveraging the genetic resources readily available from many parts of the globe. Higher water, nitrogen, and radiation-use efficiency, as well as resistance to abiotic stressors such as drought, waterlogging, and salt, makes the crop a suitable feedstock for biofuels. The crop contains sugars in the juice, a combination of glucose, sucrose, and fructose that varies by genotype. Breeding cultivars with various maturities is necessary to extend the harvest window and meet the industrial demand over a longer period (Murray et al., 2009; Burks et al., 2013). Breeding would boost annual biomass yields in tropical and subtropical areas by enabling three or four harvests per year (Ratnavathi et al., 2011). Using cultivars can increase the supply of biomass feedstock by increasing biomass maturity, extending the planting season and duration, expanding the planting area, establishing decentralized crushing facilities, and extending the harvest window. The typical characteristics of sweet sorghum are mentioned in Table 4.1. The tall plants produce grain that may be used to feed animals, and the sugars extracted from the stems can be fermented into biofuel. The resultant bagasse biomass is burned for heat and as fodder, but it can also be used to produce second-generation biofuels.

An anaerobic digester uses biomass resources to produce biogas (Molaverdi et al., 2013; Whitfield et al., 2012). Sweet sorghum's ability to fulfill food, fuel, and fodder needs means there is no conflict between the need for food and fuel when growing crops for bioethanol. In various countries, including India, the making of bioethanol from sweet sorghum biomass has been established.

TABLE 4.1
Characteristics of Sweet Sorghum

Serail Number	Characteristics	Sweet Sorghum
1	Sugars	High quantity of reducing sugar and sucrose
2	Invertase activity	High invertase
3	Purity of juice	70–90%
4	Appearance	Juice is turbid and thick
5	Density	High

4.2 BIOFUEL PRODUCTION

Sugar rice juice is found in the stalk of sweet sorghum, a plant related to sugarcane. The juice's ratio of the three sugars, sucrose, glucose, and fructose, varies depending on the type. Sweet sorghum plants develop long stalks and usually produce grains. They have numerous benefits in the debate over whether to use food or fuel, as their grain can be used as feed, and the juice from the stalks can be removed and used directly to make first-generation ethanol. After juice extraction, the leftover waste material can be used to produce second-generation biofuels by removing lignin, thereby increasing the availability of holocellulose for biogas or ethanol production. Asian countries, notably China and India, have been leaders in establishing distilleries that produce ethanol from sweet sorghum. The newest generation of bioenergy crops, sweet sorghum, has an incredibly efficient photosynthetic system and is very effective at extracting nutrients from the soil. Due to its high photosynthetic rate and its ability to survive a lack of soil nutrients and water, it is a suitable crop for bioenergy production. This crop is easily adapted to agriculture and can withstand abiotic stresses, making it ideal for growth on any terrain and for use as food, fuel, fodder, and fiber. As it readily absorbs nitrogen from the soil, it is preferred as a feedstock for biofuel production over crops such as sugarcane, maize, and sugar beet (Chohnan et al., 2011; Rohowsky et al., 2013).

4.2.1 Bioethanol

By converting sweet sorghum to produce bioethanol, we can limit the use of ever-dwindling fossil fuel supplies and greenhouse gas emissions by converting the juice and bagasse into ethanol and power, respectively. About 3500–2500 L of crude oil equivalents could be saved per hectare of sweet sorghum cultivation if the juice is converted to ethanol. The 8%, 16% and 76% of grains, leaves and stems of sweet sorghum may be combined to produce bioethanol. The chemical composition of sweet sorghum consists of moisture (73%), soluble sugars (13%), cellulose (5.3%), hemicellulose (3.7%), and lignin (2.7%). Sucrose, glucose, and fructose are the main components of the juice and can be used immediately to

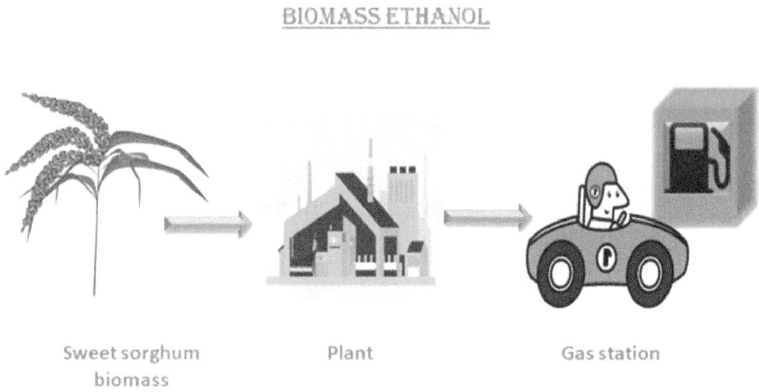

FIGURE 4.1 Biomass ethanol production by sweet sorghum.

initiate ethanol fermentation. After the delicious sorghum stalk juice is removed, the solid debris can be used to produce ethanol. Starch, which is also used in ethanol production, makes up most of the grain in sweet sorghum. Although the yield of sweet sorghum varies with genotype, temperature, location, and soil fertility, it is a potential feedstock for ethanol production (Almodares and Hadi, 2009). The schematic representation of ethanol production by sweet sorghum biomass is shown in Figure 4.1.

The efficiency of ethanol production utilizing different biomass sources from sweet sorghum is now discussed. The significant components of sweet sorghum bagasse, which may be considered lignocellulosic waste matter for ethanol fermentation, are cellulose, hemicellulose, and lignin. Bagasse needs to be pretreated using physical, chemical, or biological methods to partially remove lignin before being hydrolyzed with enzymes such as cellulases and hemicellulases to yield fermentable sugars. In contrast, sweet sorghum juice from stalks can be fermented directly into ethanol. The addition of yeast then triggers ethanol production, and the output of pentoses and hexoses requires a variety of bacteria. Before liquefaction, hydrothermal pretreatment was used to produce a high hydrolysis yield. The results showed that after 12 hr of hydrolysis, saccharification with a high solid load of around 18% dry matter yielded 41.4 g/L of ethanol. To create ethanol, the five varieties of sweet sorghum biomass were treated with H_2SO_4 at 120°C for 1 hr. Using saccharification and fermentation (SSCF), 67.5 g of ethanol was produced per kilogram of fresh sweet sorghum stalk by treating bagasse with acid (2% H_2SO_4) and sweet sorghum juice. The chemical compositions of high biomass sorghum, sweet sorghum bagasse, and Bermuda grass bagasse are provided in Table 4.2.

4.3 IDENTIFICATION OF LOCATION FOR SPECIFIC CULTIVARS OF ENERGY BIOMASS

In many countries, agriculture and forest-based bioenergy are nascent industries, and bioenergy production can reduce the energy supply-and-demand gap, reduce

TABLE 4.2
Chemical Compositions of High Biomass Sorghum, Sweet Sorghum Bagasse, and Bermuda Grass Bagasse

		Composition (%)		
Serial Number	Crop	Cellulose	Hemicellulose	Lignin
1	High biomass sorghum	25–55	15–25	5–8.5
2	Bermuda grass	30–40	25–35	10–25
3	Sweet sorghum bagasse	30–35	15–30	5–20

greenhouse gas emissions, diversify energy sources, and benefit rural communities. The tradeoffs of these emerging markets and associated ecosystem impacts have not been systematically assessed. Bioenergy certification and sustainability standards could be pivotal in deciding whether to use intensive bioenergy. Feedstock production and conversion might negatively affect the environment, aesthetics, and community relationships. In various regions of countries such as the United States, research is being conducted on the environmental and economic efficiency of using forest and agricultural biomass to generate energy. The research community is most likely to be challenged by effects on the ecosystem at the local and regional levels to create new or update existing certification systems with guidelines on how switchgrass or forest biomass-based bioenergy be generated sustainably, but applying the existing certification standards and best management practices coupled with applications of bio-economic models to a wide range of conceivable scenarios might offer insights into the breadth of possible market reactions and biomass feedstock inventory in the future (Kuzovkina and Volk, 2009).

Similar to the complex process of cultivars, the behavior of change in different agro-ecologies with the presence of the Genotype + (Genotype × Environment) [GGE] interaction interprets a cultivar's performance. Hence, to identify location/region-specific cultivars, the multilocation trials (MLT) were conducted during the rainy season with 40 energy Sorghum genotypes in four states of India (Madhya Pradesh, Gujarat, Telangana, and Tamil Nadu), comprising nine target locations: Madhya Pradesh (Gwalior, Lahar, Dewas, and Khargone); Gujarat (Khas and Modasa); Telangana (ICRISAT); and Tamil Nadu (Coimbatore and Bhavaninagar). The data on dry stalk yield were subjected to a GGE biplot analysis using R. The GGE biplot explained 72.06% of the total variation of environments. All nine target locations fall into three major environments. Gwalior, Lahar, Dewas, Khargone, Khas, and Modasa form Mega environment-1; Bhavaninagar and ICRISAT form Mega environment-II; while Coimbatore alone falls under Mega environment-III. The target environments, like Dewas, Modasa, Khas, Khargone, and Bhavaninagar, are more representative. The genotype has performed well and shown greater stability across test locations during rainy seasons. The seed of identified stable lines is provided to farmers for large-scale cultivation (Nair, 2011).

4.4 VARIABILITY FOR TRANSPIRATION EFFICIENCY IN ENERGY BIOMASS

The world economy provides approximately 14% of the total worldwide energy needs from biomass, which has become a significant contributor. Very little research on drought tolerance in biomass has been conducted, apart from the fermentation of lignocellulose biomass (cellulose and hemicellulose), which is predicted to deliver five times higher energy yields per hectare than sugar and starch (non-saturated carbohydrates). Sorghum genotypes can vary in the amount of water use (WU) required during the crop cycle and in the efficiency of converting water resources into biomass (transpiration efficiency, TE). Therefore, studying the variability in WU/TE is essential, as these represent the primary crop adaptations to water-limited environments. In glasshouse pot culture, nine superior high-sorghum genotypes and checks were analyzed for their response to progressive drought stress using a standard protocol (Burhenne et al., 2013).

Transpiration (grams per unit of time), a fraction of transpirable soil water, and transpiration efficiency were assessed; the transpiration rate was assessed gravimetrically in well-watered plants during the natural daylight cycle. The transpiration efficiency is highly variable compared to moisture stress in well-watered conditions, as the total amount of water extracted from the soil varied among genotypes. Still, the differences are minimal under progressive drought conditions. It was also observed that the transpiration rate of some biomass genotypes was generally lower than that of the selected check during the entire daylight cycle. A study showed that high biomass accumulation may not necessarily result in accelerated water exhaustion after drought imposition. This was possible only in the high biomass sorghum lines, which expressed high TE and low TR, and will be promoted for farming for farmers' cultivation in the regions of their adaptation (Kricka et al., 2014).

4.5 IDENTIFICATION OF CULTIVARS AND GERMPLASM FOR HIGH-BIOMASS FEEDSTOCKS

Biomass crops such as pearl millet are cereal crops, significant in the semiarid and arid parts of India and sub-Saharan Africa, where they are produced for food, feed, and fodder. Among cereal crops, pearl millet has the highest resistance to high temperatures during reproduction and the best salt tolerance in areas where water is scarce. It produces high biomass, primarily used as livestock fodder. Owing to its high biomass production potential in marginal environments, biomass such as pearl millet has been identified as a second-generation biofuel crop. A study identified hybrids and open-pollinated varieties with high biomass from new germplasm sources. Around 242 pearl millet biomass mini-core germplasm lines were evaluated for biomass-linked traits during the summer and rainy seasons at the ICRISAT research center in Telangana, India. The dry biomass yield of 2–13 tons/hectare at 85–90 days after planting, with green biomass varying from 6–38 tons/hectare. Based on a two-season evaluation, the 22 best germplasm accessions with high green biomass (25–34 tons/hectare) and dry biomass (9–13 tons/hectare) were identified for further utilization. Sixty-five hybrids, including single-cross and top-cross hybrids developed using high-biomass pollinators at ICRISAT, Telangana, India, were evaluated in Madhya Pradesh and Gujarat, India, along with checks in the rainy season. The five best hybrids had a dry biomass of 13–16 tons/hectare. Also, 50 entries, including earlier identified germplasm accessories and open-pollinated varieties (developed especially for high biomass), were evaluated in Madhya Pradesh and Gujarat, India, along with checks in the rainy season, with recorded green biomass of 19–52 tons/hectare and dry biomass of 4–16 tons/hectare. The 5 best entries had biomass from 15 to 16 tons/hectare. The hybrid showed an early advantage in biomass production; it matures in 100 to 110 days, while open-pollinated varieties/germplasm accessions mature in about 120 days. The identified high-biomass cultivars will be tested on a large scale at the farmer's field to identify stable cultivars, while newly identified germplasm will be utilized in breeding programs for generating high-biomass pearl millet (Hale et al., 2014; Ram et al., 2022).

4.6 IDENTIFICATION OF DROUGHT-RESISTANT BIOMASS FEEDSTOCK VARIETY FOR ENERGY AND WASTELAND RECLAMATION

Worldwide, researchers study various fields to assess the potential of wastelands, thereby identifying drought-resistant biomass for further conversion into valuable biofuels and bioproducts. In India, across multiple nurseries maintained by government organizations such as the National Bamboo Mission and Forest Development, 20 widely distributed native Indian bamboo germplasms were collected. After performing the soil sample analysis of the establishment plots, the collected bamboo germplasm was established as a mother plant at the site maintained by Abelon Agrisciences Limited in Modasa, Gujarat, India. The established mother plants were evaluated for genetic diversity using an ISSR-based molecular marker approach. The plants were multiplied through vegetative propagation after confirmation of genetic diversity among the collected bamboo germplasms. To study the effects of climatic conditions on the survival of vegetatively propagated bamboo plants, vegetative propagation was initiated in different months, with similar effects on plant growth regulators. The vegetatively propagated bamboo plants were hardened for six months before growth under artificial stress conditions. Drought stress screening was performed under drought conditions to assess broad-range salinity stress resistance. The narrow stress range was determined on the basis of the results obtained from the broad range stress resistance screening; the morphological parameters for the plant, like the number of leaves, plant height, stem girth, internodes, leaves, shoots, roots, and salt removal through leaves, were recorded (Kumar and Sharma, 2011; Achten et al., 2007).

4.7 VALUE-ADDED PRODUCTS

Fossil resources are widely used in the industrial manufacture of a wide variety of value-added products. Biomass materials are growing in popularity as a sustainable, affordable, and abundant alternative to fossil fuels in the manufacture of diverse goods with added value. Biomass can be used for various applications such as the synthesis of biodegradable plastics, chemicals, and other materials. Figure 4.2 schematically represents the conversion of biomass into value-added products and biofuels.

Bioethanol, biogas, biochar, bio-oil, and syngas are all products primarily produced from sorghum bagasse and syrup. However, additional by-products from the manufacturing of syrup or ethanol, including processed bagasse, steam, foam, and so forth, as well as leftover vinasse from the dewatering process, may be used to produce energy and produce ruminant or poultry feed (Mazumdar et al., 2012). Sorghum biomass that has been processed or discarded can be used to make briquettes, a form of solid biofuel. Briquettes made from sweet sorghum biomass had gross and net calorific values of 18.9 and 17.7 MJ/kg, respectively. Sorghum briquettes had calorific values equivalent to those of sawdust briquettes (Chaturvedi and Verma, 2013).

Biomass is used to produce biofuels, bioproducts, and crucial industrial chemicals. Some renewable fuels made from biomass include ethanol, butanol, and methanol.

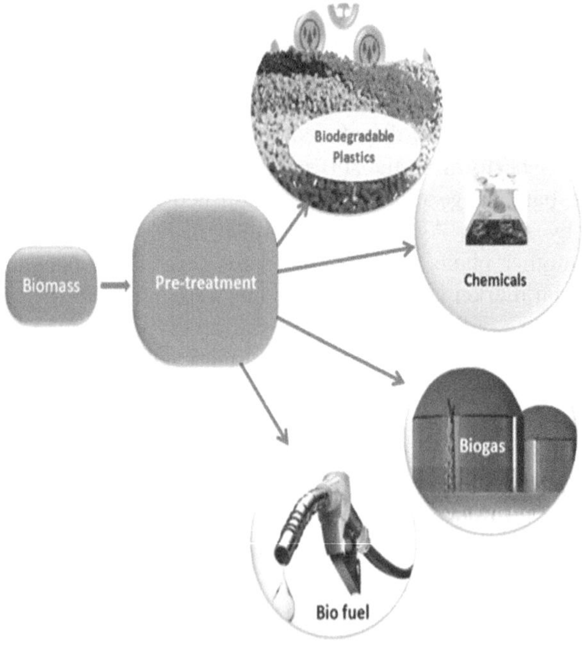

FIGURE 4.2 Conversion of biomass into value-added products and biofuels.

TABLE 4.3
The Benefits and Drawbacks of Using Biomass Resources as Raw Materials to Produce Value-Added Products

Biomass	Advantages and Disadvantages
Corn	They are edible and are widely produced in the United States. A large amount of cropland is devoted to corn, mainly used for ethanol production as a low-cost starch source.
Food biomass wastes	They are both edible and nonedible, have low values, and are released in large amounts by food industries.
Poplar trees	They are nonedible. They grow faster and produce more biomass. Poplar trees can be cultivated year-round. They have environmentally friendly applications such as reducing erosion.
Sugarcane	Sugarcane is edible and grows in the tropics and subtropics. It requires little fertilizer for any application. Sugarcane can be used directly in conversion techniques, as it doesn't require any pretreatment. Its bagasse and waste products are important feedstock for value-added products.
Switchgrass and miscanthus	They are nonedible. Usually, Miscanthus produces more biomass compared to switchgrass. They don't have to be replanted every year. They require significantly less water and low energy for production. They also need less fertilizer to use for any application.

Another popular liquid biofuel is biodiesel, which is produced independently of the lignocellulosic portion of the biomass. Through a transesterification process, vegetable or animal fat, alcohol, and a catalyst are used to create biodiesel. Biomass can be used to produce critical carbon-based compounds and materials, known as bioproducts, in addition to energy and fuel. These products include cellulose fiber and derivatives, furfurals, resins, carbonaceous materials, sugars and glycerin, sugar alcohols, and bioplastics. Treating wastewater (as an adsorbent and filter), as a catalyst, as a catalyst support, and as a storage material are only a few uses for activated carbons. Natural precursors to furan-based compounds include furfural. It has been seen as a crucial component in the manufacture of chemicals derived from nonpetroleum sources, a new generation of bioplastics, and possible biofuels or fuel additives. For instance, due to its low caloric and anticarcinogenic qualities, xylitol, a pentose sugar alcohol, is a sugar alternative in the food business. In addition, xylitol serves as a precursor for several industrial compounds. Although lignocellulosic biomass is an inedible component of plants, it is increasingly popular as a clean, sustainable energy source. Biomass resources can be used to produce products of added value such as biofuels, bioproducts, and crucial industrial chemicals (Irmak, 2017). Table 4.3 shows the advantages and disadvantages of some biomass used to produce value-added products.

4.8 OUTPUT ACROSS THE GLOBAL RESEARCH

A significant source of food and industrial goods is sorghum grain. Many sorghum-based inventions and products have recently been granted patents. With sweet sorghum, every part of the plant has a purpose. Food, feed, and drinks may be made from grain; sugar can be made from the stalk; biofuel can be made from the roots; the cover can be made from the peduncle; and brooms and pot-scouring brushes can be made from the spikes that have been through the threshing process. One of the cereal crops that can withstand drought best is sweet sorghum, which lowers irrigation and other farm expenses. A collection of patents relating to sweet sorghum has several uses in feed, food, and biofuels.

4.9 CONCLUSION

Agricultural biomass from specific germplasm can improve the development of feedstock varieties across various fields for potential utilization of wasteland, thereby identifying drought-resistant biomass for further conversion into valuable biofuels and bioproducts. The capacity to produce ethanol from lignocellulosic biomass may become significantly more economically viable with the genetic improvement of agricultural plant and tree species. In the near future, some communities' biofuel economies are projected to improve significantly through the crop species maize and sorghum. However, significant funding for genetic research will be required to improve the program's effectiveness and profitability. Combining various genetic resources and methods, such as genome sequencing initiatives, accessibility genetic analysis of complex traits, knowledge-based plant breeding, and mutants and transgenics, along with improvements in chemical analytical methods and bioprocess engineering, will benefit this effort. Effective collaboration among researchers across all areas will be essential to accelerate this envisioned energy revolution as this knowledge develops.

REFERENCES

Achten WM, Mathijs E, Verchot L, Singh VP, Aerts R, Muys B. Jatropha biodiesel fueling sustainability? *Biofuels, Bioproducts and Biorefining: Innovation for a Sustainable Economy*. 2007 Dec;1(4):283–91.

Almodares A, Hadi MR. Production of bioethanol from sweet sorghum: A review. *African Journal of Agricultural Research*. 2009 Sep 30;4(9):772–80.

Almodares A, Hadi MR, Ahmadpour H. Sorghum stem yield and soluble carbohydrates under different salinity levels. *African Journal of Biotechnology*. 2008;7:4051–5.

Appiah-Nkansah NB, Li J, Rooney W, Wang D. A review of sweet sorghum as a viable renewable bioenergy crop and its techno-economic analysis. *Renewable Energy*. 2019 Dec 1;143:1121–32.

Burhenne L, Messmer J, Aicher T, Laborie MP. The effect of the biomass components lignin, cellulose, and hemicellulose on TGA and fixed bed pyrolysis. *Journal of Analytical and Applied Pyrolysis*. 2013 May 1;101:177–84.

Burks PS, Felderhoff TJ, Viator HP, Rooney WL. The influence of hybrid maturity and planting date on sweet sorghum productivity during a harvest season. *Agron. J.*2013;105(1):263. https://doi.org/10.2134/agronj2012.0317.

Chakravorty S, Ghosh C, Joydip M. Effect of spacing on growth and yield of French bean (*Phaseolus vulgaris* L.) in red and lateritic belt of West Bengal. *Environment and Ecology*. 2009;27(2):493–5.

Chaturvedi V, Verma P. An overview of key pretreatment processes employed for bioconversion of lignocellulosic biomass into biofuels and value-added products. *3 Biotech*. 2013 Oct;3:415–31.

Chohnan S, Nakane M, Rahman MH, Nitta Y, Yoshiura T, Ohta H, Kurusu Y. Fuel ethanol production from sweet sorghum using repeated-batch fermentation. *Journal of Bioscience and Bioengineering*. 2011 Apr 1;111(4):433–6.

Dar RA, Dar EA, Kaur A, Phutela UG. Sweet sorghum—a promising alternative feedstock for biofuel production. *Renewable and Sustainable Energy Reviews*. 2018 Feb 1;82:4070–90.

Fargione J, Hill J, Tilman D, Polasky S, Hawthorne P. Land clearing and the biofuel carbon debt. *Science*. 2008 Feb 29;319(5867):1235–8.

Hale AL, Viator RP, Veremis JC. Identification of freeze-tolerant Saccharum spontaneum accessions through a pot-based study for use in sugarcane germplasm enhancement for adaptation to temperate climates. *Biomass and Bioenergy*. 2014 Feb 1;61:53–7.

Irmak S. Biomass as raw material for production of high-value products. *Biomass Volume Estimation and Valorization for Energy*. 2017 Feb 22:201–25.

Jia G, Fu Y, He C. Reversible RNA adenosine methylation in biological regulation. *Trends in Genetics*. 2013 Feb 1;29(2):108–15.

Jiang D, Hao M, Fu J, Liu K, Yan X. Potential bioethanol production from sweet sorghum on marginal land in China. *Journal of Cleaner Production*. 2019 May 20;220:225–34.

Kricka W, Fitzpatrick J, Bond U. Metabolic engineering of yeasts by heterologous enzyme production for degradation of cellulose and hemicellulose from biomass: A perspective. *Frontiers in Microbiology*. 2014 Apr 22;5:174.

Kumar A, Sharma S. Potential non-edible oil resources as biodiesel feedstock: An Indian perspective. *Renewable and Sustainable Energy Reviews*. 2011 May 1;15(4):1791–800.

Kuzovkina YA, Volk TA. The characterization of willow (Salix L.) varieties for use in ecological engineering applications: Coordination of structure, function, and autecology. *Ecological Engineering*. 2009 Aug 1;35(8):1178–89.

Maw MJ, Houx III JH, Fritschi FB. Nitrogen content and use efficiency of sweet sorghum grown in the lower Midwest. *Agronomy Journal*. 2019 Nov;111(6):2920–8.

Mazumdar SD, Poshadri A, Srinivasa Rao P, Ravinder Reddy CH, Reddy BV. Innovative use of sweet sorghum juice in the beverage industry. *International Food Research Journal*. 2012;19(4):1361–6.

Molaverdi M, Karimi K, Khanahmadi M, Goshadrou A. Enhanced sweet sorghum stalk to ethanol by fungus Mucor indicus using solid state fermentation followed by simultaneous saccharification and fermentation. *Industrial Crops and Products*. 2013 Aug 1;49:580–5.

Murray SC, Rooney WL, Hamblin MT, Mitchell SE, Kresovich S. 2009. Sweet sorghum genetic diversity and association mapping for brix and height. *Plant Genome*. 2009;2:48–62.

Nair NV. Sugarcane varietal development programmes in India: An overview. *Sugar Tech*. 2011 Dec;13:275–80.

Ram B, Hemaprabha G, Singh BD, Appunu C. History and current status of sugarcane breeding, germplasm development and molecular biology in India. *Sugar Tech*. 2022 Feb;24(1):4–29.

Ratnavathi CV, Chakravarthy SK, Komala VV, Chavan UD, Patil JV. Sweet sorghum as feedstock for biofuel production: A review. *Sugar Tech*. 2011 Dec;13(4):399–407.

Reddy DV, Elanchezhian N. Evaluation of tropical tree leaves as ruminant feedstuff based on cell contents, cell wall fractions, and polyphenolic compounds. *Cellulose (ADF-ADL)*. 2008;14(21.58):17–52.

Rohowsky B, Häßler T, Gladis A, Remmele E, Schieder D, Faulstich M. Feasibility of simultaneous saccharification and juice co-fermentation on hydrothermal pretreated sweet sorghum bagasse for ethanol production. *Applied Energy*. 2013 Feb 1; 102:211–19.

Rooney W. Sorghum breeding, 509–218. In Acquaah, G., ed., *Principles of plant genetics and breeding*. Wiley-Blackwell, London, UK. 2007.

Rosegrant MW, Msangi S. Consensus and contention in the food-versus-fuel debate. *Annual Review of Environment and Resources*. 2014 Oct 17;39:271–94.

Shen WL, Kwon Y, Adegbola AA, Luo J, Chess A, Montell C. Function of rhodopsin in temperature discrimination in Drosophila. *Science*. 2011 Mar 11;331(6022):1333–6.

Tang S, Wang Z, Chen C, Xie P, Xie Q. The prospect of sweet sorghum as the source for high biomass crop. *J. Agric. Sci. Bot*. 2018;2(3):5–11.

Tian Y, Zhao L, Meng H, Sun L, Yan J. Estimation of unused land potential for biofuels development in the People's Republic of China. *Applied Energy*. 2009 Nov 1; 86:S77–85.

Upadhyaya HD, Gowda CL, Reddy VG. Morphological diversity in finger millet germplasm introduced from Southern and Eastern Africa. *Journal of SAT Agricultural Research*. 2007;3(1):1–3.

Vermerris W, Saballos A, Ejeta G, Mosier NS, Ladisch MR, Carpita NC. Molecular breeding to enhance ethanol production from corn and sorghum stover. *Crop Science*. 2007 Dec;47:S-142.

Whitfield MB, Chinn MS, Veal MW. Processing of materials derived from sweet sorghum for biobased products. *Industrial Crops and Products*. 2012 May 1;37(1):362–75.

5 Characterization of Biomass

Nazia Shaik, Sundergopal Sridhar, and Mamilla Shyam Sunder

5.1 INTRODUCTION

Global warming has prompted a shift worldwide, with the most abundant and environmentally friendly resource increasing rapidly. Biomass is considered the fourth most commonly used energy source in the 21st century, following natural gas, coal, and oil (Liuet al., 2015). The average crude equivalent quantity of biomass feedstock is about 1.08×10^{11} tons. It is clear that, with its widespread use as an energy source, biomass continues to attract global interest due to the immense annual volumes of biomass resources, their substantial economic potential, and their rapidly growing applications (Zhou et al., 2011). The three polymers, cellulose, hemicellulose, and lignin, as well as small quantities of protein and inorganic ash, constitute most of lignocellulosic biomass.

The concentrations of different polymeric components in the cell walls of feedstocks vary widely with factors such as feedstock type, growing conditions, and the timing and processes of harvest, collection, handling, and storage (Zhu et al., 2014). Cellulose is a polysaccharide consisting of numerous linear chains of glucose units connected through glycosidic linkages. These linear chains align in parallel and are held together by hydrogen bonds, forming a crystalline structure. Due to its highly branched five- and six-carbon sugar structure, hemicellulose is more prone to enzymatic and chemical breakdown (Miyata et al., 2017). The esters of sinapyl alcohol, coniferyl alcohol, and *p*-coumaric alcohol are the precursors for lignin, a phenolic-based polymer. Lignin is a phenolic polymer composed of monomeric precursors such as *p*-coumaryl alcohol, coniferyl alcohol, and sinapyl alcohol. The cell wall's mechanical strength and chemical resistance are provided by lignin, which forms linkages with cellulose and hemicellulose (Madsen et al., 2017). As thermochemical processes have quicker reaction and conversion rates than chemical substance transformations, they are commonly used in biomass conversion, particularly pyrolysis, gasification, and hydrothermal liquefaction (Liu et al., 2017). Pyrolysis, a biomass combustion process under limited oxygen conditions, is a growing trend due to its high efficiency and low-energy requirements (García et al., 2012). The production characteristics and constituents of renewable pyrolysis debris, which are often varied, are influenced by the reaction

DOI: 10.1201/9781003327608-5

conditions and the volume of biomass feedstocks. Pyrolysis comes in two flavors: fast (200–900 K/min) and slow (4–8 K/min) (Cai et al., 2017).

One of the primary reasons for its limited utilization is the poor quality of the plant material, often determined by its inherent properties (high humidity, insufficient energy density, low bulk density, inconsistent size, and structure) (Uras et al., 2012). The yield of the product and the selective conversion of some elements present in the biomass, such as chlorine (Cl), nitrogen (N), phosphorus (P), sulfur (S), and some metals during pyrolysis, may be improved, and the risk of secondary pollution reduced by understanding the basic reaction mechanism of biomass pyrolysis. Due to the range of reactions that might happen during pyrolysis and the intricate structure of the biomass feedstock, evaluating the reaction process can be challenging (Carpenter et al., 2014).

Researchers have relied extensively on investigations of feedstock chemical composition to understand the range of materials and develop suitable conversion technologies. Various chemical fractionation and chromatographic techniques are currently used in liquid phases to determine the amounts of these polymers in feedstocks (Wang et al., 2017). The synthesis process (esterification), production of biochar and bio-oil, and the raw material, biomass, must all be thoroughly examined to understand the reaction mechanism. Energy content estimation, proximate analysis, and ultimate analysis are the main approaches for characterizing biomass feedstocks (Li and Jiang, 2017). "Energy density" refers to the amount of energy stored in a given quantity or volume of biomass. Bio-oil is typically described using physical characteristics (such as moisture content, density, heating value, and others), elemental makeup, and organic constituents. The biochar characterization processes also consider the chemical composition, surface, and structural characteristics (Al-Battashi et al., 2019).

Conventional gas chromatography (GC) can accurately quantify the gas byproducts of biomass pyrolysis. Understanding the thermochemical conversion mechanisms and intermediates involved in biomass pyrolysis is crucial. To investigate the mechanism of this process, thermogravimetric (TG) analysis is often combined with other analytical techniques such as Fourier transform infrared (FTIR) spectroscopy and gas chromatography (Kan et al., 2016). Depending on the intended application, various practical characterization techniques can be applied to biomass, including X-ray diffraction (XRD), scanning electron microscopy (SEM), FTIR, solid-state nuclear magnetic resonance (SSNMR), and transmission electron microscopy (TEM). Understanding the effects of characterization is still significantly hampered by the lack of quick, high-quality, and credible technologies for monitoring and analyzing renewable energy sources, which are crucial for energy generation and other valuable goods.

Transportation, pretreatment, and conversion are all part of the biomass-to-biofuel conversion process (Lam and Sokhansanj, 2014). The collection, handling, storage, and transportation of biomass feedstocks are all part of the logistics process. The feedstocks are crushed, dried, and filtered during the pretreatment process. The conversion process includes product collection, upgrading, collecting,

TABLE 5.1
Industrial Use of lignocellulosic Biomass's Chemical and Physical Properties

Chemical and Physical Aspects	Engineering Applications
Compactness	Selection requirements for facilities used for transforming, archiving, and carrying
Granulating	Standards of design for facilities that grind
Grain size	Standards of design for equipment for preservation and drying
Precipitation	Standards of design for facilities for storage and drying
Humidity	Design criteria for facilities and conversion procedures for drying, processing, storing, and feeding
Powder	Estimating the probability that slagging and fouling challenges could occur during the combustion or gasification of biomass
Primitive structure	Efficiency of conversion
Intensity	Capability of energy recovery
Thermal conduction	The adaptability of calorimetric modification
Synthetic compound	Conversion ability

separating intermediate, feeding, and converting. Table 5.1 lists the engineering applications of these properties (Lam and Sokhansanj, 2014;Kan et al., 2016).

5.2 PHYSICOCHEMICAL CHARACTERIZATION

5.2.1 Analysis Framework

Four types of bases of analysis are frequently employed in research to present the outcomes of a biomass study.

5.2.1.1 Received Basis

It describes a quantitative result based on the sample's total weight upon receipt at the lab, including any pretreatment.

5.2.1.2 Air-Dried Basis

It describes a scientific outcome that relies on an assumption that the material being studied is in proportion relative to the humidity of the surrounding environment. Being air-dried excludes the moisture that naturally occurs alongside it.

5.2.1.3 Dry Basis

The technique assumes that the biomass is dry and provides a quantitative consequence based on that assumption. A dry base of operations removes all moisture, both internal and external.

5.2.1.4 Dry Ash-Free Basis

It describes how the measurement result might be generated under the assumption that the sample has been thoroughly dried and ash-free. This typically happens to demonstrate that the various components included within a sample's natural mechanisms have been found in the chemical substance's sections. All biomass elements and the various analysis types are shown in Figure 5.1 (Dahlquist, 2013a).

5.3 PHYSICAL CHARACTERISTICS

Biomass made from lignin has several mechanical properties, including flowability, grindability, particle size, weight, humidity absorption, and thermal conductivity.

5.3.1 Particle Size

The mixing and fluidization, surface area for heat and mass transfer, and flow behavior of wood particles are all influenced by the shape and dimensions of the substrate granules. As a result, the conversion and energy input efficiency of various feedstocks may vary. Raw materials are typically pretreated to meet

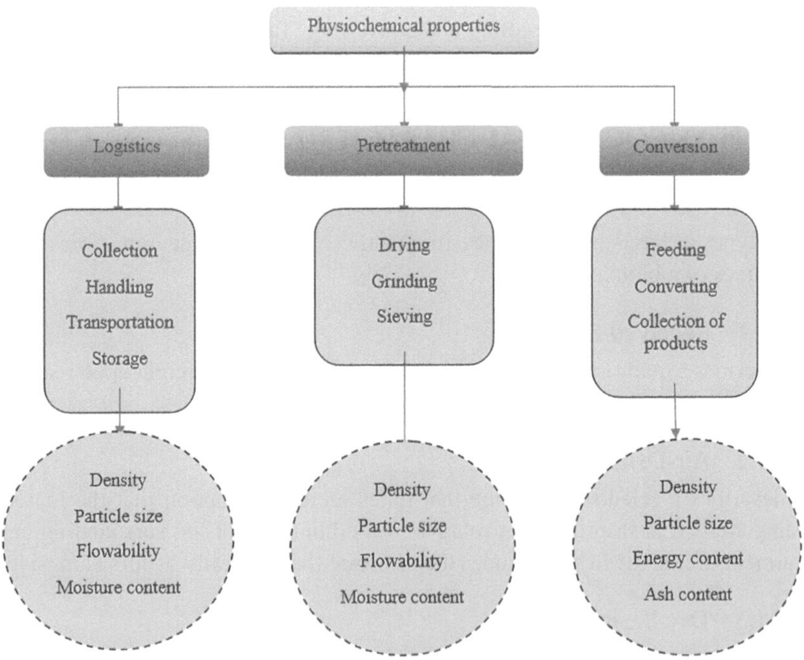

FIGURE 5.1 Biomass physicochemical characteristics.

the specific requirements of various thermal processing operations (Vidal et al., 2011). Particle size is essential for the decision-making process when choosing a thermochemical conversion technique (Lam and Sokhansanj, 2014). Lignocellulosic biomass is often amorphous, making it challenging to estimate length, breadth, and thickness accurately (Vidal et al., 2011). Accurate biomass particle dimensions and layout improvement are required for the transportation, storage, and transformation facilities.

5.3.2 Grindability

Particle size reduction is an aspect of biomass pretreatment and is closely linked to grindability, another physical characteristic. The grinding ability of a substance indicates how difficult it is to grind. Because they are both very fibrous and difficult to surface, cellulose and lignin stand out among the fibrous elements that make up wood (Capareda, 2013). Standard grindability tests for coal and petroleum coke have been developed using the Hardgrove Grindability Index (HGI) method (ASTM D409/D409M-12e1, 2012). For biomass, there isn't yet a standardized grindability test. Several research studies used the HGI test for lignite as a biofuel. The following steps can be used to empirically calculate a material's HGI using a sample mill (D5003-06a ASTM, 2011).

5.3.3 Density

Particle density and bulk density are both used to characterize biomass.

5.3.3.1 Particle Density

By dividing the mass of all substance particles by their combined area while leaving out pore space volume, the particle density for the group of components is computed as:

$$\rho_p = \frac{m_p}{v_p} \tag{5.1}$$

Particle density is indicated by the symbol ρ_p, mass by the numeral m_p, and accurate volume using the characters V_p.

5.3.3.2 Bulk Density

The volume of pore space that exists inside and between the plant matter particles is taken into consideration while determining the density of the burnside, and that between the plant matter particles is considered when calculating the thickness of bulk, which can be defined as the total weight of the cellulose fragments divided by the amount of space of the bioenergy components as a whole. It is a significant physical feature that determines a logistics framework for transporting and handling biomass. It varies through the biomass's surface properties, moisture content, particle density, and size and shape of the biomass's particles (Wang,

2014). The average thickness of a waste specimen can be determined using the American Society for Testing and Materials (ASTM) standard E873–82 (Bhagwanrao and Singaravelu, 2014). The process calls for dumping the wood material into a box with standard dimensions (305 mm × 305 mm × 305 mm) at a height of 610 mm.

5.4 FLOWABILITY

Their movement characteristics significantly influence the management, storage, and transportation of nutrients from bioenergy (Jose and Bhaskar, 2015). A common location for biomass particle bridging in conversion systems is the feeding system. As the primary flow attribute, flowability measures how easily biomass moves from one site to another (Miao et al., 2014). The inclination toward stillness is one of the measures frequently used to assess the ability to flow cellulose. The bonding factor, flexibility measure, and velocity indicator are additional factors (Ueki et al., 2011). The steepest angle at which a mass of cellulose molecules can persist stably without compressing is known as its point of repose (Dahlquist, 2013b).

Subsequently, it might be between 0° and 90°. The rotating-piston approach, the stationary-trough technique, and the tilting-box method are among the methods used to calculate the angle of repose (Sudhagar, 2015). This work explains the rigid filter method outlined in ASTM standard C144 (Szalay et al., 2015). Processed material bits are progressively fed into an opening to create a cone. Stop adding biomass particles once a biomass pile reaches a particular measurement or bottom width. The following formula is used to calculate the release position:

$$\phi = \tan^{-1}\frac{H}{R} \tag{5.2}$$

The piling cone's elevation and circumference are H and R, and the angle of repose is equal. Many flowability grades correlate to various angles of repose.

5.5 MOISTURE SORPTION

For biomass collection, processing, transmission, and preservation, it is crucial to investigate the humidity assimilation of bioenergy. Maintaining the quality of biomass feedstocks requires proper drying and storage methods. A key parameter in this context is the optimum wet percentage, which refers to the moisture content of a material at equilibrium under specific conditions of temperature and relative humidity. This value is essential for describing the fluid precipitation behavior within the material (Bridgwater and Boocock, 2013). The chemistry, permeability, structure, and specific surface region all affect the EMC of biofuel. The equilibrium moisture content can be determined using static or dynamic techniques. In the static approach, saturated salt solutions of acids with varying concentrations produce different relative humidities. In the kinetic approach, relative humidity is created by combining saturated and dry air. The dynamic approach stabilizes the sample more quickly than the traditional method. The vapor filtration isotherm often explains the relationship between optimal temperature and water content (Lin et al., 2016).

5.6 THERMODYNAMIC CHARACTERISTICS

The mechanical properties of biomass significantly impact how it is turned into energy. Two primary thermodynamic characteristics covered in this section are electrical conductivity and specific energy.

5.6.1 Thermal Conductivity

Heat conduction through the cellulose fibers of biomass particles during heating and thermochemical conversion affects how the biomass reacts (Yu et al., 2014). A method for estimating the thermal conductivity of biomass particles was developed using a specially designed research apparatus (Mason et al., 2016). Agricultural wastes (such as corn and crop fibers) showed far lower temperatures of 0.05 W/m/K compared to dry wood pellets, miscanthus, and willow, which had mechanical conductance between 0.10 and 0.12 W/m/K. An anisotropic substance is biomass. Temperature, humidity, porosity, density, and heating direction affect a material's thermal conductivity (Dahlquist, 2013a).

5.6.2 Specific Heat

Another essential thermal property of biomass frequently employed in thermodynamic calculations is assessing a material's ability to retain heat, which is determined by the degree of heat and the quantity of moisture in the biomass. The drying wood specific heat range (Basu, 2013) from 0°C to 106°C is calculated as follows:

$$C_{p\theta} = 0.266 + 0.00116\theta \tag{5.3}$$

where θ is the heat in °C and $C_{p\theta}$ is the infrared light at the temperature θ (J/g/K).

The correlation between temperature and the dehydrated object's particular temperature waste from agricultural specimens having smaller fragments than 200 μm is as follows:

$$C_{pT} = 5.340 - 299\,T \tag{5.4}$$

where T is the temperature in K, $313\ \text{K} \leq T \leq 353\ \text{K}$, and C_{pT} is the infrared energy at the boiling point T (J/kg/K).

The following equation may be used to illustrate how moisture affects latent thermal energy:

$$C_p = M_{ARB} C_W + \left(1 - M_{wet}\right) C_{p\theta} \tag{5.5}$$

Here, M_{ARB} is the amount of water determined on a receiving basis, and C_W is the water's particular temperature.

5.7 COMPOUNDS FEATURES

5.7.1 Imminent Analysis

5.7.1.1 Overall Outline

This method enables the estimation of humidity, dust, reactive matter, and carbon content in a biomass sample. The water content during production can be determined by measuring the moisture level, expressed as a percentage of the weight of each component. In addition to harvest and preparation, it strongly affects transportation, storage, processing, and end goods (Karunanithy et al., 2013). Biomass may retain moisture in both intrinsic and extrinsic forms. This section covers the amount of moisture present outside an item, which is more significant than its ideal humidity level. Usually, it develops in addition to the cell's outermost layer. The cell walls absorb the naturally occurring moisture. When the biomass sample is fully burned, the amount of solid residue left is measured as the ash. The primary elements in biomass ash include magnesium, sodium, potassium, iron, silica, aluminum, calcium, and titanium compounds (Vassilev et al., 2013). Understanding the chemistry and physics of biomass ashes helps predict the likelihood of formation in the heating system's components and the composition of the char produced by the pyrolyzer and gasifier (Nunes et al., 2016). Fixed carbon refers to the dense, combustible residue that remains after biomass is heated and its volatile components are removed.

5.8 DEPLOYING AN ASTM SPECIFICATION

The ASTM standard E1756-08 outlines the procedure for determining the moisture content of biomass (ASTM E1756-08, 2015). In this method, an appropriate sample is heated in an oven at 105 ± 3°C for a minimum of 3 hr and a maximum of 72 hr. After heating, the sample is cooled and weighed to determine its moisture content. To ensure complete drying, the process is repeated until the sample's weight remains consistent. The ash content of carbon material may be measured using ASTM standard E1755-01: a dry biomass sample is heated to 575.25°C for 3 hr in a muffle furnace, cooled, and weighed again. The ASTM standard D7582-15 for the proximate analysis of charcoal samples specifies the assessment of moisture, volatile matter, and ash by thermogravimetric analysis (TGA), which provides a continuous record of the sample's weight loss during heating. To measure volatile matter concentration, the enclosed furnace is heated to 950°C for 7 minutes in accordance with ASTM standard E872–82 (ASTM E17551-01, 2015). After the crucible is removed, it is examined after cooling in a dryer. The volatile matter content decreases in weight due to devolatilization.

5.9 THERMOGRAVIMETRIC ANALYSIS METHOD

For proximate analysis using ASTM standards, Klass (ASTM D7582-15, 2015) suggested an alternative approach using thermogravimetry to reduce time and cost. ASTM standard D7582-15 outlines the evaluation of moisture, volatile matter, and ash content using TGA. This method provides a continuous record of the sample's weight loss during heating and is used for the downstream analysis of petroleum-based samples. Several research studies employing the TGA approach included the proximate examination of bioenergy materials (García et al., 2013). The following is a description of the TGA method for proximate analysis.

5.9.1 Moisture Determination

The measured materials are heated to 105°C in furnaces with lids at an average rate of 15–50 K/min, then maintained at that temperature for 3 minutes in an inert environment (helium, argon, or nitrogen). The moisture content can be determined using the following formula:

$$M = \frac{W - B}{W} \tag{5.6}$$

where W is the weight of the sample utilized, and B is the dried mass for the moisture test.

5.9.2 Volatile Matter Determination

A cooling procedure starts with a decreasing speed ranging from 20 to 120 K/minute to 500°C, followed by a heating ramp (50–100 K/min) to 950°C. The flammable (volatile) substance content can be determined using the following formula:

$$\text{VM} = \frac{B - C}{W} \tag{5.7}$$

where VM is volatile matter and C is the specimen's density in the volatile matter test.

5.9.3 Ash Determination

After converting the flowing gas to an oxidizing gas (such as air or oxygen), the sample is heated to 800°C at a ramp rate, followed by an isothermal hold at 800°C for 3 minutes. The ash content is then determined using the following formula, where D represents the weight of the remaining residue from the waste sample.

$$A = \frac{D}{W} \tag{5.8}$$

Here, D is the weight of the leftover cake after the test.

5.10 ENERGY CONTENT

The term "heat of combustion" refers to the total energy released as heat during the complete combustion of a substance with air under normal conditions. It is often used to determine the energizing potential of biofuel and the amount of energy contained in a particular region of a feedstock collection (Dahlquist, 2013a, 2013b). The heat significance of an object, also known as the calorific value, is typically used to calculate its energy content. Higher heating value (HHV) and lower heating value (LHV) are the two heating values most commonly used in industry. The absorbed heat from the fluid dispersion in the substance being burned and the end products are included in the HHV, which is the total quantity of heat available in biomass (Ohliger et al., 2013). The LHV does not account for the energy lost in water condensation. An air explosion calorie counter that adheres to ASTM standard D5865-13 is the primary tool for calculating the HHV of biomass.

5.11 COMPOSITIONAL ANALYSIS

5.11.1 General Introduction

Lignocellulosic biomass is primarily composed of a mixture of cellulose, hemicellulose, and lignin. The recognized compound of D-glucopyranose moieties connected by (1,4) glycosidic links is called cellulose (Wu et al., 2015). A polymer composed of short, branched sugar chains is called hemicellulose. Cross-linked phenolic polymers are present in the complex, massive molecular structure known as lignin. Each of these elements has a relationship with the others and varies according to the lignocellulosic biomass type. In both biochemical and thermochemical conversion processes, these components display different behaviors and performance characteristics (Lebo et al., 2000). ASTM standard E1757-01 should be used to prepare lignocellulosic biomass samples, as it helps convert the samples into uniform, analyzable materials suitable for accurate compositional analysis. The process for creating samples with a specific dimension band and water content is defined in the standard. The following explains the preparation process. After the material has been dried at 45°C for 24–48 hr, milled to ensure that particulates pass through a 2-mm screen, and then sieved, a 20/+80 mesh fraction is selected for further analysis. Quantitative assessment techniques, near-infrared spectroscopy (NIRS), and the acid breakdown strategy are three distinct compositional analysis methods.

5.11.2 Process of Sulfate Acidification

The most widely used procedures revolve around an alternative to a more than a century-old, two-step acid hydrolysis process that has been adapted to different materials and situations. The compositional analysis techniques are based on sulfuric acid hydrolysis. Techniques of chemical hydrolysis have been stated in several comparable forms. The latest version of the Laboratory Analytical Procedure (LAP) titled *Determination of Structural Carbohydrates and Lignin in Biomass* from the National Renewable Energy Laboratory (NREL) is available (Cai et al., 2013). The procedure begins with an ethanol extraction step to remove interfering substances. This allows for the precise identification and quantification of carbohydrate-derived glucose, Klason lignin, and acid-soluble lignin, each of which can be separately measured. After extraction, the components are analyzed by high-performance anion-exchange chromatography with pulsed amperometric detection. This process typically entails an intense acid hydrolysis at room temperature, followed by a reduced-sulfuric acid hydrolysis step that converts the components into the isolated form (Sluiter et al., 2012). Soluble lignin samples may be measured by UV spectroscopy.

5.11.3 Near-Infrared Spectroscopy Method

Generally labor-intensive, costly, and requiring pre-conditioning to remove extractives, acid hydrolysis processes, however, can provide precise information on the composition of biomass (Pandey et al., 2014). The NIRS techniques can offer a reliable and affordable alternative for calculating biomass composition. The three primary benefits of the NIRS approach are (1) rapid and accurate analysis, (2) no use of dangerous chemicals, and (3) reasonably simple operation. Because various functional categories in the physical components of bioenergy may correlate with different thermal spectra, spectral characteristics can be used to examine biomass composition. Yet, infrared spectra provide information only on chemical bonds and do not yield structural data. As a result, specific statistical models that link spectral characteristics to chemical bonds are necessary. The most popular methods for qualitative analysis are principal component analysis (PCA), partial least squares (PLS), synthetic machine learning, and support vector machines (SVMs) (Roggo et al., 2007). Another independent verification of data is prepared after calibration to compare the predicted results from the standardization system with those from the reference method.

5.11.4 Methods of Analysis for Characterization of Biomass

As previously mentioned, a wide range of advanced analytical techniques is typically required to accurately determine the properties of biomass. These approaches can provide chemical data and assurance of the pretreatment process. The intended utilization of the biomass, however, determines the type of measurement procedure to be used, allowing the study's conclusions to be interpreted in light of that application. The following subsections discuss several methods of analysis frequently employed in investigations, including an overview of substances derived from biomass. An overview is represented in Figure 5.2.

5.11.5 Scanning Electron Microscope

An SEM generates an illustration of a sample by scanning an electron beam across the surface of the material. These electron interactions with the sample

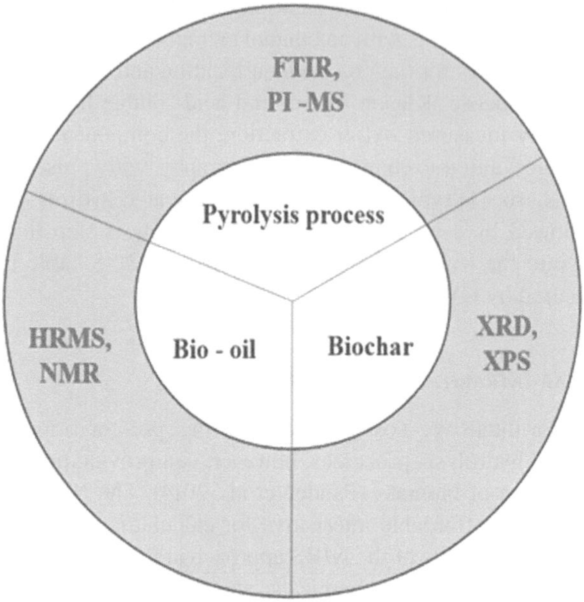

FIGURE 5.2 An overview of characterization methods.

yield a range of signals, providing additional information about its surface composition and topography. For any tiny or nanoscopic testing, biomass's macroscopic nature makes preprocessing, including dimension elimination, mandatory. The morphological characteristics of biomass relevant to its particular use can be investigated using SEM. With the knowledge gained, biomass pretreatment techniques may be improved, increasing biomass's susceptibility to biochemical or thermochemical conversion.

5.11.6 Fourier Transform Infrared Spectroscopic Analyzer

A precise method for investigating organic materials, including biomass, in terms of both quantity and quality, is FTIR. By generating a variety of infrared (IR) spectra that depict the sample's profile, it can identify molecular bonds. This analytical method can differentiate among groups that operate and is especially helpful for detecting and tracking changes in the molecular structure of biomass that may occur due to pretreatment (Gifty et al., 2016). Its utility in defining biomass materials can benefit various applications, including biochemical and thermochemical conversion. For instance, the removal of hemicellulose and lignin from chemically treated biomass during the pulping process can be studied using FTIR. It can also be used to determine which elements in plant matter are highly energetic and how they influence the conversion of organic matter to energy during thermochemical conversion. The basic principle of FTIR is that most organic compounds absorb light in the infrared wavelengths of the electromagnetic spectrum. Wave numbers, which typically range from 400/cm to 600/cm, are used to calculate the frequency of light absorption.

5.11.7 X-Ray Diffraction Analyzer

The only method of analysis capable of revealing a substance's specific structural characteristics is XRD. A layer's structural data may be gathered on factors such as its composition, bending, crystal structure, dimension, and position. An XRD device can analyze a wide range of materials, especially at the nanoscale. Investigations characterizing biomass for various applications can benefit from XRD (Binshan Mu et al., 2018). XRD is useful for investigating chemically altered renewable resources that yield a variety of biological molecules, such as carbohydrates and fatty acids, by-products of an enzyme reaction used to produce biogasoline.

5.11.8 Solid-State Nuclear Magnetic Resonance Spectroscopy

SSNMR spectroscopy is the best technology for analyzing biomass materials used to generate biofuels, charcoal, or chemicals. The major components of biomass, especially lignocellulosic biomass such as wood, can be structurally elucidated using this method. It is an addition to the XRD approach as the degree of cellulose crystallinity can also be assessed (Coyla et al., 2022). In addition to being differentiated by direction, in which dependent interactions are evident over a vast spectrum, SSNMR provides essential information on the solid-state chemistry, structure, and dynamics of materials. General access to both types of cellulose is required to produce biofuels and chemicals from lignocellulosic biomass.

5.11.9 Thermo-Gravimetric Analysis Analyzer

TGA is used to regulate the heat variables essential to the thermochemical conversion of biomass. This technique enables the sample to be combusted at controlled temperatures in a nonreactive environment of gases such as argon or nitrogen, while simultaneously monitoring its weight change during heating. It is common practice to plot the mass change of a sample as a function of temperature or time. TGA, a high-temperature analytical tool, effectively replicates the environmental conditions found in conventional power generation facilities. TGA is beneficial for studying the thermal degradation kinetics of biomass, as it provides qualitative data that helps understand process parameters and the design requirements of heat conversion systems (Bao et al., 2021).TGA must be performed under various conditions to understand the numerous peaks the thermogram produces, indicating weight shifts relative to temperature, and its derivative (DTG) must be used. This method has been developed to solve the problems mentioned in Table 5.2.

TABLE 5.2
Thermogravimetric Technique Research for Biomass

Serial Number	Biomass	Method of Analysis
1	Shell of the kernel	GC and TGA
2	Solid waste components like municipal	GC and TGA
3	Fermentation residues	TGA
4	Processing of the food waste	
5	Bamboo	
6	Bark	

5.11.10 Differential Scanning Calorimetry

Differential scanning calorimetry (DSC) measures the quantity of heat absorbed during a controlled rise or fall in temperature, using a thermodynamic approach. The approach requires heating two crucibles: one containing the sample to be examined and the other functioning as an indicator before an item is reviewed. The equipment detects phase changes that allow heat to transfer between the crucibles. Heat flow is computed as a function of temperature in the current study to evaluate the ignition characteristics that aid in determining the phase order that defines a material's thermal performance. In some cases, in addition to TGA, DSC can be used as an analytical method, particularly for determining the weakening of the temperature range where glass changes occur (Blanca et al., 2021). DSC data may help us understand how activation energy affects the rate of biomass conversion in thermal power systems, as we discuss later. DSC is beneficial for studying biomass materials intended for use as fuel in heat-treatment processes.

5.11.11 Mass Spectrometry/Pyrolysis-Gas Chromatography

Plotting the mass change of a sample against temperature or time is a standard practice. As noted earlier, TGA accurately simulates the environmental conditions typical of conventional power generation systems. It is particularly valuable for investigating the thermal degradation kinetics of biomass, providing essential qualitative data to understand process conditions and inform the design of heat conversion equipment (Bao et al., 2021). Biodegradable components designed for use as fuel in pyrolysis or liquefaction processes are particularly suitable for this approach. The generation of fuels and oils is convenient for studying the mechanisms governing these two thermochemical processes (hydrothermal liquefaction and pyrolysis). For instance, pyrolysis, an intricate process that occurs when wood is heated in an inert atmosphere, involves immediate and follow-up chemical reactions. The pyrolysis of biomass serves as the most compelling example of this reaction. Due to the compositional and structural diversity of biomass, its major components decompose via different mechanisms at varying temperatures and rates. Therefore, cutting-edge analytical instruments like Py-GC/MS are needed to analyze the complexity of this process.

5.11.12 Solid-State Nuclear Magnetic Resonance

It is a valuable tool for determining the chemical composition of a living thing's cell wall because it is nondestructive. The average distances between the main synthetic polymers in the vegetation's wall of cells can be determined. The study utilized solid-state NMR techniques, including 13C cross-polarization, along with a blending delay for circulate dispersion on highly 13C-enriched maize combustion. The distance between the carbons in lignin and the carbohydrate in the two substances typically ranges between 0.7 and 2.0 nm, according to the findings of the 13C investigation. Due to their affordability, broad applicability, and flexibility, scattering methods such as X-ray and dispersion are gaining popularity as supplementary instruments for in-situ molecular characterization of biomass.

5.12 PHYSIOCHEMICAL PROPERTIES

The Brunauer–Emmett–Teller (BET) method is widely employed to determine the surface area and porosity of a material's structure. However, at low temperatures (77 K), N_2 may accumulate throughout the tiny voids and inhibit gas passage. Hence, there is insufficient evidence to define the surface dimension of biochar. The scientific method for CO_2 and the processes of adhesion at 273 K have displaced previous methods for estimating biochar surface area, as they have improved reactivity and data accuracy. The CO_2 adsorption and desorption process produces biochar with a greater surface area than the adsorbing and subsequent decomposition method. Most biochars have a comparatively high cation exchange capacity (CEC) because conductive functional groups are abundant. The prior approach allows for the determination of CEC. Ion chromatography can quantify the Na solution after a magnesium fluid has been used to transfer and remove the deposited Na ion from the charcoal. To create Na-saturated biochar, biochar must first be combined with a solution that absorbs Na ions. Using the quantity of exchangeable ions, CEC is determined by a compulsive exchange method using barium chloride. Instead of employing ion chromatography to determine the Ba content of the extract, $MgSO_4$ was used to replace the Ba in the biochar. There is substantial variability between the CEC of biochar produced using different raw materials. Biochar's pH and electrical insulation are essential for its use in cultivation and for soil and water remediation.

5.12.1 Surface Properties

When considering biochar use, surface functionality is essential because it affects how the material interacts with soil and contaminants. Hans Peter Boehm invented the Boehm titration procedure, a quick and easy method for measuring surface functional groups, in 1966. It can be challenging to estimate the groups precisely because of the interaction between the residue in the Boehm and biochar reactants, the presence of minerals and additional chemically inert bases in the charred material, and the degradation of organic matter in the reactants. The Boehm titration process has been modified to extract the dissolved organic carbon, carbonate ions, and ash from biochar.

5.12.2 X-Ray Photoelectron Spectroscopy

This method discusses bond-energy changes that lead to an explanation of superficial sludges; this approach can characterize the interface with bioenergy. Because of the chemical conditions on it, it can detect changes in separation energy. The chemical structures on the outer layer of biochar can be extensively analyzed using XPS at a 5-nm depth to examine the surface layers of the biochar's C1 bonding environment and composition (Priya et al., 2019).

5.13 CONCLUSION

For optimal use of biomass materials in bioconversion processes, the preparation and characterization of waste are crucial steps. An evaluation of the implications of preliminary treatment on biomass using modern analytical techniques is necessary to determine the appropriate method and parameters beforehand. This evaluation will help us better understand the causes of biomass refusal and the underlying processes and effects of preliminary treatment that are important for improving various bioconversion pathways. Practical and efficient instruments for describing physical and chemical characteristics, estimating capacity and mobility, assessing nutrition efficiency, and assessing risks related to the management of biomass materials were discussed. Most challenges in characterizing biomass for handling purposes stem from the wide range of sizes and forms in which biomass fragments may be presented, as well as their heterogeneous nature.

REFERENCES

Acquah GE, Brian KV, Fasina OO, Lori GE. Rapid quantitative analysis of forest biomass using Fourier transform infrared spectroscopy and partial least squares regression. *J Anal Methods Chem*. 2016;2016:1839598. https://doi.org/10.1155/2016/1839598.

Al-Battashi HS, Annamalai N, Sivakumar N, Al-Bahry S, Tripathi BN, Nguyen QD, et al. Lignocellulosic biomass (LCB): A potential alternative biorefinery feedstock for polyhydroxyalkanoates production. *Rev Environ Sci Biotechnol*. 2019;18(1):183e205.

ASTM D409/D409M-12e1. *Standard test method for grindability of coal by the Hardgrove-machine method*. West Conshohocken, PA: ASTM International; 2012.

ASTM D7582-15. *Standard test methods for proximate analysis of coal and coke by macro thermogravimetric analysis*. West Conshohocken, PA: ASTM International; 2015.

ASTM E17551-01. *Standard test method for ash in biomass*. West Conshohocken, PA: ASTM International; 2015.

ASTM E1756-08. *Standard test method for determination of total solids in biomass*. West Conshohocken, PA: ASTM International; 2015.

Bao W, Yujie L, Jianan Z, Yi W, Xun T, Xiang Z, Weiming S. Thermogravimetric and kinetic analysis of high-temperature thermal conversion of pine wood sawdust under CO_2/Ar. *Energies*. 2021;14:5328.

Basu P. Biomass characteristics. *In: Biomass gasification, pyrolysis and torrefaction*, Second edition. Boston: Academic Press; 2013. p. 47–86.

Bhagwanrao SV, Singaravelu M. Bulk density of biomass and particle density of their briquettes. *Int J Agric Eng*. 2014;7:221–4.

Binshan Mu ID, Haigang W, Xiaolong H, Qingwen W. Morphology, mechanical properties and dimensional stability of biomass particles/high density polyethylene composites: Effect of species and composition. *Polymers*. 2018;10:308.

Blanca C, Isabel A, Liljana M, Fernandez-Anez N, Garcia-Torrent J. Study of lignocellulosic biomass ignition properties estimation from thermogravimetric analysis. *Journal of Loss Prevention in the Process Industries*. 2021 July;71:104425.

Bridgwater AV, Boocock DGB. *Developments in thermochemical biomass conversion*, Vol. 1. The Netherlands: Springer; 2013.

Cai J, He Y, Yu X, Banks SW, Yang Y, Zhang X, Yu Y, Liu R, Bridgwater AV. Review of physicochemical properties and analytical characterization of lignocellulosic biomass. *Renewable Sustainable Energy Rev*. 2017;76:309–22.

Cai J, Wu W, Liu R, Huber GW. A distributed activation energy model for the pyrolysis of lignocellulosic biomass. *Green Chem*. 2013;15:1331–40.

Capareda S. *Introduction to biomass energy conversions*. CRC Press; 2013.

Carpenter D, Westover TL, Czernik S, Jablonski W. Biomass feedstocks for renewable fuel production: A review of the impacts of feedstock and pretreatment on the yield and product distribution of fast pyrolysis bio-oils and vapors. *Green Chem*. 2014;16(2):384–406.

D5003-06a ASTM. *Standard test method for Hardgrove grindability index (HGI) of petroleum coke*. West Conshohocken, PA: ASTM International; 2011.

Dahlquist E. *Biomass as energy source: Resources, systems and applications*. CRC Press; 2013a.

Dahlquist E. *Technologies for converting biomass to useful energy: Combustion, gasification, pyrolysis, torrefaction and fermentation*. CRC Press; 2013b.

García R, Pizarro C, Lavín AG, Bueno JL. Biomass proximate analysis using thermogravimetry. *BioresourTechnol*. 2013;139:1–4.

García R, Pizarro C, Lavín AG, Bueno JL. Characterization of Spanish biomass wastes for energy use. *Bioresour Technol*. 2012;103(1):249–58.

Jose S, Bhaskar T. *Biomass and biofuels: Advanced biorefineries for sustainable production and distribution*. CRC Press; 2015.

Kan T, Strezov V, Evans TJ. Lignocellulosic biomass pyrolysis: A review of product properties and effects of pyrolysis parameters. *Renew Sustain Energy Rev*. 2016;57:1126–40.

Karunanithy C, Muthukumarappan K, Donepudi A. Moisture sorption characteristics of corn stover and big bluestem. *J Renew Energy*. 2013;2013, Article ID 939504.

Lam PS, Sokhansanj S. Engineering properties of biomass. In: Shastri Y, Hansen A, Rodríguez L, Ting KC, editors. *Engineering and science of biomass feedstock production and provision*. New York, NY: Springer; 2014. p. 17–35.

Lebo SE, Gargulak JD, Mc Nally TJ. *Lignin. Kirk-Othmer encyclopedia of chemical technology*. John Wiley & Sons, Inc; 2000.

Li DC, Jiang H. The thermochemical conversion of nonlignocellulosic biomass to form biochar: A review on characterizations and mechanism elucidation. *Bioresour Technol*. 2017;246:57–68.

Lin G, Yang H, Wang X, Mei Y, Li P, Shao J. The moisture sorption characteristics and modelling of agricultural biomass. *Biosyst Eng*. 2016;150:191–200.
Liu WJ, Jiang H, Yu HQ. Development of biochar-based functional materials: Toward a sustainable platform carbon material. *Chem Rev*. 2015l;115(22):12251–85.
Liu WJ, Li WW, Jiang H, Yu HQ. Fates of chemical elements in biomass during its pyrolysis. *Chem Rev*. 2017;117(9):6367–98.
Madsen RB, Zhang H, Biller P, Goldstein AH, Glasius M. Characterizing semivolatile organic compounds of crude from hydrothermal liquefaction of biomass. *Energy Fuels*. 2017;31(4):4122–34.
Mason PE, Darvell LI, Jones JM, Williams A. Comparative study of the thermal conductivity of solid biomass fuels. *Energy Fuels*. 2016;30:2158–63.
Miao Z, Grift TE, Hansen AC, Ting K. Flow performance of ground biomass in a commercial auger. *Powder Technol*. 2014;267:354–61.
Miyata Y, Sagata K, Hirose M, Yamazaki Y, Nishimura A, Okuda N, Arita Y, Hirano Y, Kita Y. Fe-assisted hydrothermal liquefaction of lignocellulosic biomass for producing high-grade bio-oil. *ACS Sustainable Chem Eng*. 2017;5(4):3562–9.
Munson CR, Gao Y, Mortimer JC, Murray DT. Solid-state nuclear magnetic resonance as a tool to probe the impact of mechanical preprocessing on the structure and arrangement of plant cell wall polymers. *Front Plant Sci*. 2022, January 12;12.
Nunes LJR, Matias JCO, Catalao JPS. Biomass combustion systems: A review on the physical and chemical properties of the ashes. *Renew Sustain Energy Rev*.2016;53:235–42.
Ohliger A, Förster M, Kneer R. Torrefaction of beechwood: A parametric study including heat of reaction and grindability. *Fuel*. 2013;104:607–13.
Pandey A, Negi S, Binod P, Larroche C. *Pretreatment of biomass: Processes and technologies*. Elsevier Science; 2014.
Priya S, Archit D, Chungsik J, Xuepeng D, Chung YG, Lin L-C. Surface area determination of porous materials using the Brunauer–Emmett–Teller (BET) method: Limitations and improvements. *J Phys Chem C*. 2019;123:20195–209.
Roggo Y, Chalus P, Maurer L, Lema-Martinez C, EdmondA, Jent N. A review of near infrared spectroscopy and chemometrics in pharmaceutical technologies. *J Pharm Biomed Anal*. 2007;44:683–700.
Sluiter A, Hames B, Ruiz R, Scarlata C, Sluiter J, Templeton D. *Determination of structural carbohydrates and lignin in biomass*. Laboratory Analytical Procedure: National Renewable Energy Laboratory; 2012. p. 18.
Sudhagar M. *Fuel and bulk flow properties of coal and torrefied wood mixtures for co-firing applications*. 2015 TAPPI – International Bioenergy &Bioproducts Conference. Atlanta, GA; 2015.
Szalay A, Kelemen A, Pintye-Hodi K. The influence of the cohesion coefficient (C) on the flowability of different sorbitol types. *Chem Eng Res Des*. 2015;93:349–54.
Ueki Y, Torigoe T, Ono H, Yoshiie R, Kihedu JH, Naruse I. Gasification characteristics of woody biomass in the packed bed reactor. *Proc Combust Inst*. 2011;33:1795–800.
Uras U, Carrier M, Hardie AG, Knoetze JH. Physicochemical characterization of biochars from vacuum pyrolysis of South African agricultural wastes for application as soil amendments. *J Anal Appl Pyrolysis*.2012;98:207–13.
Vassilev SV, Baxter D, Andersen LK, Vassileva CG. An overview of the composition and application of biomass ash. Part 1. phase – mineral and chemical composition and classification. *Fuel*. 2013;105:40–76.
Vidal BC, Dien BS, Ting KC, Singh V. Influence of feedstock particle size on lignocellulose conversion – a review. *Appl BiochemBiotechnol*. 2011;164:1405–21.
Wang L. *Sustainable bioenergy production*. Taylor & Francis; 2014.

Wang S, Dai G, Yang H, Luo Z. Lignocellulosic biomass pyrolysis mechanism: A state-of-the-art review. *Prog Energy Combust Sci.* 2017;62:33–86.

Wu W, Mei Y, Zhang L, Liu R, Cai J. Kinetics and reaction chemistry of pyrolysis and combustion of tobacco waste. *Fuel.* 2015;156:71–80.

Yu X, Makkawi Y, Ocone R, Huard M, Briens C, Berruti FA. CFD study of biomass pyrolysis in a downer reactor equipped with a novel gas – solid separator – I: Hydrodynamic performance. *Fuel Process Technol.* 2014;126:366–82.

Zhou CH, Xia X, Lin CX, Tong DS, Beltramini J. Catalytic conversion of lignocellulosic biomass to fine chemicals and fuels. *Chem Soc Rev.* 2011;40(11):5588–617.

Zhu Y, Biddy MJ, Jones SB, Elliott DC, Schmidt AJ. Techno-economic analysis of liquid fuel production from woody biomass via hydrothermal liquefaction (HTL) and upgrading. *Appl Energy.* 2014;129:384–94.

6 Chemical Characteristics and Chemical Interactions between Biomass Components

Boya Jithendra Sai, Rebba Sowmya, Madupathi Madhumala, Sundergopal Sridhar, and Mamilla Shyam Sunder

6.1 INTRODUCTION

Most energy-related industries examine the chemical properties of biomass to convert it into biofuel via a feasible process (Srirangan et al., 2012). Lignocellulosic biomass primarily contains cellulose (40–60%), followed by hemicellulose (20–40%) and lignin (10%–30%). The presence of cellulose in the plant cell walls helps to provide sufficient mechanical strength and chemical stability, while the hemicellulose comprises monosaccharides of pentose and hexose (Sidana and Yadav, 2022; Zhou et al., 2021). Xylan, a dominant component of hemicellulose in plants, helps to connect lignin with cellulose to form a more rigid structure. Further, the presence of monolignols indicates the presence of alcohols, especially coniferyl, sinapyl, and p-coumaryl, in lignin, which maintains the floral structure. Along with the predominant polymeric networks, the biomass includes various polysaccharides and polyphenol-based lignin (Loqué et al., 2015). The chemical characteristics of biomass vary by source material, including woody materials (soft and hard woods), grasses, rice and wheat straw, bagasse, and other wastes (Akhtar et al., 2016). The following section covers the chemical characteristics of the biomass's constituents.

6.1.1 Cellulose

Cellulose is one of the most abundant polysaccharides available in plant sources. Cellulose-based bioproducts known for their energy storage applications have worldwide importance due to their multiple uses (Marakana et al., 2021). Figure 6.1

 DOI: 10.1201/9781003327608-6

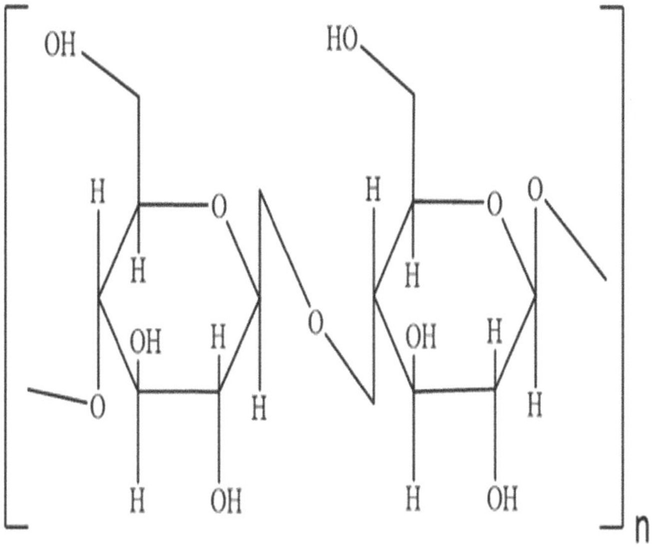

FIGURE 6.1 Structure of cellulose polymer.

shows the arrangement of cellulose polymer with replicating D-glucopyranose units bonded through β-linkages. The six-membered D-glucopyranose unit has C–H groups at the axial position, while the -OH and CH_2OH groups are positioned at the equator of the armchair. The crystalline properties of cellulose can be understood by examining its structure and interactions with surrounding groups (Vermerris and Abril, 2015; Kim et al., 2013).

The chemical properties vary with each plant source and with the downstream processing method used for isolation and purification. The insolubility of cellulose in water results in the crystallization of polymer chains, forming a flat ribbon-like structure with a density of 1.55 g/cm^3 (Klemm et al., 2005). The presence of hydroxyl groups near the edge of the ribbon forms interchain hydrogen bonds with the adjacent chains, while the -OH groups located on the flat side of the ribbon are attached through the van der Waals force of interactions (Perez and Samain, 2010).

6.1.2 Hemicellulose

The second major abundant plant source is hemicellulose, which has a branched chemical structure (Deshavath et al., 2019). Depending on the plant source, the branches within the structure are classified into polymeric sugars, such as pentoses (xylose) and hexoses (glucose, mannose, and galactose), as shown in Figure 6.2 (Howard et al., 2003). The hydrophilic nature of hemicellulose increases its solubility in alkali, thereby increasing water uptake into the fiber (John and

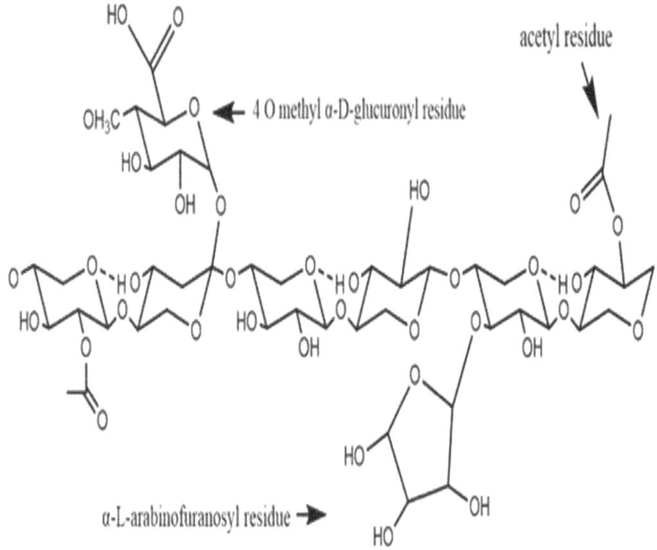

FIGURE 6.2 Hemicellulose backbone structure of arborescent plants.

Source: Scheller, H. V., and Ulvskov, P. (2010)

Anandjiwala, 2008). Among the polymeric sugars of the hemicellulose family, xylan is a commonly found polymer with 1,4 linkages between xylopyranosyl units, with α-(4-O)-methyl-D-glucuronopyranosyl units attached to anhydroxylose units. Because acetyl groups are branched and distributed along the hemicellulose polymer chain, no crystallinity is observed (Sasmal and Mohanty, 2018).

6.1.3 Lignin

The presence of dominant building blocks of phenylpropanoid units, including monolignols, that is, *p*-coumarylalcohol, coniferyl alcohol, and sinapyl alcohol, within the 3D polymer network results in the most complex nature of 3D lignin polymer (Dutta et al., 2014). The phenylpropanoid units contain the phenolic hydroxyl group, which are further connected by C—C linkage as shown in Figure 6.3. The lignin from softwood mostly contains coniferyl alcohol, whereas the hardwood lignin is majorly made of sinapyl and coniferyl alcohols, as shown in Figure 6.4 (Rai et al., 2022). Lignin in grass biomass contains three monolignols. The woody plants contain 27–32% of lignin, while herbaceous plants are made up of 14–25% lignin content. The secondary cell wall contains lignin, which further supports nutrient transport by providing cells with endurance and strength and by supporting the development of the overall plant and its fibers (Khaire et al., 2021). The binding nature of lignin enables the creation of composite materials with remarkable properties by providing resistance to compression and against

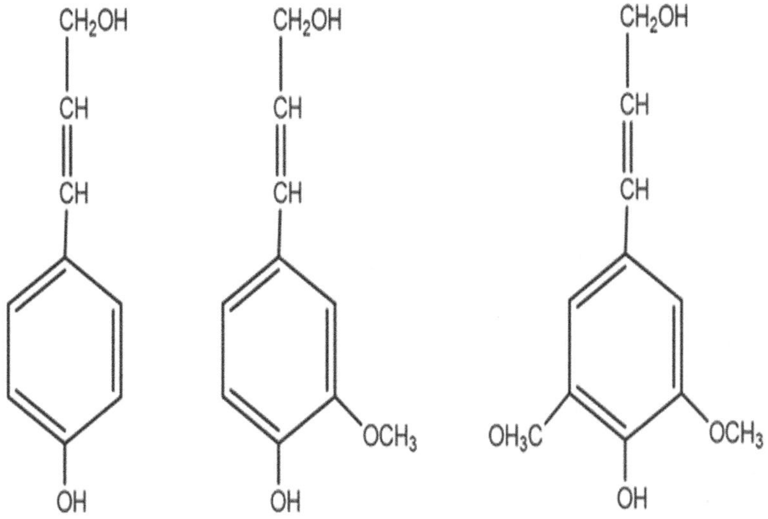

1 2 3

FIGURE 6.3 Building blocks of 3D polymer lignin: (1) *p*-coumaryl, (2) coniferyl, (3) sinapyl alcohol.

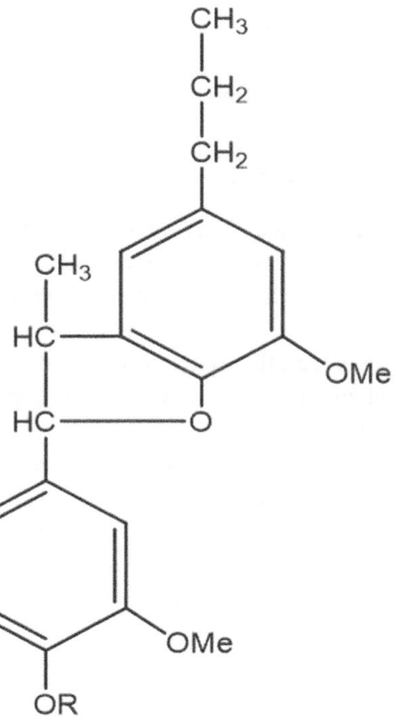

FIGURE 6.4 Two phenyl propane units connected by C—C linkages containing two chemical bonds.

harmful pathogens that hinder plant growth (Kai et al., 2016). The composition of elements C, O, and H and the ash content within lignin vary from plant to plant. Lignin finds applications as a chelating agent in metallurgy, as an adhesive precursor, as a surfactant, and so forth (El-Salamony and El Shafey, 2021).

6.1.4 Chemical Analysis of Lignocellulose Constituents

The quantity of lignocellulosic constituents is generally determined by the National Renewable Energy Laboratory method, whereas electron dispersive X-ray analysis determines the percentage mass of organic elements in biomass stock (González-García, 2018). The morphological study of biomass is carried out using field-emission scanning electron microscopy, which evaluates surface morphology (Verma et al., 2021). Fourier transform infrared spectroscopy measures band intensities and the relationship between structure and function, whereas Fourier transform ion cyclotron resonance provides structural elucidation of polymers and their respective oligomers (Lupoi et al., 2015). Nuclear magnetic resonance spectroscopy studies the molecular structure and composition of constituents and their derivatives, while the average molecular weight distribution is analyzed using gel permeation chromatography and gas chromatography-mass spectrometry (Wang et al., 2015).

6.2 CHEMICAL INTERACTIONS BETWEEN COMPONENTS

Lignocellulose contains mainly four bonds: ester/ether bonds, carbon-carbon bonds, and hydrogen bonds, which are formed within lignocellulose derivatives and with other components, resulting in a complex structure (Korányi et al., 2020).

6.2.1 Intra-Polymer Linkages

The ether bonds associated with aryl- or phenyl-ether groups and carbon-carbon-carbon bonds of bio-phenyls are found within the building molecules of lignin, while ether and ester bonds are present within the hemicellulose structure (Figure 6.5). The bondage between allylic-aryl, aryl-aryl, and allylic-allylic carbon atoms represents the ether and carbon bond linkages. It has been found that ether bonds predominate over carbon-carbon bonds in lignin molecules in biomass (Hossain et al., 2022).

Hydrogen bonds form within the cellulose structure between the hydroxyl groups of glucose monomers and other polymer chains (Figure 6.6). This bond significantly influences the properties of cellulose and its byproducts. Due to the strong reactivity of hydroxyl groups, cellulose appears to have a 3D crystalline structure with limited solubility in usual solvents (Sasmal and Mohanty, 2018).

6.2.2 Interpolymer Linkages

The breakdown of lignocellulose into its constituent polymers is mainly achieved through various treatment methods. These polymers are interconnected via ester,

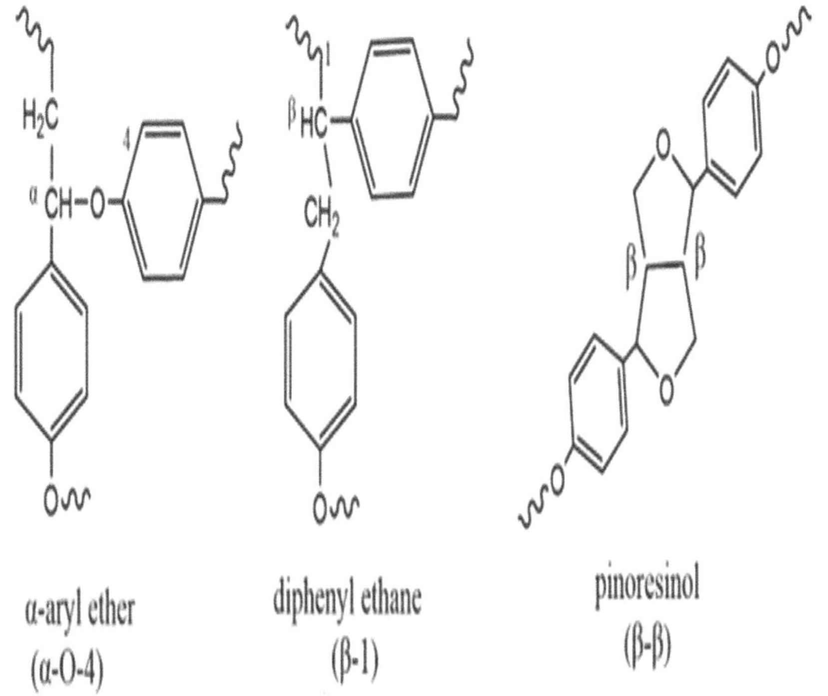

FIGURE 6.5 Major ether and carbon linkages in lignin.

Source: Alzagameem et al. (2019)

ether, and hydrogen linkages. The hemicelluloses and lignin are connected by ether or ester or hydrogen bonding, while cellulose and lignin and hemicellulose are interconnected by ether or hydrogen bonds (Sasmal and Mohanty, 2018). For example, the hydrogen bonds in cellulose molecules connect the hydroxyl groups of C6 with the oxygen of the adjacent C3 chain. However, it is not clear whether the $R\text{-}O\text{-}R^1$ group is strongly bonded to lignin or to cellulose or hemicellulose. Comparatively, the hydrogen bond between the hemicellulose and the cellulose is weaker due to a lack of external bonding with -OH functional group over the pyranoside moiety ring in hemicelluloses (Chen et al., 2022).

6.2.3 Promising Functional Groups in the Lignocellulose Biomass

The lignocelluloses metabolize into sugar monomers, and, eventually, the production of biofuel and other byproducts involves reaction between the functional groups during (a) hydrolysis of polysaccharides to monomers and further monomer degradation to produce furfural sugar and (b) lignin depolymerization to phenolic compounds to enable easy accessibility of cellulose with an enzyme.

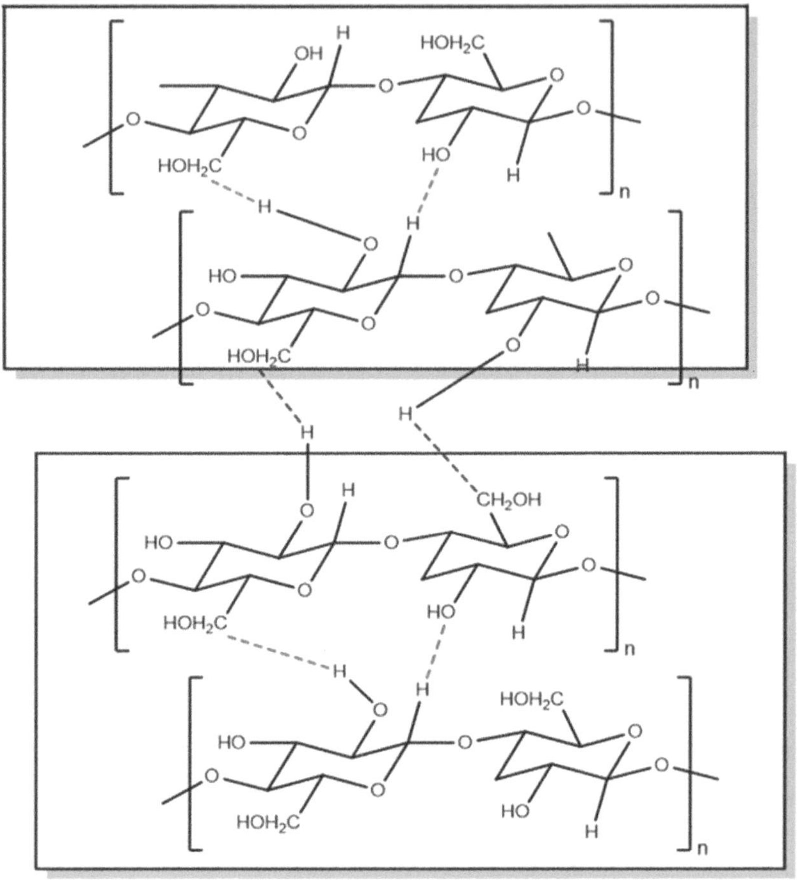

FIGURE 6.6 Hydrogen bonding within the cellulose polymer chain.

The major functional groups in lignin are aromatic rings, hydroxyl groups, carbon-carbon, and ether linkages (Suchy and Argyropoulos, 2002). The aromatic ring in lignin polymer is subject to electrophilic chlorination and nitration substitution reactions to result in Cl_2 or NO_2groups. The oxidation reaction in the presence of chlorine and compounds, that is, ClO_2 and O_2, converts the aromatic ring to cyclic moieties of mono and di-carboxylic acids. The addition of sulfonic acid converts the carboxyl group to ether or an allylic ether, facilitating the solubility of lignin in water. The ether bond is considered the most prevalent bond in lignin due to the presence of glucosidic linkages, which stabilize the glucose monomer within the polymer chain (Xie et al., 2020). Cellulose contains an ether linkage and a hydrogen bond. The hydrogen bond is observed between the CH_2OH group glucose moiety and the -OH group of another glucose sugar in the cellulose chain, resulting in its insolubility in water. Further, the hemicellulose contains ester and hydrogen bonds within the structure. The ester bond is formed due to the reaction between the acetyl group and the hydroxyl group of the polysaccharide chain. However, there are unproven interpretations of hydrogen bonding within lignin, hemicellulose, and cellulose polymers (Xie et al., 2020).

6.3 CONCLUSION

The study of the chemical characteristics of lignocellulosic biomass, their interactions among components, and their polymer structure is important for further converting the constituents into biofuels and value-added products. The polymer linkages within the lignocellulose connect the compounds to form a complex organic matrix. Further, the analysis using various characterization methods determines structure-property relationships and elucidates the functional properties and molecular distribution of lignocellulosic constituents.

REFERENCES

Akhtar N, Gupta K, Goyal D, Goyal A. Recent advances in pretreatment technologies for efficient hydrolysis of lignocellulosic biomass. *Environmental Progress & Sustainable Energy*. 2016, 35(2):489–511.

Alzagameem A, Elisabeth Klein S, Bergs M, Tung Do X, Korte I, Dohlen S, Hüwe C, Kreyenschmidt J, Kamm B, Larkins M, Schulze M. Antimicrobial activity of lignin and lignin-derived cellulose and chitosan composites against selected pathogenic and spoilage microorganisms. *Polymers*. 2019, 11(4):670–87.

Chen WH, Nižetić S, Sirohi R, Huang Z, Luque R, Papadopoulos AM, Sakthivel R, Nguyen XP, Hoang AT. Liquid hot water as sustainable biomass pretreatment technique for bioenergy production: A review. *Bioresource Technology*. 2022, 344:126207.

Deshavath NN, Veeranki VD, Goud VV. Lignocellulosic feedstocks for the production of bioethanol: Availability, structure, and composition. In *Sustainable Bioenergy*. 2019 (pp. 1–19). Elsevier.

Dutta S, Wu KC, Saha B. Emerging strategies for breaking the 3D amorphous network of lignin. *Catalysis Science & Technology*. 2014, 4(11):3785–99.

El-Salamony RA, El Shafey AM. Extraction of silica and lignin-based nanocomposite materials from agricultural waste for wastewater treatment using photocatalysis technique. *Waste Recycling Technologies for Nanomaterials Manufacturing*. 2021, 363–84.

González-García P. Activated carbon from lignocellulosics precursors: A review of the synthesis methods, characterization techniques and applications. *Renewable and Sustainable Energy Reviews*. 2018, 82:1393–414.

Hossain S, Afrin S, Anika S, Sultana S, Haque P, Shahruzzaman M. Synthesis, characterization, and modification of natural polysaccharides. In *Radiation-Processed Polysaccharides*. 2022 Jan 1 (pp. 29–74). Academic Press.

Howard RL, Abotsi EL, Van Rensburg EJ, Howard S. Lignocellulose biotechnology: Issues of bioconversion and enzyme production. *African Journal of Biotechnology*. 2003, 2(12):602–19.

John MJ, Anandjiwala RD. Recent developments in chemical modification and characterization of natural fiber-reinforced composites. *Polymer Composites*. 2008, 29(2):187–207.

Kai D, Tan MJ, Chee PL, Chua YK, Yap YL, Loh XJ. Towards lignin-based functional materials in a sustainable world. *Green Chemistry*. 2016, 18(5):1175–200.

Khaire KC, Moholkar VS, Goyal A. Bioconversion of sugarcane tops to bioethanol and other value-added products: An overview. *Materials Science for Energy Technologies*. 2021, 4:54–68.

Kim SH, Lee CM, Kafle K. Characterization of crystalline cellulose in biomass: Basic principles, applications, and limitations of XRD, NMR, IR, Raman, and SFG. *Korean Journal of Chemical Engineering*. 2013, 30:2127–41.

Klemm D, Heublein B, Fink HP, Bohn A. Cellulose: Fascinating biopolymer and sustainable raw material. *Angewandte Chemie International Edition*. 2005, 44(22):3358–93.

Korányi TI, Fridrich B, Pineda A, Barta K. Development of 'Lignin-First' approaches for the valorization of lignocellulosic biomass. *Molecules*. 2020, 25(12):2815.

Loqué D, Scheller HV, Pauly M. Engineering of plant cell walls for enhanced biofuel production. *Current Opinion in Plant Biology*. 2015, 25:151–61.

Lupoi JS, Singh S, Parthasarathi R, Simmons BA, Henry RJ. Recent innovations in analytical methods for the qualitative and quantitative assessment of lignin. *Renewable and Sustainable Energy Reviews*. 2015, 49:871–906.

Marakana PG, Dey A, Saini B. Isolation of nanocellulose from lignocellulosic biomass: Synthesis, characterization, modification, and potential applications. *Journal of Environmental Chemical Engineering*. 2021, 9(6):106606.

Perez S, Samain D. Structure and engineering of celluloses. *Advances in Carbohydrate Chemistry and Biochemistry*. 2010, 64:25–116.

Rai R, Kumar V, Dhar P. Recalcitrance of lignocellulosic biomass and pretreatment technologies: A comprehensive insight. In *Thermochemical and Catalytic Conversion Technologies for Future Biorefineries: Volume 1*. 2022 Sep 2 (pp. 13–52). Singapore: Springer Nature Singapore.

Sasmal S, Mohanty K. Pretreatment of lignocellulosic biomass toward biofuel production. *Biorefining of Biomass to Biofuels: Opportunities and Perception*. 2018, 203–21.

Scheller, HV, Ulvskov, P. Hemicelluloses. *Annual Review of Plant Biology*. 2010, 61:97–122.

Sidana A, Yadav SK. Recent developments in lignocellulosic biomass pretreatment with a focus on eco-friendly, non-conventional methods. *Journal of Cleaner Production*. 2022, 335:130286.

Srirangan K, Akawi L, Moo-Young M, Chou CP. Towards sustainable production of clean energy carriers from biomass resources. *Applied Energy*. 2012, 100:172–86.

Suchy M, Argyropoulos DS. Catalysis and activation of oxygen and peroxide delignification of chemical pulps: A review. *Tappi J*. 2002, 1(2):1–8.

Verma C, Chhajed M, Gupta P, Roy S, Maji PK. Isolation of cellulose nanocrystals from different waste biomass, collating their liquid crystal ordering with morphological exploration. *International Journal of Biological Macromolecules*. 2021, 175:242–53.

Vermerris W, Abril A. Enhancing cellulose utilization for fuels and chemicals by genetic modification of plant cell wall architecture. *Current Opinion in Biotechnology*. 2015, 32:104–12.

Wang Y, Wang S, Leng F, Chen J, Zhu L, Luo Z. Separation and characterization of pyrolytic lignins from the heavy fraction of bio-oil by molecular distillation. *Separation and Purification Technology*. 2015, 152:123–32.

Xie Y, Zhang K, Cui S, Liu Y. A review on the structure and biodegradation of cellulose-lignin complexes. *Paper and Biomaterials*. 2020, 5(4):44–50.

Zhou Z, Liu D, Zhao X. Conversion of lignocellulose to biofuels and chemicals via sugar platform: An updated review on chemistry and mechanisms of acid hydrolysis of lignocellulose. *Renewable and Sustainable Energy Reviews*. 2021, 146:111169.

7 Composition of Lignocellulosic Biomass
An Overview

Rebba Sowmya, Boya Jithendra Sai, Mamilla Shyam Sunder, and Sundergopal Sridhar

7.1 INTRODUCTION

Presently, the combustion of fossil fuels provides 80% of the world's energy, 58% of which is used in the transportation industry (Vohra et al., 2014). Yet, conventional fuels face three main difficulties that vary by country. First, due to the rapid growth of industrialization, the consumption of fossil fuels has led to the depletion of nonrenewable resources (Menon and Rao, 2012). Second, greenhouse gas emissions can cause changes in climate and sea levels, thereby increasing pollution (Taha et al., 2016). A lack of oil might result in an emphasis on petroleum products. These crises have caused unrest in the energy sector in developed and developing nations (Zabed et al., 2016). To create alternative energy sources for business and society, it is vital to use energy that is sustainable, renewable, efficient, and cost-effective (Sarkset al., 2016). Consequently, one must choose materials that emit fewer greenhouse gases, such as bioethanol, but its fuel grade is denatured which creates toxicity and handling concerns (Lin et al., 2016).

Biomass materials include lignocellulosic materials, which store energy in chemical bonds and are generated from corn cobs, corn stover, rice, wheat straw, and cotton stalks (Rangabhashiyam and Balasubramanian, 2019). Breakage between the bonds occurs biologically and chemically so that the energy is stored in those bonds (Saritha et al., 2012). To maintain the high-energy-consuming lifestyle people have grown accustomed to, the prospect of converting renewable biomass into biofuels such as ethanol, methanol, and biodiesel must be investigated. (Arijanaet al., 2012). The biomass contains mainly cellulose, hemicellulose, and lignin, which differ significantly among biomass species. Their composition affects the yield of biomass conversion into biofuels, biochemicals, and by-products, as well as the chemical composition and structures of the biomass's biopolymers (Furkan et al., 2015).

The biomass contains cellulose, hemicellulose, and lignin, and the challenge in utilizing this available lignocellulosic biomass as a source for bioethanol production is separating lignin from cellulose and hemicellulose (Devendra Prasad

DOI: 10.1201/9781003327608-7

et al., 2015). Ethanol can be produced from the fermentation of sugars, and these are glucose and pentose, which can be obtained from the cellulose and hemicellulose parts of biomass found in plant matter, particularly in the lignocellulosic biomass (Larissa et al., 2012). Pretreatment of the biomass reduces cellulose fiber crystallinity and increases porosity, thereby enhancing enzyme accessibility. It can be achieved through physical, physiochemical, chemical, and biological pretreatment methods. Figure 7.1 shows a typical composition of lignocellulosic biomass.

The production of bioethanol from biomass fermentation – biomass that contains sugars or carbohydrates – might convert it into soluble sugars. These feedstocks can be divided into sugars, starch, and lignocellulosic biomass (LCB) (Kumar et al., 2016). Although it may be slightly more straightforward to produce alcohol materials such as starch and glucose than those derived from LCBs, the high cost of the components and environmental concerns make the former approach unviable (McIntosh et al., 2016). In addition, bioethanol production is limited to 3% of the total fuel used in the transportation industry, regardless of commercialization. For this reason, research has focused on LCB, which offers advantages such as the use of waste materials, low prices, rich carbohydrate content, and non-competitiveness in the food chain (Lin et al., 2016). LCB also reduces greenhouse gas emissions and environmental pollution. The major challenge in energy consumption is the pretreatment process, which requires multiple steps to ferment both pentose and hexose sugars. To overcome these problems, numerous research studies have been conducted on ethanol production (Jönsson et al., 2016).

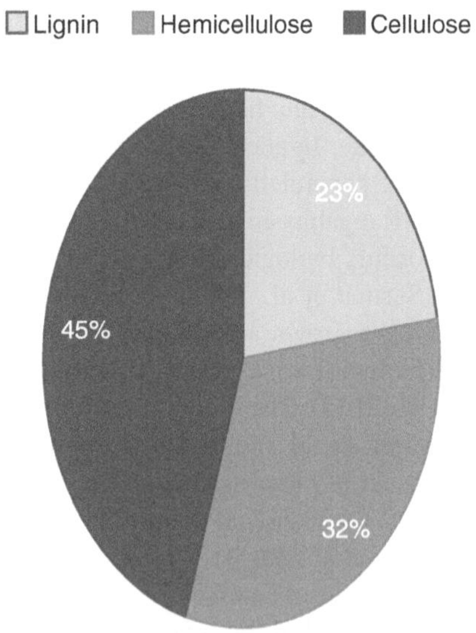

FIGURE 7.1 Lignocellulose biomass composition.

One of the most significant technological challenges to commercializing lignocellulosic biomass into ethanol is how well the process scales up from the lab to manufacturing. Significant technological advancements before treatment, breakdown, and production of biofuel technologies are essential for large-scale, inexpensive ethanol production. Even though numerous strategies for all these problems have been suggested recently, there are some technical, environmental, and economic issues in implementing them on an industrial scale (Lin et al., 2016; Hellsmark et al., 2016). The fermentation of LCB into ethanol by microorganisms relies heavily on consuming coupled peptides (sugar) and pentoses (xylose). Commonly used indigenous microbes have been engineered to express heterologous metabolic pathways, enabling them to ferment both xylose and glucose and create synthetic microorganisms. This has been done because local microbes can utilize both types of sugar (Zhao et al., 2016; Wei et al., 2015).

The species and availability of biomass materials determine each biomass's composition. The diversity of this biomass can change the solubilization efficiency of plant material components during hydrolysis and alter the yield of the target compound and byproducts (Gabriela et al., 2020). The distribution of molecular weights of the hydrolysates affects the conversion into biofuel and other significant chemical production. Low-weight oxygenated compounds derived from biofuel hydrolysates, used as feed in the aqueous phase, may be used to produce biomass with high hydrogen gas yields. A factor that can influence more degraded organics is favored for product conversion. (Hu et al., 2012).

7.2 STRUCTURE AND SOURCES OF LIGNOCELLULOSIC BIOMASS

Figure 7.2 illustrates the three different forms of lignocellulosic biomass, as well as trace amounts of minerals, phenolic substituents, and acetyl groups. Along with different biomass composition ratios, these are arranged into uniform three-dimensional structures to varying degrees (Abdellatif et al., 2013). The matrix of the lignin-hemicellulose to lignocellulose, which can be more resilient, can be influenced by the crystallinity of cellulose, the hydrophobicity of lignin, and the packaging of cellulose in nature (Moraïs et al., 2012). Cellulose is a key component of lignocellulosic biomass, and when additional units of cellulose are repeated, a compound referred to as disaccharide cellobiose is created (Esben et al., 2011). Inter and intra-molecular and hydrogen bonds, which are strongly linked with sugar units, make up this structure.

Hemicellulose is the second most common molecule in biomass. This consists of several heteropolymers, including xyloglucan, arabinoxylan, glucuronoxylan, galactomannan, and xylan, which are organized randomly in an amorphous form, as illustrated in Figure 7.2. The hemicellulose composition of hard and soft woods mainly consists of xylans and glucomannans (Moraïs et al., 2012). The hemicellulose heteropolymers, however, are composed of C5 and C6 monosaccharide molecules, including acetylated sugars, pentoses, as well as xylose, all the sugar

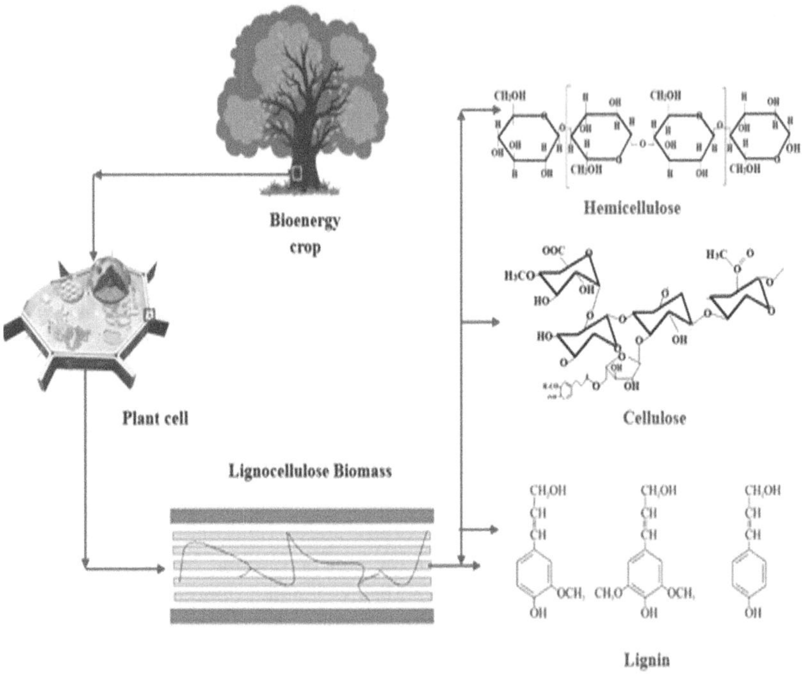

FIGURE 7.2 Representation of the bioenergy crop for lignocellulosic biomass.

arabinose, and peptides (mannose, glucose, and galactose). A complicated web of connections is created when the components of cellulose fibers, tiny fragments, and lignin hemicellulose are combined. Cross-linking gives the plant cell walls their structural strength (Valery et al., 2011).

Phenylpropanoid monomers make up part of the three-dimensional polymer known as lignin. The structural adhesive gives plant matter and individual fibers compressive strength, strength to their cell barriers, and resistance to insects and diseases (Abdellatif et al., 2013).

On the contrary, the distribution of the components of the three substances within the growing cell walls depends on the tissue and species. Typically, lignocellulosic biomass is composed of 10–25% lignin, 35–50% cellulose, and 20–35% hemicellulose (Ahmed et al., 2013). The remaining percentage is made up of proteins, oils, and ash. Table 7.1 lists several material types and their chemical compositions (Vishnu and Mala, 2012).

7.3 PLANT CELL WALL AND ITS CONSTITUENTS

The rigid cell wall of renewable residues serves as a mechanism for food storage, secretion, protection, and expansion control, and its intracellular space provides mechanical strength.

TABLE 7.1
The Chemical Structure of Various Plant Species

Lignocellulosic Biomass	Biomass Source	Cellulose (%)	Hemicellulose (%)	Lignin (%)
Hardwood	Popular	48–55	25–29	15–17
	oak	40.4	30–35	25
	Eucalyptus	50–55	17	21
Softwood	Pine	35–55	24.0–27.0	22
	Spruce	30–50	11.0	29
	Douglas fir	40–48	22.9	28
Agriculture pollution	Oat straw	30–40	20.0–26.0	16
	Barley hull	35	36.0	22
	Ray straw	32–50	19.0–24.5	25
	Corn stalks	30–40	16.8–35.0	20
	Wheat straw	35–45	24.0–33.0	10
	The substance of grain	30–40	24.0–27.0	25
Grasses	Leaves	20–45	25.0–50.0	40
	Switchgrass	30–50	25.0–30.0	25

Primary and secondary cell walls are produced from the preexisting cell wall, with some cells, such as fiber cells in wood, forming a further cell wall within the primary cell wall (da Costa et al., 2019).

7.3.1 Lignocelluloses

Biomass is mainly composed of cellulose, hemicellulose, and lignin, and it also contains small amounts of nitrogen based molecules and other chemical compounds (Collard and Blin, 2014; Mori et al., 2015). The most common substance with a unique polymer crystalline structure is cellulose, and the required packing classifications give it its stable characteristics. Because lignin is a challenging hydrophobic polymer, it impedes hydrolysis, being a polyphenolic chemical and a 3-D heterogeneous, polycrystalline, reticulated polymer (Balat, 2011). Hence, the repeating units are not adequately regularly arranged and ordered.

Unlike hemicellulose, which contains crystalline regions and branched and straight polysaccharides, the latter is easily converted into monosaccharides such as sugar, glucose, cellulose, fructose, and nutrients (Karimi and Taherzadeh, 2016). The difficulty of the cell wall deteriorating depends on various factors. Highly crystalline zones and numerous binding interactions between cell wall components are examples of these characteristics. To effectively use cellulose and lignocellulose, the network structure of lignin must be degraded by pretreatment (Chaula et al., 2014). There are significant challenges in producing and distributing ethanol from lignocellulosic biomass because lignin surrounds the cellulose.

Biomass must be pretreated to make it more receptive to pathogens, enzymes, and microbes. Therefore, the lignocellulosic biomass pretreatment procedure is quite costly for the generation of bioethanol (Mupondwa et al., 2016). The chosen process must maintain the fiber percentage, prevent a reduction in the dimensions of material fragments, require less energy, produce lignin with high value as a coproduct, and minimize the formation of degradation products. (Studeret al., 2011).

7.4 METHODS OF LIGNOCELLULOSIC BIOMASS PREREQUISITE TREATMENT

The main objective of this processing technique is to improve the biological characteristics, macrostructure, and microstructure of the lignocellulose. The natural lignocellulosic macromolecule is, therefore, susceptible to bacterial breakdown (An et al., 2015). A pretreatment method is needed to increase the substance's number of pores, diminish the substance's crystal structure, and eliminate the substance. A suitable pretreatment should be cost-effective, provide substantial cellulose support, and produce a minimal barrier (Mumtaz et al., 2016). It should focus on the fact that pretreatment efficiency is a key factor in achieving a better fuel yield.

Improved biomass surface area, cellulose and/or phenol breakdown, and smaller biomass molecule sizes are the three primary objectives of the pretreatment procedure. The structure of LCB may be altered physically or chemically, improving the ability of nutrients or enzymes to access the cellulose surface and enhancing cellulose hydrolysis (Kumari and Singh, 2018). The most commonly employed techniques in earlier investigations were physical, chemical, biological, and combined pretreatments. To produce bioenergy from feedstocks, the majority of new pretreatment methods for LCB are chemical, physical, or biological (Halderet al., 2019). As seen in Figure 7.3, many materials have been employed for these techniques.

7.5 CHEMICAL METHODS

The current strategy emphasizes the employment of chemicals for pretreatment, which may be carried out with one of four primary LCBs.

7.5.1 Alkaline Pretreatment

Due to its high efficiency and relatively simple procedure, this type of treatment is among the most reliable pretreatments. Eliminating lignin precisely without diminishing the number of carbs or sugars, increasing the porosity and surface area of biomass, and enhancing enzymatic hydrolysis are the primary advantages of the alkaline examination (Kimet al., 2016). Longer response instances (a few hours up to a day) are this method's principal drawback compared to other

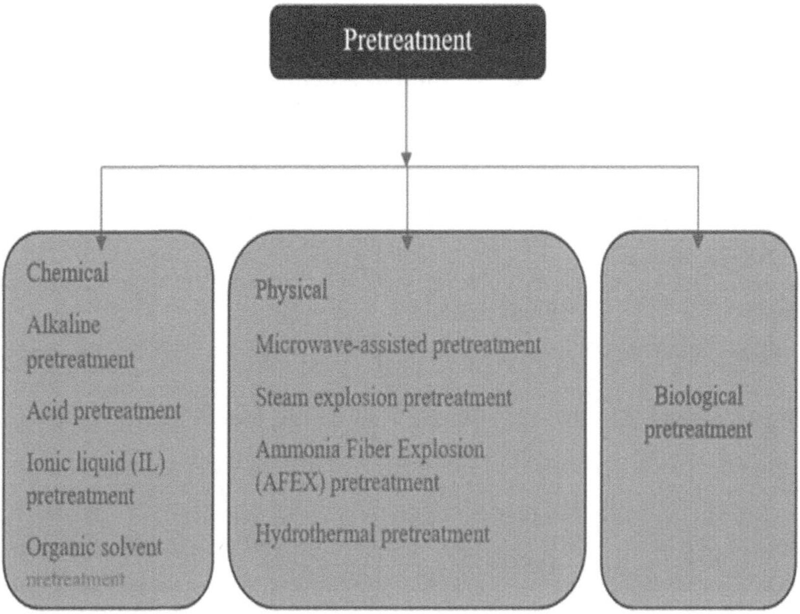

FIGURE 7.3 Different techniques for pretreatment.

pretreatment addresses (Bali et al., 2015). By delignifying biomass, this method primarily enhances enzymatic digestibility. In lignin, alkyl-aryl bonds are easily disrupted in an alkaline environment. Table 7.2 summarizes current research on the production of bioethanol from LCB using diverse alkaline pretreatment approaches.

7.5.2 Acid Pretreatment

A commonly employed method to produce bioethanol from LCBs is acid pretreatment. Treatment of the LCB with acid results in greater hemicellulose breakdown. The three most commonly encountered acids are sulfuric acid, acetic acid, and phosphoric acid (Gonzales et al., 2016). Solids loading, acid concentration, temperature, and residence period are the most important and effective factors for acid pretreatment (Solarte-Toroet al., 2019). Additionally, acids can dissolve all polysaccharide-lignin bonds, aiding in the recovery of most monomeric sugars. By rearranging the LCB structure, hemicelluloses have been converted into soluble sugars throughout this process. In diluted-acid pretreatment, raising the temperature may accelerate the conversion of hemicelluloses (Putro et al., 2016). The advantages of the lignocellulosic material over alternative approaches can be attributable to the acid preparation procedure.

TABLE 7.2
Current Research on the Generation of Bioethanol from LCB

New Component	Type of Hydroxides	Pretreatment Condition	Reducing Sugars	Delignification Rate (%)	Environment for Hydrolysis	Bioethanol Productivity	Reference
Sugarcane bagasse	NaOH (15%)	175°C; 1.5 hr	5.29 g/L	22–90	37°C; 10 hr	8.8 g/L	Carvalho et al. (2016)
Sugarcane bagasse	NaOH (0.5%)	60°C; 20 min	269.30 g/kg	48.31	30°C; 96 hr	17.26 g/L	Teran Hilareset al. (2017).
Eucalyptus	NaOH (10%)	NA	2.70 g/L	11–51	NA	3.4 g/L	Carvalhoet al. (2016)
Rice straw	NaOH (1%)	60°C; 72 hr	94 g/L	NA	35°C; 144 hr	13.8 g/L	Liet al. (2018)
Rice straw	Na_2CO_3	93°C; 3–10 hr	77.4 g/L	54.5–62.7	37°C; 120 hr	83.1 g/L	Molaverdiet al. (2019)
Bagasse	NaOH	50°C; 1 hr	NA	NA	30°C; 72 hr	7.05 g/L	Yuanet al. (2018)
Wheat straw	$NaOH/H_2O_2$	50°C; 3–15 hr	61.9 g/L	48.31	30°C; 96 hr	17.26 g/L	Liet al. (2018)

Diluted acid pretreatment is one of the most widely used techniques for LCB preparation, but it creates unfavorable conditions for extracting monomer sugars from biomass (Loow et al., 2016). Dilute acid hydrolysis offers some advantages over concentrated acid hydrolysis, as it requires fewer chemicals while still yielding a sufficient proportion of glucose from crystalline cellulose (Rabemanolontsoa and Saka, 2016). To improve the feasibility of processing cellulosic material into ethanol, sulfuric acid was used as a pretreatment. Acid pretreatment changed the structure of the biomass, and the cracking of the lignin structure reduced crystallinity (Rezania et al., 2018). Table 7.3 displays recent studies on the synthesis of ethanol from lignin using acid pretreatment.

7.5.3 Ionic Liquid Pretreatment

Using ILs as the initial treatment yielded high levels of sugars and carbohydrates due to their excellent biomass dissolution (Moniruzzaman and Goto, 2018). Cellulase activity and stability are maintained after pretreatment with ILs, which improves enzymatic delignification. Additionally, during IL pretreatment, temperature and biomass composition affected the rate of hydrolysis (Elgharbawy et al., 2016). Imidazolium-based products are some of the pretreated chemicals utilized in LCB (Zhang et al., 2017). The breaking of ether linkages significantly impacts lignin depolymerization, and alkaline liquids (AILs), a subclass of ILs, hold great promise for the pretreatment of LCB.

TABLE 7.3
Recent Studies of Acid Pretreatment of LCB for Bioethanol Production

RawMaterial	Acid Type	Pretreatment Condition	Reducing Sugars	Delignification Rate (%)	Fermentation Condition	Bioethanol Yield (g/L)	Ref.
Wheat straw	H_2SO_4(2%)	180°C; 10 min	43 g/L	NA	30°C; 72 hr	0.44	Prasad et al. (2018)
Wheat straw	H_2SO_4 and Na_2SO_3	121°C; 60 min	440 mg/kg	92	35°C; 72 hr	17.25	Jaisamutet al. (2016)
Rice straw	H_2SO_4	200°C; 1 min	NA	NA	30°C; 48 hr	2.3	Linet al. (2016)
Rice straw	H_2SO_4	120°C; 30 min	NA	NA	45°C; 24 hr	11.77	Castroet al. (2015)
Rye	H_2SO_4	121°C; 60 min	47.2 mg/g	NA	35°C; 72 hr	20.63	Mikulskiet al. (2018)
Wheat	H_2SO_4	131°C; 60 min	42.8 mg/g	NA	35°C; 72 hr	17.86	-
Maize	H_2SO_4	131°C; 60 min	134.4 mg/g	NA	35°C; 72 hr	17.26	-

7.5.4 Organic Solvent Pretreatment

A few advantages of organic solvent pretreatment include the ability to efficiently separate LCB into three categories and to regenerate the fluid. Studies on the application of biological solvents for the pretreatment of LCB are numerous and have significantly improved biomass conversion to sugars (Shuai and Luterbacher, 2016). A variety of biodegradable chemicals, including formaldehyde and amine with and without catalysts, are being utilized for conditioning LB (Zhao et al., 2009). Due to their affordability and ease of recovery, ethanol and methanol have been chosen as low-boiling-point alcohols (Espinoza-Acosta et al., 2014).

Organosolv is an organic pretreatment that uses a synthetic or deionized organic solvent at temperatures ranging from 100°C to 250°C. The two benefits of this technology are the separation of good cellulose with minimum degradation and exceptionally effective hemicellulose fractionation. The high-purity phenol and cellulose constituent chemicals, as well as a high-value by-product of organic pretreatment, pose the main economic challenges for this technology compared to dilute acid pretreatment. (Zhang et al., 2016). Recent research on bioethanol production from LCB using organic solvent pretreatment is shown in Table 7.4.

7.6 PHYSICAL METHODS

Physical/mechanical pretreatment can be carried out to open the structure of LCBs by degrading their surface and reducing their size to 10–30 mm (Prussi

TABLE 7.4
Recent Research on LCB Pretreatment with Chemical Solvents for the Production of Bioethanol

Raw Material	Pretreatment Type	Pretreatment Condition	Reducing Sugars	Delignification Rate (%)	Fermentation Condition	Bioethanol Yield (g/L)
Rice straw	Choline chloride-based solvent	60–121°C; 30 min – 12	Xylose:88	57.273.6	37°C; 72 hr	36.7 g/L
Wheat straw	Organosolv	180°C; 40 min	89.2	76.4	35°C; 72 hr	67%
Sugarcane bagasse	$FeCl_3$-catalyzed organosolv	160°C; 72 hr	Glucose: 93	62.7	50°C; 72 hr	NA
Cotton stalks	Organosolv	80°C; 1 hr	NA	81	30 hr	52%
Sorghum bagasse	Organosolv	200°C; 1 hr	Glucose: 90 Xylose:70	15.3	35°C; 72 hr	61.9 g/L
Wheat straw	Eutectic solvents	70°C; 9 hr	Glucose: 79.7	71.4	50°C; 72 hr	89.8%

et al., 2019). Incremental milling in the LCB pretreatment process accounts for a sizable portion of the overall operating cost. The primary considerations for physical pretreatment are the biomass's characteristics and its final particle size. Meanwhile, this method's major limitations are its substantial power consumption and low efficiency. There are several other types of physical pretreatment, including grinding, elevated uniformity, electromagnetic radiation treatments, heat enlargement, and photographic catalysis, which have been shown to encourage enzymatic hydrolysis but are frequently used (Tsapekoset al., 2017).

In a recent study, various types of equipment were used to pretreat maize stover: pneumatic filtration, an automated cylindrical process, and a high-speed mill. These methods reduced biomass by 100–230 mm, increasing the surrounding area available for the metabolite's action. In addition to these, the reduction of biomass may end in an increase in glucose in the range of 29–44%, showing the outstanding pretreatment efficiency of the air classifier mill and high-speed mill (Gu et al., 2019). Although LCB milling increases biofuel yield, it is not cost-effective due to its high energy consumption at large scales. The next section discusses the most popular physical pretreatment techniques for LCBs, such as moisture explosion, boiling warm water, and organosolv.

7.6.1 Microwave-Assisted Pretreatment

Microwave-assisted pretreatment has been one of the most widely used techniques for LCBs. It uses irradiation and has been used for 30 years to achieve an unheard-of yield of bioethanol. The microwave pretreatment approach offers several advantages, including a faster response and a lower activation energy for the reaction (Kang et al., 2019). Tolerant structures in LCB were disrupted by

TABLE 7.5
Current Research of LCB Pretreatment with Microwave Assistance for Bioethanol

Raw Substance	Pretreatment Type	Pretreatment Condition	Reducing Sugars	Delignification Rate (%)	Fermentation Condition	Bioethanol Yield (g/L)
Wheat straw	Microwave-associated NaOH	160°C; 15 min	718	69.48	30°C; 108 hr	6.82
Wheat straw	Microwave-associated alkali	80°C; 20 min	610.35	11.2	72 hr	6.84
Rice straw	Microwave-associated alkali	60°C; 25min	NA	NA	30°C; 24 hr	0.551
Maize	Microwave-associated H_2SO_4	50°C; 20 min	104	NA	50°C; 48 hr	NA
Eucalyptus sawdust	Microwave-associated	180°C; 17 min	104.4	112.1	50°C; 48 hr	NA
Cotton stalks	Microwave-associated acid	21°C; 10 min	NA	81	210°C; 10 min	15.9

microwave heating, which overcame the material's rigid structure (Chen et al., 2011). According to Zheng et al., the elimination of hydroxide and neutral metals via electromagnetic processing may be regarded as an effective technique to increase the corncob's sugar production. According to another study, microwave pretreatment with $CaCl_2$ increased hemicellulose breakdown to 85–90% and the corresponding dimension to 168.93% when compared to untreated maize stover. Table 7.5 presents recent research on the production of bioethanol from LCB via heat-up-assisted pretreatment.

7.6.2 Steam Explosion Pretreatment

In this thermophysical-chemical approach, vapor cracking and explosive decompression phases can mechanically disassemble LCBs. In this process, elevated heated steam is applied to the biomass. The cell wall structure is then suddenly disrupted by pressure release, mostly solubilizing the hemicellulose and lignin components (Maniet et al., 2017). Steam explosion is one of the strategies with the highest potential for eradicating lignin and hemicellulose from biomass. By rendering cellulose more crystalline and disrupting lignin structure, steam explosion can alter the physicochemical characteristics of LCBs.

The primary benefits of moisture treatments are minimal environmental impact, high energy efficiency, fragmentation of the biomass form, defibrillation, dissolution of significant parts, and reduction of the hemicellulosic fraction.

However, this strategy's disadvantages are inadequate lignin removal and the production of numerous hazardous substances (Bonfiglioet al., 2019).

7.6.2.1 Ammonia Fiber Explosion Pretreatment

This process provides a perfect imitation of combustion. Ammonia fiber explosion (AFEX) pretreatment techniques include expanding the material to enhance the readily accessible surface area, dissolving biomass fibers to release cellulose, and inhibiting the lignin-carbohydrate complex (Behera et al., 2014). While hemicellulose is broken down into deacetylated oligomeric sugars, lignin works with aqueous ammonia to break down and rupture the lignin-carbohydrate bonds. For instance, during the processing of maize stover with diluted acid and AFEX, the high AFEX efficiency resulted in substantial cellulose accessibility. The diluted acid largely destroyed the hemicellulosic component of biomass (xylan), even though AFEX revealed no loss of hemicellulose or lignin.

Even with a feedstock such as maize, the cost advantages of urea processing and reprocessing are a concern for large-scale usage. Stover treated with AFEX demonstrated enhanced enzymatic activity (Kumar et al., 2009). Recent research on steam explosion pretreatment for producing bioethanol from LCB is shown in Table 7.6.

TABLE 7.6
Challenges and Additional Approaches for Biological Pretreatment Methods

Pretreatment Type	Limitations	Recommendations
Organic solvent	Low rate of biomass recovery.	Enhance preprocessing variables such as the environment, time, alcohol concentration, and catalyst type.
Biological (fungal)	Rising prices and contamination as a result of very long pretreatment time, low downstream yields, and loss of carbohydrates.	Initial treatment for microorganisms, when combined, can improve enzymatic digestibility and shorten the pretreatment time.
Microwave irradiation (MWI)	Prior treatment is prohibitively costly, and large-scale equipment is in short supply. Due to the high energy demand, MWI's impact on various biomass forms was unknown.	Design more energy-efficient microwave systems. Investigate the impact of MWI on the biomass microstructure. Scaling up our microwave decontamination reactors becomes essential.
Ionic liquid (IL)	Lack of an economical solution for IL recycling.	Instead of relying solely on experimental levels, conduct preliminary-scale studies. Utilize adequate IL in relation to interactions with biomass. New and creative methods must be developed for recycling and reusing ILs.
Hydroxide and acids	Expensive adverse byproducts require enormous energy.	Elucidation of the structure and other characteristics of biomass.

7.6.3 Hydrothermal Pretreatment

The LCB is heated using hot water in hydrothermal pretreatment to prepare it for bioethanol production. This technique accelerates the breakdown of the lignocellulosic matrix at temperatures between 160°C and 240°C by using hot water under high pressure to retain it in a liquid state (Mosier et al., 2005). It offers a significant cost-saving advantage and is widely recognized as a green approach because it doesn't use chemicals. Low sugar concentrations, heavy water use, high energy consumption, and the presence of fermentation inhibitors are the main downsides. The severity factor is an essential factor because hemicellulose removal is more effective at higher values (up to 97%). The main component of hemicellulose, along with certain lignin, is eliminated with this strategy by being broken down into soluble fractions, which causes the cell wall's intolerant structure to be damaged.

Safflower straw, for instance, has been pretreated hydrothermally at 120°C, 150°C, and 180°C. In addition to the outcome, cellulose and hemicellulosic monomers, the primary solid and liquid polymers, were produced. The least unfavorable condition yields a maximum biofuel yield of 191.4 NmL/g VS after 1 hr at 120°C. The authors concluded that low-severity hydrothermal pretreatment increases biogas output. The results show that pretreatment removed lignin and altered the composition of the cell membrane. Additionally, the surface area increased after LHW pretreatment, but the amount of lignin and hemicellulose fractions removed decreased (Zhanget al., 2018).

7.7 BIOLOGICAL TREATMENT

Biological treatment is one of the most crucial methods for processing LCB to produce bioethanol. Because it can deliver relatively quick responses, this method, which primarily uses yeast and bacteria or their enzymes, is gaining more attention (Sindhu et al., 2016). Numerous fungi and a few bacteria have been used frequently in biological pretreatment. Cellulose is more susceptible to enzymatic or microbial attack after biological pretreatment because it has lost its crystalline structure, the lignin barrier, and some of its molecules.

Therefore, cellulose and hemicellulose are frequently hydrolyzed into isolated sugars by hemicellulolytic bacteria. The main advantages of biological methods include their low energy consumption, limited chemical recycling after pretreatment, minimal inhibitor formation, low downstream processing costs, and operational flexibility (Millati et al., 2011). However, the extremely slow rate of matter breakdown is the main difficulty with biological pretreatment methods. Additionally, oxidative and hydrolytic enzymes produced by bacteria and fungi can dissolve the hard exterior of LCBs (enzymatic method).

7.8 PRETREATMENT LIMITATIONS

By identifying the variables that inhibit LCBs' enzymatic hydrolysis, a few pretreatment methods are used to overcome their strong inherent resistance.

The following list includes the most essential requirements for successful pretreatment:

- High levels of sugar storage are preserved.
- Inhibitory formation is avoided.
- Low energy consumption.
- Cost-effective process.
- Environmental friendliness.

The original biomass size is preserved, while high levels of sugars and low levels of lignin are also produced.

Although several techniques, including microwaves, acids, alkalis, ILs, organic solvents, steam explosions, hydrothermal processes, and biological processes, have been developed to process LCBs, using them on an industrial scale involves overcoming numerous obstacles. Based on the literature, each approach has certain drawbacks; suggestions are provided in Table 7.6.

7.9 CONCLUSION AND FUTURE RECOMMENDATIONS

In this work, the most effective treatment methods for LCBs, including physical, chemical, biological, and combined methods for bioenergy generation, have been investigated. All individual methods have benefits and drawbacks, but further study is required to identify a successful combination of the currently used approaches. Furthermore, the effectiveness of pretreatment may be increased by conducting additional research on how it works or on the practical uses of the by-products produced. However, the pretreatment process has to be improved in terms of energy use and made more environmentally friendly. Therefore, the focus of future research should be on addressing several difficulties, such as the rise in large-scale commercialization, by examining economic factors and implementing an appropriate approach.

REFERENCES

Abdellatif, B., Hugo, D.V., Xavier, R. Dry fractionation process as an important step in current and future lignocellulose biorefineries: A review. *Bioresource Technology*. 2013;134:362–73.

Ahmed, M., Abdel, H., Jose, O.S., Cann, I.K.O. Insights into lignin degradation and its potential industrial applications. *Adv Appl Microbiol*. 2013;82:1–28.

An, Y.X., Zong, M.H., Wu, H., Li, N. Pretreatment of lignocellulosic biomass with renewable cholinium ionic liquids: Biomass fractionation, enzymatic digestion and ionic liquid reuse. *Bioresource Technology*. 2015;192:165–71.

Arijana, B., Nenad, M., Semjon, K., Galina, M., Halina, B., Mirela, I.S., Drazenka, K., Srdan N., Bozidar, S. Bioethanol production from renewable raw materials and its separation and purification: A review. *Food Technology Biotechnology*. 2012;56(3):289–311.

Balat, M. Production of bioethanol from lignocellulosic materials via the biochemical pathway: A review. *Energy Conversion and Management*. 2011;52:858–75.

Bali, G., Meng, X., Deneff, J.I., Sun, Q., Ragauskas, A.J. The effect of alkaline pretreatment methods on cellulose structure and accessibility. *ChemSusChem*. 2015;8(2):275–9.

Behera, S., Arora, R., Nandhagopal, N., Kumar, S. Importance of chemical pretreatment for bioconversion of lignocellulosic biomass. *Renew Sustain Energy Rev*. 2014;36:91–106.

Bonfiglio, F., Cagno, M., Rey, F., Torres, M., Bothig, S., Menendez, P. Pre-treatment of switchgrass by steam explosion in a semi-continuous pre-pilot reactor. *Biomass Bioenergy*. 2019;121:41–7.

Canilha, L., Chandel, A.K., Milessi, T.S.D.S., Antunes, F.A.F., Freitas, W.L.D.C., Felipe, M.D.G.A., da Silva, S.S. Bioconversion of sugarcane biomass into ethanol: An overview about composition, pretreatment methods, detoxification of hydrolysates, enzymatic saccharification, and ethanol fermentation. *J Biotechnol Biomed*. 2012;15:989572.

Carvalho, D.M., Queiroz, J.H., Colodette, J.L. Assessment of alkaline pretreatment for the production of bioethanol from eucalyptus, sugarcane bagasse and sugarcane straw. *Ind Crop Prod*. 2016;94:932–41.

Castro, R.C., Roberto, I.C. Effect of nutrient supplementation on ethanol production in different strategies of saccharification and fermentation from acid pretreated rice straw. *Biomass Bioenergy*. 2015;78:156–63.

Chaula, Z., Said, M., John, G., Manyele, S., Mhilu, C. Modelling the suitability of pine sawdust for energy production via biomass steam explosion. *Smart Grid and Renewable Energy*. 2014;5: 1.

Chen, W.H., Tu, Y.J., Sheen, H.K. Disruption of sugarcane bagasse lignocellulosic structure by means of dilute sulfuric acid pretreatment with microwave-assisted heating. *Appl Energy*. 2011;88(8):2726–34.

Collard, F.X., Blin, J. A review on pyrolysis of biomass constituents: Mechanisms and composition of the products obtained from the conversion of cellulose, hemicelluloses and lignin. *Renewable and Sustainable Energy Reviews*. 2014;38:594–608.

da Costa, R.M.F., Pattathil, S., Avci, U., Winters, A., Hahn, M.G., Bosch, M. Desirable plant cell wall traits for higher-quality miscanthus lignocellulosic biomass. *Biotechnology for Biofuels*.2019;12:85.

Devendra Prasad, M., Ankit, S., Sangeeta, N. An overview of key pretreatment processes for biological conversion of lignocellulosic biomass to bioethanol. *3 Biotech*. 2015;5:597–609.

Elgharbawy, A.A., Alam, M.Z., Moniruzzaman, M., Goto, M. Ionic liquid pretreatment as emerging approaches for enhanced enzymatic hydrolysis of lignocellulosic biomass. *Biochem Eng J*. 2016 (109)252–67.

Espinoza-Acosta, J.L., Torres-Chavez, P.I., Carvajal-Mill, E., Ramírez-Wong, B., Bello-Perez L.A., Montano-Leyva, B. Ionic liquids and organic solvents for ~ recovering lignin from lignocellulosic biomass. *BioResources*. 2014;9(2):3660e–87.

Gabriela, V., Regis Teixeira, M., George, A. Lignocellulosic biomass as a substrate for oleaginous microorganisms: A review. *Appl Sci*. 2020;10(21):7698. https://doi.org/10.3390/app10217698.

Gonzales, R.R., Sivagurunathan, P., Kim, S.H. Effect of severity on dilute acid pretreatment of lignocellulosic biomass and the following hydrogen fermentation. *Int J Hydrogen Energy*. 2016;41(46):21678–84.

Gu, Y.M., Kim, S., Sung, D., Sang, B.I., Lee, J.H. Feasibility of continuous pretreatment of corn stover: A comparison of three commercially available continuous pulverizing devices. *Energies*. 2019;12(8):142.

Halder, P., Kundu, S., Patel, S., Setiawan, A., Atkin, R., Parthasarthy, R. Progress on the pre-treatment of lignocellulosic biomass employing ionic liquids. *Renew Sustain Energy Rev*. 2019;105:268–92.

Hellsmark, H., Mossberg, J., Söderholm, P., Frishammar, J. Innovation system strengths and weaknesses in progressing sustainable technology: The case of Swedish biorefinery development. *J Clean Prod.* 2016;131:702–15.

Isikgor, F.H., Remzi Becer, C. Lignocellulosic biomass: A sustainable platform for the production of bio-based chemicals and polymers. *Polymer Chemistry.* 2015;6:4497–559.

Jaisamut, K., Paulova, L., Patakova, P., Kotú, C.S., Rychtera, M. Effect of sodium sulfite on acid pretreatment of wheat straw with respect to its final conversion to ethanol. *Biomass Bioenergy.* 2016;95:1e7.

Jönsson, L.J., Martín, C. Pretreatment of lignocellulose: Formation of inhibitory by-products and strategies for minimizing their effects. *BioresourceTechnology.* 2016;199:103–12.

Kang, K., Nanda, S., Sun, G., Qiu, L., Gu, Y., Zhang, T. Microwave-assisted hydrothermal carbonization of corn stalk for solid biofuel production: Optimization of process parameters and characterization of hydrochar. *Energy.* 2019;186:115795.

Karimi, K., Taherzadeh, M.J. A critical review of analytical methods in pretreatment of lignocelluloses: Composition, imaging, and crystallinity. *Bioresource Technology.* 2016;200:1008–18.

Kim, J.S., Lee, Y.Y., Kim, T.H. A review on alkaline pretreatment technology for bioconversion of lignocellulosic biomass. *Bioresource Technology.* 2016;199:42–8.

Kumar, P., Barrett, D.M., Delwiche, M.J., Stroeve, P. Methods for pretreatment of lignocellulosic biomass for efficient hydrolysis and biofuel production. *Ind Eng Chem Res.* 2009;48(8):3713–29.

Kumar, R., Tabatabaei, M., Karimi, K., Sárvári, H.I. Recent updates on lignocellulosic biomass-derived ethanol – a review. *Biofuel Res J.*2016;3:347–56.

Kumari, D., Singh, R. Pretreatment of lignocellulosic wastes for biofuel production: A critical review. *Renew Sustain Energy Rev.* 2018;90:877–9.

Li, J., Chi, X., Zhang, Y., Wang, X. Enhanced coproduction of hydrogen and butanol from rice straw by a novel two-stage fermentation process. *Int BiodeteriorBiodegrad.* 2018;127:62–68.

Lin, T.H., Guo, G.L., Hwang, W.S., Huang, S.L. The addition of hydrolyzed rice straw in xylose fermentation by Pichia stipitis to increase bioethanol production at the pilot scale. *Biomass Bioenergy.* 2016;91:204–9.

Loow, Y.L., Wu, T.Y., Jahim, J.Md., Mohammad, A.W., Teoh, W.H. Typical conversion of lignocellulosic biomass into reducing sugars using dilute acid hydrolysis and alkaline pretreatment. *Cellulose.* 2016;23(3):1491–520.

Maniet, G., Schmetz, Q., Jacquet, N., Temmerman, M., Gofflot, S., Richel, A. Effect of steam explosion treatment on chemical composition and characteristic of organosolv fescue lignin. *Ind Crop Prod.* 2017;99:79–85.

McIntosh, S., Zhang, Z., Palmer, J., Wong, H.H., Doherty, W. O, Vancov, T. Pilot-scale cellulosic ethanol production using eucalyptus biomass pre-treated by dilute acid and steam explosion. *Biofuels Bioprod Biorefining.* 2016;*10*(4):346–58.

Menon, V., Rao,M. Trends in bioconversion of lignocellulose: Biofuels, platform chemicals & biorefinery concept. *Progress in Energy Combust Sci.*2012;38:522–50.

Mikulski, D., Kłosowski, G. Efficiency of dilute sulfuric acid pretreatment of distillery stillage in the production of cellulosic ethanol. *Bioresource Technology.* 2018;268:424–33.

Millati, R., Syamsiah S, Niklasson, C., Cahyanto, M.N., Ludquist, K., Taherzadeh, M.J. Biological pretreatment of lignocelluloses with white-rot fungi and its applications: A review. *BioResources.* 2011;6(4):5224–59.

Molaverdi, M., Karimi, K., Mirmohamadsadeghi, S. Improvement of dry simultaneous saccharification and fermentation of rice straw to high concentration ethanol by sodium carbonate pretreatment. *Energy.* 2019;167:654.

Moniruzzaman, M., Goto, M. Ionic liquid pretreatment of lignocellulosic biomass for enhanced enzymatic delignification. In: Itoh, T., Koo, Y.M. (eds) *Application of Ionic Liquids in Biotechnology. Advances in Biochemical Engineering/Biotechnology*, Vol. 168. Springer, Cham; 2018.

Moraïs, S., Barak, Y., Caspi, J., Hadar, Y., Lamed, R., Shoham, Y., Wilson, D.B., Bayera, E.A. Deconstruction of lignocellulose into soluble sugars by native and designer cellulosomes. *Microbiology Careers Salary Survey*. 2012;3(6).

Mori, T., Tsuboi, Y., Ishida, N., Nishikubo, N., Demura, T., Kikuchi, J. Multidimensional high-resolution magic angle spinning and solution-state NMR characterization of 13C-labeled plant metabolites and lignocellulose. *Scientific Reports*. 2015;5.

Mosier, N., Wyman, C., Dale, B., Elander, R., Lee, Y.Y., Holtzapple, M. Features of promising technologies for pretreatment of lignocellulosic biomass. *Bioresource Technology*. 2005;96(6):673–86.

Mumtaz, M.W., Mukhtar, H., Dilawer, U.A., Hussain, S.M., Hussain, M., Iqbal, M., Adnan, A., Nisar, J. Biocatalytic transesterification of Eruca sativa oil for the production of biodiesel. *Biocatalysis and Agricultural Biotechnology*. 2016;5:162–7.

Mupondwa, E., Li, X., Tabil, L., Sokhansanj, S., Adapa, P. Status of Canada's lignocellulosic ethanol: Part II: Hydrolysis and fermentation technologies. *Renewable and Sustainable Energy Reviews*. 2016;79:1535–55.

Prasad, S., Malav, M.K., Kumar, S., Singh, A., Pant, D., Radhakrishnan, S. Enhancement of bio-ethanol production potential of wheat straw by reducing furfural and 5-hydroxymethylfurfural (HMF). *Bioresource Technology*. 2018;4:50e6.

Prussi, M., Padella, M., Conton, M., Postma, E.D., Lonza, L. Review of technologies for biomethane production and assessment of Eu transport. *J Clean Prod*. 2019;222:565–72.

Putro, J.N., Soetaredjo, F.E., Lin, S.Y., Ju, Y.H., Ismadji, S. Pretreatment and conversion of lignocellulose biomass into valuable chemicals. *RSC Adv*. 2016;6(52) 46834–52.

Rabemanolontsoa, H., Saka, S. Various pretreatments of lignocellulosics. *Bioresource Technology*. 2016;199:83–91.

Rangabhashiyam, S., Balasubramanian, P. The potential of lignocellulosic biomass precursors for biochar production: Performance, mechanism and wastewater application – A review. *Industrial Crops and Products*. 2019;128:405–23.

Rezania, S., Din, M.F.M., Taib, S.M., Mohamad, S.E., Dahalan, F.A., Kamy, H. Ethanol production from water hyacinth (Eichhornia crassipes) using various types of enhancers based on the consumable sugars. *Waste Biomass Valori*. 2018;9(6):939e46.

Saritha, M., Arora, A., Lata. Biological pretreatment of lignocellulosic substrates for enhanced delignification and enzymatic digestibility. *Indian Journal of Microbiology*. 2012;52(2):122–30.

Sarks, C., Bals, B.D., Wynn, J., Teymouri, F., Schwegmann, S., Sanders, K. Scaling up and benchmarking of ethanol production from pelletized pilot-scale AFEX-treated corn stover using Zymomonas mobilis. *Biofuels*. 2016;1–15.

Shuai L, Luterbacher J. Organic solvent effects in biomass conversion reactions. *ChemSusChem*. 2016;9(2):133–55.

Sindhu, R., Binod, P., Pandey, A. Biological pretreatment of lignocellulosic biomass e an overview. *BioresourTechnol*. 2016;199:76–82.

Solarte-Toro, J.C., Romero-García, J.M., Martínez-Patino, J.C., Ruiz-Ramos, E., Castro-Galiano, E., Cardona-Alzate, C.A. Acid pretreatment of lignocellulosic biomass for energy vectors production: A review focused on operational conditions and techno-economic assessment for bioethanol production. *Renew Sustain Energy Rev*. 2019;107:587–601.

Studer, M. H, DeMartini, J. D, Davis, M. F, Sykes, R. W, Davison, B., Keller, M., Tuskan, G. A, Wyman, C.E. Lignin content in natural Populus variants affects sugar release. *Proceedings of the National Academy of Sciences*. 2011;108:6300–6305.

Taarning, E., Osmundsen, C.M., Yang, X., Voss, B., Andersen, S.I., Christensena, C.H. Zeolite-catalyzed biomass conversion to fuels and chemicals. *Energy Environ Sci.* 2011;4:793–804.

Taha, M., Foda, M., Shahsavari, E., Aburto-Medina, A., Adetutu, E., Ball, A. Commercial feasibility of lignocellulose biodegradation: Possibilities and challenges. *Curr OpinBiotechnol.* 2016;38:190–7.

Teran Hilares, R., Ienny, J.V., Marcelino, P.F., Ahmed, M.A., Antunes, F.A.F., da Silva, S.S. Ethanol production in a simultaneous saccharification and fermentation process with interconnected reactors employing hydrodynamic cavitation-pretreated sugarcane bagasse as raw material. *Bioresource Technology.* 2017;243:652–9.

Tsapekos,P., Kougias, P.G., Egelund, H., Larsen, U., Pedersen, J., Trenel, P. Mechanical pretreatment at harvesting increases the bioenergy output from marginal land grasses. *Renew Energy.* 2017;111:914–21.

Valery, B.A., Nazim, C., Richard, S., Alex, B., David, B.L. Biomass pretreatment: Fundamentals toward application. *Biotechnology Advances.* 2011;29(6):675–85.

Vishnu, M., Mala, R. Trends in bioconversion of lignocellulose: Biofuels, platform chemicals & biorefinery concept. *Progress in Energy and Combustion Science.* 2012;38(4):22–550.

Vohra, M., Manwar, J., Manmode, R., Padgilwar, S., Patil, S. Bioethanol production: Feedstock and current technologies. *J Enviro Chem Eng.* 2014;2:573–84.

Wei, N., Oh, E.J., Million, G., Cate, J.H., Jin, Y.S. Simultaneous utilization of cellobiose, xylose, and acetic acid from lignocellulosic biomass for biofuel production by an engineered yeast platform. *ACS Synth Biol.* 2015;4:707–13.

Yuan, Z., Wen, Y., Kapu, N.S., Beatson, R. Evaluation of an organosolv-based biorefinery process to fractionate wheat straw into ethanol and co-products. *Ind Crop Prod.* 2018;121:294–302.

Zabed, H., Faruq, G., Sahu, J., Boyce, A., Ganesan, P. A comparative study on normal and high sugary corn genotypes for evaluating enzyme consumption during dry-grind ethanol production. *Chem Eng J.* 2016;287:691–703.

Zhang, K., Pei, Z., Wang, D. Organic solvent pretreatment of lignocellulosic biomass for biofuels and biochemicals: A review. *Bioresource Technology.* 2016;199:21–33.

Zhang, Q., Hu, J., Lee, D-J. Pretreatment of biomass using ionic liquids: Research updates. *Renew Energy.* 2017;111:77–84.

Zhang,Y., Nakagawa, K., Shibuya, M., Sasaki, K., Takahashi, T., Shintani, T. Improved permselectivity of forward osmosis membranes for efficient concentration of pretreated rice straw and bioethanol production. *J Membr Sci.*2018;566:15–24.

Zhao, H., Lu, D., Wang, J., Tu, W., Wu, D., Koh, S.W., Gao, P., Xu, Z.J., Deng, S., Zhou, Y., You, B., Li, H. Raw biomass electroreforming coupled to green hydrogen generation. *Nature Communications.* 2012;12.

Zhao, X., Cheng, K., Liu, D. Organosolv pretreatment of lignocellulosic biomass for enzymatic hydrolysis. *Appl MicrobiolBiotechnol.* 2009;82(5):815.

Zhao, X., Xiong, L., Zhang, M., Bai, F. Towards efficient bioethanol production from agricultural and forestry residues: Exploration of unique natural microorganisms in combination with advanced strain engineering. *Bioresource Technology.* 2016;209:265–76.

8 Biomass Components

Sundergopal Sridhar and
Mamilla Shyam Sunder

8.1 INTRODUCTION

Biomass refers to any organic material derived from plant or animal sources, including municipal and industrial waste, trees, crops, grasses, as well as agricultural and forestry residues (Fantini, 2017). This substance can be used directly as an energy source or converted into fuels such as biogas, biofuels, and bio-oil. The significance of biomass lies in its potential to support the global shift toward cleaner, more sustainable energy sources. Unlike fossil fuels, biomass is renewable because it can be replenished over time (Parmar, 2017). Additionally, biomass can help reduce fossil fuel dependency and associated greenhouse gas emissions, while enhancing energy security. Moreover, biomass is an abundant energy resource containing various substances that can be utilized for numerous applications, including energy generation, biofuel production, and so forth. Biomass components refer to various types of organic matter which differ in composition, characteristics, and potential applications (Overend, 2019). Biomass components are classified into cellulose, hemicellulose, and lignin. All three are referred to as lignocellulosic biomass, and each constituent has unique features that can be used in various ways to harness their energy content. Figure 8.1 represents the primary classification and brief role of each biomass component.

Lignocellulosic biomass is the most widely available biomass component and serves as a vital energy source and structural support for plant bodies. It is mainly found in substances such as crop stalks, straw, wood waste, and switchgrass. Cellulose and hemicellulose are carbohydrates that can be converted to glucose and fermented to produce biofuels such as ethanol and butanol (Wei et al., 2017). On the other hand, lignin is a complex polymer that provides structural support to plant cells and is resistant to degradation (Sahay, 2022). Moreover, it can be processed using several chemical technologies for energy extraction or utilized as a raw material for producing bio-oil and other chemicals (Merklein et al., 2016).

8.2 CELLULOSE AND ITS STRUCTURE

Cellulose is the main compound of various plants, bacteria, algae, fungi, and animals. French chemist Anselme Payen discovered and isolated a white, fibrous substance from the plant, which he called cellulose, meaning "small cells." Cellulose is widely available in nature and is the primary structural component of

DOI: 10.1201/9781003327608-8

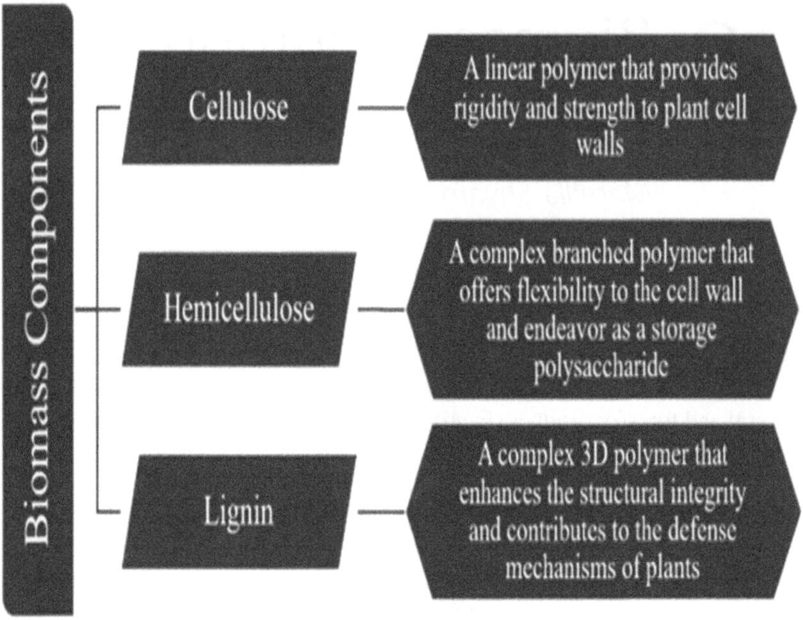

FIGURE 8.1 Biomass components and their features.

plant cell walls, providing rigidity and strength to the plant (O'Sullivan, 1997). Cellulose is a polysaccharide having the formula $(C_6H_{10}O_5)$, which entails thousands of β(1–4) linked D-glucose units in a linear chain model (Crawford, 1981).

In 1920, Hermann Staudinger determined the structure of the cellulose polymer (Figure 8.2) (Crawford, 1981), while Kobayashi and Shoda were the first to chemically synthesize cellulose without using any biologically derived enzymes in 1992 (Nishiyama et al., 2002; King, 1982). Cellulose is abundant, with an annual yield of approximately 1.3×10^9 metric tons of organic matter.

The linear chains of the molecule are attached by hydrogen bonding to form strong, fibrous, and insoluble microfibrils. These microfibrils are bundled together to form cellulose fibers. The arrangement of these microfibrils gives cellulose fibers their characteristic strength and flexibility. Microfibrils that undergo hydrogen bonding determine whether crystalline or amorphous bonds are introduced into the cellulose structure. Stabilizing the long chains in a structured arrangement enables functional groups to interact. These groups are the hydroxyl molecules linked to each glucopyranose molecule, which are accountable for supramolecular structure and cellulose's physical and chemical properties through hydrogen bonding (H-bond) (Kobayashi et al., 1991). Cellulose is a biodegradable polymer with a wide range of industrial and commercial applications, including its use in paper and textile production, as well as a renewable energy source for biofuel generation.

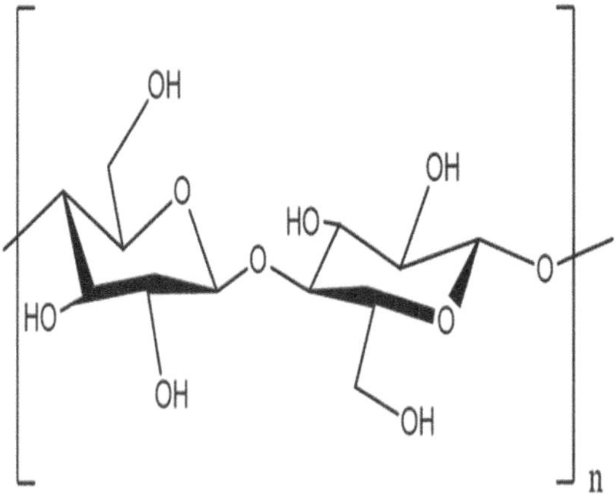

FIGURE 8.2 Structural representation of cellulose.

8.2.1 Properties of Cellulose

a. **Insolubility in water:** Cellulose is relatively insoluble in water and other ordinary organic solvents, which makes it an excellent material for specific applications such as papermaking, where it can form a robust and stable network of fibers.
b. **High tensile strength:** Cellulose has high tensile strength because of its firm hydrogen bonds, which are resistant to breaking or stretching. This makes it useful for various applications, including textiles and construction materials.
c. **Biodegradability:** Cellulose is biodegradable, meaning natural processes can break it down into simpler compounds. This makes it a more environmentally friendly material compared to many synthetic alternatives.
d. **Hydrophilicity:** Cellulose is hydrophilic and capable of forming hydrogen bonds with water molecules, enabling it to absorb moisture and swell. This property is essential in various biological systems and industrial applications.
e. **Chemical resistance:** Cellulose is highly resistant to many chemicals, including acids and bases. It is helpful in various industrial applications, such as filtration and purification.
f. **Electrical conductivity:** In its pure form, cellulose is not a good conductor of electricity. However, it can be modified to improve electrical conductivity, making it useful in some electronic applications.

8.2.1.1 Physical Properties

a. Its molar mass is 162.1406 grams/mole.
b. Its density is 1.5 grams/cm^3.
c. Its melting point is 260–270°C.

8.2.1.2 Chemical Properties

a. It has a strong affinity to itself and compounds containing hydroxyl groups, mainly water.
b. It is highly reactive to water and promotes those reactions with cellulose chains that immediately form hydrogen bonds.
c. It reacts with concentrated mineral acids at high temperatures and breaks into smaller glucose molecules.
d. It is more crystalline than starch.

8.2.2 Uses of Cellulose

Cellulose has a wide variety of uses and applications in numerous industries, such as the following:

a. Cellulose is the primary raw material used to produce paper and various other products, including writing paper, newspapers, cardboard, and tissue paper.
b. Cellulose-based fibers such as cotton, linen, and rayon are widely used in the textile industry to make clothing, bedsheets, and other textiles.
c. Cellulose is often used as a food additive to provide texture and bulk to food products and dietary fiber supplements.
d. Cellulose is used in the pharmaceutical industry to make capsules, tablets, and other dosage forms.
e. Cellulose-based feedstocks such as wood chips, grasses, and agricultural waste are further processed to produce biofuels, an alternative to fossil fuels.
f. Cellulose-based materials, such as insulation and fiberboard, are used in the construction industry to provide insulation and soundproofing.
g. Cellulose is commonly used in cosmetics to enhance texture and viscosity. It functions as a thickener or stabilizer in products such as creams, lotions, and other personal care formulations.

8.2.3 Morphology

Cellulose is synthesized at the plasma membrane of plant cells, where its microfibrils are composed of 36 cellulose chains, aligned in parallel and held together by hydrogen bonds. They have a hierarchical structure with strong crystalline regions on their surfaces and along their length. The hierarchical structure is necessary to deconstruct plant fibers into new materials by chemical or mechanical means (Krumm et al., 2016).

At the microscopic level, cellulose exhibits a fibrous structure composed of long chains of glucose units that align to form flat, ribbon-like structures known as cellulose microfibrils. These microfibrils can be 10–100 nm in diameter and several micrometers in length. The overall morphology of cellulose is hierarchical, with structures at the micro-, meso-, and macro-scales all contributing to the unique properties of this vital biomaterial.

Cellulose can exist in several crystalline forms, including cellulose I, II, III, and IV. Among these, cellulose I primarily exists in two crystal phases: triclinic (Iα) and monoclinic (Iβ). The monoclinic form (Iβ) is more stable and predominant, characterized by two parallel chains oriented upward and tightly packed in a sheet-like arrangement. Triclinic cellulose contains a single chain and has similar glycosyl linkages and hydroxymethyl groups.

Cellulose II is formed by liquefying cellulose I in a solvent and then precipitating it or using an alkali to swell cellulose I fibers. Cellulose II is monoclinic and contains anti-parallel chains. Cellulose III is formed by treating celluloses I and II with ammonia and further heating them, which results in the formation of cellulose IV.

8.3 HEMICELLULOSE AND ITS STRUCTURE

Hemicellulose consists of short, highly branched sugar chains, including D-xylose, L-arabinose, and uronic acids. Unlike cellulose, hemicellulose has a branched structure, rendering it amorphous and relatively easier to hydrolyze into its constituent sugars. Hardwood hydrolysis produces hemicellulose sugars and materials rich in xylose (a five-carbon sugar). Figure 8.3 shows the structure of hemicelluloses (Krishnamachari et al., 2011).

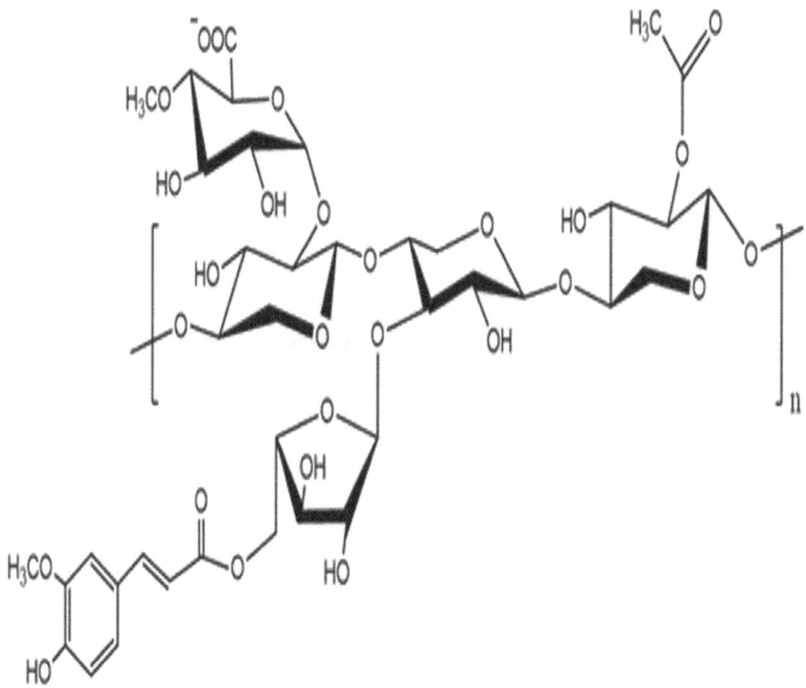

FIGURE 8.3 Structural representation of hemicellulose.

Hemicellulose polysaccharides can interact with cellulose via many hydrogen bonds and with lignin via covalent bonds and are soluble in diluted alkali. Hemicellulose is a family of polysaccharides that includes arabinoxylans, glucomannans, galactan, and others that are generated in different ways in plant cell walls. The most prevalent hemicellulose is xylan, and its structure depends on availability and source.

The cellulose fibrils that make up plant cell walls are coated with hemicellulose, a thermochemically sensitive lignocellulosic substance. Hemicelluloses are usually categorized as xylans, mannans, and glucans.

8.3.1 Xylans

Xylan is a polysaccharide with β(1–4) linkage between D-xylose and its related branches, as illustrated in Figure 8.4 (Hu et al., 2020). It is the most prevalent group of hemicellulose, and many plant cell walls comprise around one-third of all plant biomass. It is the secondary cell wall where xylan is primarily found, and as the cellulose synthase complex extrudes the microfibril, xylan appears to collect on its surface. By forming hydrogen bonds with the other polysaccharides and covalent couplings with the ferulic and coumaric acids found in lignin, xylans create cross-links between other hemicellulose components, cellulose, lignin, and pectin (Correia et al., 2011).

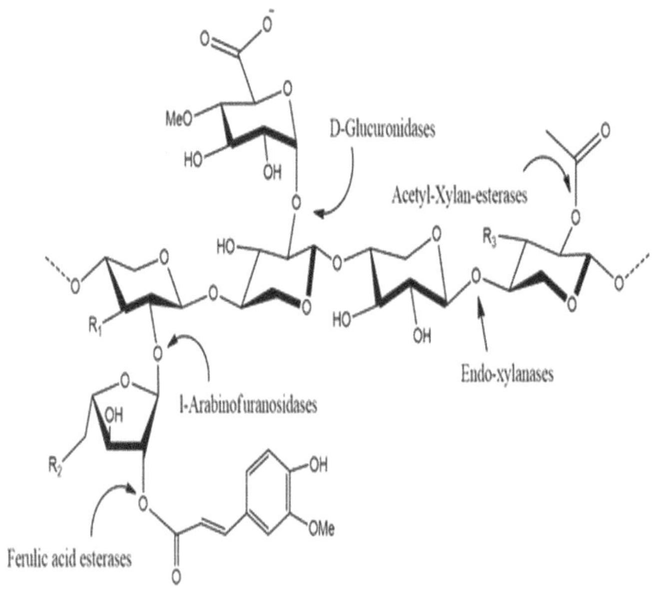

FIGURE 8.4 Structure of xylans.

8.3.2 Mannans

Mannan refers to a linear polymer of β-(1,4)-linked mannopyranosyl residues. Mannan and cellulose are both linear β-(1,4)-linked monosaccharide polymers, and as a result, their structures and degradation processes are similar. The mannan polymer can be branched by making groupings of various galactose residues and glucose, which give rise to glucomannans, galactomannans, gluconic acid mannans, and so forth. The structure of mannans and their derivatives is illustrated in Figure 8.5 (Wyman et al., 2004).

A storage polysaccharide, glucomannan, is present mainly in the roots of the *Amorphophallus konjac* plant. It has a 1.6:1 ratio of mannopyranose and glucopyranose, linked by β-(1,4). Galactomannans, known as extracellular carbohydrate storage, consist of β-(1,6) bonds of galactose units. Gluconic acid, prevalent in the cell wall, is composed of mannose and gluconic residues linked by β(1–4) and β(1–2) bonds, respectively, in the main chain (Correia et al., 2011).

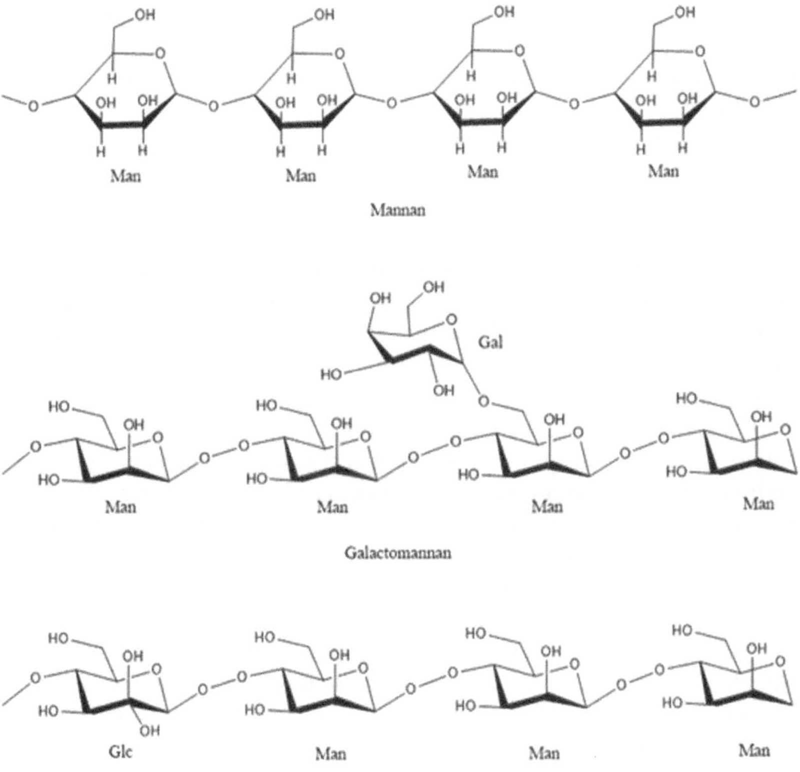

FIGURE 8.5 Structure of mannans and their derivatives.

8.3.3 Galactans and Arabinogalactans

Galactans comprise galactose residues joined by a polymer widely present in larch bark. In molar bonds, galactose and arabinose coexist, and the skeleton is built of galactan with lateral chains made of glucose, arabinose, and arabinogalactan in a ratio of 6:1.

8.4 LIGNIN COMPONENTS AND THEIR STRUCTURES

Lignin (or lignen) is a biomass component introduced by De Candolle in 1819 from the word "lignum," which means wood (Crawford, 1981). It is a complex compound with abundant biomass that plays a significant role in plant functioning. It is the third largest, after cellulose and hemicellulose. It is a rigid, impermeable compound that is principally found in the cell walls of vascular plants. The lignin content of biomass varies with plant species and age, constituting 15–20% of the total plant material.

Lignin is a chemically complex, three-dimensional polymer composed of phenylpropane units, namely *p*-coumaryl alcohol, sinapyl, and coniferyl (King, 1982). These monomer units participate in the oxidation reactions and form a cross-linked 3D structure within plant cell walls. The distinctive structure of lignin enables its unique characteristics, including strength and resistance to degradation.

Overall, lignin is a natural binder that links proteins and polysaccharides in the plant cell walls and is constructed to resist microbial attack. Moreover, the lignin structure is established by strong intramolecular and intermolecular hydrogen bonds. Lignin is obtained through the irreversible dehydration reaction of sugars. This aromatic compound is greatly insoluble in any solvent except alkaline solutions. Further, during condensation, total lignin is converted into two lignin fractions, soluble and insoluble lignin, leading to cell wall alteration; this phenomenon is called lignification. Figure 8.6 shows the structure of various types of monomers.

The central role of lignin is to provide structural support for plants, allowing them to stand upright and withstand external stresses. Additionally, lignin acts as a primary barrier against pests and pathogens and assists in water transport and storage. Moreover, lignin has distinct chemical properties that can be extracted for various applications.

Scientists and scholars are keenly exploring approaches to effective lignin breakdown, empowering the exploitation of lignocellulosic biomass as a renewable feedstock. These include chemical and biological treatments such as microbial degradation and enzymatic and other catalytic depolymerization reactions. The conversion of lignin into minor-value-added products enables the production of high-value chemicals, biofuels, and other valuable compounds.

The researchers found that the global lignin availability is around 300 billion tons, with an annual increase of 20 billion tons. There are a few novel technologies for converting lignin into value-added products that could boost the

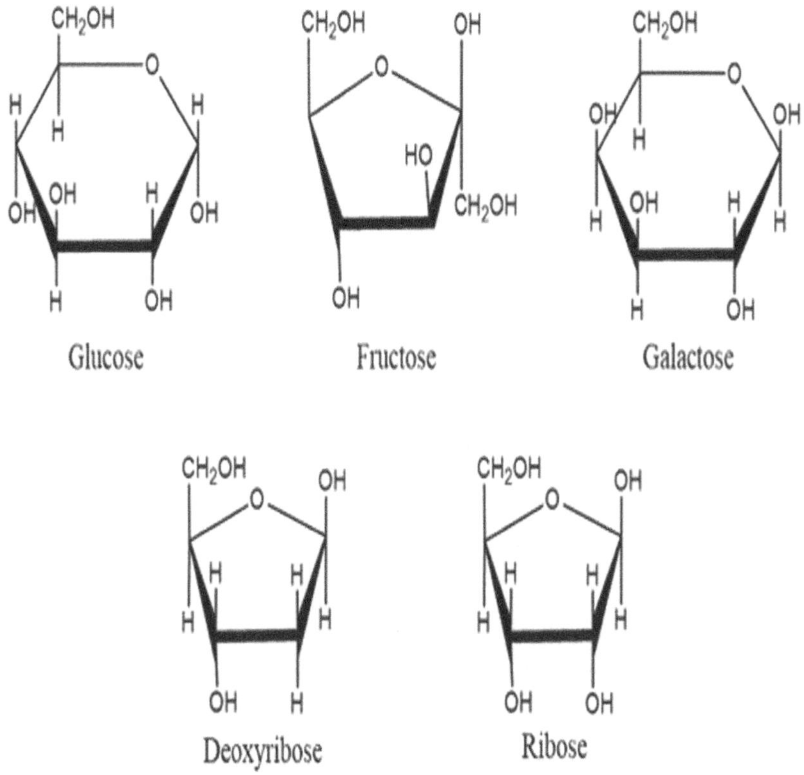

FIGURE 8.6 Structures of different types of glucose monomers.

global economy. Until today, lignin has been burned as a low-value fuel, and its higher calorific value has not been explicitly considered for utilization. Moreover, many valuable products are derived from lignin, including macromolecular materials, biofuels, and aromatics. The key value-added use of lignin in the past has been as a flavoring product, such as vanilla, and for drilling oil wells. Lignosulfonate demand will more likely be met by conventional wood pulping sources in the foreseeable future, as vanilla production uses only a small fraction of the overall lignin market.

8.5 OTHER COMPONENTS OF LIGNOCELLULOSIC COMPONENTS

Lignocellulosic biomass mainly consists of cellulose, hemicellulose, and lignin, besides a few minor components that are actively available, which are explained in the next subsections.

8.5.1 Starch

Starch appears in different morphological forms depending on plant species, as granules that contain millions of amylopectin molecules. The common representation of starch is $(C_6H_{10}O_6)_n$, where *n* indicates the number of residues of α-D-glucose units linked together to create the polymer. Starch has two forms: amylase, which constitutes 25–27% and is soluble in hot water, and amylopectin, which constitutes 73–75% and is insoluble in water. Amylose is a single, non-branched chain polymer, while amylopectin is highly branched. The ratio of amylose to amylopectin varies among plant species, resulting in different types of starch with distinct properties.

8.5.2 Extractives

These are organic substances, such as lipids, resins, tannins, waxes, and other phenolic compounds, which can be extracted using solvents. These valuable compounds contribute to the overall composite of lignocellulosic biomass and can be further utilized and processed.

8.5.3 Ash

Biomass contains traces of ash, the quantity of which varies depending on the biomass source. Ash is an inorganic substance composed of minerals, including calcium, magnesium, potassium, silica, and trace elements. The quantity of ash content can significantly affect biomass properties, especially during thermal conversion processes.

8.5.4 Proteins

Lignocellulosic biomass also contains proteins, which are present in different amounts depending on the source of biomass. The quantity of protein components is predominantly high in agricultural residues such as pine, reeds, birch, spruce, and wheat straw.

8.5.5 Pectin

Pectin is a complex polysaccharide found in certain types of lignocellulosic biomass. It is found in the middle lamella and primary cell walls of plants and contributes to the overall structure and properties of biomass.

8.5.6 Minerals

In addition to the previously mentioned ash content, lignocellulosic biomass can contain other metals such as copper, iron, manganese, and zinc. The presence of these minerals in biomass can affect the biomass conversion process either positively or negatively.

TABLE 8.1
Key Characteristics of Lignocellulosic Biomass

Characteristics	Cellulose	Hemicellulose	Lignin
Structure	• A linear, structured polymer consisting of glucose molecules. • Glucose units are arranged in a straight chain. • Strong intermolecular hydrogen bonding between adjacent cellulose chains.	• Complex branched polymer. • Comprises different sugar molecules linked by various glycosidic bonds.	• Complex 3D aromatic structure. • Composed of phenylpropane molecules. • It forms a matrix filling the spaces between cellulose and hemicellulose within the plant cell wall.
Solubility	Insoluble in water and most organic solvents.	Comparatively more soluble than cellulose, mostly in alkaline solutions.	Insoluble in water and most organic solvents and can be partially solubilized under particular process conditions.
Functionality	• Provides rigidity and strength to the plant cell wall. • Enables maintaining plant structural integrity. • Contributes to the overall mechanical strength of plant tissues. • Acts as a barrier against pathogens and external stresses.	• It plays a key role in the plant cell wall by interacting with cellulose and lignin. • It provides flexibility to the cell wall and allows for the expansion and growth of plant tissues. • It provides a source of energy for plants.	• Enhances mechanical strength and firmness. • Enhances the structural integrity of plant tissues. • Acts as a physical barrier against microbial attack.

8.6 STRUCTURAL AND FUNCTIONAL ATTRIBUTES OF LIGNOCELLULOSIC BIOMASS

Table 8.1 lists the important characteristics of biomass components: structure, solubility, and functionality.

8.7 CONCLUSION

Biomass has various components depending on its source, availability, and environmental and climatic conditions, among which cellulose, hemicellulose, and lignin are the most important. Cellulose is a bountiful and structurally robust polysaccharide in biomass, whereas hemicellulose is a complex mixture of polysaccharides, which contributes to plant structural integrity. Lignin is a highly cross-linked complex polymer of great significance, as it is biomass's second most abundant component. These three components are the central drivers of the production of various value-added substances, precursors, biofuels, and other chemicals that meet human needs worldwide. These biomass components include diverse organic compounds that can be harnessed for renewable energy production. Moreover, biomass composition significantly affects energy production rates, which depend on the specific plant species, growing conditions, and the processing technique employed. Therefore, the presence and quantity of these components may vary based on the biomass source.

Ongoing research is needed to develop and optimize biomass conversion technologies that enhance the sustainability and productivity of biomass resources. In conclusion, cellulose, hemicellulose, and lignin together form integral constituents of biomass, which play crucial roles in maintaining the structure and functionality of the plant. The combined presence of these components represents a valuable energy resource for various applications, highlighting their significance in renewable energy and environmental sustainability.

REFERENCES

M. A. S. Correia *et al.*, "Structure and Function of an Arabinoxylan-specific Xylanase," *J. Biol. Chem.*, vol. 286, no. 25, pp. 22510–22520, Jun. 2011, https://doi.org/10.1074/jbc.M110.217315.

R. L. Crawford, "Lignin Biodegradation and Transformation," *Lignin Biodegrad. Transform.*, pp. 1–10, 1981.

M. Fantini, "Biomass Availability, Potential and Characteristics," in *Lecture Notes in Energy*, vol. 57, Springer Verlag, 2017, pp. 21–54.

L. Hu, X. Fang, M. Du, F. Luo, and S. Guo, "Hemicellulose-Based Polymers Processing and Application," *Am. J. Plant Sci.*, vol. 11, pp. 2066–2079, Jan. 2020, https://doi.org/10.4236/ajps. 2020.1112146.

H. K. King, "Lignin Biodegradation and Transformation," *Biochem. Soc. Trans.*, vol. 10, no. 3, p. 192, Jun. 1982, https://doi.org/10.1042/bst0100192.

S. Kobayashi, S. Ichiro Shoda, and K. Kashiwa, "Enzymatic Polymerization. The First in Vitro Synthesis of Cellulose Via Non-biosynthetic Path Catalysed by Cellulase," *American Chemical Society, Polymer Preprints, Division of Polymer Chemistry*, vol. 32, no. 1, pp. 417–418, Feb. 1991, https://doi.org/10.1002/masy. 19920540138.

P. Krishnamachari, R. Hashaikeh, and M. Tiner, "Modified Cellulose Morphologies and Their Composites; SEM and TEM Analysis," *Micron*, vol. 42, no. 8, pp. 751–761, 2011, https://doi.org/10.1016/j.micron.2011.05.001.

C. Krumm, J. Pfaendtner, and P. J. Dauenhauer, "Millisecond Pulsed Films Unify the Mechanisms of Cellulose Fragmentation," *Chem. Mater.*, vol. 28, no. 9, pp. 3108–3114, May 2016, https://doi.org/10.1021/acs.chemmater.6b00580.

K. Merklein, S. S. Fong, and Y. Deng, "Biomass Utilization," in *Biotechnology for Biofuel Production and Optimization*, Elsevier Inc., 2016, pp. 291–324.

Y. Nishiyama, P. Langan, and H. Chanzy, "Crystal Structure and Hydrogen-bonding System in Cellulose Iβ from Synchrotron X-ray and Neutron Fiber Diffraction," *J. Am.*

Chem. Soc., vol. 124, no. 31, pp. 9074–9082, Aug. 2002, https://doi.org/10.1021/ja0257319.

Antoinette C. O'Sullivan, "Cellulose: The Structure Slowly Unravels," *Cellulose*, vol. 4, pp. 173–207, 1997.

R. P. Overend, "Biomass Energy Heat Provision for Cooking and Heating in Developing Countries," in *Energy from Organic Materials (Biomass)*, Springer, New York, NY, 2019, pp. 513–531.

K. Parmar, "Biomass - An Overview on Composition Characteristics and Properties," *IRA-International J. Appl. Sci.*, vol. 7, no. 1, p. 42, 2017, ISSN: 2455-4499, https://doi.org/10.21013/jas.v7.n1.p4.

S. Sahay, "Deconstruction of Lignocelluloses: Potential Biological Approaches," in *Handbook of Biofuels*, Elsevier, 2022, pp. 207–232.

H. Wei, Y. Yingting, G. Jingjing, Y. Wenshi, and T. Junhong, "Lignocellulosic Biomass Valorization: Production of Ethanol," in *Encyclopedia of Sustainable Technologies*, Elsevier, 2017, pp. 601–604.

C. Wyman, S. Decker, M. Himmel, J. Brady, C. Skopec, and L. Viikari, "Hydrolysis of Cellulose and Hemicellulose," *Polysaccharides*, vol. 186, pp. 5–68, 2004.

9 Importance of Various Methods for Pretreatment of Lignocellulosic Biomass

Mamilla Shyam Sunder, Nishnat Muley, and Sundergopal Sridhar

9.1 INTRODUCTION TO PRETREATMENT AND ITS NECESSITY

Exhaustion of fossil fuels led to the search for new, sustainable resources. This paved the way for the use of lignocellulosic biomass as a substitute. Due to its surplus nature, lignocellulosic biomass has become the focus and is also economically and environmentally feasible. Thus, it has dominated the energy field and is emerging in other fields (Kucharska et al., 2018). Despite various sources, lignocellulosic biomass is classified mainly into herbaceous and wood-based, with many subcategories. It comprises polysaccharides (linear-chain celluloses and branched hemicelluloses) and lignin (a three-dimensional phenylpropane polymer) to a greater extent, as shown in Figure 9.1 (McMillan, 1994). It also contains trace amounts of extractives like resins and tannins, ash, proteins, minerals, and pectin (Kucharska et al., 2018).

The utilization of biomass for wealth as an energy source or as bioproducts occurs in two ways (Anukam et al., 2020).

1. Biochemical conversion – enzymatic and microbial-based conversion
2. Thermochemical conversion – use of heat

It is a milestone with multiple successes in converting agricultural waste into value-added products, but efficient and complete utilization remains a significant challenge. Unrefined biomass cannot be used in its native form because of its inherent biomass recalcitrant structure, creating both physical and chemical hindrances like high moisture content, irregular size (Anukam et al., 2016, 2020), complexity in hydrolysis, fermentation of pentose sugars, presence of inhibitors, and formation of intermittent compounds (Galbe and Zacchi, 2012).

 DOI: 10.1201/9781003327608-9

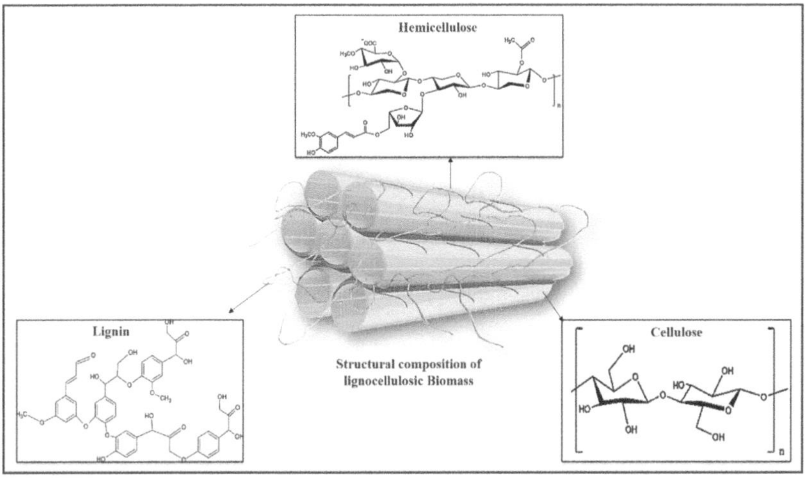

FIGURE 9.1 Major components of lignocellulosic biomass.

Source: Anukam et al. (2020)

The unyielding nature of the lignocellulosic biomass is due to the following reasons (Shafiei et al., 2015):

1. Deposition of thick cell wall layers oriented with cellulose microfibrils linked with amorphous hemicellulose held together with the help of lignin, which acts as an obstacle for the degradation of holocellulose (cellulose and hemicellulose) polysaccharides into monosaccharides.
2. The different sources of lignocellulose, like agricultural remnants, woody biomass, and municipal wastes, have different compositions of cellulose, hemicellulose, and lignin content.
3. The hydrogen bonding at the surface of microfibrils is stronger inside the crystalline core, whereas these bonds in amorphous regions are weaker and therefore easier to hydrolyse. The crystalline cellulose fibers result from H-bonding in cellulose, which is 100 times stronger than the van der Waals forces (Karimi et al., 2013).
4. Direct linkage of high molecular weight cellulose with the Xyloglucans of hemicellulose increases the cell wall rigidity.
5. Lignin degradation is complex under normal conditions except under low-nitrogen levels (Lee, 1997).
6. Hemicellulose-lignin matrix limits the diffusivity of water or any cellulolytic enzymes.

Hence, the pretreatment of the lignocellulosic biomass is crucial before processing into commercial commodities. Pretreatment of lignocellulosic biomass

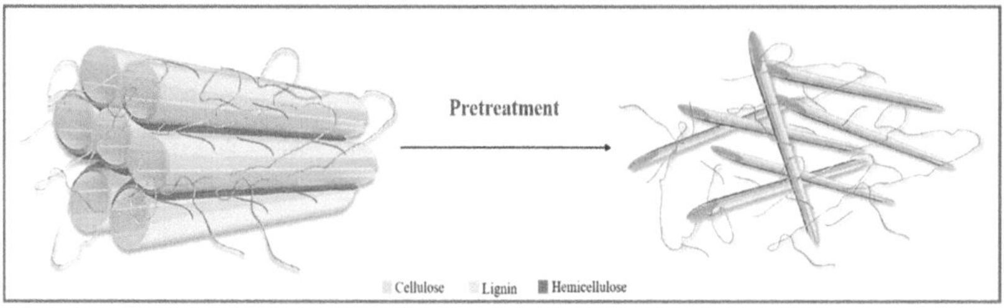

FIGURE 9.2 Lignocellulosic biomass pretreatment.

Source: Muley and Boldor (2017)

is nothing but the preparatory step to make it suitable for easy access of polysaccharides for further and efficient processing, as shown in Figure 9.2. These preparatory steps facilitate the growth of microbes on biomass as substrates for fermentation, enzymatic reactions, and hydrolysis by improving surface area and simplifying the organic matter present in municipal waste-based lignocellulosic biomass (Preethi et al., 2023).

Preprocessing of lignocellulosic biomass is primarily classified into chemical, physical, and biological pretreatments, as shown in Figure 9.3. The pretreatment methods are determined by identifying the sources of lignocellulosic biomass, the final desired product, production scale, capital investment, and income.

1. Physical pretreatment primarily deals with size reduction and homogeneity, decreasing crystallinity, and mechanizing mass transfer, thereby reducing power consumption. The type of application of the lignocellulosic biomass determines the particle size. Some methods include grinding, ball milling, extrusion, microwave irradiation, acoustic treatment, and freezing (Mankar et al., 2021).
2. Chemical pretreatment is predominantly used for small-scale processing of lignocellulosic biomass with low lignin content by disrupting the polymeric linkages (intra and inter) with suitable organic or inorganic substances. The various chemical pretreatment processes are acid hydrolysis (weak acid, intensive acid treatment), alkaline hydrolysis (sodium hydroxide), organosolv, oxidative delignification (ozonolysis, H_2O_2), ionic liquids, and so on (Norrahim et al., 2021).
3. Biological pretreatment is a selective-based pretreatment method using the potential microorganisms or a mixture of enzymes to degrade lignocellulosic biomass. This green preprocessing reduces the use of power and chemicals, reduces the emission of toxins, and increases efficient digestion. The most commonly used microorganisms are the bacterial genera Aspergillus, Bacillus, and Streptomyces, as well as white-rot

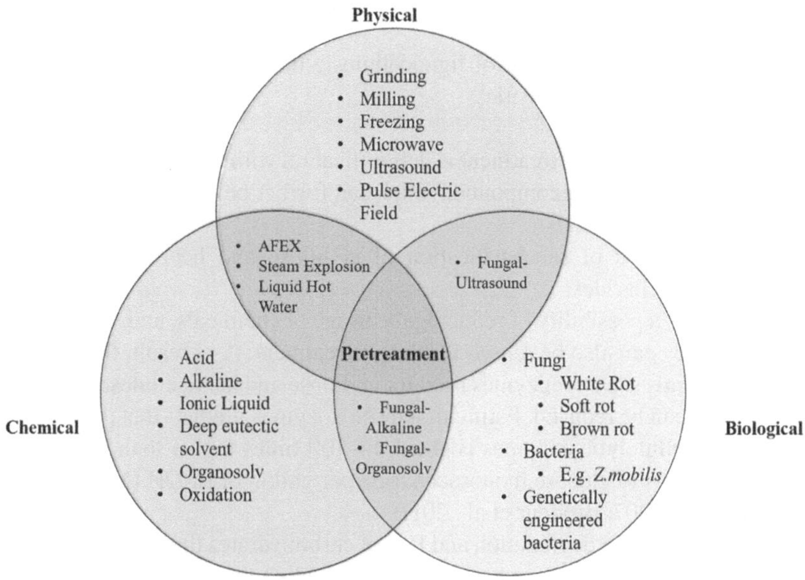

FIGURE 9.3 Pretreatment techniques of lignocellulosic biomass.

fungi that synthesize enzymes such as lignin peroxidases and laccases. The significant concerns regarding this method are the selection of suitable microorganisms based on the substrate, the adaptability of the microbial consortia for growth and function, and the long-term process (Ummalyma et al., 2019).

4. Considering the advantages and drawbacks of the types mentioned earlier, the integration strategy is currently being investigated, for example, AFEX (ammonia fiber expansion) NaOH pretreatment of oak, *Pennisetum sinese* (herbaceous wood), and camphorwood (Zhang et al., 2022); the use of ultrasonic irradiation to enhance enzymatic hydrolysis (Subhedar and Gogate, 2013); preprocessing of corncob by hydrothermal-mechanical method (Phojaroen et al., 2022), and pretreatment of soybean, straws of wheat, and corn stover by *Ceriporiopsissubvermispora*, followed by hot water extraction method (Wan and Li, 2011). Rice hull preprocessing by hydrogen peroxide, a strong oxidant, followed by *Pleurotus ostreatus* (a white rot fungus) decreased the preprocessing time from 60 days by fungal pretreatment to combined treatment of 18 days, simultaneously increasing the sugar yield (Yu et al., 2009).

The upcoming sections discuss each preprocessing technique's mechanism and its pros and cons in detail.

9.2 EFFICACY OF LIGNOCELLULOSIC BIOMASS PRETREATMENT

As the preliminary treatment of lignocellulosic biomass is necessary, it should achieve the following necessities:

1. The goal of the pretreatment is delignification with lower chemical alteration of the lignin compound, which can further be used to produce value-added chemicals.
2. Higher yield of saccharification of cellulose and hemicellulose into monosaccharides.
3. There is a possibility of reducing the usage of chemicals, and, if applicable, they can also be reused for the pretreatment. As a result, the cost of chemicals such as enzymes used for cellulose and hemicellulose fermentation can be reduced. Estimation by Novozymes predicts that the cost of holo-cellulolytic enzymes is about 40–100 times higher than for starch hydrolysis to glucose monosaccharide per gallon of Et-OH (Merino and Cherry, 2007; Brodeur et al., 2011).
4. Preventing the degradation and loss of carbohydrates that affect the final yield of the desired product, as well as avoiding the production of inhibitory byproducts impacting saccharification and fermentation.
5. Reducing the strength of hydrogen bonds to minimize the crystallinity of cellulose and improving the porosity for easier access by hydrolytic enzymes and fermentative microbes.
6. Minimizing the cost and energy consumption in the pretreatment of lignocellulosic biomass. For example, preliminary steps of pretreatment, like size reduction, require high energy.
7. Less production of waste and hazardous by-products.

The pretreatment of lignocellulosic biomass should aim to achieve all the aforementioned goals for efficient utilization, not entirely but significantly (Shafiei et al., 2015; Kumar et al., 2009; Agbor et al., 2011; Bajpai, 2016).

9.3 CHARACTERIZATION OF PRETREATED BIOMASS

The theoretically estimated performance may not match the actual performance; thus, the pretreated biomass must be evaluated. It is crucial to analyze the composition of lignocellulosic biomass, its interactions, and the effects of different pretreatments on the biomass structure. The characterization of pretreated biomass helps determine and optimize the appropriate pretreatment method for various lignocellulosic biomass sources. The efficiency of pretreated biomass is analyzed on the basis of its composition and physicochemical characteristics. Various advanced analytical techniques are used, for example, FTIR for the analysis of chemical bonding and identifying the changes of biomass structure after pretreatment, XRD for determining the hydrolysis efficiency as a result of chemical pretreatment, and SEM and TEM analyses for the comparative studies of raw and pretreated biomass surface morphology (Anukam et al., 2020).

Analyzing changes in biomass composition before and after pretreatment helps optimize the process and is a basis for biofuel production. Estimating moisture, ash, total solids, and carbon content helps determine the utility of biomass in its native form or whether it should be preprocessed. For example, biomass with a low moisture content is preferred in the production process over higher-moisture biomass. The elemental composition of the biomass is also analyzed to determine C, H, O, N and very low concentrations of sulfur. Higher levels of sulfur dioxide lead to the formation of ash (Daramola and Ayeni, 2020). Leaching dried biomass samples with a benzene-ethanol mixture determines the concentration of extractives that interfere with further analysis of downstream processing (Milne et al., 1992). The ash content of kernel shells and mesocarp fibers of palm and their fresh fruit residues after leaching with different solutions was estimated by a thermogravimetric analyzer.The comparison between pretreated and raw biomass indicated a reduction in ash concentration, thereby minimizing deposition, slagging, and high-temperature corrosion during subsequent thermochemical steps (Asadieraghi and Wan Daud, 2016). The composition of lignocellulosic biomass can also be analyzed using NREL (National Renewable Energy Laboratory) standard practices.

When selecting a pretreatment, the biomass's crystalline structure, particle size, and mass transfer properties should be considered (Singh et al., 2009). They utilized the plant cell wall's autofluorescence to determine the switchgrass's solubilizing mechanism during ionic liquid (IL) pretreatment. Upon pretreatment of biomass, it can be inferred that the IL treatment has enhanced the conversion of polysaccharides into glucose, indicating significant disruption of the biomass's recalcitrant structure (Singh et al., 2009). Characterization of alkaline-pretreated, pressed oil palm leaf oil was compared with the native form using SEM, XRD, and FTIR. The results indicated that the former has distorted cell walls, decreased amorphous hemicellulose, and reduced lignin concentration compared to the latter native form (Syazwana Hashim et al., 2017). NMR analysis for the determination of porosity of three different biomasses (poplar, wheat straw, and miscanthus) by different pretreatment methods (ionic liquid, diluted acid, sodium chlorite, and hot water) showed an increase in pore size of about 10–15 nm compared to native forms of wheat straw. The other two biomasses showed no significant changes (Herbaut et al., 2018).

9.4 ECONOMIC ASSESSMENT OF PRETREATMENT OF LIGNOCELLULOSIC BIOMASS

The implementation and efficiency of lignocellulosic biomass pretreatment determine the revenue and economic performance of the entire process. Depending on the application of the lignocellulosic biomass, the pretreatment method differs. Subsequently, depending on the pretreatment process, the economy will gain profit or loss. For example, energy-intensive techniques such as crushing, milling, and drying require higher costs for preliminary treatments to achieve particle size homogeneity and low moisture content (Patel et al., 2016). The pretreatment method should achieve economic feasibility while considering operation and maintenance utility costs because capital cost is a fixed expenditure (equipment, construction cost). In contrast, expenditure on operational costs (labor charges, chemicals, catalysts, energy, and electricity) is common (Preethi et al., 2023). Based on Eggeman and Elander's estimates, investing in pretreatment processes yields higher annual capacity with lower total fixed expenditure per gallon than in the case of no pretreatment (Eggeman and Elander, 2005). According to Baral and Shah (2016), sugar production price per unit with ionic liquid pretreatment was lower in corn stover by about 2.7 $/kg compared to switchgrass (3.2 $/kg) and poplar (3.0$/kg), which was due to the former having low raw material necessity and operating costs annually as a consequence of higher conversion rates during pretreatment; thereby, IL pretreatment method can be considered economically and environmentally suitable for ethanol fermentation. Comparative analysis of organosolv pretreatment with the diluted acid method indicated that, in defiance of enhanced ethanol production, less consumption of water, and reduction in equipment costs, a significant part of the total annual cost is invested in utilities due to a vast amount of energy requirement (Rodrigues Gurgel da Silva et al., 2018). The economic feasibility of fungal pretreatments of different biomasses indicated that this treatment is more expensive than conventional preprocessing due to decreased sugar yield, longer processing time, and sterilization. Hence, this pretreatment must be optimized to achieve a higher yield in less time (Vasco-Correa and Shah, 2019). The various economic feasibility studies demonstrate the need to account for preprocessing costs, yield efficiency, and environmental sustainability.

9.5 APPLICATION

Considering the sustainability of the lignocellulosic biomass, its applications are vast. Proper pretreatment of lignocellulosic biomass is essential for the production of value-added commodities. The different processed products obtained from lignocellulosic biomass are commonly biofuels and value-added chemicals. Second-generation biofuels like syngas, bioethanol, bio-oil, biogas, and biohydrogen obtained by the hydrolysis and depolymerization of lignocellulose (Kumar and Sharma, 2017) and the extraction of biopolymeric substances like bio-composites and nanocellulose require chemical preprocessing before further processing. Alterations in lignocellulosic biomass structure enhance cellulose fibrillation. Also, it reduces the recalcitrant nature of the biomass, enhancing ethanol production (Norrrahim et al., 2021): value-added chemicals like furfural and its derivatives from carbohydrates for the production of polyethylene terephthalate-based plastics (Alam and Saha, 2015); glycerol in cosmetics and surfactants (Choi et al., 2015); production of cinnamyl and syringyl phenolic derivative from lignin; vanillin as a petroleum substitute obtained from lignin; biosorbents for separation; active carbon material in supercapacitors; and production of cellulose nanofibrils by ultrasonic pretreatment of lignocellulosic biomass weakening the van der Waals interaction (Putro et al., 2016).

9.6 CONCLUSION

Pretreatment of lignocellulosic biomass is pivotal in efficiently converting biomass into biofuels and bioproducts. Various pretreatment methods, including physical, chemical, and biological techniques, play a crucial role in enhancing the accessibility of cellulose and hemicellulose. This enhancement increases yields of fermentable sugars, which are essential for subsequent biofuel production processes. The efficacy of these pretreatment methods is vital for improving conversion efficiency and ensuring the economic viability of large-scale biorefineries. Effective pretreatment processes can significantly reduce production costs, making biofuels more competitive with traditional fossil fuels. Additionally, the characterization of pretreated biomass is essential for optimizing downstream processing steps and ensuring the consistent quality of the final products. Beyond the production of biofuels, pretreated lignocellulosic biomass has a wide range of applications, including the production of biochemicals, bioplastics, and other value-added products. These applications contribute to developing a sustainable economy, which is crucial for reducing our reliance on nonrenewable resources. In conclusion, the selection and optimization of pretreatment methods are fundamental to the successful utilization of lignocellulosic biomass. Continued research and development in this field will enhance the efficiency and economic viability of biomass conversion technologies, paving the way for a greener, more sustainable future.

REFERENCES

V. B. Agbor, N. Cicek, R. Sparling, A. Berlin, and D. B. Levin, "Biomass Pretreatment: Fundamentals toward Application," *Biotechnol. Adv.*, vol. 29, no. 6, pp. 675–685, Nov. 2011, https://doi.org/10.1016/j.biotechadv.2011.05.005.

M. I. Alam and B. Saha, "Catalysis for the Production of Sustainable Chemicals and Fuels from Biomass," *Sustain. Catal. Process.*, pp. 99–123, Jan. 2015, https://doi.org/10.1016/B978-0-444-59567-6.00004-2.

A. Anukam, J. Berghel, A. Anukam, and J. Berghel, "Biomass Pretreatment and Characterization: A Review," *Biotechnol. Appl. Biomass*, Sep. 2020, https://doi.org/10.5772/INTECHOPEN.93607.

A. Anukam, S. Mamphweli, P. Reddy, E. Meyer, and O. Okoh, "Pre-processing of Sugarcane Bagasse for Gasification in a Downdraft Biomass Gasifier System: A Comprehensive Review," *Renew. Sustain. Energy Rev.*, vol. 66, pp. 775–801, Dec. 2016, https://doi.org/10.1016/J.RSER.2016.08.046.

M. Asadieraghi and W. M. A. Wan Daud, "Characterization of Lignocellulosic Biomass Thermal Degradation and Physiochemical Structure: Effects of Demineralization by Diverse Acid Solutions," *Energy Convers. Manag.*, vol. 82, pp. 71–82, Jun. 2014, https://doi.org/10.1016/j.enconman.2014.03.007.

P. Bajpai, "Pretreatment of Lignocellulosic Biomass for Biofuel Production," in SpringerBriefs in Molecular Science, pp. 17–70, 2016, Springer Nature. https://doi.org/10.1007/978-981-10-0687-6_4.

N. R. Baral and A. Shah, "Techno-economic Analysis of Cellulose Dissolving Ionic Liquid Pretreatment of Lignocellulosic Biomass for Fermentable Sugars Production," *Biofuels, Bioprod. Biorefining*, vol. 10, no. 1, pp. 70–88, Jan. 2016, https://doi.org/10.1002/BBB.1622.

G. Brodeur, E. Yau, K. Badal, J. Collier, K. B. Ramachandran, and S. Ramakrishnan, "Chemical and Physicochemical Pretreatment of Lignocellulosic Biomass: A Review," *Enzyme Res.*, vol. 2011, no. 1, 2011, https://doi.org/10.4061/2011/787532.

S. Choi, C. W. Song, J. H. Shin, and S. Y. Lee, "Biorefineries for the Production of Top Building Block Chemicals and Their Derivatives," *Metab. Eng.*, vol. 28, pp. 223–239, Mar. 2015, https://doi.org/10.1016/j.ymben.2014.12.007.

M. O. Daramola and A. O. Ayeni, Eds., *Valorization of Biomass to Value-Added Commodities* in Green Energy and Technology. Cham: Springer International Publishing, 2020. https://doi.org/10.1007/978-3-030-38032-8.

T. Eggeman and R. T. Elander, "Process and Economic Analysis of Pretreatment Technologies," *Bioresour. Technol.*, vol. 96, no. 18, pp. 2019–2025, Dec. 2005, https://doi.org/10.1016/j.biortech.2005.01.017.

M. Galbe and G. Zacchi, "Pretreatment: The Key to Efficient Utilization of Lignocellulosic Materials," *Biomass and Bioenergy*, vol. 46, pp. 70–78, Nov. 2012, https://doi.org/10.1016/J.BIOMBIOE.2012.03.026.

M. Herbaut *et al.*, "Multimodal Analysis of Pretreated Biomass Species Highlights Generic Markers of Lignocellulose Recalcitrance," *Biotechnol. Biofuels*, vol. 11, no. 1, pp. 1–17, Feb. 2018, https://doi.org/10.1186/s13068-018-1053-8/figures/9.

K. Karimi, M. Shafiei, and R. Kumar, "Progress in Physical and Chemical Pretreatment of Lignocellulosic Biomass," *Biofuel Technol. Recent Dev.*, vol. 9783642345197, pp. 53–96, Aug. 2013, https://doi.org/10.1007/978-3-642-34519-7_3.

K. Kucharska, P. Rybarczyk, I. Hołowacz, R. Łukajtis, M. Glinka, and M. Kamiński, "Pretreatment of Lignocellulosic Materials as Substrates for Fermentation Processes," *Molecules*, vol. 23, No. 11, p. 2937, Nov. 2018, https://doi.org/10.3390/molecules23112937.

A. K. Kumar and S. Sharma, "Recent Updates on Different Methods of Pretreatment of Lignocellulosic Feedstocks: A Review," *Bioresour. Bioprocess.*, vol. 4, no. 1, pp. 1–19, Jan. 2017, https://doi.org/10.1186/S40643-017-0137-9.

P. Kumar, D. M. Barrett, M. J. Delwiche, and P. Stroeve, "Methods for Pretreatment of Lignocellulosic Biomass for Efficient Hydrolysis and Biofuel Production," *Ind. Eng. Chem. Res.*, vol. 48, no. 8, pp. 3713–3729, Apr. 2009, https://doi.org/10.1021/ie801542g/asset/images/large/ie-2008-01542g_0010.jpeg.

J. Lee, "Biological Conversion of Lignocellulosic Biomass to Ethanol," *J. Biotechnol.*, vol. 56, no. 1, pp. 1–24, Jul. 1997, https://doi.org/10.1016/S0168-1656(97)00073-4.

A. R. Mankar, A. Pandey, A. Modak, and K. K. Pant, "Pretreatment of Lignocellulosic Biomass: A Review on Recent Advances," *Bioresour. Technol.*, vol. 334, p. 125235, Aug. 2021, https://doi.org/10.1016/j.biortech.2021.125235.

J. D. McMillan, "Pretreatment of Lignocellulosic Biomass," *Bioenergy*, pp. 292–324, Oct. 1994, https://doi.org/10.1021/BK-1994-0566.CH015.

S. T. Merino and J. Cherry, "Progress and Challenges in Enzyme Development for Biomass Utilization," *Adv. Biochem. Eng. Biotechnol.*, vol. 108, pp. 95–120, Apr. 2007, https://doi.org/10.1007/10_2007_066.

T. A. Milne, H. L. Chum, F. Agblevor, and D. K. Johnson, "Standardized Analytical Methods," *Biomass and Bioenergy*, vol. 2, no. 1–6, pp. 341–366, Jan. 1992, https://doi.org/10.1016/0961-9534(92)90109-4.

P. D. Muley and D. Boldor, "Advances in Biomass Pretreatment and Cellulosic Bioethanol Production Using Microwave Heating," Proceedings of SEEP2017, 27–30 June 2017, Bled, Slovenia, pp. 173–180, https://doi.org/10.18690/978-961-286-048-6.18.

M. N. F. Norrrahim, R. A. Ilyas, N. M. Nurazzi, M. S. A. Rani, M. S. N. Atikah, and S. S. Shazleen, "Chemical Pretreatment of Lignocellulosic Biomass for the Production of Bioproducts: An Overview," *Appl. Sci. Eng. Prog.*, vol. 14, no. 4, pp. 588–605, Oct. 2021, https://doi.org/10.14416/j.asep.2021.07.004.

M. Patel, X. Zhang, and A. Kumar, "Techno-economic and Life Cycle Assessment on Lignocellulosic Biomass Thermochemical Conversion Technologies: A Review," *Renew. Sustain. Energy Rev.*, vol. 53, pp. 1486–1499, Jan. 2016, https://doi.org/10.1016/j.rser.2015.09.070.

J. Phojaroen, T. Jiradechakorn, S. Kirdponpattara, M. Sriariyanun, J. Junthip, and S. Chuetor, "Performance Evaluation of Combined Hydrothermal-Mechanical Pretreatment of Lignocellulosic Biomass for Enzymatic Enhancement," *Polymers*, vol. 14, no. 12, p. 2313, Jun. 2022, https://doi.org/10.3390/POLYM14122313.

Preethi, M. Gunasekaran, and R. Banu. J, "Indexing Energy and Cost of the Pretreatment for Economically Efficient Bioenergy Generation," *Front. Energy Res.*, vol. 10, p. 1060599, Jan. 2023, https://doi.org/10.3389/fenrg.2022.1060599/bibtex.

J. N. Putro, F. E. Soetaredjo, S. Y. Lin, Y. H. Ju, and S. Ismadji, "Pretreatment and Conversion of Lignocellulose Biomass into Valuable Chemicals," *RSC Adv.*, vol. 6, no. 52, pp. 46834–46852, May 2016, https://doi.org/10.1039/C6RA09851G.

A. Rodrigues Gurgel da Silva, M. Errico, and B. G. Rong, "Techno-economic Analysis of Organosolv Pretreatment Process from Lignocellulosic Biomass," *Clean Technol. Environ. Policy*, vol. 20, no. 7, pp. 1401–1412, Sep. 2018, https://doi.org/10.1007/s10098-017-1389-y/metrics.

M. Shafiei, R. Kumar, and K. Karimi, "Pretreatment of Lignocellulosic Biomass," pp. 85–154, 2015, https://doi.org/10.1007/978-3-319-14033-9_3.

S. Singh, B. A. Simmons, and K. P. Vogel, "Visualization of Biomass Solubilization and Cellulose Regeneration during Ionic Liquid Pretreatment of Switchgrass," *Biotechnol. Bioeng.*, vol. 104, no. 1, pp. 68–75, Sep. 2009, https://doi.org/10.1002/BIT.22386.

P. B. Subhedar and P. R. Gogate, "Intensification of Enzymatic Hydrolysis of Lignocellulose Using Ultrasound for Efficient Bioethanol Production: A Review," *Ind. Eng. Chem. Res.*, vol. 52, no. 34, pp. 11816–11828, Aug. 2013, https://doi.org/10.1021/ie401286z/asset/images/large/ie-2013-01286z_0006.jpeg.

F. Syazwana Hashim, H. Wan Yussof, M. Ahmad Khushairi Mohd Zahari, R. A. Rahman, and R. Md Illias, "Physicochemical and Morphological Characterisation of the Native and Alkaline Pretreated Fibre Pressed Oil Palm Frond for Fermentable Sugars Production," *Chem. Eng. Trans.*, vol. 56, 2017, https://doi.org/10.3303/CET1756182.

S. B. Ummalyma *et al.*, "Biological Pretreatment of Lignocellulosic Biomass – Current Trends and Future Perspectives," *Second Third Gener. Feed. Evol. Biofuels*, pp. 197–212, Jan. 2019, https://doi.org/10.1016/B978-0-12-815162-4.00007-0.

J. Vasco-Correa and A. Shah, "Techno-Economic Bottlenecks of the Fungal Pretreatment of Lignocellulosic Biomass," *Fermentatiom*, vol. 5, no. 2, p. 30, Mar. 2019, https://doi.org/10.3390/fermentation5020030.

C. Wan and Y. Li, "Effect of Hot Water Extraction and Liquid Hot Water Pretreatment on the Fungal Degradation of Biomass Feedstocks," *Bioresour. Technol.*, vol. 102, no. 20, pp. 9788–9793, Oct. 2011, https://doi.org/10.1016/j.biortech.2011.08.004.

J. Yu, J. Zhang, J. He, Z. Liu, and Z. Yu, "Combinations of Mild Physical or Chemical Pretreatment with Biological Pretreatment for Enzymatic Hydrolysis of Rice Hull," *Bioresour. Technol.*, vol. 100, no. 2, pp. 903–908, Jan. 2009, https://doi.org/10.1016/j.biortech.2008.07.025.

J. Zhang *et al.*, "Effect of Ammonia Fiber Expansion Combined with NaOH Pretreatment on the Resource Efficiency of Herbaceous and Woody Lignocellulosic Biomass," *ACS Omega*, vol. 7, no. 22, pp. 18761–18769, Jun. 2022, https://doi.org/10.1021/acsomega.2c01302/asset/images/large/ao2c01302_0005.jpeg.

10 Physical Pretreatment of Biomass

Mamilla Shree Veena, Sundergopal Sridhar, and Mamilla Shyam Sunder

10.1 INTRODUCTION

The disposal of lignocellulosic biomass is abundant and will be renewed as a helpful resource. Significant study and understanding are required for resourceful conversion. Extracting these high-value-added compounds is challenging because they are confined within the plant cell, with limited resistance to mass transfer across the cell membrane and cell wall. Lignocellulosic biomass is a plant material composed of lignin, cellulose, and hemicellulose. These feedstocks pose an ample renewable resource for manufacturing biofuels and bio-based essentials. They include various plant materials such as wood, agricultural residues, and energy crops. Different tree parts have varying lignin contents: shoots have low lignin content, while wood has high lignin content. There are three subunits of lignin, namely, guaiacyl units and their polymers stemming from the monomeric units of coniferyl alcohol (common in softwood), syringyl units, and p-hydroxyphenyl phenylpropanoid (familiar in hardwood with varying ratios of guaiacyl and syringyl units), which is a mixed unit of guaiacyl and syringyl units. Lignin is a complex organic natural polymer that can persist in the environment for a long time and is tough to break down. It provides strength and stiffness to plant cell walls. It can impede the interaction of enzymes or other catalysts with cellulose.

Cellulose and hemicellulose are the polysaccharides that contribute to a significant part of the plant cell. The complex and heterogeneous structure of lignocellulosic biomass makes it difficult to convert into useful products: weak van der Waals forces and hydrogen bonding hold lignin, cellulose, and hemicellulose together. Through enzymatic hydrolysis, a process that breaks down the cellulosic components (cellulose and hemicellulose) of biomass into fermentable sugars, biomass can be further processed into an array of bio-based products. The major structural features can be categorized as chemical and physical. The chemical features constitute the compositions and structures of cellulose, hemicellulose, and lignin. In contrast, bodily features include cellulose crystallinity, cellulose polymerization level, accessible surface area, lignin, hemicellulose shield, and acetylating hemicellulose. To make these cellulosic compounds more accessible to enzyme hydrolysis, the biomass must be pretreated. Biomass recalcitrance (resistance to chemical and biological breakdown) is pivotal in pretreatment

DOI: 10.1201/9781003327608-10

efficiency. In addition to structural alteration, pretreatment procedures aim to remove hemicellulose and lignin from biomass. For biomass to be hydrolyzed, the carbohydrate component must be available. A study Amusa et al. (2020) provides a clear understanding of the importance of biomass pretreatment in membrane preparation, as it requires organic/inorganic materials to be incorporated into the membrane matrix for versatile applications. The cellulose obtained from organic agro-based materials can be used to prepare mixed-matrix membranes by integrating it with polymers. In such a case, the polymer serves as the continuous phase, and the cellulose as the dispersed phase. Many research studies are being initiated to develop polymer solutions combined with extracted cellulose from lignocellulosic biomass to leverage its remarkable properties for gas separation, water purification, food packaging, tissue engineering, and so forth (Amusa et al., 2020). Physical pretreatment increases enzyme hydrolysis efficiency and reduces the required enzyme dosage. It entails using mechanical, thermal, or chemical techniques to alter biomass's physical properties, making it more accessible for subsequent processing.

Physical pretreatment involves both irradiation and mechanical treatment. Roller crushing, hammer crushing, colloid crushing, ball crushing, and vibro-energy crushing are typical mechanical pretreatment methods used during milling (Figure 10.1). Chipping, grinding, and coarse size reduction are a few other methods that are employed as mechanical pretreatments (Putro et al., 2016). Milling is a specific type of mechanical grinding that uses coarse cutting tools to reduce cellulose's crystallinity. A vibratory ball mill is an effective piece of equipment for increasing the lignocellulosic biomass's ability to be digested compared to standard milling types of equipment. The wet disk milling method is another piece of equipment used for machine-driven pretreatment due to its low energy consumption, high suitability for enzymatic hydrolysis, and inhibitor prevention. A study states that wet milling is superior to dry milling for the pretreatment of corn stover. The

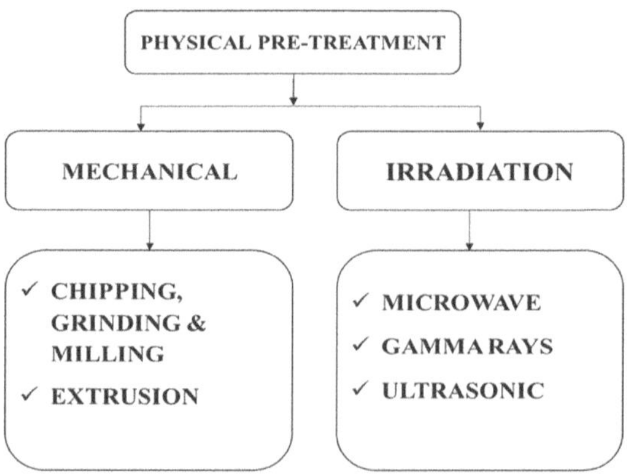

FIGURE 10.1 Classification of physical pretreatment processes.

essential elements include the type of milling and time; the type of biomass to be treated determines the effectiveness of the intensification in specific surface contact, polymerization level, and a net decrease in the rate of cellulose crystallinity.

Pretreatment lays the groundwork for disrupting the lignocellulosic biomass's highly organized structure with little or no chemical modification of its individual components. During delignification, lignin is removed from the biomass. Physical pretreatment is essential in producing biofuels and biochemicals from lignocellulosic feedstocks. As woody feedstocks consume more energy for size reduction, the milling method would be economically feasible. It improves the hydrolysis process for better heat and mass transfer. Some of the benefits of mechanical pretreatment include increased surface area, reduced chemical waste, reduced particle size, increased bulk and energy densities, and decreased crystallinity and level of polymerization. The two major drawbacks of this treatment are its inability to discard lignin, which limits access to cellulose, and its high energy usage, which leads to prohibitive costs for scale-up operations.

10.2 MECHANICAL PRETREATMENT

10.2.1 Comminution

Comminution refers to the process of reducing the size of solid material. It is an essential process in many industries, including chemical, pharmaceutical, mining, and other manufacturing. The comminution process involves applying mechanical forces to break solid materials into smaller particles. Size reduction may be classified (on the basis of the type of force being applied) as compression, impact, attrition, and cutting. Compression and impact apply identical forces but differ in the amount of energy transferred to the materials. Attrition is the force (a surface mechanism) caused by friction between the walls and particles or beads (Mayer-Laigle et al., 2018). Size reduction has been considered the single pretreatment method that enhances the degradability of biomass for the manufacture of biogas, bio-based ethanol, and hydrogen. It is essential to recognize the limitations of the positive effect of size reduction.

Excessive size reduction can lead to variations in chemical composition, potentially inhibiting the production of the desired product. Mechanical comminution commonly includes shredding, chipping, milling, grinding, and coarse size reduction. Other methods of physical pretreatment of biomass include high-pressure electrical pulses, irradiation (e.g., different types of radiation), and pyrolysis. These methods help cleave β-1,4 glycosidic bonds, resulting in lower cellulose crystallinity and increased surface area. The major drawbacks of these methods are that they are costly and present substantial environmental and safety concerns. Extrusion is a rare pretreatment method that combines heating, shearing, and mixing, resulting in physical and chemical changes in the biomass after it passes through the steam extruder. In pyrolysis, the biomass is open to heating at 300°C with further chemical pretreatment, giving high-value-added sugar with

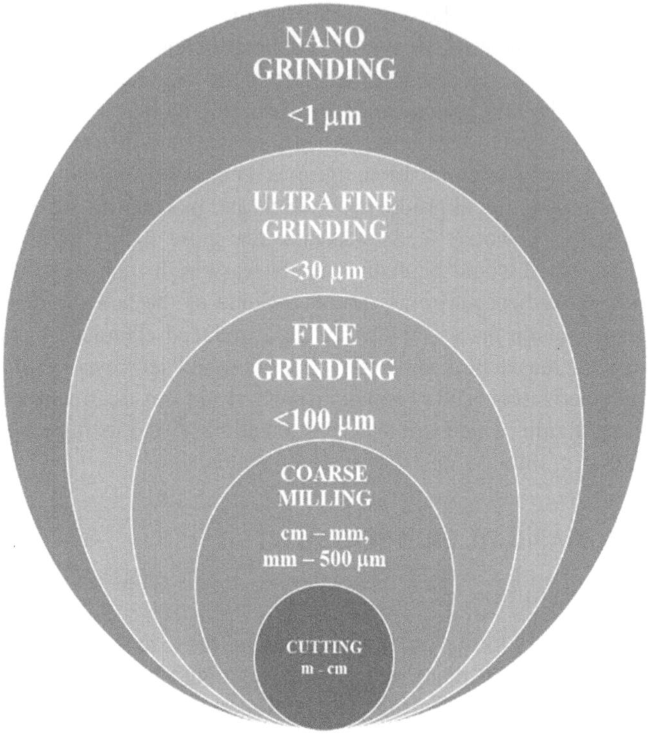

FIGURE 10.2 Size range of elements of comminution.

Source: Barakat et al. (2014)

up to 90% yield. It is also a nonmechanical process in which oxygen can accelerate the breakdown of cellulosic materials, yielding gaseous products and residual char. As shown in Figure 10.2, the comminution process involves several steps, from organ dissociation to size reduction below the cell wall, where the biomass can be reduced to less than 1 μm (Barakat et al., 2014).

10.2.2 Chipping and Shredding

In the chipping process, sharp edges and corners are separated, leaving the remainder of the parent particle intact. The biomass can be chipped down to 10–30 mm. However, it has little-to-no effect on the hydrolysis rate (Sun and Cheng, 2002). Shredding is a coarse-size reduction approach for challenging-to-handle feedstocks such as waste paper and grass. Feedstock fragmentation is achieved using equipment such as knives, hammers, and screw shredders. Biomass shredding is carried out by applying linear shear (Kratky and Jirout, 2011).

10.2.3 Milling

Size reduction is predominantly carried out by milling. Milling involves different types of equipment, which can be differentiated by the mechanical stresses they impart (e.g., impact, compression, shear force, and friction), such as ball mills, hammer mills, knife mills, disc mills, rod mills, roll mills, centrifugal mills, and cylindrical mills. Many studies show that physical pretreatment of biomass using milling increases bioproduct yield. Grinding and milling methods can reduce the biomass particle to about 0.2–2.0 mm. Figure 10.3 categorizes the different types of equipment used in the milling process by operational management and size-reduction mechanism. For example, hardwood requires a higher energy input than other agricultural residues; in such cases, mechanical comminution is not economically viable for industrial-scale up. Moisture content (MC) is also an essential factor to consider when selecting an appropriate milling method for optimal outcomes. In the case of dry biomass (MC < 15%, wet basis), hammer or knife milling is suitable, whereas colloid milling is appropriate for damp biomass (MC > 15%). Both wet and dry biomass can be ground using ball and vibratory milling methods (Zheng et al., 2017).

10.2.4 Hammer Mill

A hammer mill is a piece of machinery with hammers mounted onto a rotor. An essential parameter in hammer milling is screen size, which ranges from 1.6 to 30 mm. Screen opening size significantly affects the mean particle size and milling performance. Hammer mills operating at high speed with reduced-diameter rotors efficiently process fine or challenging-to-grind materials. Ball milling is appropriate for producing fermented sugars from straw under mild hydrolytic conditions; it dramatically reduces the crystallinity index from 4.9% to 72.4% (Bitra et al., 2008).

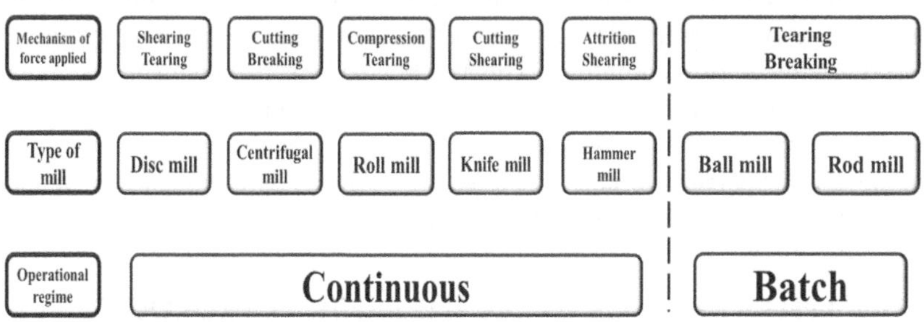

FIGURE 10.3 Classification of mills.

10.2.5 Ball Mill

Ball mills are of different types (categorized on the basis of the motion of balls): tumbler, vibratory, attritor, and planetary ball mills. Tumbler ball mills use gravity to grind particles, resulting in multiple collisions. To obtain the desired efficiency, an equilibrium must be maintained between the centrifugal and gravitational forces. Vibratory ball mills contain vessels loaded with agri-feedstocks and operate at the maximum vibrational recurrence rate.

Attrition mills consist of a vertically held tank and a spinning shaft with attached horizontal arms. Due to the erratic motion of the grinding balls, both shear and frictional forces are produced. A benefit-producing factor of the attrition mill is self-agitation (i.e., it does not use power to rotate the grinding chamber). Planetary ball mills combine various mechanical forces (specifically, frictional, shear, and impaction). This piece of machinery consists of grinding pots mounted on a base disk. The pots rotate around two parallel axes, causing uneven acceleration. The ball-milling technique consumes high energy; therefore, it is expensive. However, these methods do not produce any toxic or inhibitive substances and, thus, are suitable for a wide range of lignocellulosic biomass. A knife cutter or knife mill is best used for straw, stalk, and grass feed. Particle size and other available biomass features determine the energy required for mechanical comminution (Sitotaw et al., 2021).

10.2.6 Disc Mill

Disc mills work on the principle of frictional force between the two discs, which move relative to each other and the particle. Fibrous feedstocks can be ground easily using a disc milling process (Arce and Kratky, 2022). They can be constructed with single or double discs with straight or contoured blades. At high temperatures, the specific energy decreases rapidly. Compression and shear forces are observed in the operation of disc mills (Kratky and Jirout, 2011).

10.2.7 Grinding

In the modern era, grinding is the most widely used technology among the processes involved in mechanical comminution. This process consumes the most energy. The grinding process is carried out in two stages, involving the grinding of feedstocks by collision or impact. This is followed by screening using the moving parts of a rotor press, which crushes the materials. Many grinding devices operate by mechanical action. The hammer mill is considered a preliminary grinding equipment for plant materials. The crushing operation is unsuitable for lignocellulosic biomass, as it is best suited for brittle materials (Lomovsky et al., 2016).

10.3 EFFECT OF MILLING ON THE PARTICLE PROPERTIES

The milling process affects particle properties such as size, shape, and surface area. The type of grinder and other parameters, such as the velocity of the grinder and residence time, influence the size distribution. Under mechanical stress, particle properties change. The force applied due to compression results in a constricted size distribution with similar diameters. The mechanical stress from the impact results in a wide range of particle sizes. Studies have shown that the particle shape after grinding is difficult to predict, as it depends on the biomass form and its moisture content. The particle shape has a substantial impact on particle flowability. Size reduction directly affects the bulk density and rheological characteristics of biomass, as bulk density depends on pores and interspecific voids. The powder becomes denser as porosity is reduced and the interparticular specific gap closes. However, links among particles (through van der Waals forces) can form new interparticle cavities – comminution results in increased cohesiveness, a balance between inter-particle and gravity forces, and reduced flowability. In the case of specific surface contact, we can consider ultrafine grinding, which modifies particle surfaces by opening cell walls and trapping some constituents within the cell (Mayer-Laigle et al., 2018).

10.4 EXTRUSION

Extrusion is a conventional pretreatment technique in which treatment is carried out under shear mixing and at high temperatures (>300°C). Screw blades cause shear force by maintaining the high temperatures in the barrel. Shear force and temperature are essential for disrupting the cellulose matrix in biomass residues. Materials with a 14–20% moisture content are suitable for comminuting via extrusion. The high energy needs of this approach make it costly and challenging to scale up for industrial use. Extruders come in two varieties: single-screw and twin-screw extruders. A single-screw extruder operates on three motions: forward, kneading, and reverse. A twin-screw extruder can perform multiple operations simultaneously, such as mixing, grinding, reaction, drying, shearing, and separation (Zheng and Rehmann, 2014). The key parameters of this process include the screw model used, compression ratio, screw speed, and barrel temperature, all of which are affected by feedstock pretreatment. High shearing forces are generated with the contact of one or two rotating barrels. This method's speedy heat transmission and efficient mixing are well known. Challenges related to extrusion include high energy consumption, high investment costs, and process scale-up (Konan et al., 2022). Extrusion was used to improve the nutritional value and digestibility of maize used as livestock feed. Researchers found that ethanol production increased from 0.21 to 0.76 kg/kg biomass, and glucose output rose from 0.23 to 0.69 kg/kg biomass. This process is extensively employed on an industrial scale, subjected to anaerobic digestion for biogas production. Extruders are advantageous for continuous processing, large-scale applications, and ease of online adjustment.

10.5 ULTRASOUND IRRADIATION

The ultrasound method is employed to treat solid organic waste, disrupting cell structure, improving surface contact, reducing polymerization levels, and enhancing lignocellulosic feedstock fragmentation. One of the essential features of this method is that the transport of enzyme macromolecules toward the substrate surface has been dramatically improved by diffusive effects induced by the ultrasound field. The consequence caused by cavitation is hundred times superior in heterogeneous systems than in homogeneous systems; the mechanical impact is a significant benefit of opening up the surface of the substrate for enzyme hydrolysis, and the maximum effect of cavitation is observed at the temperature of 50°C, which is considered the ideal temperature for enzyme growth. A few studies were conducted to define the efficiency of ultrasound pretreatment for the manufacture of bio-based products (from grape pomace and agave leaves), which conclude that this technique has positive effects on both chemical structure and yield due to the development of cavitation bubbles, which can automatically disintegrate the cell wall structure of lignocelluloses (Yachmenev et al., 2009; Jędrzejczyk et al., 2019).

10.6 MICROWAVE-ASSISTED PRETREATMENT

A microwave is an electromagnetic, nonionizing wave whose frequency ranges from 300 MHz to 300 GHz. Three main properties exhibited by microwave irradiation are penetration, reflection, and absorbance. For example, microwaves pass through glass and plastics, are absorbed by water, and are reflected by metals. Based on these properties, microwave reactors are divided into two types: those that permit the flow of microwaves and those that reflect microwaves. The reasons for its wide range of use are ease of operation, low energy consumption, rapid increase in heating capacity, limited inhibitor generation, and the structural organization of cellulose being degraded. By applying this treatment method, the orientation of molecules in the substrate changes repeatedly, leading to a more vigorous collision between the molecules of the polymer causing their degradation (Bikash Kumar et al., 2020). A study mentioned that microwave pretreatment with lactic acid effectively eliminated lignin and hemicellulose within 45 seconds. The molecular polarity of different eutectic solvents increased when combined with microwave radiation, thereby enhancing the efficacy of the pretreatment. A research study found that biogas yield from wheat straw increased by 28% after microwave pretreatment (Jędrzejczyk et al., 2019). It is often used with chemical pretreatments to reduce the severity and temperature of the pretreatment. The disadvantage of this method is that microwave-assisted pretreatment may generate inhibitors for the downstream bioprocess due to its high-temperature operation.

10.7 PULSED ELECTRIC FIELD PRETREATMENT

Pulsed electric field (PEF) pretreatment is a short, high-voltage pulse that hits the samples positioned between the electrodes. The PEF system is the most effective way to speed up the hydrolysis step. The compound's bioavailability is increased by cracking the raw substrate's cell structure. A high-voltage power source, a generator, an oscilloscope, and a treatment chamber make up the PEF system. A PEF reactor is equipped with a collinear plate on the left panel and a parallel plate on the right panel, and the pulse generator is coupled to this electrode configuration. When a system's orientation is either parallel to the flow or in the opposite direction, it helps us to determine the type of grounding. If the electric field is parallel to the material flow, grounding one pole of the pulse circuit is advantageous. In the middle of the pulse generator, the pulse circuit delivers positive and negative voltages for the electrode system. The PEF system is simple in design because it lacks movable elements. In this process, the electric field strength and pulse interval are essential factors that interact and determine the electroporation rate. During pretreatment, the treatment zone, or the gap between the electrodes, is chosen to be smaller to achieve a strong, uniform electric field. The substrate is provided with a shielding material that prevents undesired effects and reduces ohmic losses. Typical insulating materials include PVC, polyethylene, polysulfone, polypropylene, and so forth (Kovačić et al., 2020). PEF treatment offers benefits such as low energy requirements and consistent process conditions (temperature and pressure). This technique is commonly used to process pine chips and switchgrass, and a significant increase in porosity and a decrease in crystallinity were observed. This method is in a preliminary phase of development. PEF pretreatment is also used for microalgae.

10.8 PYROLYSIS

Pyrolysis involves thermal decomposition, in which biomass is heated to 500–800°C in the absence of an oxidizing agent. Based on the heating rate, the pyrolysis process is divided into slow and fast pyrolysis processes. Due to high-temperature operation, rapid cellulose decomposition occurs, leading to the formation of the end product. Based on the type of pyrolysis process selected, biomass physical characteristics, reaction limitations, and the amount of the end product vary. Fast pyrolysis generally produces liquid products. This process is widely adopted across many thermal industries due to its significant advantages, such as simple transportation management, storage, combustion, flexibility in production and marketing, and retrofitting. The pyrolysis process resulted in higher efficiency when operated at low temperatures in the presence of oxygen (as maximum bonds were fragmented in the presence of oxygen) (Kumar and Sharma, 2017). A comparative study was conducted to assess the efficacy of hydrolysis rate or cellulose bond cleavage in the presence of oxygen and nitrogen. The bond-breaking rate in the presence of oxygen was 7.8×10^9 bonds/min; in the presence of nitrogen, it was 1.7×10^8 bonds/min/g. Pretreatment of biomass is not economically viable, posing a significant drawback. Therefore, pyrolysis can be combined with microwave-assisted pretreatment, leveraging microwave dielectric heating, to achieve better results. Pyrolysis is commonly used to produce bio-oil (a mixture of polar organics and water) (Kumar et al., 2009). Torrefaction is an emerging technique in which partial decomposition of biomass occurs at temperatures between 200 and 300°C. This process is also called mild pyrolysis (Abomohra, 2019).

10.9 ENERGY EFFICIENCY DURING COMMINUTION

The crucial parameters that affect energy efficiency are mill type; mill operation factors (such as motor speed); and biomass properties (such as chemical composition, moisture, and temperature). The interrelation between these parameters must be well understood to improve the particle size distribution and shape (Eisenlauer and Teipel, 2017). The mechanical grinding method requires less energy for fibrous materials than for brittle materials. A study showed that the ratio of the final mean particle size to the original mean particle size was directly correlated with the energy consumed (Miao et al., 2011). A comparative study was initiated on the energy consumption of barley straw, corn stover, wheat, and switchgrass. The study concluded that corn stover consumed the least specific energy, and switchgrass used the most energy due to its high calorific value and low ash content (Mani et al., 2004).

10.10 RELATION BETWEEN PLANT MATERIAL AND MECHANICAL STRESS DURING COMMINUTION

Two types of failure occur when plant material breaks at the microscale under different mechanical stresses: intercellular failure and intracellular failure. Intercellular failure is considered peeling in which cells are separated from one another due to fracture propagation between them. Intracellular failure disrupts the secondary cell walls through fractures and cell wall intersections. For example, the milling of cork results in intracellular failure, and the mechanical stress generated by impact causes intercellular failure (Mayer-Laigle et al., 2018; Miao et al., 2011).

10.11 CONCLUSION

The versatility of physical and physicochemical pretreatment techniques for converting lignocellulosic feedstocks into bio-based goods is studied. This multiproduct biorefinery infrastructure offers a route to lower energy and second-generation fuels. Cellulosic biofuels have emerged as possible alternatives due to their economic and widespread availability. However, the recalcitrant composition of lignocellulosic biomass is a major obstacle to the production of bio-based products. The major challenges include feedstock costs, feedstock variability, production, environmental impact, enzyme costs, preprocessing, new technology development, transportation, and the successful operation of lignocellulosic valorization. The primary need for pretreatment is to provide accessible carbohydrates for biodegradation by reducing crystallinity, removing lignin and hemicellulose, reducing pore size, and increasing the accessible specific surface area. The most commonly suggested particle size for easy access to the hydrolysis of lignocellulosic substrates is about 3 mm. The substrate surface contact directly affects the approachability to cellulose, as it is a mass transfer constraint. Mechanical pretreatments significantly reduce particle size, making the feedstock easier to handle, limit the generation of waste products, reduce the use of chemicals, and increase the surface-to-volume ratio. Despite the increase in pretreatment techniques, multiple drawbacks still significantly affect the pretreatment process and need special attention. The economics of the overly expensive physical pretreatment process are an important issue. The integration of a few pretreatment methods can attain a potential solution. Mechanical and chemical pretreatment methods can be combined to reduce the energy requirements and improve the enzyme's effectiveness for hydrolysis. Therefore, further research can be carried out to develop multidisciplinary processes that are efficient, cost-competitive, and aligned with an improved environmental footprint.

REFERENCES

Abomohra AE, editor. *Biomass for bioenergy: Recent trends and future challenges*, 2019. IntechOpen, London.

Amusa AA, Ahmad AL, Adewole JK. Mechanism and compatibility of pretreated lignocellulosic biomass and polymeric mixed matrix membranes: A review. *Membranes*. 2020 Nov 26;10(12):370.

Arce C, Kratky L. Mechanical pretreatment of lignocellulosic biomass towards enzymatic/fermentative valorization. *iScience*. 2022 Jun 16:104610.

Barakat A, Mayer-Laigle C, Solhy A, Arancon RAD, de Vries H, Luque R. Mechanical pretreatments of lignocellulosic biomass: Towards facile and environmentally sound technologies for biofuels production. *RSC Advances*. 2014;4:89.

Bitra VS, Womac AR, Chevanan N, Sokhansanj S. Comminution properties of biomass in hammer mill and its particle size characterization. In *2008, Providence, Rhode Island, June 29–July 2, 2008*, 2008 (p. 1). American Society of Agricultural and Biological Engineers.

Eisenlauer M, Teipel U. Comminution of biogenic materials. *The Canadian Journal of Chemical Engineering*. 2017 Jul;95(7):1236–44.

Jędrzejczyk M, Soszka E, Czapnik M, Ruppert AM, Grams J. Physical and chemical pretreatment of lignocellulosic biomass. In *Second and third generation of feedstocks*, 2019 Jan 1 (pp. 143–96). Elsevier. https://doi.org/10.1016/B978-0-12-815162-4.00006-9.

Konan D, Koffi E, Ndao A, Peterson EC, Rodrigue D, Adjallé K. An overview of extrusion as a pretreatment method of lignocellulosic biomass. *Energies*. 2022 Apr 20;15(9):3002.

Kovačić Đ, Rupčić S, Kralik D, Jovičić D, Spajić R, Tišma M. Pulsed electric field: An emerging pretreatment technology in biogas production. *Waste Management*. 2021;120:467–83. https://doi.org/10.1016/j.wasman.2020.10.009.

Kratky L, Jirout T. Biomass size reduction machines for enhancing biogas production. *Chemical Engineering & Technology*. 2011 Mar;34(3):391–9.

Kumar AK, Sharma S. Recent updates on different methods of pretreatment of lignocellulosic feedstocks: A review. *Bioresources and Bioprocessing*. 2017 Dec;4(1):1–9.

Kumar B, Bhardwaj N, Agrawal K, Chaturvedi V, Verma P. Current perspective on pretreatment technologies using lignocellulosic biomass: An emerging biorefinery concept. *Fuel Processing Technology*. 2020;199:106244. ISSN: 0378-3820.

Kumar P, Barrett DM, Delwiche MJ, Stroeve P. Methods for pretreatment of lignocellulosic biomass for efficient hydrolysis and biofuel production. *Industrial & Engineering Chemistry Research*. 2009 Apr 15;48(8):3713–29.

Lomovsky O, Bychkov A, Lomovsky I. Mechanical pretreatment. *Biomass Fractionation Technologies for a Lignocellulosic Feedstock-Based Biorefinery*. 2016 Jan 1:23–55.

Mani S, Tabil LG, Sokhansanj S. Grinding performance and physical properties of wheat and barley straws, corn stover and switchgrass. *Biomass and Bioenergy*. 2004 Oct 1;27(4):339–52.

Mayer-Laigle C, Blanc N, Rajaonarivony RK, Rouau X. Comminution of dry lignocellulosic biomass, a review: Part I. From fundamental mechanisms to milling behaviour. *Bioengineering*. 2018 Jun 2;5(2):41.

Miao Z, Grift TE, Hansen AC, Ting KC. Energy requirement for comminution of biomass in relation to particle physical properties. *Industrial Crops and Products*. 2011 Mar 1;33(2):504.

Putro JN, Soetaredjo FE, Lin SY, Ju YH, Ismadji S. Pretreatment and conversion of lignocellulose biomass into valuable chemicals. *RSC Advances*. 2016;6(52):46834–52.

Sitotaw YW, Habtu NG, Gebreyohannes AY, Nunes SP, Van Gerven T. Ball milling as an important pretreatment technique in lignocellulose biorefineries: A review. *Biomass Conversion and Biorefinery*. 2021 Aug 12:1–24.

Sun Y, Cheng J. Hydrolysis of lignocellulosic materials for ethanol production: A review. *Bioresource Technology*. 2002 May 1;83(1):1–11.

Yachmenev V, Condon B, Klasson T, Lambert A. Acceleration of the enzymatic hydrolysis of corn stover and sugar cane bagasse celluloses by low-intensity uniform ultrasound. *Journal of Biobased Materials and Bioenergy*. 2009;3:25e31.

Zheng J, Rehmann L. Extrusion pretreatment of lignocellulosic biomass: A review. *International Journal of Molecular Sciences*. 2014 Oct 20;15(10):18967–84.

Zheng Y, Shi J, Tu M, Cheng YS. Principles and development of lignocellulosic biomass pretreatment for biofuels. *Advances in Bioenergy*. 2017 Jan 1;2:1–68.

11 Physicochemical Pretreatment Methodologies

Mamilla Shyam Sunder and Mamilla Shree Veena

11.1 INTRODUCTION

Commonly used fossil fuels are nonrenewable. Researchers are focusing more on pathways to sustainable energy in this modern era. Lignocellulosic biomass is a significant source, unlike fossil fuels, for producing high-value chemicals such as ethanol, bio-oil, phenols, aldehydes, and cellulose acetate. Lignocellulosic biomass comprises cellulose, hemicellulose, polymer lignin, and other polar and nonpolar substances. Pretreatment of lignocellulosic biomass is a crucial step in breaking down complex lignin structures and facilitating access to cellulose for subsequent hydrolysis. In an ideal case of pretreatment, the factors that meet the pretreatment requirements improve the formation of sugars, prevent carbohydrate degradation and the formation of other inhibitors that would impede subsequent hydrolysis and fermentation, minimize energy consumption, and be economically feasible (Sun and Cheng, 2002). Pretreatment can be categorized into physical pretreatment, which mainly includes size reduction, autoclaving, and ultrasonication, and chemical processes, such as the use of acids, alkalis, and solvents, which are combined with biological and physicochemical processes to ensure the digestion of lignocellulose constituents. The physicochemical pretreatment process for various lignocellulosic biomass feedstocks is essential for subsequent processes that produce eco-friendly, nontoxic products. Typically, the pretreatment method requires high energy consumption, whereas chemical methods offer efficient biomass fractionation and yield good sugars during enzymatic hydrolysis. Therefore, green solvent-based pretreatment techniques are viable for disrupting lignin and enhancing digestibility. In most agricultural residual biomass, cellulose is abundantly present in the cell walls of plants. It is responsible for mechanical strength, whereas the composition of lignocellulose constituents varies across different sources. The pretreatment process involves partial breakdown of cellulose and hemicellulose into pseudo-lignin, which is subsequently converted into acid-insoluble lignin. This pseudo-lignin comprises functional groups such as —COOH, —CO—, C_6H_5, and aliphatic groups, which significantly hinder cellulose-hydrolytic enzymes due to their presence on the surface

DOI: 10.1201/9781003327608-11

of the biomass remnant. Lignocellulosic biomass fractionation is crucial for producing bio-based products. Therefore, various green processes, such as liquid hot water, steam explosion, supercritical fluids, and ammonia fiber explosion, have been developed to convert the lignocellulose components described subsequently. The steam explosion method is the most broadly used for biomass pretreatment. A comparative study was conducted between mechanical processes and steam explosion methods, concluding that the steam explosion process consumes less energy to achieve the equivalent particle size.

11.2 STEAM EXPLOSION

The steam explosion method is a commonly used physicochemical pretreatment process and is widely used in today's technology for treating lignocellulosic biomass. Depending on the amount of available biomass for pretreatment, lignocellulosic biomass is treated at extreme pressures, followed by saturated steam at elevated temperatures between 160°C and 260°C for a short period. This causes the release of partially hydrolyzed biomass fibers, increasing the enzyme's accessibility to the first cellulose when the pressure is released to atmospheric conditions. Applying the steam explosion technique to lignocellulosic biomass can be broadly categorized into uncatalyzed and catalyzed methods. Uncatalyzed steam explosion, also known as auto-hydrolysis, is a combination of chemical and physical pretreatment processes. This process involves high-pressure, high-temperature conditions in which biomass particles are saturated for several seconds to a few minutes, then rapidly depressurized. The process occurring in the catalyzed steam explosion is equal to the process of auto-hydrolysis, with the significant difference being the impregnation of lignocellulosic biomass with acidic gases or liquids like sulfur dioxide (SO_2), sulfuric acid (H_2SO_4), nitric acid (HNO_3), and hydrochloric acid (HCl), which act as catalysts (Sohail Toor et al., 2013). The aspects that affect steam explosion include temperature, pressure, residence time, moisture content, and biomass size. During preprocessing, the carbohydrate fraction predominates, followed by the solubilization of hemicellulose in the liquid phase, where lignin conversion occurs as temperature increases. Additionally, the cellulose portion provides more readily available biomass for digestion. This method involves removing moisture and volatiles, increasing the biomass's calorific value and further thermal degradation of hemicellulose. The severity of the steam explosion affects the decrease in the number of hydroxyl groups. Steam explosion pretreatment can turn biomass from being a flexible, tenacious material to a brittle, rigid material. Biomass treated by steam explosion exhibits properties similar to those of coal (Stelte, 2013). Hardwood and grassy biomass are suitable feedstocks for steam explosion pretreatment.

The advantages of steam explosion include the use of limited chemicals, adaptability to large particle sizes, a low environmental impact, no recycling costs, high energy efficiency, and the total recovery of sugars, compared to other pretreatment processes. The steam explosion treatment efficiency can be enhanced using catalysts such as sulfuric acid, phosphoric acid, and carbon dioxide, which minimize residence time, decrease temperature, and yield minimal inhibitory compounds, thereby allowing enzymes to undergo hydrolysis.

The disadvantages of this process include incomplete disruption of the lignin-carbohydrate matrix, formation of inhibitors at high temperatures, and reduced final product yield.

11.3 HOT WATER TREATMENT

The process of hot water treatment was first applied by two scientists, Bobleter and Pape. It is also known as autohydrolysis, aqueous liquefaction, liquid hot water pretreatment, aqueous per-hydrolysis, hydrothermal pretreatment, and cooking under pressure with water (Mosier et al., 2005). Liquid hot water technology is a prominent preprocessing method that reduces the formation of toxic substances and by-product inhibitors. The process of this method is more similar to steam explosion, with pressure and temperature used to maintain water in the liquid phase without adding chemicals. The high-temperature, high-pressure conditions cause in-situ autoionization of water, leading to the generation of hydronium ions and the formation of acetic acid from the acetyl group of hemicelluloses. This process plays a dynamic role in the disintegration of biomass and the cleavage of uronic acids. Water acts as an acid catalyst during pretreatment, possessing acid properties at higher temperatures. This method renders cellulose more accessible to biodegradation and recovers hemicellulose as monosaccharides and oligosaccharides by allowing water to penetrate the biomass cell walls, thereby promoting cellulose hydration, hemicellulose solubilization, and a slight lignin removal. However, complete lignin removal is not possible with hot-water treatment. Moreover, this method of pretreatment offers several advantages; for example, it requires low temperature, excludes any catalyst or chemical, does not need a further neutralization or washing step, uses a cost-effective solvent for large applications, and biomass size reduction is not required as pretreatment breaks down particles, making the process more attractive on a large scale. A study has characterized liquid hot water pretreatment as the most effective method for extracting hemicellulose from wood used in the pulp and paper industry. Auto-hydrolysis pretreatment of sugarcane bagasse resulted in an 80% recovery of xylose by controlling the pH between 4 and 7 to prevent sugar degradation and the formation of inhibitory compounds (Kumar et al., 2020).

11.4 AMMONIA FIBER EXPLOSION

The preprocessing of biomass materials, such as lignocellulose, with ammonia fiber explosion is similar to the steam explosion method, but the primary difference lies in the use of ammonia. The pretreatment process involves elevated temperatures and a pressure range of 0.7–2.7 MPa. After heating the biomass with liquid ammonia in a specific, closed reactor, the reactor is opened when a particular temperature and pressure are reached; the ammonia explosion results in evaporation and a decline in the reactive system's temperature. The design of a reactive system resembles a steam explosion, wherein an ammonia solution is used instead of water. The anhydrous ammonia dissociates to form ammonium and hydroxide ions, which cause the swelling of biomass, deacetylation of hemicellulose to oligomeric sugars, disruption of lignin-carbohydrate linkage, and a decrease in crystallinity of cellulose. The ammonia fiber explosion method is more effective at high temperatures for biomass with low lignin content than for biomass with high lignin content. It breaks down the bonds between cellulose and lignin, making the biomass more accessible to enzymes and microorganisms that can convert it into valuable products. Additionally, the process enhances the biomass's water-holding capacity and improves the digestibility of the feedstock.

Key characteristics, including ash, volatile, and moisture content, as well as heating values, remain the same before and after pretreatment. Biochar and bio-oil yield production increased to 42–46% after ammonia fiber explosion pretreatment compared to pyrolysis treatment (22–26%) (Sundaram et al., 2017). The lignocellulosic biomass should be soaked before AFEXAFEX reprocessing to improve glucan metabolism and increase moisture content to approximately 10%. This moisture content plays a significant role in enzymatic hydrolysis, making the biomass more accessible to enzymes and thereby enhancing the conversion efficiency compared to other methods. This process facilitates the cleavage of ester-acetylated linkages, thereby increasing biomass porosity and enhancing enzymatic and fermentation processes. The characteristics that determine the process's effectiveness are time, temperature, moisture content, and the ammonia-to-biomass ratio. A higher ratio of ammonia to biomass, combined with a low moisture content, yields the highest conversion of monomeric units of gluten. However, a higher ammonia level is not economically desirable.

The ideal pretreatment method offers multiple benefits, such as eliminating the need to reduce biomass particle size or remove toxic materials and avoiding the need to condition fermenting microbes. Additionally, this process does not require a nitrogen source during fermentation and allows for the recovery of almost 99% of the sugars. The ammonia used in the process can also be recycled, making it a more sustainable and cost-effective solution. However, this method may not be effective for processing woody biomass and feedstocks with a high lignin content.

Moreover, the ammonia soaking preprocessing technique works similar to the other two processes, ammonia recycles percolation (ARP) and AFEX, in which ammonia is used, but biomass is treated at low temperatures, which requires less energy. This makes the process less cost-effective, depending on the available biomass for the pretreatment.

11.5 PRETREATMENT OF AMMONIA RECYCLE PERCOLATION AND SOAKING IN AQUEOUS AMMONIA

Ammonia recycles percolation; the soaking egg process is a liquid-ammonia-based pretreatment method for biomass. In contrast, ARP involves high temperatures, while soaking in aqueous ammonia is conducted at lower temperatures. Another approach, ammonia recycle percolation with ammonia fiber expansion pretreatment, employs the same ammonia basis for both processes.

Nevertheless, this process exhibits unique features that necessitate a thorough evaluation, given the availability of different pretreatment options. With ARP, a specific ammonia concentration is circulated through a biomass bed at a particular flow rate of the order of milliliters per minute, along with a specified temperature and residence time. Despite the small liquid volume, ARP preprocessing has been effectively employed with no reduction in efficiency.

Furthermore, ammonia recycling percolation offers several advantages over APEX, including the removal of up to 85% of cellulose while maintaining 50–60% solubilization of hemicellulose. This specifies ammonia's ability to degrade lignin through ammonolysis and solubilize hemicelluloses over extended retention times. The said process is an attractive alternative, as it can maintain a high cellulose content post-treatment.

11.6 SUPERCRITICAL FLUID

The process of supercritical fluid involves a liquid above its critical temperature and pressure, and supercritical fluids exhibit properties that combine the density of liquids and the compressibility of gases. These fluids include three types: liquids at room temperature and pressure, gases at ambient conditions, and binary and ternary fluid mixtures. Gases used in the pretreatment of supercritical fluids include CO_2, ethylene, nitrous oxide, and butane. A study stated that treating aspen wood chips for 4 hr at 130°C improved enzymatic hydrolysis rates (61% lignin was removed, maintaining 83% of total carbohydrate) (McMillan, 1994). Supercritical fluids aim to enhance the substrate availability to enzymatic hydrolysis. The biomass to be treated is pre-wetted for solvent dissolution. It involves elevated temperature and pressure. Under supercritical conditions, lignin is fragmented into low-molecular-weight phenolic compounds and other compounds, as well as relative aldehydes (Escobar et al., 2020). Carbon dioxide is used as a common supercritical fluid, a natural chemical with environmentally friendly characteristics, including a low critical temperature and pressure (31.1°C and 7.36 MPa), nonhazardous properties, and biodegradability. Key parameters considered during the treatment are biomass moisture, temperature, pressure, and pretreatment time. In this pretreatment process, carbon dioxide combines with the water that is available in the water. It produces a carbonic acid mixture, which creates a weakly acidic environment that promotes hemicellulose hydrolysis and increases mass transfer rates. Other solvents, such as ethanol and hexane, can also be used. Ethanol promotes an improved solubility of lignin fragments. High-pressure conditions facilitate a better interaction between the solvent mixtures and promote the dissociation of lignin from the lignocellulosic matrix (Serna et al., 2016).

The significant drawbacks of this process include specialized reaction environments, expensive instrumentation, and high temperatures. Research showed that glucose conversion varies significantly with temperature and pressure. It was also observed that lignocellulosic biomass with a higher moisture content, approximately 40–70%, improved enzymatic digestibility. The pretreatment process, followed by the integration of carbon dioxide and ethanol-water, increased the biomass digestibility. A mixture of ethanol and water can dissolve lignin by increasing the surface area and, to a lesser extent, reducing the inhibition of cellulose hydrolysis (Roy et al., 2020).

11.7 ORGANOSOLV

The organosolv or organosolvation method has gained popularity for biomass preprocessing. Organic solvents break down linkages within lignin and hemicellulose, leaving a pure form of cellulose remnant. Acids like oxalic and salicylic acids further enhance the reactions, and methanol, ethylene glycol, tetrahydrofurfuryl alcohol, and ethanol are commonly used. Methanol and ethanol are preferred because they are less expensive than other solvents such as ethylene glycol. This pretreatment process is used to extract lignin and sugars from the biomass. Many researchers have studied various solvents and have shown that an acid catalyst, such as sulfuric acid, is the most powerful due to its high reactivity. Still, it has drawbacks in terms of recovery and recycling.

The solvent must be carefully removed to prevent any detrimental effects on microbial development, as microbes break down enzymes through hydrolysis and fermentation. The risk of handling extremely combustible organic solvents also renders them undesirable choices.

The advantages of this technology are particularly prominent in emerging pretreatment applications, thanks to convenient solvent recovery via distillation, which enables recycling in the preprocessing stage, and the ability to isolate sufficient lignin to generate value-added products for industrial applications.

Despite its many benefits, it has a few drawbacks. For instance, using costly solvents necessitates their recovery to the fullest extent possible, which can be a high-energy process. Furthermore, the highly combustible and volatile nature requires strict control and safety measures.

11.8 IONIC LIQUIDS

Ionic liquid preprocessing is a comparatively recent physicochemical procedure in which green solvents are safe and noncombustible for lignocellulose biomass pretreatment. This solvent consists of ions with melting points below 100°C. It has a high velocity, low vapor pressure, and high temperature resistance. It tends to liquefy unprocessed biomass. It can also develop biopolymers from unprocessed biomass. It can primarily be achieved by breaking the intra- and intermolecular hydrogen bonds in the biological polymers of lignocellulosic biomass.

Ionic liquids are a new type of solvent that have anions and cations with melting points below 100°C, strong polarity, high thermal stability, and negative vapor pressure. The categories encompass both organic and inorganic ions under the term "anion," including imidazolium, pyridinium, and aliphatic ammonium.

Cellulose and lignin are solubilized during the pretreatment procedure due to the action of cations and anions. Although ionic liquids with lower viscosities are more straightforward, viscosity is not a significant issue in cellulose solubilization.

11.9 CARBON DIOXIDE EXPLOSION

This is the process technique where carbon dioxide (CO_2) is used as a supercritical fluid to perform liquid hot water splitting at high pressure, with temperatures about 120°C to 180°C, and moisture content up to 80%, with different residence times. In this supercritical CO_2 explosion, using the greener alternative with lower energy requirements appears to be an available alternative to ammonia. Supercritical CO_2 has mass conversion properties of a "gas-like" substance with a "liquid-like" solvating power, and it can enter spaces as a gas and later dissolve in water to produce carbonic acid, which increases the hydrolysis of hemicellulose. Its components can also penetrate lignocellulose residues. Thereafter, the complex structure, composed of hemicelluloses and lignin, is fragmented. This technique is inappropriate for biomass with low or no moisture content, as excessive moisture can increase the likelihood of splitting. In this pretreatment procedure, CO_2 is used as a supercritical fluid, and liquid hot water is split at pressures ranging from 3,050 to 4,000 psi, with a moisture content of up to 80%, reaching a temperature of 170°C. Biomass disruption was due to high carbon dioxide pressure. Similarly, the available carbon dioxide dissolves in water, forming carbonic acid, which enhances the hydrolysis of hemicellulose and releases pressurized gas, causing structural damage to the biomass and increasing the surface area available to enzymes. When the temperature used in this process is low, sugars are stabilized, preventing them from denaturing, unlike those processed by other methods.

This process is more appealing because it utilizes carbon dioxide at a low cost. It requires a reduced temperature, high solid volume, and no generation of toxins. However, the high economic cost of the reactor and its inability to withstand high-pressure conditions are significant barriers to its use in scale-up processes.

The process has numerous limitations, including the inability of expensive equipment to withstand high-pressure conditions. Numerous studies have examined the scale-up of high-pressure CO_2 pretreatment processes for industrial implementation, demonstrating their effectiveness in penetrating cellulosic pores and enabling complete glucose saccharification through enzymatic hydrolysis. While the overall process has been shown to be economically viable, further optimization is necessary to facilitate large-scale deployment.

11.10 OZONOLYSIS

Ozone (O_3) treatment has been reported to effectively isolate lignin at room temperature and standard pressure (Shatalov and Pereira, 2008). O_3 degrades lignin to a lesser extent than hemicellulose and cellulose. Therefore, lignin yields are higher than those of hemicellulose and cellulose via ozonolysis. The high moisture content of lignin, when treated with O_3, lowers the oxidation rate. Many studies have focused on lignocellulosic raw materials such as wheat straw and rye straw (Garcı´a-Cubero et al., 2009), cotton straw (Silverstein et al., 2007), bagasse, and poplar, among others (Kumar and Wyman, 2009). Furthermore, the experiment requires pretreating lignocellulosic constituents with ozone to produce ethanol.

The advantage of this pretreatment is that ozone doesn't yield harmful inhibitors; rather, it initiates another chemical process. However, the process is expensive, as ozonolysis requires a significant amount of ozone.

11.11 CONCLUSION

Pretreatment of biomass is essential to enhance enzymatic hydrolysis and convert biomass into bioenergy and biofuels. The parameters that hinder biomass's digestibility are biomass's surface area, cellulose crystallinity, and low hemicellulose solubility. Physical, chemical, and other commercially available pretreatment methods were used. Therefore, an approach has been initiated toward green pretreatment, a blend of physical and chemical treatments. This green approach exhibited exceptional performance, reducing the use of toxic chemicals and eliminating harsh reaction conditions. Despite its advantages, the green pretreatment method requires specialized instruments, making it economically unfeasible. Therefore, further studies are necessary to enhance the economic viability of green pretreatment.

REFERENCES

Escobar EL, Da Silva TA, Pirich CL, Corazza ML, Pereira Ramos L. Supercritical fluids: A promising technique for biomass pretreatment and fractionation. *Frontiers in Bioengineering and Biotechnology*. 2020 Apr 23;8:252.

Kumar B, Bhardwaj N, Agrawal K, Chaturvedi V, Verma P. Current perspective on pretreatment technologies using lignocellulosic biomass: An emerging biorefinery concept. *Fuel Processing Technology*. 2020;199:106244. ISSN: 0378-3820.

Kumar R, Wyman CE. Effects of cellulase and xylanase enzymes on the deconstruction of solids from pretreatment of poplar by leading technologies. *Biotechnology Progress*. 2009;25:302–14. doi: 10.1002/btpr.102.

McMillan JD. Pretreatment of lignocellulosic biomass. *Biomass*. 1994;292–324.

Mosier N, Wyman C, Dale B, Elander R, Lee YY, Holtzapple M, Ladisch M. Features of promising technologies for pretreatment of lignocellulosic biomass. *Bioresource Technology*. 2005 Apr 1;96(6):673–86.

Roy R, Rahman MS, Raynie DE. Recent advances in greener pretreatment technologies of lignocellulose. *Current Research in Green and Sustainable Chemistry*. 2020. 1;3:100035.

Serna LD, Alzate CO, Alzate CC. Supercritical fluids as a green technology for the pretreatment of lignocellulosic biomass. *Bioresource Technology*. 2016 Jan 1;199:113–20.

Shatalov AA, Pereira H. Arundo donax L. reed: New perspectives for pulping and bleaching. 5. Ozone-based TCF bleaching of organosolv pulps. *Bioresource Technology*. 2008;99(3):472–78.

Silverstein RA, Chen Y, Sharma-Shivappa RR, Boyette MD, Osborn JA. A comparison of chemical pre-treatment methods for improving saccharification of cotton stalks. *Bioresource Technology*. 2007;98:3000–11.

Sohail Toor S, Rosendahl L, Hoffmann J, Holm-Nielsen JB, Augustine Ehimen E. lignocellulosic biomass – thermal pre-treatment with steam. *Pretreatment Techniques for Biofuels and Biorefineries*. 2013:59–75.

Stelte W. Steam explosion for biomass pre-treatment. *Danish Technological Institute*. 2013 Sep 20:1–5.

Sun Y, Cheng J. Hydrolysis of lignocellulosic materials for ethanol production: A review. *Bioresource Technology*. 2002 May 1;83(1):1–1.

Sundaram V, Muthukumarappan K, Gent S. Understanding the impacts of AFEXt pretreatment and densification on the fast pyrolysis of corn stover, prairie cord grass, and switchgrass. *Appl. Biochem. Biotechnol.* 2017;181(3):10601079.

12 Micro Biological Pretreatment of Lignocellulosic Biomass

Manideep Pabba, Sundergopal Sridhar, and Mamilla Shyam Sunder

12.1 INTRODUCTION

Society demands more energy yearly, so we must consider new options beyond traditional fossil fuels. One solution lies in lignocellulosic biomass, an abundant source found in agricultural and forestry byproducts, which can be used to produce bioethanol sustainably and at low cost (Maurya et al., 2015). Lignocellulosic biomass has great potential to meet our biofuel, biochemical, and bioproduct needs. Its renewable nature makes it an attractive source of energy and chemicals as this complex mixture of lignin and polysaccharides is readily accessible (Cheng et al., 2008). The nature of converting lignocellulosic biomass into practical products adds complexity due to high lignin concentrations and complex structural features, further impeding effective transformation. Added constraints are imposed by the inherent recalcitrance arising from the close association of cellulose, hemicellulose, and lignin, yet their distinct crystalline or amorphous nature creates significant challenges for enzyme accessibility and effective hydrolysis.

Lignin's role as an obstacle blocks enzymes and other compounds from penetrating the biomaterial matrix. This means that pretreatment of lignocellulosic biomass is a crucial step, with several techniques applied to alter its composition and structure, including physical, chemical, or biological processes that aim to improve enzyme accessibility to the material's matrix. Achieving such successful pretreatments that allow practical product formation requires removing hemicelluloses and lignin from this material to enhance enzymatic saccharification. Various approaches exist for prepping biomass before processing; however, none are without trade-offs. Given the distinct attributes of each type of biomass, using a universal prep method isn't feasible. One promising route worth exploring is biological pretreatment, which uses microorganisms or their enzymes to break down or modify lignin and hemicellulose components, enabling easier cellulase access. A vital advantage of this green approach over traditional chemical treatments is that no dangerous compounds or high heat input is required (Chen et al., 2014). In recent research on biological pretreatment, scientists examined

 DOI: 10.1201/9781003327608-12

an approach that uses microbial communities or enzymes with selective breakdown capabilities to degrade lignin and hemicellulose while leaving cellulose unchanged. By doing so, they can harness value-added products such as biofuels, biochemicals, and biopolymers from various sources, including different biomasses.

There's been considerable interest in exploring microorganisms, including bacteria, fungi, and actinomycetes, for their ability to optimize degradation pathways during biological pretreatment procedures. At the same time, all three types show promise; fungal species appear especially promising for breaking down complex components like lignin, thanks in part to their production of valuable enzymes such as laccase, manganese peroxidase, and lignin peroxidase, which can facilitate enzymatic hydrolysis by improving accessibility levels for both cellulose and hemicellulose (Saha et al., 2016). It's worth noting that some microorganisms can produce specific enzymes that aid in biodegradation. Bacteria and actinomycetes are examples of such organisms, as they produce cellulases and hemicellulases that target cellulose and hemicellulose, respectively. Meanwhile, white-rot fungi like Phanerochaete chrysosporium have a reputation for being formidable biological pretreatments due to their arsenal of enzymes – laccase, lignin peroxidase (LiP), and manganese peroxidase (MnP) (Kirk and Farrell, 2003). One major issue with biological pretreatment is optimizing settings while identifying appropriate microbes or enzymes for specific types of biomass. Evaluating how effective bioprocessing is at breaking down plant tissue into usable components, such as lignin or cellulose, requires careful consideration of factors, including the microbial consortia present during processing, the chemical composition, physical structure, temperature, pH, and moisture content throughout the treatment. Figure 12.1 shows the structure and composition of the lignocellulosic biomass. This information enables to design biological pretreatment methods efficiently and effectively overall (Sharma et al., 2019).

While significant advances have been made over the past few years in using biological processes to convert lignocellulosic biomaterials, there remain hurdles to optimizing these processes. Identifying which microbes or enzyme combinations perform best on specific materials remains a challenge. Despite setbacks, integrating bio-processing into industry practices represents an exciting new frontier for improving our use of natural resources. Recent studies suggest that biological pretreatment techniques can yield more efficient, higher-quality conversions of lignocellulosic biomass into biofuels and other high-value products. The search for innovative methods to convert lignocellulosic biomass into biofuels and other valuable products continues, with biological pretreatment as one potential avenue. Nevertheless, researchers must continue their efforts to identify optimal treatment conditions and select appropriate microbes or enzymes based on the type of biomass at hand. This chapter presents a general review of recent achievements, including biological pretreatments such as microbial consortia, enzyme use, and optimization methodologies (Sharma et al., 2019; Sindhu et al., 2016; Millati et al., 2011).

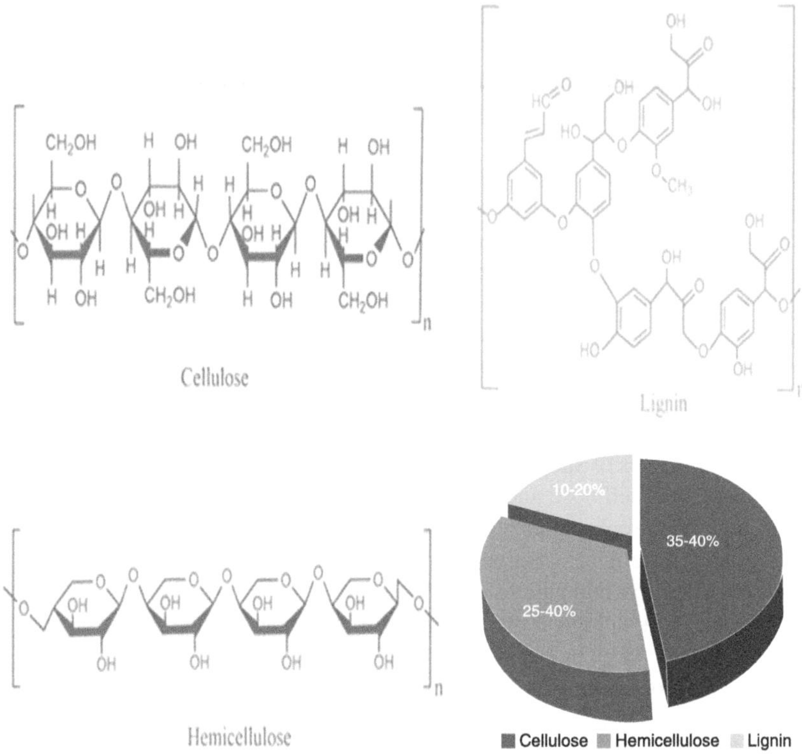

FIGURE 12.1 Structure and composition of lignocellulosic biomass.

Source: Amin et al. (2017)

12.2 VARIOUS BIOLOGICAL PRETREATMENT PROCESSES

To successfully convert lignocellulose into polysaccharides through enzymatic hydrolysis, prior treatment of the biomass is necessary. The most common methods include chemical-intensive techniques, such as acid and alkaline processes, as well as energy-intensive techniques, such as autohydrolysis or steam explosion. However, amid growing environmental concerns about chemical use, biological pretreatments are becoming increasingly popular because they improve enzyme digestion without harsh chemicals (Machado and Ferraz, 2017). Although there may have been limited awareness of how best to prepare various types of biomass for their intended use, advancements in biological pretreatment techniques are helping change that, as is the recognition that not every strategy can work across the board due to differences in element composition or percentages. As such, relying on cost-effective yet effective strategies such as enzyme-based microbial consortia to enhance cellulose accessibility is emerging as a popular approach with fewer drawbacks than traditional chemical or physical methods (Sindhu et al., 2016). It is widely accepted among scientists, based on extensive research documented in countless articles, that various types of bacteria and fungi can decompose organic matter. Specific examples include *Bacillus* and *Actinomycetes*. Likewise, it has been shown through experimentation involving cellulolytic bacterial communities (e.g., *Candida*, *Aspergillus*, *Streptomyces*, or *Bacillus*) that an expansive assortment of materials can be readily broken down (Poszytek et al., 2016; Mahamadi et al., 2017).

For example, Zhong et al. and Wang et al. described using a fungal consortium and a bacterial strain, respectively, to pretreat sugarcane bagasse and maize stover, resulting in higher digestibility and better biofuel yields, as well as enhanced cellulose hydrolysis and bioethanol production. Many biological pretreatment techniques for lignocellulosic biomass have been proposed to improve enzymatic digestibility and minimize recalcitrance (Figure 12.2). This section will review some of the most commonly adopted biological pretreatment procedures.

12.2.1 Fungal Pretreatment

Fungi possess significant potential to release ligninolytic enzymes that degrade lignin, thereby enhancing enzymatic hydrolysis of cellulose and hemicellulose. These enzymes include laccases, peroxidases, and manganese peroxidases, which aid in degrading lignin while improving access to the material's substrate for other enzymes. Implementing efficient fungal pretreatment requires using a fungal strain with greater capacity to improve polysaccharide digestibility while consuming less; this is key to maintaining total mass balance in sugar release during biotreatment. While numerous species are known for their remarkable ability to enhance polysaccharide digestion alone, only some have what it takes to completely degrade substantial amounts of lignin while preserving significant amounts of cellulose and some hemicellulose (Salvachúa et al., 2011).

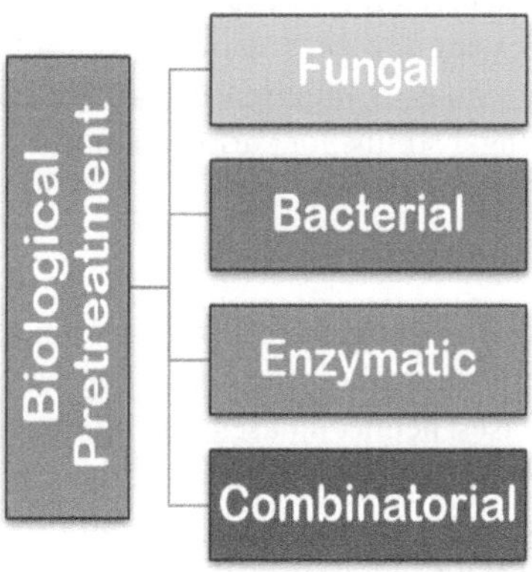

FIGURE 12.2 Types of biological pretreatment.

According to recent research, fungal pretreatment can improve the enzymatic digestibility of several lignocellulosic materials such as wheat straw, corn stover, and sugarcane bagasse. In particular, the selective white-rot fungus Ceriporiopsis subvermispora effectively preserved the glucan fraction while enhancing cellulose digestion during biological pretreatment of sugarcane bagasse. When studying mass balance statistics following a 60-day course of *C. subvermispora* biotreatment combined with enzymatic digestion processes, researchers observed a sugar-rich syrup with an impressive 47% potential glucose content (Machado and Ferraz, 2017). Fungal pretreatment of lignocellulosic biomass can be an efficient and long-term approach for increasing enzymatic digestibility and decreasing recalcitrance. In this section, we will examine some of the fungi used in the pretreatment of lignocellulosic biomass. *C. subvermispora is a white-rot fungus widely examined for its capacity to break down lignin and increase the enzymatic digestibility of lignocellulosic biomass.* According to research, applying *C. subvermispora* during the pretreatment of maize stover increased glucose and xylose release. *Pleurotus ostreatus*, often called the oyster mushroom, is another white-rot fungus examined for its potential to break down lignin and increase the enzymatic digestibility of lignocellulosic biomass. Researchers evaluated the usage of *P. ostreatus* for pretreating wheat straw.

The investigators found that pretreatment with *P. ostreatus* increased cellulose conversion compared to unprocessed wheat straw. *Phanerochaete chrysosporium* is a white-rot fungus that has been demonstrated to be efficient in digesting lignin and enhancing lignocellulosic biomass enzymatic digestibility. Researchers studied the application of *P. chrysosporium* for pretreating sugarcane bagasse. According to the authors, pretreatment with *P. chrysosporium* increased glucose and xylose release compared to non-treated sugarcane bagasse. *Trametes versicolor*, often known as the turkey tail fungus, is a white-rot fungus examined for its capacity to break down lignin and increase lignocellulosic biomass enzymatic digestibility. The application of *T. versicolor* for pretreating maize stover showed that pretreatment with *T. versicolor* increased cellulose hydrolysis compared to untreated maize stover. Therefore, we can consider fungal pretreatment a potential technique for increasing the enzymatic digestibility of lignocellulosic biomass. However, further study is required to optimize pretreatment parameters and identify suitable fungal strains for various lignocellulosic biomass types.

12.2.2 Bacterial Pretreatment

Enzymatic digestibility is improved by using bacteria to pretreat various plant-based materials such as switchgrass, sugarcane bagasse, or maize stover. This is because different cellulases, hemicellulases, and ligninases are created by bacteria that work together to break down the structure of these plant-based fibers. Instead of traditional methods involving chemicals or heat, this ecologically sound process uses bacteria's natural processes, enabling a sustainable, eco-friendly operation (Kumar et al., 2009). Researchers studied the use of cellulase-producing bacteria for pretreating wheat straw and found that pretreatment with *Bacillus licheniformis* increased cellulose breakdown by 22% (Kumar et al., 2009).

Bacteria are at the forefront of biorefinery research, as they produce enzymes such as cellulases, hemicellulases, and ligninases that can effectively degrade lignocellulosic biomass. Here, we will analyze some gram-positive bacteria used for bacterial pretreatment. One prominent bacterium is *Bacillus subtilis.* This type of bacteria has a proven track record in breaking down the rigid materials found in biomass. Observations showed increased glucose and xylose release following pretreatment with B. subtilis compared with untreated sugarcane bagasse.

Another impressive bacterium is *Streptomyces* sp., which is again classified as a gram-positive strain. *Streptomyces* sp. was effective in degrading rigid polymers, such as those found in lignin, while also improving enzymatic digestion of various types of biomass – including rice straw, which showed a clear improvement after treatment. Researchers have been seeking to enhance the natural breakdown process through innovative biotechnological solutions to efficiently convert biomass resources, such as rice straw or maize stover, into valuable materials or energy sources. One such approach involves using the gram-positive bacterium cellulomonas sp., which has attracted attention for its ability to digest cellulose and hemicellulose in plant cell walls.

Experiments on the pretreatment of rice straw and maize stover samples with Cellulomonas sp. resulted in a significant increase in glucose and xylose release compared to untreated samples. Similarly, *Pseudomonas putida*, a gram-negative bacterium found in natural environments such as soil and water, has shown promise for improving the enzymatic digestion of lignocellulosic biomass by degrading lignin. Tests conducted with wheat straw samples showed that pretreatment with this bacterium resulted in higher cellulose hydrolysis rates than in untreated samples. Bacterial pretreatment might significantly enhance the enzymatic digestibility of lignocellulosic biomass. Still, we must conduct extensive research to optimize pretreatment conditions and identify the most effective bacterial strains for various lignocellulosic materials (Table 12.1).

12.2.3 Enzymatic Pretreatment

Enzymatic pretreatment involves utilizing synthetic or microbial enzymes to modify or break down the structure of lignocellulosic materials. The application of this process improves enzymatic digestibility, especially of materials such as sugarcane bagasse, corn stover, and wheat straw. It's emerging as a viable substitute for traditional physicochemical methods used for the same purpose. The class of enzymes, including ligninases alongside cellulases and hemicellulases, has shown enormous potential for breaking down plant-derived biomass, thereby improving its enzymatic digestibility. Polysaccharides break down into sugars; proteins break down into amino acids; lipids break down into glycerol and long-chain fatty acids, facilitated by diverse classes of enzymes like cellulase, cellobiose, xylanase, amylase, protease, and lipases, which form the basis on which

TABLE 12.1
Biological Pretreatment Conditions for Various Feedstocks

Feedstock	Microorganism	Process Condition	Effect on Biomass	References
Sugarcane bagasse	*Ceriporiopsis subvermispora*	27 ± 2°C for 60 days	47% sugar was recovered as sugar-rich syrup	Machado and Ferraz (2017)
Sawdust	*Pleurotus pulmonarius*	28°C for 30 days	Sugar concentration increased from 2.51mol/ml	Castoldi et al. (2014)
Wheat straw	*Ceriporiopsissubvermispora*	7 weeks of solid-state fermentation incubated at 24°C	In-vitro gas production of 297.0 ml/g	Nayan et al. (2018)
Paddy straw	*Pleurotus florida*	25–29°C for 28 days	Maximum saccharification efficiency up to 75.3%	Manickam et al. (2018)
Straw	Fungal consortium	Incubated at 30°C and 55°C for 6 days	7-fold increase in hydrolysis	Taha et al. (2015)
Corn stover	Fungal consortium	Pretreatment for 42 days with fungi	43.8% lignin removal and 7-fold increase in hydrolysis	Song et al. (2013)
Corn stalks	*Irpexlacteus*	28 days incubation	82% hydrolysis yield observed	Du et al. (2011)
Bamboo clums	*Punctularia* sp. TUFC20056	Not specified	50% of lignin removed	Suhara et al. (2012)
Corn stover	*Ceriporiopsis subvermispora*	Solid state fermentation at 28°C for 42 days	57–67% glucose yield increase	Wan and Li, (2010)
Rice straw	*Pholiotaadiposa*	Saccharification for 48 hr	Releases 716 mg sugar/g substrate	Jagtap et al. (2013a)
Aspen biomass	*Armillaria gemina* SKU2114	48 hr of hydrolysis	Maximum saccharification yield of 62%	Jagtap et al. (2013b)

Source: Baruah et al. (2018)

complex biomolecules are dismantled during enzymatic pretreatment (Indrasith et al., 1988).

Zhu et al. analyzed the use of a commercial enzyme combination for pretreating maize stover. They discovered that such enzymatic treatment led to a noteworthy 25% increase in cellulose conversion rates. This section will review some of the latest studies on enzymatic pretreatment methods for lignocellulosic biomass (Zhu et al., 2008).

12.2.3.1 Cellulase Pretreatment

Cellulase is an enzyme that breaks down tough-to-break-down substances like cellulose into something more useful, like glucose. During enzymatic saccharification, this enzyme often binds to larger chunks of structured cellulose while floating in the water. These glycosyl hydrolase family 3 enzymes are key factors in breaking down biomass, specifically cellulases (Figure 12.3). Together, they work as a team to break apart the complicated cellulose structure into a sugar treasure trove. For this reason, *Trichoderma viride and Aspergillus niger are excellent sources of cellulase for biomass hydrolysis, and even commercially available enzyme mixtures rely on their power in* their blends (Passos et al., 2009).

12.2.3.2 Hemicellulase Pretreatment

Hemicellulases are enzymes that can hydrolyze hemicellulose into different sugars. Breaking down complex components, such as plant biomass, requires specialized enzymatic activity, such as that provided by hemicellulases. These enzymes play a pivotal role in the natural carbon cycle, catalyzing the hydrolysis of polysaccharides, such as hemicellulose, into simpler sugars. Hydrogen bonds facilitate the linkage between hemicelluloses and cellulose microfibrils, with xylose being the most prevalent pentose sugar found in xylan, an essential constituent of hemicellulosic polysaccharides. The enzyme xylanase hydrolyzes this pentose sugar (Binod et al., 2011).

12.2.3.3 Ligninase Pretreatment

Breaking down lignocellulosic biomass requires a targeted approach to degrading the compound known as "lignin." While essential for the structure of plant cell walls, excess lignin can inhibit the breakdown of other key components such as cellulose and hemicellulose. Fortunately, "ligninases" like MnP, LiP, and laccases are highly specialized in degrading this compound and improving access to other materials. Certain microorganisms produce these enzymes with unique mechanisms of degradation that influence the types and amounts of enzyme products available (Sahadevan et al., 2023).

12.2.3.4 Multi-Enzyme Pretreatment

A mixture of cellulases, hemicellulases, and ligninases can be used to pretreat lignocellulosic biomass (Figure 12.4). In their study, Guo et al. evaluated the application of multi-enzyme pretreatment for rice straw. The scientists discovered

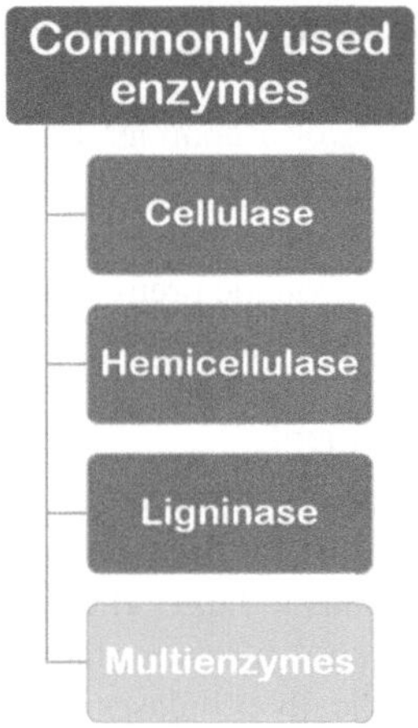

FIGURE 12.3 Common enzymes used in enzymatic pretreatment.

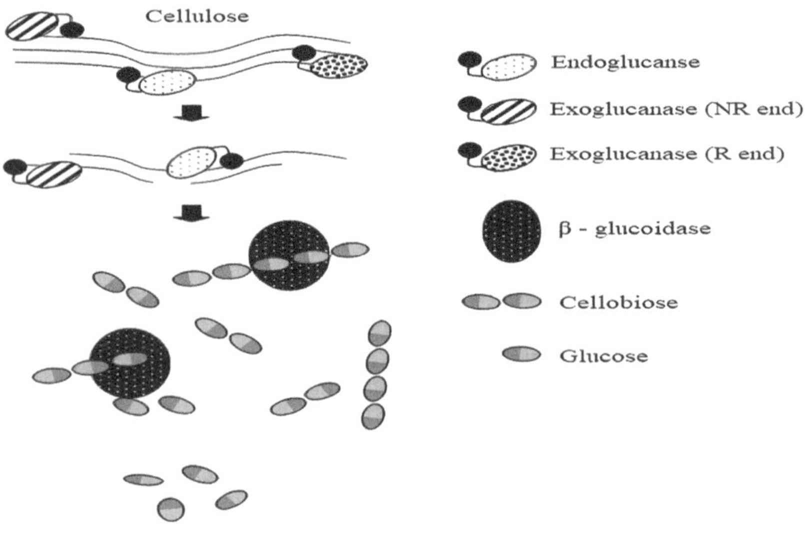

FIGURE 12.4 Mechanism of cellulase.

Source: Ferdeş et al. (2020)

that pretreatment with a mixture of enzymes increased glucose release by 77% compared to untreated rice straw.

Enzymatic pretreatment is emerging as an exciting avenue for improving the conversion of lignocellulosic biomass into fermentable sugars. Researchers use cellulases, hemicellulases, and ligninases to determine optimal enzyme mixtures for pretreatment. One such study, conducted by Guo et al., found that using multiple enzymes on rice straw resulted in a remarkable 77% increase in glucose release compared to untreated samples. As promising as these findings are, additional investigation is necessary before applying this method to different forms of biomass (Haldar and Banerjee, 2022).

12.2.3.5 Combinatorial Pretreatment

A combinatorial approach holds promise for lignocellulosic biomass, as it significantly increases enzymatic digestibility by leveraging synergies among methods. Both switchgrass and maize stover are prime examples that can benefit from this approach by improving their overall efficiency during processes such as fermentation or hydrolysis. Current research has investigated possible combinations of fungal and bacterial treatments for switchgrass. However, using a combination of fungi, bacteria, and enzymes has recently gained momentum as an efficient technique for achieving optimal lignocellulosic biomass treatment outcomes. This section will discuss noteworthy research into implementing these three elements together (Kirk and Farrell, 2003).

Researchers exploring lignocellulosic biomass have identified three pretreatment methods: sequential treatment with fungi, bacteria, and enzymes; simultaneous treatment with these agents; and integrated pretreatment, which combines them all at once. One such study focused on rice straw as a model substrate to test sequential treatments with Aspergillus terreus, Bacillus pumilus, and cellulase, resulting in higher glucose release than in untreated samples. In another project, Zhang et al. looked at maize stover samples treated simultaneously with *Trametes hirsute*, *Bacillus subtilis*, and cellulase, which exhibited outcomes similar to those observed after sequential treatment – higher levels of glucose release than in controls. Meanwhile, Wang et al.'s work examined an integrated approach combining *Phanerochaete chrysosporium*, Bacillus subtilis, and cellulase to treat maize stover. Bio-based pretreatment methods have demonstrated impressive promises in enhancing the enzyme-mediated digestibility of lignocellulosic materials. Yet, further inquiry is needed to optimize pretreatment conditions and identify optimal microbial strains or enzymes for diverse lignocellulose substrates.

12.3 EFFECT OF INHIBITORS ON MICROBIAL PRETREATMENT

Lignocellulosic materials contain abundant polysaccharides that require pretreatment to produce biofuels or other valuable products successfully. During this treatment process, various challenges arise as inhibitors, such as furfural, 5-hydroxymethylfurfural, and acetic acid, which can hinder effective treatment. Additionally, intermediate by-products generated during pretreatment might challenge the downstream processing of pretreated biomass. Here, we explore how biological pretreatment mechanisms for lignocellulosic biomaterials are affected by inhibitors produced during the breakdown and solubilization of hemicelluloses and lignin (Jönsson and Martín, 2016).

As we understood from the previous sections, fungi, bacteria, and enzymes can carry out biological pretreatment or a combination of them.In this section, we shall explore the influence of inhibitors on microbial pretreatment processes of lignocellulosic biomass. To effectively break down lignocellulosic biomass, many researchers rely on fungal pretreatment. Nonetheless, Martin Sampedro et al. identified inhibitors that impede this process in their research on the effects of these inhibitors on eucalyptus wood chips. Specifically, their findings demonstrate that acetic acid, furfural, and hydroxymethylfurfural reduce the success rate of fungal pretreatment and subsequent enzymatic hydrolysis (Martín-Sampedro et al., 2012). Sathitsuksanoh et al. examined the effect of inhibitors on the fungal pretreatment of switchgrass with *Ceriporiopsis subvermispora*. According to scientists, inhibitors such as acetic acid and furfural lowered the efficacy of fungal pretreatment and subsequent enzymatic hydrolysis.

Another potential microbial pretreatment approach for lignocellulosic biomass is bacterial pretreatment. According to scientists, the effect of inhibitors on bacterial pretreatment of maize stover and the presence of inhibitors, such as acetic acid and furfural, hindered the efficacy of bacterial pretreatment and subsequent enzymatic hydrolysis (Sivagurunathan et al., 2017). Enzymatic pretreatment is a common approach for lignocellulosic biomass. In their study, researchers evaluated the influence of inhibitors on the enzymatic pretreatment of maize stover (Wojtusik et al., 2017). Inhibitors such as acetic acid and furfural can hinder the enzymatic pretreatment's ability to efficiently hydrolyze lignocellulosic biomass. Another method currently under investigation for dealing with this type of biomass is combinatorial pretreatment, which involves combining different enzymes, fungi, and bacteria. For example, a study by Singh et al. evaluated how adding Aspergillus oryzae, *Bacillus coagulans*, and cellulase influenced rice straw treatment in the presence of inhibitors. Among alternative approaches to convert lignocellulosic biomass into a viable biofuel source, biological pretreatments, such as fungal or bacterial methods, can be used. These treatments hold much promise, but there is a hurdle: their execution is inhibited by acetic acid and furfural, which reduce their efficiency.

12.4 POSSIBLE METHODS TO OVERCOME INHIBITORS

Biological pretreatment of lignocellulosic biomass typically involves using microbes to break down or modify the biomass, but various inhibitors can sometimes hamper this process. Because biological pretreatment is performed under modest circumstances, the by-products generated do not generally inhibit further hydrolysis. The following are a few methods for dealing with inhibitors during biological pretreatment:

- Enzyme optimization: Enzymes are essential in the biological pretreatment technique. Optimizing enzyme mixtures, including selecting appropriate enzyme types and amounts, can help overcome inhibitors. Employing enzymes that are more resistant to inhibitors, for example, or altering enzyme doses can enhance the efficiency of lignocellulosic biomass breakdown (Galbe and Zacchi, 2012).

- Microorganism selection: Selecting microorganisms inherently more resistant to inhibitors can help overcome inhibitory activity. Certain bacteria have evolved tolerance or detoxification mechanisms such as producing particular enzymes or transporters that may neutralize or pump out inhibitors from their cells. Screening and choosing such microbes can be advantageous.
- Process conditions: Changing the operating state can also help remove inhibitors. For instance, adjusting pH, temperature, and oxygen levels can create a more suitable environment for microbes and enzymes to function efficiently, even in the presence of inhibitors. To reduce the antagonistic effect, process modification may also include changing the timeframe and intensity of the pretreatment procedure (Mosier et al., 2005; Palmqvist and Hahn-Hägerdal, 2000).
- Detoxification techniques: Detoxification procedures can eliminate or minimize inhibitors from lignocellulosic biomass. Washing, soaking, or leaching the biomass with water, solvents, or chemicals, for example, can help eliminate or minimize inhibitors such as lignin, phenols, and furans. This may improve the biomass's suitability for biological treatments (Liu et al., 2005).
- Co-culturing and microbial consortia: Employing co-cultures or microbial consortia, in which numerous microorganisms work together, can improve inhibitor elimination. Certain microbes, for example, can work together to break down inhibitors, while others can use the released sugars to degrade further. This synergistic effect can help remove inhibitors and increase the overall effectiveness of the biological pretreatment process.
- Genetic modification: Genetic engineering approaches may create microbes or enzymes that are more resistant to inhibitors. For instance, incorporating genes encoding detoxifying enzymes or transporters into microbes can assist them in surviving inhibitors during pretreatment (Liu et al., 2005).
- Feedstock selection: Selecting lignocellulosic biomass with a reduced inhibitor percentage can also counteract inhibitors throughout biological pretreatment. Some biomass or source materials may have lower inhibitor levels, enabling a more effective pretreatment.

It is important to note that the best solutions for eliminating inhibitors during biological pretreatment of lignocellulosic biomass may vary depending on the biomass type, microorganisms, enzymes used, and processing parameters. As a result, a detailed understanding of the inhibitory chemicals and their properties and meticulous process optimization is required for efficient biological pretreatment.

12.5 CONCLUSION

Biological pretreatment holds immense potential for efficiently converting lignocellulosic biomass into biofuels and value-added products. The biological pretreatment process has potential advantages over physical, chemical, and other pretreatment processes, as it is mainly associated with the action of microorganisms, such as fungi and bacteria, which can produce enzymes to degrade hemicelluloses, lignin, and polyphenols present in the biomass, thereby achieving higher yields of desired products. Although the process can be slow, using a combined approach, fine-tuning process variables, and developing specific microbial consortia and reactors can significantly improve the process economics. Furthermore, metabolic and genetic engineering can enhance lignin degradation and reduce sugar loss. More research is needed to understand the changes in lignocellulose structure during the process and optimize the use of specific microbial strains and reactors to realize the full benefits of biological pretreatment.

REFERENCES

F. R. Amin *et al.*, "Pretreatment methods of lignocellulosic biomass for anaerobic digestion," *AMB Express*, vol 7, no. 1, p. 72, 2017, https://doi.org/10.1186/s13568-017-0375-4.

J. Baruah *et al.*, "Recent trends in the pretreatment of lignocellulosic biomass for value-added products," *Front. Energy Res.*, vol. 6, no. DEC, pp. 1–19, 2018, https://doi.org/10.3389/fenrg 2018.00141.

P. Binod, K. U. Janu, R. Sindhu, and A. Pandey, "Hydrolysis of lignocellulosic biomass for bioethanol production," *Biofuels Altern. Feed. Convers. Process.*, pp. 229–250, Jan. 2011, https://doi.org/10.1016/B978-0-12-385099-7.00010-3.

R. Castoldi, M. L. T. M. Polizeli, G. de Cassia-Pereira, and C. G. Boer, "Biological pretreatment of Corn Stover by pleurotus pulmonarius and its effect on the successive saccharification," *J. Sci. Food Agric.*, vol. 94, no. 11, pp. 2243–2250, 2014.

S. Chen, X. Zhang, D. Singh, H. Yu, and X. Yang, "Biological pretreatment of lignocellulosics: Potential, progress and challenges," *Biofuels*, vol. 1, no. 1, pp. 177–199, Jan. 2014, https://doi.org/10.4155/bfs.09.13.

K. K. Cheng *et al.*, "Sugarcane bagasse hemicellulose hydrolysate for ethanol production by acid recovery process," *Biochem. Eng. J.*, vol. 38, no. 1, pp. 105–109, Jan. 2008, https://doi.org/10.1016/j.bej.2007.07.012.

W. Du, H. Yu, L. Song, J. Zhang, C. Weng, F. Ma, and X. Zhang, "The promoting effect of byproducts from Irpex lacteus on subsequent enzymatic hydrolysis of bio-pretreated cornstalks," *Biotechnol. Biofuels*, vol. 4, p. 37, 2011.

M. Ferdeş, M. N. Dincă, G. Moiceanu, B. Ş. Zabava, and G. Paraschiv, "Microorganisms and enzymes used in the biological pretreatment of the substrate to enhance biogas production: A review," *Sustainability*, vol. 12, no. 17, pp. 2–25, 2020, https://doi.org/10.3390/su12177205.

M. Galbe and G. Zacchi "Pretreatment: The key to efficient utilization of lignocellulosic materials," *Biomass and Bioenergy*, vol. 46, pp. 70–78, Nov. 2012, https://doi.org/10.1016/j.biombioe.2012.03.026.

S. Haldar and S. Banerjee, "Enzyme technology for the degradation of lignocellulosic waste," *Biotechnol. Zero Waste*, pp. 143–153, Mar. 2022, https://doi.org/10.1002/9783527832064.ch10.

L. S. Indrasith, T. Sasaki, and O. Yamashita, "A unique protease responsible for selective degradation of a yolk protein in Bombyx mori. Purification, characterization, and cleavage profile," *J. Biol. Chem.*, vol. 263, no. 2, pp. 1045–1051, Jan. 1988, https://doi.org/10.1016/S0021-9258(19)35459-6.

L. J. Jönsson and C. Martín, "Pretreatment of lignocellulose: Formation of inhibitory by-products and strategies for minimizing their effects," *Bioresour. Technol.*, vol. 199, pp. 103–112, Jan. 2016, https://doi.org/10.1016/j.biortech.2015.10.009.

T. K. Kirk and R. L. Farrell, "Enzymatic 'Combustion': The microbial degradation of lignin," *Annual Review of Microbiology*, vol. 41, pp. 465–505, Nov. 2003, https://doi.org/10.1146/annurev.mi.41.100187.002341.

P. Kumar, D. M. Barrett, M. J. Delwiche, and P. Stroeve, "Methods for pretreatment of lignocellulosic biomass for efficient hydrolysis and biofuel production," *Ind. Eng. Chem. Res.*, vol. 48, no. 8, pp. 3713–3729, Apr. 2009, https://doi.org/10.1021/ie801542g.

Z. L. Liu, P. J. Slininger, and S. W. Gorsich, "Enhanced biotransformation of furfural and hydroxymethylfurfural by newly developed ethanologenic yeast strains," *Appl. Biochem. Biotechnol.*, vol. 121, no. 1, pp. 451–460, 2005, https://doi.org/10.1385/ABAB:121:1-3:0451.

A. da S. Machado and A. Ferraz, "Biological pretreatment of sugarcane bagasse with basidiomycetes producing varied biodegradation patterns," *Bioresour. Technol.*, vol. 225, pp. 17–22, Feb. 2017, https://doi.org/10.1016/j.biortech.2016.11.053.

N. Mahamadi et al., "Production of efficient microbial complex for organic fraction of municipal organic solid waste pretreatment upstream anaerobic digestion," *Int. J. Environ. Bioremediation Biodegrad.*, vol. 5, no. 3, pp. 77–85, 2017, https://doi.org/10.12691/ijebb-5-3-1.

R. Martín-Sampedro, M. E. Eugenio, J. C. García, F. Lopez, J. C. Villar, and M. J. Diaz, "Steam explosion and enzymatic pretreatments as an approach to improve the enzymatic hydrolysis of Eucalyptus globulus," *Biomass and Bioenergy*, vol. 42, pp. 97–106, Jul. 2012, https://doi.org/10.1016/j.biombioe.2012.03.032.

D. P. Maurya, A. Singla, and S. Negi, "An overview of key pretreatment processes for biological conversion of lignocellulosic biomass to bioethanol," *3 Biotech*, vol. 5, no. 5, pp. 597–609, Oct. 2015, https://doi.org/10.1007/s13205-015-0279-4/tables/1.

R. Millati, S. Syamsiah, C. Niklasson, M. Nur Cahyanto, K. Lundquist, and M. J. Taherzadeh, "Biological pretreatment: Review," *BioResources*, vol. 6, no. 4, pp. 5224–5259, 2011.

N. Mosier, R. Hendrickson, N. Ho, M. Sedlak, and M. R. Ladisch, "Optimization of pH-controlled liquid hot water pretreatment of corn stover," *Bioresour. Technol.*, vol. 96, no. 18, pp. 1986–1993, Dec. 2005, https://doi.org/10.1016/j.biortech.2005.01.013.

N. Nayan et al., "Screening of white-rot fungi for bioprocessing of wheat straw into ruminant feed," *J. Appl. Microbiol.*, vol. 125, no. 2, pp. 468–479, Aug. 2018, doi: 10.1111/jam.13894. Epub 2018 May 23.

E. Palmqvist and B. Hahn-Hägerdal, "Fermentation of lignocellulosic hydrolysates. II: Inhibitors and mechanisms of inhibition," *Bioresour. Technol.*, vol. 74, no. 1, pp. 25–33, Aug. 2000, https://doi.org/10.1016/s0960-8524(99)00161-3.

C. P. Passos, S. Yilmaz, C. M. Silva, and M. A. Coimbra, "Enhancement of grape seed oil extraction using a cell wall degrading enzyme cocktail," *Food Chem.*, vol. 115, no. 1, pp. 48–53, Jul. 2009, https://doi.org/10.1016/j.foodchem.2008.11.064.

K. Poszytek, M. Ciezkowska, A. Sklodowska, and L. Drewniak, "Microbial Consortium with High Cellulolytic Activity (MCHCA) for enhanced biogas production," *Front. Microbiol.*, vol. 7, no. MAR, p. 324, Mar. 2016, https://doi.org/10.3389/fmicb.2016.00324/bibtex.

B. C. Saha, N. Qureshi, G. J. Kennedy, and M. A. Cotta, "Biological pretreatment of corn stover with white-rot fungus for improved enzymatic hydrolysis," *Int. Biodeterior. Biodegradation*, vol. 109, pp. 29–35, Apr. 2016, https://doi.org/10.1016/j.ibiod.2015.12.020.

L. Sahadevan, C. M.-U. J. of, and undefined 2013, "Ligninolytic enzymes for application in treatment of effluent from pulp and paper industries," *environmentaljournal.org*, 2249, Accessed: May 09, 2023. [Online]. Available: http://environmentaljournal.org/3-1/ujert-3-1-2.pdf

D. Salvachúa, A. Prieto, M. López-Abelairas, T. Lu-Chau, Á. T. Martínez, and M. Jesús Martínez, "Fungal pretreatment: An alternative in second-generation ethanol from wheat straw," *Elsevier*, vol. 102, pp. 7500–7506, 2011, https://doi.org/10.1016/j.biortech.2011.05.027.

H. K. Sharma, C. Xu, and W. Qin, "Biological pretreatment of lignocellulosic biomass for biofuels and bioproducts: An overview," *Waste and Biomass Valorization*, vol. 10, no. 2, pp. 235–251, Feb. 2019, https://doi.org/10.1007/s12649-017-0059-y/metrics.

R. Sindhu, P. Binod, and A. Pandey, "Biological pretreatment of lignocellulosic biomass – An overview," *Bioresour. Technol.*, vol. 199, pp. 76–82, Jan. 2016, https://doi.org/10.1016/j.biortech.2015.08.030.

P. Sivagurunathan *et al.*, "Fermentative hydrogen production using lignocellulose biomass: An overview of pretreatment methods, inhibitor effects and detoxification experiences," *Renew. Sustain. Energy Rev.*, vol. 77, pp. 28–42, Sep. 2017, https://doi.org/10.1016/j.rser.2017.03.091.

L. Song, H. Yu, F. Ma, and X. Zhang, "Biological pretreatment under non sterile conditions for enzymatic hydrolysis of Corn Strover," *Bioresources*, vol. 8, no. 3, pp. 3802–3816, 2013.

H. Suhara, S. Kodama, I. Kamei, N. Maekawa, and S. Meguro, "Screening of selective lignin-degrading basidiomycetes and biological pretreatment for enzymatic hydrolysis of bamboo culms," *Int. Biodeterior. Biodegrad.*, vol. 75, pp. 176–180, 2012.

M. Taha, E., Shahsavari, K. Al-Hothaly, A. Mouradov, A. T. Smith, A. S. Ball, and E. M. Adetutu, "Enhanced biological straw saccharification through coculturing of lignocellulose-degrading microorganisms," *Appl. Biochem. Biotechnol.*, vol. 175, pp. 3709–3728, 2015.

C. Wan and Y. Li, "Microbial delignification of corn stover by Ceriporiopsis subvermispora for improving cellulose digestibility," *Enzyme Microb. Technol.*, vol. 47, no. 1–2, 5, pp. 31–36, 2010.

M. Wojtusik, J. C. Villar, M. Zurita, M. Ladero, and F. Garcia-Ochoa, "Study of the enzymatic activity inhibition on the saccharification of acid pretreated corn stover," *Biomass Bioenergy*, vol. 98, pp. 1–7, Mar. 2017, https://doi.org/10.1016/j.biombioe.2017.01.010.

L. Zhu, J. P. O'Dwyer, V. S. Chang, C. B. Granda, and M. T. Holtzapple, "Structural features affecting biomass enzymatic digestibility," *Bioresour. Technol.*, vol. 99, no. 9, pp. 3817–3828, Jun. 2008, https://doi.org/10.1016/j.biortech.2007.07.033.

13 Biological Pretreatment for Available Biomass

Sundergopal Sridhar and Mamilla Shyam Sunder

13.1 INTRODUCTION

Biological pretreatment also is one of the most effective pretreatments, which uses wood-degrading microorganisms, such as fungi and bacteria, to modify the chemical composition of lignocellulosic biomass by altering or disrupting its structure. It is an eco-friendly and low-cost pretreatment technique, with no inhibitor formation and lower energy consumption, resulting in an attractive process (Sindhu et al., 2016; Bhatia et al., 2017). This process has potential advantages over physical, chemical, and other pretreatment processes as it is mainly associated with the action of fungi that are capable of producing enzymes to degrade hemicelluloses, lignin, and polyphenol present in the biomass, thereby getting high yields of desired products (Ria-Millati et al., 2011; Saritha et al., 2012). However, it also has disadvantages, as the process is very slow and requires a careful control of growth conditions and ample space to perform. Additionally, most lignocellulolytic microorganisms stabilize and consume not only lignin but also cellulose and hemicellulose (Singh et al., 2008; Kuhar et al., 2008).

The biological pretreatment method involves treating various white, brown, and soft-rot fungi, as well as certain bacteria, to hydrolyze lignocellulosic biomass and facilitate its subsequent degradation (Chen et al., 2010). For instance, fungi-like brown and soft-rot fungi attack cellulose, while white-rot fungi target lignin. However, white-rot fungi primarily participate in biological pretreatment, which is associated with high sugar yields and enzymatic saccharification (Yesilada et al., 2018). Table 13.1 summarizes the various biological processes and pretreatment conditions for different biomass feedstocks.

13.2 VARIOUS BIOLOGICAL PRETREATMENT PROCESSES

Lignocellulosic biomass, including forest and agricultural residues, is an abundant, inexpensive, and renewable energy source for many useful products in our day-to-day lives. Pretreatment is necessary for the further processing of biomass into value-added products. Several pretreatment strategies are available, each with advantages and limitations. The pretreatment process cannot be used as a standard for all biomasses, as they have different compositions and constituent

DOI: 10.1201/9781003327608-13

TABLE 13.1
Various Biological Pretreatment Process Conditions That Have Been Used in the Treatment of Different Biomass Feedstocks Using Bio-Catalysts

Feedstock	Microorganism	Process Condition	Effect on Biomass	References
Sugarcane bagasse	*Ceriporiopsis subvermispora*	27 ± 2°C for 60 days	47% sugar is recovered as sugar-rich syrup	Machado and Ferraz (2017)
Sawdust	*Pleurotus pulmonarius*	28°C for 30 days	Sugar concentration increased from 2.51 mol/ml	Castoldi et al. (2014)
Wheat straw	*Ceriporiopsis subvermispora*	7 weeks of solid-state fermentation incubated at 240°C	In-vitro gas production of 297.0 ml/g	Nayan et al. (2018)
Paddy straw	*Pleurotus florida*	25–290°C for 28 days	Maximum saccharification efficiency up to 75.3%	Manickam et al. (2018)
Straw	Fungal consortium	Incubated at 30°C and 55°C for 6 days	7-fold increases in hydrolysis	Taha et al. (2015)
Corn stover	Fungal consortium	Pretreatment for 42 days with fungi	43.8% lignin removal and 7-fold increase in hydrolysis	Song et al. (2013)
Corn stalks	*Irpexlacteus*	28 days of incubation	82% hydrolysis yield observed	Du et al. (2011)
Bamboo clums	*Punctularia* sp. TUFC20056	Not specified	50% of lignin removed	Suhara et al. (2012)
Corn stover	*Ceriporiopsis subvermispora*	Solid state fermentation at 28°C for 42 days	57–67% glucose yield increase	Wan and Li (2010)
Rice straw	*Pholiotaadiposa*	Saccharification for 48 hr	Releases 716 mg sugar/g substrate	Jagtap et al. (2013a)
Aspen biomass	*Armillaria gemina* SKU2114	48 hr of hydrolysis	Maximum saccharification yield of 62%	Jagtap et al. (2013b)

percentages, and costly chemicals and other pretreatment sources cannot be used every time.

In this context, biological pretreatment was adopted to alter lignocellulose degradation by microorganisms and enzymes during the pretreatment process (Table 13.1). The potent microbes involved in the biological pretreatment are essential for environmental benefits, as they do not interfere with hydrolysis or fermentation, which are carried out under mild conditions. This process is environmentally friendly, as it does not use any chemicals and employs a recycling method that does not produce toxic or hazardous compounds.

Microorganisms involved in biological pretreatment: Biological pretreatments primarily rely on microorganisms that produce enzymes and organisms that can effectively increase productivity at a cost. Studies have reported that many bacterial cultures, including bacilli and actinomycetes, can degrade organic matter. Other researchers have shown that microbial consortia of cellulolytic bacteria, such as those of *Bacillus*, *Candida*, and *Streptomyces*, exhibit broad-spectrum biodegradation. At least 30 predominant rumen cellulolytic bacterial species produce high cellulolytic activity, degrading the cellulolytic material. Some bacterial strains, such as *Bacillus subtilis* and *Azospirillum lipoferum*, produce bacterial laccases that catalyze lignin polymerization. Microbes and fungi are also well known for their effective degradation of lignocellulosic residues through enzymes widely distributed in nature. The lignolytic and lignocellulolytic fungi include species of *Ascomycota such as Penicillium, Aspergillus*, and *Trichoderma reesei. Basidiomycetes*, on the other hand, include white-rot fungi, such as *Phanerochaete chrysosporium* and *Schizophyllum*, and brown-rot fungi, such as *Forrtilopsis palustris.*

Besides fungi and bacteria, there are several microorganisms such as insects, gastropods, ruminants, gut flora, or combinations of these organisms. More than 20 families, representing 10 orders, such as beetles (*Coleoptera*), wood wasps (*Hymenoptera*), termites (*Isoptera*), crickets (*Orthoptera*), and silverfish (*Thysanura*), can digest cellulosic biomass, including leaf litter, wood, and forage. Many studies have been conducted on microbial isolation, which is used for biomass pretreatment via biological processes and for bioproduct production.

Enzymes involved in biological pretreatment: Enzymes play a crucial role in the pretreatment of biomass produced by potent microbes, which degrade lignocellulose. Varieties of enzymes, such as lignin peroxidases, laccases, and manganese peroxidases (MnP), are involved. Other enzymes that act on lignocellulosic biomass are arabinases, pectinases, galactinases, lyases, and esterases. The lignocellulosic biomass hydrolysis process depends on enzyme efficiency and concentration, thermal inactivation, adsorption, end-point inhibition, and interference from lignin. Different types of enzymes play various roles in the pretreatment processes. Some enzymes are helpful in the commercial process of converting biomass into value-added products.

1. **Cellulases:** These are key enzymes for the hydrolysis of biomass. They act on cellulose, hydrolyzing it into monomers.

2. **Hemicellulases:** These key enzymes act on hemicelluloses, which are a mixture of glucose and other sugar monomers. Hemicellulose contains pentose sugar (xylose) as xylan, and the enzyme xylanase catalyzes the hydrolysis of xylan, which is formed by *Aspergillus niger, Trichoderma reesei*, and *Bacillus* species.
3. **Ligninases:** These enzymes are highly in demand in the industry, and fungi are reported to be good producers of ligninases, which play a crucial role in lignin degradation. Fungi that produce ligninolytic enzymes are *Trichoderma versicolor*, Dichotomous *squealers*, and *Phanerochaete radiata.*
4. **Pectinases:** These complex enzymes degrade pectin in lignocellulosic biomass. Pectinases are characterized into three main clusters.
5. **Other accessory enzymes:** α-L-arabinofuranidase for breaking down arabinose into monomers of furanose and pyranose.

13.3 EFFECT OF INHIBITORS ON MICROBIAL PROCESSES

The chemical pretreatment of biomass involves several thermochemical treatments that convert the phenolic compounds and sugars present in plant materials into degradable compounds. The further presence of these compounds inhibits the fermentation process (Talebnia et al., 2010). The type of raw material; conditions applied such as pH, temperature time, residence time, and pressure (Cardona et al., 2010, Redding et al., 2011); and the pretreatment method exhibit the nature and concentration of the degradation compounds, and these compounds are, namely, furan derivatives (furfural and 5-hydroxymetyl-2-furaldehyde, or HMF), phenol derivatives, carboxylic acids, and heavy metal ions which are released by corrosion of the digester.

The inhibitory effects of degradation products on aldehyde dehydrogenase, pyruvate dehydrogenase, and alcohol dehydrogenase from Saccharomyces cerevisiae were found to cause further DNA breakdown, resulting in the inhibition of RNA and protein synthesis (Modig et al., 2002). It was evident that *S. cerevisiae* and *Panellus stipticus* strains were more sensitive to inhibition by furfural than HMF at the same concentration, and the presence of both furfural and HMF suppressed the cell growth (Liu et al., 2004).

Some studies have found that furan derivatives damage cell walls and membranes; however, the inhibitory effect of these compounds depends on the concentration of the inhibitor in the broth. Some concentrations of furfural interfered with the respiration and growth of ***Pichia stipitis***, and their development was reduced to 40%, 70%, and 100% with concentrations of 0.5, 0.75, and 1.5 g/L of HMF, respectively (Delgenes et al., 1996).

13.3.1 Formation of Inhibitors

This formation occurs during the pretreatment process, leading to additional by-products and presenting many hurdles due to specific side reactions.

Furthermore, these by-products may hinder the downstream processing of pretreated biomass. These inhibitors are formed during the pretreatment process due to the degradation and solubilization of hemicelluloses and lignin, as well as during downstream hydrolysis and fermentation, which contribute to their inhibitory effects. Water processing, which is further recycled, and inhibitor concentration increase due to accumulation. Some of the inhibitors formed during the pretreatment process include furans, phenolic compounds, uric acids, and aliphatic carboxylic acids (Jönsson, 2016; Larsson et al., 1999).

The feedstock composition and the type of pretreatment employed express the mechanism behind inhibitor formation. During acid pretreatment, the hemicellulose portion is degraded to furfural, which is volatile and has a high boiling point (161.7°C). Furfural thus formed further degrades to formic acid and resinous tars, which polymerize to form different products (Danon et al., 2013). Alternatively, hexoses can be broken down into HMF, and lignin degradation can yield phenolic compounds. Acetic acid is formed due to the hydrolysis of acetyl groups present in hemicelluloses (Danon et al., 2013). This distinct group of inhibitory compounds affects the enzymatic hydrolysis or microbial activity. Carbohydrate degradation leads to the formation of carboxylic acids and furan aldehydes. The low concentrations of acetic acid, formic acid, and carbonic acid indicate an inhibitory effect (Larsson et al., 1999).

To handle the inhibitors, a detoxification technique is applied by adding reducing agents, chemical additives, and polymers to convert them into less harmful compounds. However, it is a time-consuming process, and designing an accurate method can eliminate these inhibitors.

13.3.2 How to Overcome Inhibitors?

During fermentation, to overcome the inhibitory effect, the hydrolysate needs to be detoxified (Zhang et al., 2011), or microorganisms can be adapted to these inhibitory compounds. Detoxification appears to be an expensive process, but adapting microorganisms to remove inhibitory compounds may be an effective alternative.

Removal of inhibitors or detoxification: The inhibitors formed during the various pretreatment methods have to be removed to improve the efficiency of hydrolysate fermentation, and the effectiveness of a detoxification process can be decided by the type of inhibitors present in the hydrolysate and the microorganisms used for fermentation of the hydrolyzed material (Yu et al., 2011). Many detoxification methods are available to convert the inhibitory compounds into inert materials or reduce their concentration. One physical method, by evaporation, removes the volatile compounds (like vanillin, acetic acid, and furfural) (Mussatto and Roberto, 2004); other chemical methods of detoxification of the toxins can be neutralized by activated charcoal or tin oxides, calcium hydroxide over liming, and use of ion exchange resins (Yang and Wyman, 2008, Chandel et al., 2007), and further detoxification by biological methods using enzymes such as laccase and peroxidase obtained from fungi such as *Aspergillus nidulans, Trichodrmaresseae*, and *Trametesversicolar.*

Adaptation of microorganisms: Adapting microorganisms can eliminate inhibitors in the hydrolysate and enhance fermentation, thereby improving product yields (Parawira and Tekere, 2011). Some studies have reported that *P. stipitis* participates in the formation of HMF and furfural by reducing the aldehyde groups (Liu et al., 2004). *P. stipitis* is also unaffected by furfural factors such as low concentration (Mussatto and Roberto, 2004). Thus, using microorganisms resistant to strain would be preferable (Larsson et al., 2001).

13.4 CONCLUSION

Biological pretreatment is an effective method that utilizes wood-degrading microorganisms, such as fungi and bacteria, to modify the chemical composition of lignocellulosic biomass by altering its structure. It is an eco-friendly, low-cost pretreatment technique that consumes less energy. This process has more advantages than chemical and other pretreatment processes, as it primarily relies on fungal action, which can produce enzymes that degrade hemicelluloses, lignin, and polyphenols in the biomass, resulting in high yields of desired products.

REFERENCES

Bhatia SK, Kim SH, Yoon JJ, Yung Hun Yang. Current status and strategies for second-generation biofuel production using microbial systems. *Energy Conver Manag*. 2017;148:1142–56. https://doi.org/10.1016/j.enconman.2017.06.073

Cardona CA, Quintero JA, Paz IC. Production of bioethanol from sugarcane bagasse: Status and perspectives. *Bioresour Technol*. 2010;101:475466.

Castoldi R, Bracht A, Morais GD, Baesso ML, Correa RCG, Peralta RA, et al. Biological pretreatment of Eucalyptus grandis sawdust with white-rot fungi: Study of degradation patterns and saccharification kinetics. *Chem Eng J*.2014;258:240–6. https://doi.org/10.1016/j.cej.2014.07.090

Chandel AK, Kapoor RK, Singh AK, Kuhad RC. Detoxification of sugarcane bagasse hydrolysate improves ethanol production by Candida shehatae NCIM 3501. *Bioresour Technol*. 2007;98:194750.

Chen S, Zhang X, Singh D, Yu H, Yang X. Biological pretreatment of lignocellulosics: Potential, progress, and challenges. *Biofuels*.2010;1:177–99. https://doi.org/10.4155/bfs.09.13

Danon B, Van der Aa L, De Jong W. Furfural degradation in a dilute acidic and saline solution in the presence of glucose. *Carbohydr Res*.2013;375:145–52.

Delgenes J, Moletta R, Navarro J. Effect of lignocellulose degradation products on ethanol fermentations of glucose and xylose by Saccharomyces cerevisiae, Zymomonas mobilis, Pichia stipitis, and Candida shehatae. *Enzyme Microb Technol*.1996;19:220–5.

Du W, Yu H, Song L, Zhang J, Weng C, Ma F, et al. The promising effects of by-products from Irpex lacteus on subsequent enzymatic hydrolysis of bio-pretreated corn stalks. *Biotechnol Biofuels*. 2011;4:37. https://doi.org/10.1186/1754-6834-4-37

Jagtap SS, Dhiman SS, Kim TS, Li J, Kang YC, Lee JK. Characterization of a β-1,4-glucosidase from a newly isolated strain of Pholiota adiposa and its application to the hydrolysis of biomass. *Biomass Bioenergy*.2013a;54:181–90. https://doi.org/10.1016/j.biombioe.2013.03.032

Jagtap SS, Dhiman SS, Kim TS, Li J, Lee JK, Kang YC. Enzymatic hydrolysis of aspen biomass into fermentable sugars by using lignocellulases from Armillariagemina. *Bioresour Technol.* 2013b;133:307–14. https://doi.org/10.1016/j.biortech.2013.01.118

Jönsson LJ, Martín C. Pretreatment of lignocellulose: Formation of inhibitory by-products and strategies for minimizing their effects. *Bioresour Technol.* 2016;199:103–12.

Kuhar S, Nair LM, Kuhad RC. Pretreatment of lignocellulosic material with fungi capable of higher lignin degradation and lower carbohydrate degradation improves substrate acid hydrolysis and the eventual conversion to ethanol. *Can J Microbiol.* 2008;54:305–13.

Larsson S, Cassland P, Jonsson LJ. Development of a Saccharomyces cerevisiae strain with enhanced resistance to phenolic fermentation inhibitors in lignocellulosic hydrolysates by heterologous expression of laccase. *Appl Environ Microbiol.* 2001;67:1163–70.

Larsson S, Palmqvist E, Hahn-Hägerdal B, Tengborg C, Stenberg K, Zacchi G, Nilvebrant N-O. The generation of fermentation inhibitors during dilute acid hydrolysis of softwood. *Enzyme Microb Technol.* 1999;24:151–9.

Liu ZL, Slininger PJ, Dien BS, Berhow MA, Kurtzman CP, Gorsich SW. Adaptive response of yeasts to furfural and 5-hydroxymethylfurfural and new chemical evidence for HMF conversion to 2,5-bis-hydroxymethylfuran. *J Ind Microbiol Biotechnol.*2004;31:345–52.

Machado ADS, Ferraz A. Biological pretreatment of sugarcane bagasse with basidiomycetes producing varied patterns of biodegradation. *Bioresour Technol.*2017;225:17–22. https://doi.org/10.1016/j.biortech.2016.11.053

Manickam NK, Rajarathinam R, Muthuvelu KS, Senniyappan T. New insight into the effect of fungal mycelia present in the bio-pretreated paddy straw on their enzymatic saccharification and optimization of process parameters. *Bioresour Technol.*2018;267:291–302. https://doi.org/10.1016/j.biortech.2018.07.003

Modig T, Lidén G, Taherzadeh MJ. Inhibition effects of furfural on alcohol dehydrogenase, aldehyde dehydrogenase, and pyruvate dehydrogenase. *Biochem J.* 2002;363:769–76.

Mussatto SI, Roberto IC. Alternatives for detoxification of diluted-acid lignocellulosic hydrolyzates for use in fermentative processes: A review. *Bioresour Technol.* 2004;93:1–10.

Nayan N, Sonnenberg ASM, Hendriks WH, Cone JW. Screening of white-rot fungi for bioprocessing of wheat straw into ruminant feed. *J. Appl. Microbiol.* 2018;125:468–79. https://doi.org/10.1111/jam 13894

Parawira W, Tekere M. Biotechnological strategies to overcome inhibitors in lignocellulose hydrolysates for ethanol production: Review. *Crit Rev Biotechnol.* 2011;31:20–31.

Redding AP, Wang Z, Keshwani DR, Cheng JJ. High temperature dilutes acid pretreatment of coastal Bermuda grass for enzymatic hydrolysis. *Bioresour Technol.* 2011;102:1415–24.

Ria-Millati I, Syamsiah S, Niklasson C, Cahyanto MN, Lundquist K, Taherzadeh MJ. Biological pretreatment of lignocelluloses with white-rot fungi and its applications: A review. *Bioresources.* 2011;6:1–36.

Saritha M, Arora A, Lata. Biological pretreatment of lignocellulosic substrate for enhanced delignification and enzymatic digestibility. *Ind J Microbiol.* 2012;52:122–30.

Sindhu R, Binod P, Pandey A. Biological pretreatment of lignocellulosic biomass – an overview. *Bioresour Technol.*2016;199:76–82. https://doi.org/10.1016/j.biortech.2015.08.030

Singh P, Suman A, Tiwari P, Arya N, Gaur A, Shrivastava AK. Biological pretreatment of sugarcane trash for its conversion to fermentable sugars. *World J MicrobiolBiotechnol.* 2008;24:667–73.

Song L, Yu H, Ma F, Zhang X. Biological pretreatment under nonsterile conditions for enzymatic hydrolysis of corn stover.*Bioresources*.2013;8:3802–16. https://doi.org/10.15376/biores.8.3.3802-3816

Suhara H, Kodama S, Kamei I, Maekawa N, Meguro S. Screening of selective lignin-degrading basidiomycetes and biological pretreatment for enzymatic hydrolysis of bamboo culms. *Int Biodeter Biodegr.* 2012;75:176–80. https://doi.org/10.1016/j.ibiod.2012.05.042

Taha M, Shahsavari E, Hothaly KA, Mouradov A, Smith AT, Ball AS, et al. Enhanced biological straw saccharification through coculturing of lignocellulose-degrading microorganisms. *Appl Biochem Biotechnol.* 2015;7:6. https://doi.org/10.1007/s12010-015-1539-9

Talebnia F, Karakashev D, Angelidaki I. Production of bioethanol from wheat straw: An overview on pretreatment, hydrolysis and fermentation. *Bioresour Technol.* 2010;101:4744–53.

Wan C, Li Y. Microbial delignificant of corn strover with Ceriporiopsis subvermispora for improving cellulose digestibility. *Enzyme Microb Technol.* 2010;47:31–6. https://doi.org/10.1016/j.biortech.2010.03.070

Yang B, Wyman CE. Pretreatment: The key to unlocking low-cost cellulosic ethanol. *Biofuels BioprodBiorefining*. 2008;2:26–40.

Yesilada O, Birhanli E, Geckil H. Bioremediation and decolorization of textile dyes by white rot fungi and laccase enzymes. In *Mycoremediation and Environmental Sustainability, Fungal Biology*, ed. R. Prasad. Cham: Springer; 2018, 121–53.

Yu Y, Feng Y, Xu C, Liu J, Li D. Onsite bio-detoxification of steam-exploded corn stover for cellulosic ethanol production. *Bioresour Technol.* 2011;102:5123–8.

Zhang K, Agrawal M, Harper J, Chen R, Koros WJ. Removal of the fermentation inhibitor, furfural, using activated cellulosic-ethanol production. *Ind Eng Res.* 2011;50:14054–60.

14 Pretreatment Processes for Lignocellulosic Biomass

Sundergopal Sridhar and Mamilla Shyam Sunder

14.1 INTRODUCTION

The primary goal of the pretreatment process for lignocellulosic biomass is to enhance surface area by decrystallizing cellulose while also facilitating the removal and reduction of lignin and hemicellulose. Table 14.1 summarizes the effect of different pretreatments. Researchers conducted studies on various pretreatment technologies for other firms, embedding each pretreatment process within a comprehensive bioethanol facility model and performing further economic analysis. Different pretreatment processes using the same biomass feedstock were employed in the study, which involved characterizing the solid and liquid phases and further obtaining data for an energy balance and other economically viable processes. Table 14.2 presents the analytical results examining the impact of pretreatment approaches on operating and capital costs, as well as product yields (sugar). The low cost of the pretreatment process is outweighed by the high expenses of solvent removal and the additional costs of alternative catalysts or ethanol use, ultimately leading to a costly product recovery process. Thus, there is a variation in the economics of the projected performance of the pretreatment process.

A new research study (Sendich and Dale, 2009) developed a tool to produce ethanol from cellulosic biomass. The model was integrated, leveraging bio-refinery technologies to assess economic viability and reduce emissions. However, process improvements to identify the optimal enzyme blend for each hydroxylate's pretreatment and conditioning requirements may lead to more significant differentiation in projected process economics.

A novel integrated approach has been developed that combines green solvent-based pretreatment with established methods, such as enzymatic hydrolysis and fermentation, to optimize the production of value-added products from lignocellulosic biomass. This process requires an in-depth understanding of the structural characteristics of lignocellulosic biomass, as well as the chemical and physical aspects of pretreatment, enzymatic conversion, and fermentation. Furthermore, advancements in genetic engineering have enabled the development of

DOI: 10.1201/9781003327608-14

TABLE 14.1
Various Pretreatment Methods for Lignocellulosic Biomasses

Pretreatment Method	Increase in Accessible Surface Area	Cellulose Decrystallization	Hemicellulose Removal	Lignin Removal	Structural Alteration
Steam explosion	High (H)	No (–)	High (H)	No (–)	Low (L)
Liquid hot water	High (H)	No Data (ND)	High (H)	No (–)	Low (L)
Dilute acid	High (H)	No (–)	High (H)	No (–)	High (H)
AFEX (ammonia fiber expansion)	High (H)	High (H)	Low (L)	High (H)	High (H)
ARP (ammonia recycle percolation)	High (H)	High (H)	Low (L)	High (H)	High (H)
Lime	High (H)	No data (ND)	Low (L)	High (H)	High (H)
Green solvents (NMMO/ionic liquids)	High (H)	High (H)	Low (L) or high (H)	Low (L) or high (H)	Low (L)
Supercritical fluid	High (H)	High (H)	High (H)	No (–)	Low (L)

Abbreviations: H: high; L: low; ND: not detectable
Source: Mosier et al. (2005)

TABLE 14.2
Capital Costs of Various Pretreatment Technologies

Pretreatment Method Capital, $MM	Pretreatment Direct Fixed (% Other)	Pretreatment Breakdown (%Reactor) [millions of dollars (USD), $MM]	Total Fixed Capital (Million Gallons Per Year, MMgal/yr)	Ethanol Production Annual Capacity	Total Fixed Capital ($/gal)
Dilute acid	25.0	64/36	208.6	56.1	3.72
Hot water	4.5	100/0	200.9	44.0	4.57
AFEX	25.7	26/74	211.5	56.8	3.72
ARP	28.3	25/75	210.9	46.3	4.56
Lime	22.3	19/81	163.6	48.9	3.35
No pretreatment	0	–	200.3	9.0	22.6
Ideal pretreatment	0	–	162.5	64.7	2.51

Source: Eggeman and Elander (2005)

microbial strains capable of performing fermentation at elevated temperatures, significantly boosting the efficiency of sugar conversion into biofuels and resulting in higher product yields.

14.2 PROCESS DESCRIPTION AND MODE OF ACTION

Methods of pretreatment: Pretreatment can be performed using four methods, as follows.

1. **Physical pretreatment**
   i. Mechanical communication: Lignocellulose and other waste materials can undergo comminution by methods such as chipping, grinding, and milling to reduce cellulose crystallinity. The raw material will typically be 10–30 mm after chipping and reduced to 0.2–4.0 mm after milling and grinding.
   ii. Nonmechanical pretreatment: Pyrolysis is also used to pretreat lignocellulosic materials. When heated above 300°C, cellulose decomposes rapidly, producing a gaseous product and a residual char.
2. **Physicochemical pretreatment**
   i. Steam explosion (auto-hydrolysis): In this method, chipped and ground biomass is treated by high-pressure saturated steam for a short period, and then the pressure is rapidly reduced, causing the materials to undergo explosive decompression. Equal solubilization of hemicelluloses can be achieved at high temperatures (up to 270°C) and low residence times or at low temperatures (190°C) and longer residence times. The steam explosion pretreatment process offers the benefit of lower energy consumption than mechanical comminution, while avoiding environmental impacts and eliminating the need for recycling.
   ii. Ammonia fiber explosion: Ammonia fiber explosion (AFEX) pretreatment is another type of pretreatment process in which lignocellulosic materials are exposed to liquid ammonia at high temperatures and pressures for a short period, followed by rapid pressure reduction. The liquid ammonia dosage is 1–2 kg/kg dry material at 90°C, with a residence time of 30 minutes, resulting in increased accessible surface area and reduced cellulose crystallinity, thereby increasing enzymatic digestibility (Elizabeth, Sendich et al., 2008). To protect the environment and ensure the economic cost-effectiveness of the pretreatment process, ammonia should be recycled.
   iii. Carbon dioxide explosion: Similar to steam and ammonia explosion pretreatment, carbon dioxide pretreatment is also used as a pretreatment process. Carbon dioxide was hypothesized to form carbonic acid, thereby increasing the rate of hydrolysis.
3. **Chemical pretreatment**
   Many chemicals are used to pretreat lignocellulosic biomass, removing lignin and disrupting the crystalline structure.

i. Alkaline hydrolysis: This pretreatment method depends on the available lignin content of the material. The alkaline hydrolysis mechanism involves the saponification of intermolecular ester bonds, breaking the cross-links between xylan hemicellulose and other components, thereby releasing them. The cell porosity of lignocelluloses increases with the removal of the cross-links. Dilute sodium hydroxide treatment of lignocellulosic materials resulted in swelling, increasing the internal surface area, decreasing crystallinity, and separating saturated linkages between lignin and carbohydrates, further disrupting the lignin structure.

ii. Lime pretreatment: Plane (1984) studied and treated sugarcane bagasse biomass for up to 192 hr at ambient conditions to improve the digestibility of cellulose from 20% to 72% with enzyme pretreatment. Higher temperatures and shorter reaction times were also found to be more effective in pretreating lignocelluloses with lime.

iii. Acid hydrolysis: Dilute acids, such as sulfuric and hydrochloric acid, have been used to treat lignocellulosic materials. However, dilute sulfuric acid pretreatment has achieved high reaction rates and significantly improved cellulose hydrolysis, as well as processes that achieve high xylan-to-xylose conversion with high xylan-to-xylose yields. Archiving high xylan-to-xylose yields is necessary to achieve favorable overall process economics. Pretreatment with concentrated sulfuric acid and hydrochloric acid may not yield favorable results compared to dilute acids, and the process economics are also higher than those of the dilute acid pretreatment process.

iv. Oxidative delignification: Oxidative delignification, achieved through hydrogen peroxide pretreatment, showed encouraging results. By this method, the peroxidase enzyme can facilitate liquid biodegradation, and pretreating cane bagasse with hydrogen peroxide significantly enhances its susceptibility to enzymatic hydrolysis.

v) Organosolv process: In this organosolv process, an organic mixture is mixed with aqueous inorganic catalysts, including methanol, ethanol, glycol, acetone, ethylene, trimethylene glycol, and tetrahydrofurfural alcohol. Organic acids such as oxalic and acetylsalicylic acid can also be used as acids in the organosolv process. The addition of acid can yield a high xylose content.

4. **Biological pretreatment**

The principal biological sources include fungi and enzymes. Certain enzymes produced by fungi can break down lignin and/or hemicellulose constituents and leave the cellulose part. The advantage of biological pretreatment is that it requires minimal energy input and is environmentally friendly. However, the pretreatment rate is very slow in most processes and needs to be optimized to make it an effective pretreatment method. White-rot fungi, such as *Phanerochaete chrysosporium*, are primarily used microbes for delignification, degrading 48–58% of lignin, 5.3% cellulose, and 19.72% of cellulose in grape cluster stems over 10–12 days.

Other fungi, specifically *Cyathus* sp., increased digestibility by 3–6.9 times the control values over 29 days. Compared with chemical and physical pretreatments, the biological pretreatment is not feasible.

5. **Other pretreatments**

   Other pretreatment methods include radiation and supercritical carbon dioxide. A rice straw pretreatment process using 240 W microwave irradiation was found to release 2.4% of reducing sugars; 100 MR of irradiation increased the effectiveness of enzymatic and acid hydrolysis by factors of 2 and 4, respectively. In sugarcane bagasse biomass, supercritical carbon dioxide pretreatment is above its critical point of 31°C and 73 atm, and supercritical carbon dioxide did not affect the yield of sugar or the subsequent enzymatic fermentation process conversion of lignocellulosic biomass.

14.2.1 Advantages and Disadvantages

Pretreatment methods are categorized into four main types: physical, chemical, physicochemical, and biological approaches. The main aim for the treatment process is the reduction of available biomass size and breakdown of its crystallinity by grinding or milling process, which enhances the hydrolysis process (due to its crystallinity breakdown) and improves the mass transfer required for the pretreatment process of biomass material (depending on the particle size of biomass and its crystallinity), which may be advantageous for physical pretreatment.

The main limitation of the pretreatment process is that, although it is often regarded as the only viable option, it typically requires more energy than the theoretical minimum and would be expensive for further scale-up, which is a disadvantage.

The chemical pretreatment process involves adding dilute or concentrated acids or bases to the biomass. Common acids include sulfuric acid, hydrochloric acid, phosphoric acid, and nitric acid. The most widely used bases (alkalis) are calcium hydroxide, potassium hydroxide, sodium hydroxide, and ammonium hydroxide. These acids and bases break down the biomass structure to produce an appropriate product, which is advantageous. However, using them requires a neutralization step to remove inhibitors and requires more energy input. It may be expensive, which is disadvantageous.

In the physical-chemical pretreatment, physical treatment, biomass size reduction, and chemical hydrolysis are required. This is advantageous for achieving high sugar yields through enzymatic and other processes for biofuel conversion. However, the use of high-energy processes, as in some processes, and the neutralization of chemicals used may be expensive, which is disadvantageous.

In biological pretreatment, microorganisms are typically used to degrade lignin, hemicelluloses, and lignin components, while leaving the cellulose intact (Kumar and Wyman, 2009; Sánchez, 2009). This pretreatment method is less cost-effective than alternative approaches due to the rigid nature of using microorganisms and the potential formation of inhibitory compounds, which pose additional challenges. A summary of the key advantages and disadvantages of different pretreatment methods is presented in Table 14.3.

TABLE 14.3
The Different Benefits and Limitations Associated with Pretreatment Methods for Lignocellulosic Biomass Materials

Pretreatment Method	Advantages	Disadvantages
Alkaline treatment	(i) Effectively removes lignin (ii) Produces fewer inhibitors	(i) Expensive alkaline catalysts (ii) Alters lignin structure
Acid recovery	(i) High glucose yield (ii) Efficient hemicellulose solubilization	(i) High acid costs (ii) Requires corrosion-resistant equipment (iii) Inhibitor formation
Green solvents	(i) Breaks down lignin and hemicellulose (ii) Can process various biomass types at high loadings	(i) High cost of solvents (ii) Requires solvent recovery and recycling (iii) Operates at low temperatures
Steam explosion	(i) Economical process (ii) Transforms lignin and solubilizes hemicellulose (iii) High yields in two-step processing	(i) Partial hemicellulose degradation (ii) Requires an acid catalyst for high-lignin biomass (iii) Generates toxic by-products
Liquid hot water (LHW)	(i) Separates hemicellulose with high purity (ii) Catalyst-free process	(i) High energy and water consumption (ii) Residual solid waste (cellulose/lignin) (iii) Hemicellulose hydrolysis
AFEX (ammonia fiber expansion)	(i) Highly effective for herbaceous and low-lignin biomass (ii) Enhances cellulose accessibility (iii) Reduces lignin-enzyme interactions (iv) Minimal inhibitor formation	(i) Requires ammonia recycling (ii) Less efficient for lignin-rich biomass (iii) Alters lignin structure (iv) High ammonia cost
ARP (ammonia recycle percolation)	(i) Removes most lignin (ii) Leaves with high cellulose content post-treatment (iii) Most effective on herbaceous biomass	(i) High energy consumption (ii) Generates significant liquid waste
Supercritical fluid process	(i) Minimal sugar degradation (ii) Economical in operation (iii) Improves cellulose accessibility	(i) Requires high pressure (ii) Less effective on lignin and hemicellulose

Source: Gary Brodeur et al. (2011). https://doi.org/10.4061/2011/787532.

14.3 ECONOMIC ASSESSMENT OF PRETREATMENT PROCESS TECHNOLOGIES

Economic assessment of any pretreatment process is an integral part of the research and development of a product, as it involves the application of raw materials, such as various biomass, to convert them into valuable products and biofuels. Table 14.4 provides a detailed economic assessment of sorghum biomass for 1 kilogram.

14.4 APPLICATIONS

Every pretreatment method has its specific application method for producing value-added products and biofuels. Various researchers have studied many pretreatment methods; some are still in development. Evaluating the pretreatment method is challenging, as each process operates differently and involves factors such as upstream and downstream costs, capital investment costs, chemical recycling, waste treatment, and the use of biomass, which has a rigid structure that requires a specific pretreatment process. There are many applications for the pretreatment process, which are discussed next:

Physical pretreatment: Physical pretreatment leads to a reduction in the size of the biomass material such as aspen chips, lodge pole pine, Salix, and bamboo; olive tree pruning, wheat straw, eucalyptus chips, corn fiber, sweet sorghum bagasse, Bermuda grass, and rice straw can be applied for pretreatment through steam explosion and liquid hot water process. This physical pretreatment method reduces the crystallinity and degree of polymerization of lignocellulosic biomass while enhancing its surface area and pore size accessibility.

TABLE 14.4
Economics of Pretreatment per Kilogram of Sorghum Biomass

Economic Costing for Pretreatment Sorghum Biomass of 1 Kg

Serial Number	Name of the Biomass Material	Sorghum
1	Quantity taken	1 kg
2	Particle size of the biomass material particles	200–600 μm
3	Cost of biomass sizing	Rs. 1.10
4	Chemicals used for pretreatment	Alkali (NaOH)
5	Cost of chemicals/kg biomass	Rs. 0.20 (10 g NaOH/kg biomass)
6	Time of treatment	1 hr
7	Pretreatment conditions	140°C; 10% solid loading
8	Quantity of steam used	1.52 kg of steam used
9	Steam cost/kg biomass	1.52 (kg steam) × Rs. 1.50 (coal-based) = Rs. 2.28.

Chemical pretreatment: Chemicals, such as acids and bases, were used to improve the biodegradability of cellulose, hemicelluloses, and lignin. Primarily, the hemicelluloses and alkali treatment degrade cellulose by removing lignin and hemicellulose. In the chemical pretreatment process, the crystallinity and degree of polymerization of the cellulose component in lignocellulosic biomass are enhanced, thereby improving enzymatic saccharification and yielding high sugars for further fermentation into biofuels. The biomass used for this process includes Bermuda grass, rice straw, wheat straw, eucalyptus chips, corn fiber, sweet sorghum bagasse, aspen chips, lodgepole pine, Salix, bamboo, and olive tree pruning, among others.

Physicochemical pretreatment: This process employs physical and chemical methods to dissolve hemicelluloses and alter the lignin structure, thereby enhancing cellulose accessibility for downstream processes and facilitating the production of desired products. The various biomasses used for this pretreatment process include corn stover, *Miscanthus giganteus*, aspen, switch grass, softwood pine, Avicel, sugarcane bagasse, wheat straw, hybrid poplar chips, beech wood chips, rye straw, and *Picea abies* (softwood). The various pretreatment processes are steam explosion, liquid hot water, wet oxidation, ammonia fiber, recycle percolation, aqueous ammonia, organosolv, and green solvents. These pretreatments alter the physical and chemical properties of lignocellulosic biomass by removing most of the lignin, thereby forming accessible cellulose that facilitates lower inhibitor formation, improved sugar degradation, and greater cost-effectiveness.

14.5 CONCLUSION

In the pretreatment process of lignocellulosic biomass, it's challenging to evaluate each method, as this is also considered in upstream and downstream processes, along with pretreatment cost economics and chemical recycling. By characterizing the different pretreatment processes using the same feedstock and further analyzing the data, the results show that bioconversion technologies are economically viable for improving cost economics and reducing gas emissions.

REFERENCES

G. Brodeur, E. Yau, K. Badal, J. Collier, K. B. Ramachandran, S. Ramakrishnan, "Chemical and physicochemical pretreatment of lignocellulosic biomass: A review," *Enzyme Research*, vol. 2011, no. 1, pp. 1–17, 2011.

T. Eggeman and R. T. Elander, "Process and economic analysis of pretreatment technologies," *Bioresource Technology*, vol. 96, no. 18, pp. 2019–2025, 2005.

R. Kumar and C. E. Wyman, "Effects of cellulase and xylanase enzymes on the deconstruction of solids from pretreatment of poplar by leading technologies," *Biotechnology Progress*, vol. 25, no. 2, pp. 302–314, 2009.

N. Mosier, C. Wyman, B. Dale et al., "Features of promising technologies for pretreatment of lignocellulosic biomass," *Bioresource Technology*, vol. 96, no. 6, pp 673–686, 2005.

C. Sánchez, "Lignocellulosic residues: Biodegradation and bioconversion by fungi," *Biotechnology Advances*, vol. 27, no. 2, pp. 185–194, 2009.

E. Sendich, M. Laser, S. Kim et al., "Recent process improvements for the ammonia fiber expansion (AFEX) process and resulting reductions in minimum ethanol selling price," *Bioresource Technology*, vol. 99, no. 17, pp. 8429–8435, 2008.

E. D. Sendich and B. E. Dale; "Environmental and economic analysis of the fully integrated biorefinery," *Global Change Biology Bioenergy*, vol. 1, no. 5, pp. 331–345, 2009.

15 Pretreatment of Lignocellulosic Biomass for Bioprocess Evaluation

Thangsei Nengneilhing Baite, Vikonoksh, Bishnupada Mandal, and Mihir Kumar Purkait

15.1 INTRODUCTION: IMPORTANCE OF VARIOUS PRETREATMENT TECHNIQUES OF LIGNOCELLULOSIC BIOMASS

15.1.1 Introduction to Pretreatment and Its Necessity

The depletion of fossil fuel reserves has driven an increasing demand for sustainable, viable energy sources such as lignocellulosic biomass (LCB). This demand is further intensified by factors such as rapid global industrialization, oil supply disruptions due to ongoing geopolitical tensions, supply-demand imbalances, greenhouse gas emissions, and various environmental concerns. LCB, a plant-derived biomass, encompasses hardwood, softwood, agricultural residues, and grasses. Agro-based byproducts, which are produced in abundance in the form of bagasse, spent grains, cotton stalks, salvageable miscellaneous water from various food processing industries, and so forth, can be utilized as a potential source from which second-generation biofuels (ethanol, biogas, biohydrogen, butanol, etc.) and chemical products can be manufactured on a large scale without hampering the food supply while also ensuring proper waste management (Taghizadeh et al., 2013; Haldar, 2020).

LCB comprises 30–50%, 15–35%, and 10–30% cellulose, hemicellulose, and lignin, respectively (Duarah et al., 2020; da Costa Sousa et al., 2009). These components can either be hydrolyzed or be microbiologically converted to yield desirable end products (Debnath et al., 2021). However, native LCB is recalcitrant owing to its intrinsic compositional, physicochemical, and structural factors. The crystallinity, high degree of polymerization, and complex network of inter- and

 DOI: 10.1201/9781003327608-15

intra-hydrogen bonds of the hydroxyl groups in cellulose contribute significantly to LCB recalcitrance. The lignin fraction, comprising highly complex methoxylated phenylpropanoid units, also contributes to recalcitrance; hemicellulose has a lower degree of polymerization and, due to its amorphous and hydrophilic nature, exerts comparatively less influence.

It alters the biomass matrix by linking the cellulose and lignin fractions. Valuable chemical products can be derived from reducing sugars present in cellulose and hemicellulose (Duarah et al., 2022). Simultaneously, a range of enriched aromatic compounds can be obtained through the catalytic conversion of the lignin fraction (Mankar et al., 2021). Thus, some pretreatment becomes a prerequisite to disrupting the covalent and non-covalent bonds linking hemicelluloses and lignin to convert LCB to biofuels efficiently (Ummalyma et al., 2019). In their native form, the components of LCB are only moderately fermentable. Pretreatment can efficiently convert them into fermentable sugars by modifying the physical and chemical attributes of the plant cell wall (Figure 15.1). The physical and chemical properties of pretreated biomass are significantly influenced by both the type of pretreatment technique employed and the specific lignocellulosic material used. This, in turn, will decide the choice of downstream processes (enzyme and microbial selection), pre-conditioning (if any), the utility of by-products, waste residue handling, and the recovery of desired products. Pretreatment will also affect the economic costs of each stage of the bio-refining process. Lately, two or more pretreatment techniques have been combined to improve their efficiency (Hassan et al., 2018).

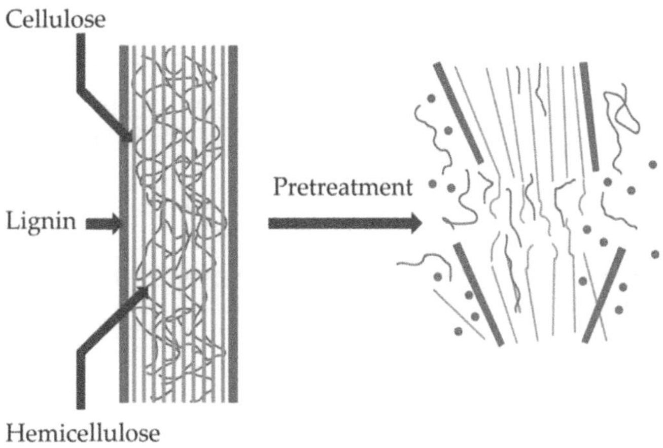

FIGURE 15.1 Breakdown of lignocellulosic biomass following pretreatment.

Source: Haq et al. (2021)

15.2 GOALS OF PRETREATMENT

In addition to the physicochemical conversion, pretreatment must also serve the following purposes (McMillan et al., 1994):

- The pretreatment process must be chemically and energetically efficient. It must be economical enough to render biofuel and chemical production profitable.
- The selected pretreatment method should facilitate the efficient conversion of biomass components into fermentable sugars, aiming for a high yield of fermentable sugars.
- Additionally, the destruction and loss of carbohydrates must be minimized with sufficient lignin recovery.
- The pretreated biomass must be readily digestible and not inhibit cell metabolism or enzymatic hydrolysis. The formation of inhibitory compounds and the subsequent requirement to detoxify or wash the pretreated biomass are undesirable outcomes.
- Pretreated materials must be hydrolyzed most effectively at low enzyme levels; thus, reducing the possibility of enzymes binding nonspecifically to lignin and other pretreated fractions is desirable.

All of these highlight the significance of pretreatment in biorefineries for generating value-added biofuels and chemicals. Commonly employed pretreatment techniques include physical, chemical, physicochemical, and biological processes (Figure 15.2).

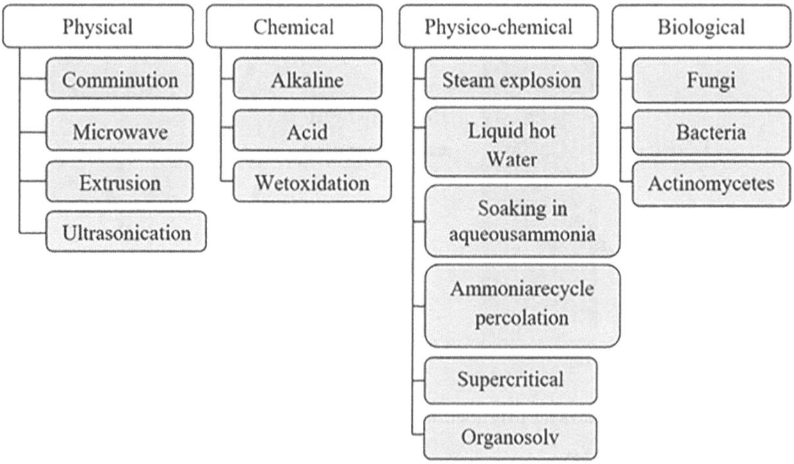

FIGURE 15.2 Classification of pretreatment methods.

15.2.1 Efficacy of Pretreatment

Studies indicate that pretreatment accounts for over 40% of the total processing cost (Bhutto et al., 2017). Hence, it is crucial to choose correct type of pretreatment to be employed.

The efficacy of a pretreatment technique can be assessed on the basis of the following (Gupta and Verma, 2015):

- Direct hydrolysis of monomeric sugars or after enzymatic hydrolysis/fermentation
- Minimal loss and/or degradation of monomeric sugars
- Reduction in the production of inhibitory byproducts
- Minimization of cost

None of the commonly used pretreatment methods satisfies all the listed ideal attributes. A balanced decision should be made on the basis of factors such as biomass type, targeted end product, available equipment, and capital investment. Figure 15.3 depicts the distinctive features of bioethanol's efficient and effective production.

15.2.2 Assessment of Pretreatment

To determine feasibility, any pretreatment method must be assessed on the basis of technological, economic, and environmental factors. The financial feasibility

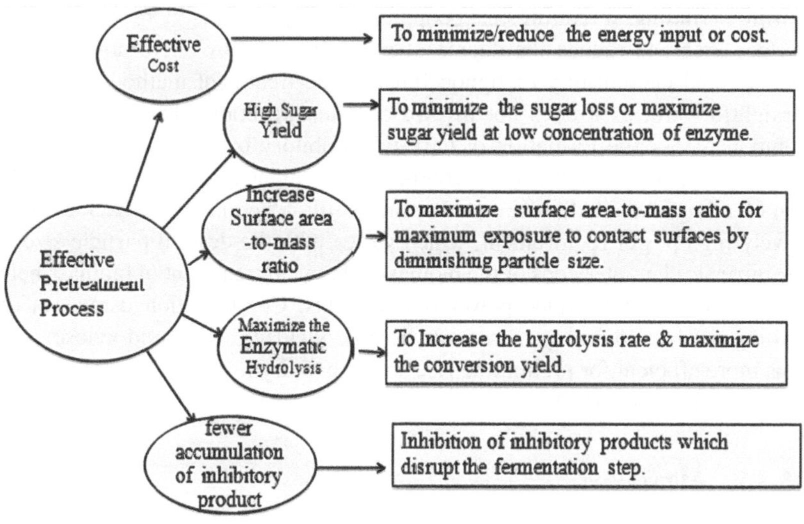

FIGURE 15.3 Features of the effective pretreatment process.

of a particular biorefining method is highly dependent on the monosaccharide concentration and yield and the effectiveness of the pretreatment. For instance, the former will play a role in determining the reactor volume, sufficient to process the amount of monosaccharide generated. Simultaneously, this will help determine the appropriate bioconversion method and the related costs. Additionally, environmental factors such as land use and waste management influence the overall economics of the bioconversion process. The energy demand of a pretreatment technique is determined by a range of factors, including operating conditions (temperature, pressure, time, etc.); materials used (chemicals, solvents, water, etc.); and unit operations (recycling, mixing, pre-conditioning, etc.). The choice of each factor and its use will affect energy requirements and bioconversion efficiency, with or without adverse environmental effects. All these will subsequently impact the economics of the bioconversion process (da Costa Sousa et al., 2009).

Lignin recovery is also an essential aspect of evaluating a pretreatment process. High lignin recovery ensures two crucial things: its removal, leading to a reduction in nonspecific binding with hydrolytic enzymes, and its possible utilization for chemical production. Lignin, considered a waste in biorefinery, is a valuable source from which many chemicals (benzene, toluene, xylene, styrene, etc.) can be manufactured. Lignin utilization can improve the economics of the biorefining process (Kumare et al., 2011).

15.3 PHYSICAL PRETREATMENT

15.3.1 Comminution

Comminution includes several environmentally friendly unit operations such as milling, grinding, shredding, and chopping. These processes increase the specific surface area and reduce the degree of polymerization by decreasing the particle size and crystallinity of lignocellulose. The treatment method is relatively straightforward, as it does not involve chemical reactions, loss of fermentable components, or the formation of harmful inhibitory byproducts. Comminution is predominantly carried out in a continuous dry mode operation with up to 90% solid loading in the ball, disk, and hammer mills. The main drawback is the relatively high power requirement, which varies with the desired particle size and the intrinsic characteristics of the biomass. Chemical treatment of biomass before comminution could reduce power requirements. Comminution using wet disk milling has been found to increase hydrolysis yields (glucose and xylose) and is thus more efficient for pretreating rice straw than dry milling (Tomás-Pejó et al., 2011; Zhang et al., 2016).

15.3.2 Microwave

Microwaves are nonionizing electromagnetic radiations with wavelengths between 1 mm and 1 m, corresponding to frequencies between 300 and 300,000 MHz on the electromagnetic spectrum. They can selectively transfer energy based on the type of substance involved. Dielectric materials absorb microwaves, and the electromagnetic energy is converted into heat at the molecular level, thus uniformly distributing the power within the material. Generally, biomass is regarded as a low-loss material, which may require supplementation with materials such as graphite, charcoal, activated carbon, and pyrites to promote rapid healing (Salema et al., 2017). Nonetheless, the ionic crystallinity and nonionic amorphous zones within the LCB get polarized in the microwave, resulting in intense molecular collision and formation of hot spots, which disrupts cellulosic components and degradation of lignin and hemicelluloses. The rapid and uniform heating of biomass fragments by microwaves has been reported to cause fiber swelling and disintegration, thereby improving their enzymatic susceptibility (Diaz et al., 2015). Increased rates of hydrolysis, oxidation, alkylation, and esterification characterize an efficient microwave pretreatment. Its satisfactory performance has enabled microwaves to evolve from the laboratory to pilot scale as a reliable, green thermal process for pretreating LCB in biorefineries. However, before it can be scaled up for industrial implementation, issues such as high energy consumption, high investment and operational costs, and limited knowledge of the dielectric properties of biomass must be addressed (Salema et al., 2017).

At present, LCB pretreatment by microwave can be broadly grouped under the following categories (Hassan et al., 2018):

- Microwave-assisted solvolysis at relatively lower temperatures (<200°C) for depolymerization of the biomass.
- Microwave-assisted pyrolysis of lignin at elevated temperatures (> 400°C) for biomass conversion to biofuels. In this, after microwave irradiation as a pretreatment, biofuels are obtained from biomass, in addition to thermochemical pyrolysis.

15.3.3 Extrusion

Extrusion is a thermo-mechanical process characterized by high temperature and pressure, generated when high shear forces act as biomass is forced through an extruder. An extruder primarily consists of a barrel fitted with single or twin screws. High shear forces are generated between the barrel, feedstock, and the screw, subjecting the LCB to rapid heating, mixing, and shearing. Elevated temperature and pressure induce beneficial physical changes – such as fiber defibrillation and shortening, along with increased specific surface area – and modify the chemical structure to enhance enzyme accessibility during hydrolysis (Kumar et al., 2019). The efficiency and output of the process depend on the screw type, rotational speed of the screw, working temperature, moisture, and so forth. This process also allows certain modifications such as adding chemicals, applying high pressure, and performing expansion treatment with steam or other solvents. However, this process is better suited to herbaceous biomass, it involves high energy expenditure, and its effect is not well pronounced without the aid of chemical agents (Duque et al., 2017).

15.3.4 Ultrasonication

Ultrasound is a mechanical wave that produces zones of rarefaction (low density) and zones of compression (high density) as it propagates through a medium. This generates acoustic cavitation that promotes the formation of microbubbles, which in turn expand and contract during rarefaction and compression cycles, respectively. When bubbles approach a critical size, they collapse, forming hotspots accompanied by a rise in temperature and pressure (~5,000°C, ~50 MPa). This can break the α-O-4 and β-O-4 ether linkages, splitting the structural polysaccharides and lignin fractions (Hassan et al., 2018). An alternative theory proposes that the high-frequency acoustic waves (≥20 kHz) promote the formation of oxidizing radicals, which assist in breaking the bonds within lignocellulosic biomass components. Recently, this approach has been combined with other pretreatment methods to enhance lignin degradation and improve enzymatic digestibility. Some examples include ultrasound-assisted acidification, ultrasonication, microwave-assisted techniques and exposure to organic solvents, alkalis, or ionic liquids. This green technique has been hailed for its benefits, such as short treatment time, high activation energy, and effective mass transfer (Cho et al., 2011). The available findings on applying acoustic energy to LCB must be thoroughly scrutinized and analyzed to elevate this method to an industrial level.

15.4 CHEMICAL PRETREATMENT

15.4.1 Alkaline Hydrolysis

In this method, LCB is hydrolyzed with bases like NH_4OH, KOH, NaOH, $Ca(OH)_2$, NH_3, and $(NH_4)_2SO_3$ to obtain a desirable modification in the structure of LCB such as cellulose swelling, fractional depolymerization, decrystallization of cellulose, partial solvation of hemicellulose portion, and structural impairment of lignin (Akhtar et al., 2016). Generally, it is carried out at ambient temperature, with residence times ranging from a few seconds to days. Still, lower temperature treatment has recently been explored for NaOH/urea (–20°C) or NaOH solutions (–5°C). Alkali hydrolysis is reportedly more efficient on agro-based waste than on wood materials. An increase in cellulose digestibility and lignin solubilization, with a minimal effect on cellulose and hemicellulose, is reported for alkali pretreatments compared with acid or hydrothermal processes. Additionally, less sugar degradation is reported for alkali hydrolysis than for acid pretreatment (Tomás-Pejó et al., 2011). The high economics of the alkali used and the structural alteration of lignin may limit the utilization of this method.

15.4.2 Acid Hydrolysis

In acid pretreatment, sulfuric acid, acetic acid, and phosphoric acid are used in diluted or concentrated form to liquefy the lignin-hemicellulose network, allowing enzymes to more easily access the cellulose fraction for catalysis. Dilute acid hydrolysis (1–3%) can be performed either at high temperatures (above 160°C) with low substrate concentrations (5–10 wt%) and short residence times or at lower temperatures (up to 160°C) with higher substrate concentrations (10–40 wt%) for longer durations (30–90 minutes) (Akhtar et al., 2016). In contrast, concentrated acid hydrolysis (30–70%) requires low temperatures (below 50°C) to be effective (Den et al., 2018).

The dilute acid treatment is superior to concentrated acid treatment in terms of the low formation of inhibiting compounds, higher chemical recovery, and lower risk of equipment corrosion. Nonetheless, it involves higher operating costs due to the requirement for elevated temperatures and higher maintenance charges. Using concentrated acid may decrease energy requirements and thus operating costs, but at the risk of forming inhibitory compounds (furfural, 5-hydroxymethylfurfural), which can have an antagonistic effect on the microorganisms used for fermentation and pose a high risk of corrosion (Mankar et al., 2021). The wheat straw, pretreated with dilute organic acids (maleic acid, fumaric acid, etc.), reported lesser furfural content than that pretreated with sulfuric acid (Akhtar et al., 2016).

15.4.3 Wet Oxidation

Wet oxidation (WO) is an oxidative hydrothermal process that utilizes water and an oxidizer (air, O_2, H_2O_2, etc.) at higher temperatures (125–300°C) and pressure (0.5–20 MPa) conditions to treat biomass. Oxygen utilization can accelerate reaction rates but generates free radicals, which require considerable energy when using pure oxygen. It solubilizes and hydrolyses the hemicellulose fraction, breaking it into monosaccharides and forming organic acids. Consequently, acidification leads to delignification while cellulose undergoes decrystallization and partial degradation, making it more susceptible to enzymatic attack and fermentation. Process temperature, pressure, reaction duration, and water content are important factors for any WO treatment (Devi et al., 2021). One advantage of the WO technique is that it eliminates the need for a dewatering step before treatment. However, as a nonselective process, WO can cause significant loss of organic matter such as hemicellulose (Rahmati et al., 2020). Additionally, the high demand for catalysts and oxygen, the requirement for high-pressure equipment, and the formation of inhibitory compounds (such as furfural and soluble aromatic compounds) resulting from lignin oxidation restrict the commercial scalability of the WO process (Devi et al., 2021).

15.5 PHYSICOCHEMICAL PRETREATMENT METHODOLOGIES

15.5.1 Steam Explosion

Steam explosion (SE) is a hydrothermal process in which biomass is exposed to rapid heating with high-pressure saturated steam (0.69–4.83 MPa) at temperatures ranging from 160°C to 260°C and held for a short duration, varying from seconds to several minutes. High-pressure steam readily condenses and penetrates the biomass, triggering autohydrolysis as organic acids are generated from acetyl groups in hemicelluloses. This causes breakage of glycosidic bonds, leading to solubilization of hemicellulose. On the other hand, the abrupt release of pressure causes the condensed moisture within the fibers to reevaporate, disrupting the fiber matrix. All of these lead to enhanced accessibility of enzymes to cellulose. For lignin, the high temperature of SE induces homolytic cleavage of the β-O-4 ether and other acid-sensitive bonds, resulting in lignin reallocation and removal. This is of concern as lignin byproducts are known to inhibit microbial growth. Also, reallocating modified lignin may hinder enzyme accessibility by increasing the number of nonspecific binding sites.

Initially, it was operated only in batch mode, but it has transitioned into continuous mode over the years. Continuous SE can achieve lower inhibitor pile-up and better control of operating variables and heat transfer (Duque et al., 2016). The origin of the biomass, particle size, temperature, reaction time, and moisture are significant factors that decide the technique's efficacy. SE is comparatively cost-effective, requires less than 70% less energy consumption than conventional mechanical processes), uses little to no chemicals, and poses a minor environmental threat (D. Kim, 2018).

15.5.2 Liquid Hot Water Treatment

Liquid hot water (LHW) treatment, also known as autohydrolysis of biomass, is a hydrothermal process in which hot water is added to LCB, and the temperature increases. Consequently, ionization of water releases carboxylic acid, primarily acetic acid. This, in conjunction with the effects of high pressure and temperature, results in auto-hydrolysis, deconstructing the internal structure of the biomass and thereby increasing the accessible surface area and enabling subsequent processes such as enzymatic digestion and fermentation (Jimenez-Gutierrez et al., 2021). Studies show that the severity of pretreatment methods not only correlates with the amount of carbohydrate release but also increases the rate of degradation reactions, leading to the formation of more inhibitors. In this regard, LHW pretreatment stands out as a promising technique compared to many physical, chemical, physicochemical, and biological methods, as it avoids the use of harmful chemicals and operates under moderate conditions. However, the need for a large amount of water, high energy requirements, further processing requirements of diluted products so obtained, and large machinery may pose a considerable challenge in upscaling. Combining LHW with other pretreatment techniques, such as aqueous ammonia treatment, step-change flow rate LHW, and step-change temperature LHW, can mitigate the adverse effects of high water intake and energy input. Additionally, the combined production of ethanol and other enriched products can make LWH more suitable for industry (Zhuan et al., 2016).

Systematic comparative studies between laboratory and pilot scales are underway to understand mass transfer and heat scalability for biomass of similar composition and temperature profile (Aguilar et al., 2018). Subsequent examinations for upscaling to industrial levels should be conducted to maximize the merits of LHW treatment.

15.5.3 Ammonia Fiber Expansion Treatment

Ammonia fiber expansion (AFEX) treatment is a thermochemical pretreatment method that employs volatile ammonia to treat lignocellulosic biomass (LCB) at moderately high temperatures for a controlled duration. In contrast to most aqueous-based physicochemical pretreatment techniques, AFEX is a dry-to-dry method; i.e., it generates a pretreated solid product with minimal change in the biomass makeup. This eliminates the need for a washing step, the burden of waste management, and its accompanying expenses. Using ammonia in vapor form offers high diffusivity into the biomass, resulting in rapid, consistent ammonia distribution. Also, ammonia vapor can quickly dissolve into the wet biomass, generating heat that uniformly heats the biomass. Ammonia causes lignocellulose to swell, leading to the physical disintegration of the intricate network of fibers, partial decrystallization of cellulose, and breakdown of lignin-carbohydrate bonds. The deconstruction of biomass ultrastructure by AFEX increases the accessibility of hydrolytic enzymes and accelerates hydrolysis several-fold. AFEX is comparatively more efficient on graminoid monocot-derived biomass, such as straws, grasses, bagasse, and corn stover, than on dicot and gymnosperm-derived biomass, such as native forbs, softwoods, and hardwoods. This can be attributed to the process's ability to target lignin-carbohydrate ester linkages, which are inherently abundant in lignin (Chundawat et al., 2020).

Some crucial factors that determine the effectiveness of AFEX are initial water and ammonia loading, pressure, temperature, reaction time, and the number of treatments (Aggarwal et al., 2022). AFEX pretreatment is a promising alternative that can produce easily digestible plant biomass for biofuels and chemicals. Advanced and detailed studies must be continued before attempting the industrial-scale-up of this promising alternative.

15.5.4 Soaking in Aqueous Ammonia and Ammonia Recycle Percolation

Soaking in aqueous ammonia (SAA) is performed at low temperatures (30–75°C), and soaking times range from a few hours to days. It allows the conservation of glucan and xylan in the solids, making the pretreated material suitable for pentose-fermenting microbes. The high xylose recovery observed in SAA reflects minimal sugar degradation, leading to lower formation of inhibitory compounds. A study highlighted that increasing the processing temperature from room temperature to 60°C can reduce the soaking duration from 60 days to 12 hr and reduce the ammonia and water requirements, but at the cost of lignin removal and glucan conversion (T.H. Kim and Lee, 2007). Recently, SAA was used with other pretreatment techniques for higher recovery of fermentable sugars. Examples of these are ozone and SAA-based pretreatments and aqueous ammonia with glycerol mixture (Zhao et al., 2020).

In ammonia recycle percolation (ARP), the LCB is treated with aqueous ammonia solutions, which flow continuously through a percolation reactor where the biomass is loaded. For the same effect, replacing SAA with ARP can halve the ammonia and water requirements. Conventional ARP is characterized by high liquid throughput and a long reaction time. A low-liquid ARP with low energy input and brief reaction times can be used to overcome this. This is reported to result in lignin removal and hemicellulose retention of 59–70% and 48–57%, while the glucan and xylan conversions reached 95% and 86%, respectively. ARP combined with dilute acid treatment (ARP-DA) can reduce lignin content and thereby prevent lignin's irreversible adsorption of cellulases. Combining LHW treatment with ARP can enhance glucan recovery to 78–85% (Zhao et al., 2020). A significant challenge in ARP is reducing energy costs, which can be addressed by either lowering the liquid load or decreasing the process temperature.

15.5.5 Supercritical Fluid (SCF)

Supercritical fluids (SFs) possess the desirable attributes of both gas and liquid, allowing them to quickly diffuse into the solid matrix like a gas while solubilizing the target biomolecule like a liquid solvent when maintained above their respective critical temperatures and pressures. Using SCF, lignin can be selectively removed, thereby increasing the substrate digestibility of the treated LCB. Supercritical extraction can be supplemented with co-solvents such as ethanol and methanol to enhance lignin removal (Tomás-Pejó et al., 2011). Different types of SCFs, such as water, CO_2, and ammonia, are being investigated for non-extraction purposes. CO_2 is the most commonly used solvent for supercritical extraction due to its low cost, nontoxic nature, nonflammability, and ease of removal from the final product. In addition, it has a moderate critical temperature (31.1°C) and pressure (73.8 bar). It is also flexible and versatile because the solvent power/selectivity can be altered by manipulating the process parameters, such as pressure and temperature, to obtain diverse extract compositions. CO_2 can form carbonic acid in aqueous solution, thereby favoring hydrolysis. However, the high cost of the setup often limits its applicability.

15.5.6 Organosolv Process

This technique utilizes organic solvents (ethanol, methanol, acetone, glycerol, tetrahydrofurfuryl alcohol) or their mixtures, with or without a catalyst (organic or inorganic acids or bases) (Kumar et al., 2019). The biomass is mixed with an aqueous solution of the organic solvents and heated to about 100–250°C. Acids such as H_2SO_4, HCl, salicylic acid, or oxalic acid can be incorporated when the processing temperature is below 185–210°C. The addition of acid increases delignification and yields greater xylose. The disruption of various aryl and ester bonds liberates lignin and hemicellulose from the LCB matrix, making cellulose more available for further processing (Kumar et al., 2019). The fractions obtained after this pretreatment are cellulosic fibers, pure lignin after solvent removal, and a solution of xylose and minute traces of other hemicellulosic sugars. An essential step after this pretreatment is the removal of the solvents initially used by suitable extraction and separation techniques. If not separated, the solvent may impede enzymatic digestion or disrupt the fermentative culture. A significant issue for industrial applications is the significantly high cost of solvents. Recycling can help reduce operational costs. Alcohols like ethanol and methanol, with lower molecular weights and boiling points, are preferred for further cost-cutting. Benefits such as the production of easily digestible cellulose substrate from most types of LCB and the recovery of high-purity lignin make this technique desirable. Moreover, removing lignin allows for easier enzyme absorption, as evidenced by the lower enzyme dosage requirements for the treated LCB. However, generating a notable quantity of furfural, HMF, and soluble phenols from lignin may curtail the quality of the treated LCB (Tomás-Pejó et al., 2011).

15.5.7 Ionic Liquids

As the name implies, ionic liquids (ILs) are ionic salts composed mainly of large organic cations and small inorganic anions, which remain liquid at relatively low temperatures. ILs facilitate the solubilization of cellulose, hemicellulose, and lignin by disrupting their existing hydrogen-bond networks and forming new hydrogen bonds with cellulose and lignin, all while minimizing the formation of inhibitory compounds (Ninomiya et al., 2012).To improve the enzymatic saccharification of LCB, *N*-methyl morpholine-*N*-oxide monohydrate (NMMO), 1-allyl-3-methylimidazolium chloride (AMICl), 1-butyl-3-methylimidazolium chloride (BMIMCl), 1-ethyl-3-methylimidazolium acetate, and 3-methyl-*N*-butylpyridinium chloride (MBPCl) can be employed. NMMO can be applied to increase methane production from microalgae and to pretreat wheat straw. The disruption of the intricate non-covalent interactions depends on the cation structure, the degree of anion charge delocalization in ILs, the residence period, and the temperature. Its notable attributes include thermal and chemical stability, elastic solvating properties, low toxicity, viscosity and hydrophobicity, nonflammability, and a broad liquid temperature range. ILs are regarded as green solvents as no toxic or explosive gases are generated. However, constraints such as high operational costs, an energy-intensive recycling process, and IL's toxicity to enzymes and yeasts limit its industrial applications. Advanced studies to improve energy-intensive recycling methods and techniques to mitigate the toxic effects of ILs on enzymes and fermentative microorganisms should be pursued if ILs are used for biomass pretreatment at the industrial level. Additionally, the potential production of ILs from carbohydrates can be investigated to offset the high cost of using ILs (Kumar et al., 2019; Tomás-Pejó et al., 2011).

15.5.8 Carbon Dioxide Explosion

In a carbon dioxide explosion (CDE), high-pressure CO_2 gas is released, causing the disintegration of the cellulose and hemicellulose matrix. This increases the substrate's specific surface area, consequently enhancing enzymatic hydrolysis (Tomás-Pejó et al., 2011). Of late, supercritical Na_2CO_3 has been explored for non-extractive applications due to its many benefits such as non-toxicity, non-flammability, low cost, environmental acceptability, and easy recovery after extraction. Supercritical combines gas-like mass transfer characteristics with liquid-like solvating abilities. In contrast, subcritical CO_2 is less effective because it cannot diffuse into and penetrate biomass pores as efficiently, nor disrupt the structure through rapid pressure release. When used in combination with water, supercritical has been shown to enhance the enzymatic digestibility of both aspen (hardwood) and southern yellow pine (softwood). The efficacy of delignification using pressurized can be further enhanced when co-solvents like ethanol-water or acetic acid-water are employed. Although supercritical CO_2 offers many advantages, its industrial implementation is impractical due to its high operating costs (Taherzadeh and Karimi, 2008). The need for extreme pressure is concerning, but on the flip side, using CO_2 produced during ethanolic fermentation may help cut costs.

15.5.9 Ozonolysis

Ozone is known as one of the most potent oxidizing agents. Being electron-deficient at the terminal oxygen, ozone exhibits high delignification efficiency because it specifically targets lignin, an electron-rich substrate (Travaini et al., 2016). Ozonolysis is an effective oxidative pretreatment for lignin degeneration with minimum impact on the hemicellulose and no impact on the cellulose fraction. The inhibitors produced from hemicellulose and cellulose are minimal. Ozonolysis is typically performed at atmospheric pressure and ambient temperature. Several biomasses have been successfully treated with ozone, including wheat straw, rye straw, cotton straw, bagasse, poplar, grass, macroalgae, and municipal solid waste (Tomás-Pejó et al., 2011).

Despite demonstrating effectiveness and efficiency with high delignification capability (~80%), high total sugar release yields (~75%), and minimal carbohydrate losses, ozone generation is a significant limitation due to its high production cost and the enormous quantity required for ozonolysis. Although recent technological advancements have reduced production costs, pretreatment by ozonolysis must be optimized (minimization of ozone consumption and maximization of process efficiency), which will ultimately impact the process economy. Hemicellulose and degradation products of lignin (e.g., phenols and benzene) can also be recovered to improve the economic balance. The generation of degradation products during ozonolysis is a suitable pretreatment for the subsequent production of lignin-derived products (Travaini et al., 2016).

15.6 BIOLOGICAL PRETREATMENT

Although physicochemical techniques are widely used for biomass pretreatment, they have several drawbacks, including technical, environmental, and economic issues. In this regard, biological pretreatment (BP) may be more appealing than traditional pretreatment procedures as it employs natural bacteria or their enzymes under moderate conditions (Zabed et al., 2019). The ligninolytic capability of some microorganisms (fungi and bacteria) is used to minimize feedstock recalcitrance during the biological pretreatment of LCB and to improve digestibility by hydrolytic enzymes (Jayasekara et al., 2019). The primary benefits of BP include economical and easy operation, minimal inhibitor production, cheap downstream processing costs, and no need for chemical recycling after pretreatment. Consequently, BP provides a green, safe, and cost-effective method for biomass pretreatment. Furthermore, BP may offer the potential to produce a variety of enriched products from byproducts or mainstream chemicals generated after pretreatment, thereby promising an economically and technologically viable BP process. Despite its potential, large-scale adoption of BP is currently hampered by critical challenges, including extended pretreatment times, carbohydrate losses, and low downstream yields (Wyman et al., 2017).

15.6.1 Biological Pretreatment Processes

15.6.1.1 Whole-Cell Pretreatment

Research has demonstrated that several bacteria, including *Bacillus*, *Actinomycetes* and certain recognized fungi, may decompose organic materials (Poszytek et al., 2016). Consortia composed of cellulose-hydrolyzing bacteria from the genera *Aspergillus*, *Streptomyces*, *Candida*, and *Bacillus* demonstrate broad-spectrum biodegradation. Microbial pretreatment outperforms enzymatic pretreatment in anaerobic digestion due to its superior functional diversity and tolerance to temperature, pH, and other environmental conditions (Nikiema et al., 2017). Fungi facilitate simultaneous saccharification and fermentation, boosting ethanol output (Chen et al., 2017).

Different fungi, such as *Phanerochaete chrysosporium, Gloeophyllumtrabeum*, and *Trichoderma reesei*, have been employed in conjunction with mild alkali and steam pretreatment of wet-milled corn fiber for rapid fermentation of hydrolysates. The findings reveal a significantly higher ethanol yield than commercial cellulase-aided saccharification and fermentation. Traditional physicochemical approaches require substantial energy; thus, biomass pretreatment using fungi is more efficient and environmentally friendly (Ummalyma et al.). Several white-rot fungi, including *Pleurotus ostreatus*, *P. chrysosporium*, *Cyathus stercoreus*, *Ceriporiopsis lacerata*, and *Ceriporiopsis subvermispora*, have been shown to produce enzymes capable of delignifying various lignocellulosic biomasses (Madadi and Abbas, 2017). Consortia of diverse microbial species have evolved to tolerate inconsistent temperatures and pH and exhibit greater tolerance to inhibitory substances such as hazardous chemicals, heavy metals, and pollution. Microorganisms found in soil, manure, agricultural byproducts, animal rumen, or other ecological niches are prospective consortia capable of digesting lignocellulose (Ummalyma et al., 2018).

15.6.1.2 Enzymatic Pretreatment

BP with delignifying enzymes is often performed under moderate conditions and substantially affects lignin removal (Nijuet al., 2019). Enzymatic hydrolysis, in particular, involves the conversion of cellulose into glucose. This is accelerated by the activity of different fungi and enzymes, specifically cellulases, which release glucose by breaking the glycosidic bonds of cellulose microfibrils. This, in turn, serves as an ideal substrate for microbial fermentation (Ferdeş et al., 2020). Various bacteria and fungi produce hydrolytic and oxidative enzymes like laccase, glucanases, peroxidases, cellobiose, pectinase, xylanase, amylase, and proteases. The pretreatments achieved with these enzymes are superior to those achieved with the microbial treatments derived from them. Cellulase is the most often utilized enzyme in biological pretreatment, followed by β-glucosidase and xylanase (Ferdeş et al., 2020). While laccase is the most widely used lignocellulosic enzyme, oxidase and peroxidase are the most prevalent. Laccases enhance biomass conversion efficiency through lignin breakdown and offer the advantage of lower energy requirements and zero residual toxic by-products (Niju et al., 2019).

The enzymatic pretreatment approach is gaining popularity owing to the comparatively fast reaction time and the minimal feed requirement. Furthermore, the enzymatic pretreatment does not necessitate using costly processing equipment. The impact of enzymes on LC biomass depends on the type of enzymes used and the composition of the treated biomass. Microbial enzymes such as proteases, pectinases, and cellulases are commonly produced by solid-state fermentation (SSF) and submerged fermentation (SF). SF provides benefits in terms of facile process control, enzyme recovery, and a standardized technological foundation for extending processes to an industrial scale (Ferdeş et al., 2020).

However, the enzymes' activity and their associated reaction efficiency are affected by several parameters, including the biomass composition, incubation duration, temperature, pH, and bioreactor layout. Furthermore, the economic barrier posed by the high enzyme costs persists, impacting the viability of these pretreatment approaches for large-scale biogas generation.

15.6.2 Effect of Inhibitors on Microbial Processes

The primary goal of pretreatment is to fractionate the biomass's primary constituents and release cellulose for enzymatic saccharification. However, this results in undesirable byproducts derived from the feedstock, which hinder the downstream processes. Inhibition issues become more severe as derivatives are collected from the water's recirculation and as high solid loadings are used to achieve high-product titers and concentrated sugar streams (Jönsson et al., 2016).

15.6.2.1 Formation of Inhibitors

Most of the inhibitors obtained from the lignocellulosic complex during pretreatment are created by the solubilization and degradation of hemicellulose and/or lignin (Behera et al., 2014). The inhibitory compounds generated during pretreatment include organic acids such as levulinic acid, acetic acid, and formic acid. Additionally, lignin degradation produces compounds like 4-hydroxybenzaldehyde, vanillin, and syringaldehyde, while sugar degradation leads to furfural (from xylose) and 5-hydroxymethylfurfural (from hexoses). To minimize the formation of formic acid and levulinic acid – which occurs at the expense of fermentable sugars – it is essential to optimize pretreatment conditions (Figure 15.4) (Kordala et al., 2021). The lignin derivatives impede the fermentation of lignocellulosic hydrolysates even at lower concentrations and are considered the most hazardous inhibitors. The precise mechanism of their fermentation-inhibiting activity is unclear; nevertheless, it has been shown that it may be attributed to a discontinuity in the plasma membrane, with a consequent reduction in cell growth and sugar absorption (Kordala et al., 2021; D. Kim, 2018).

Inhibitors are produced from LCB mostly during the acidic pretreatment. Acidic substances hinder enzymatic hydrolysis, leading to the inactivation of metabolic activity in most alcoholic fermentation yeast strains (Hasunuma and Kondo, 2012). Their concentration influences the toxicity of the inhibitors; the type of microbes used for fermentation; the culture technique; and conditions such as pH, temperature, and oxygen content (van der Polet al., 2015). Lower sugar yields result from furan aldehydes like formic and levulinic acids; hence, limiting their production during pretreatment is desirable. Quinones and small aliphatic aldehydes are inhibitory chemicals that can form during acidic pretreatment (Figure 15.4) (Jönsson et al., 2015).

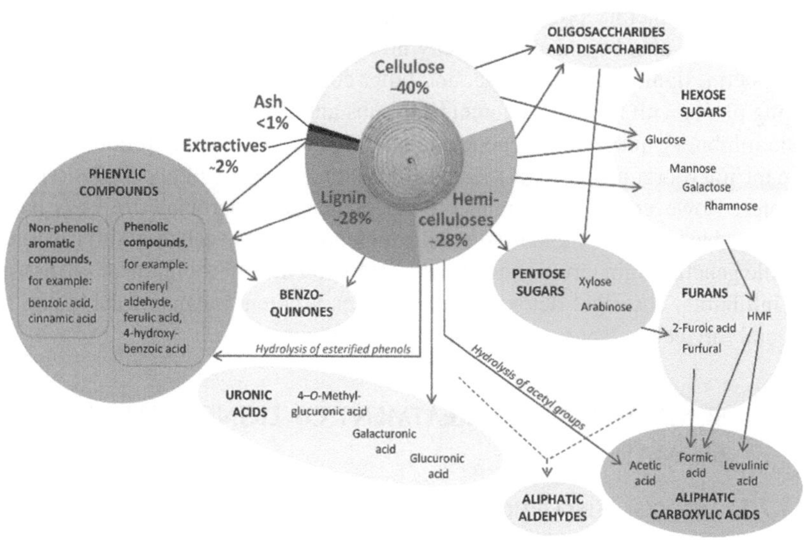

FIGURE 15.4 Acidic pretreatment degradation products from lignocellulosic biomass.

Soluble carbohydrates and aromatic compounds also inhibit cellulases in the pretreatment medium. The inhibitory effects of oligosaccharides produced from xylan and mannan have been studied. The existence of such oligosaccharides is determined by the pretreatment technique and the presence of enzymes that break down hemicellulose-derived oligosaccharides. Phenolics and related solubilized aromatics may deleteriously impact enzymatic saccharification (Purkait et al., 2005). This suggests that aromatic chemicals contribute primarily to the inhibition of cellulolytic enzymes; the issue is also caused by hydrophobic interactions between aromatic compounds and cellulolytic enzymes.

15.6.2.2 Overcoming Inhibitors

One effective strategy to combat inhibition issues is detoxifying or conditioning lignocellulosic hydrolysates and slurries. This method utilizes chemical additives such as polymers, alkali, and other reducing agents. Many detoxification procedures have the disadvantage of requiring a separate process step. Microbial strains having high inhibitor resistance can be identified by screening groups of microorganisms sourced from industrial or natural locations. The specific productivity of the microbe is a crucial consideration, as resistance to inhibitors is insufficient to qualify a bacterium for industrial-scale production. The sugars and inhibitors' quantities in hydrolysates are affected by the biomass sample and the conditions during pretreatment and hydrolysis (Galbe and Zacchi, 2007). As a result, one option is to use a less resistant feedstock, enabling pretreatment under moderate conditions. However, the generation of chemicals from renewable sources is expected to significantly influence the markets for chemicals, fuels, and materials. In that case, it is preferable to use a variety of lignocelluloses.

Furthermore, because manufacturing bulk chemicals is yield-dependent, tolerating a low sugar yield is not realistic. This will lead to a low total product yield due to unsatisfactory pretreatment conditions. The recalcitrance associated with the LCB can also be reduced, thereby minimizing inhibitor release by engineering pectin, lignin, hemicellulose, and other components. The selection of developing plants with low acetyl content can substantially reduce the danger of acetic acid inhibitory quantities. Genetic engineering has successfully produced recombinant microorganisms with increased resistance toward lignocellulosic hydrolysates. However, the performance of the generated microbial strains is hardly comparable to that of standard detoxification procedures such as alkali treatment. While genetic engineering dramatically improved the microorganism's resistance to inhibitors, chemical detoxification remains a potent means of achieving fermentability equivalent to that in an inhibitor-free medium.

15.7 SUMMARY OF PRETREATMENT OF LIGNOCELLULOSIC BIOMASS

15.7.1 Process Description

In biorefining, pretreatment is vital for efficiently converting LCB into value-added products, including biofuels (ethanol, butanol, etc.), monomeric sugars, and other chemicals. Pretreatment can modify the recalcitrance of LCB and facilitate its deconstruction into individual components, namely cellulose, hemicellulose, and lignin. The choice of pretreatment and the type and state of the pretreated LCB will, in turn, determine the downstream process (enzyme hydrolysis/fermentation) to be implemented, preconditioning requirements (if any), the utility of by-products, waste management, and the recovery of desired products. It also impacts each process economically. A single pretreatment method does not apply to all LCBs, as each type has its own complexities and compositional differences.

Table 15.1 summarizes the different types of pretreatment methods and their advantages and disadvantages. Physical pretreatment methods primarily focus on modifying biomass's physical attributes, such as reducing crystallinity, decreasing particle size, increasing surface area, and altering fiber structural properties. Although these processes offer the benefits of ease of operation and reduced production of inhibitory compounds, they may be power- and energy-intensive, incur high costs, and be suitable only for specific biomass types (Devi et al., 2021). The remaining pretreatment methods, namely, chemical, physicochemical, and biological processes, emphasize the fractionation of the major components and lignin removal (Bajpai et al., 2022). These methods can achieve high efficiency and selectivity. However, some techniques, such as ILs or SCF, still entail high capital and operating costs. In addition, the risk of inhibitor formation is higher with these techniques, though there are a few exceptions. In general, the industrial adoption of any pretreatment process is relatively rare due to the significant limitations associated with each unit operation (Hassan et al., 2018). The major challenge is to develop a low-cost, industry-friendly method for LCB pretreatment. Due to the significant constraints associated with each unit activity, industrial adaptations of any one of the pretreatment processes are often reasonably uncommon. Hybrid processes involving two or more processes specific to the end application may help increase pretreatment's overall efficiency with minimal waste and cost (Akhtar et al., 2016).

15.7.2 Economic Assessment

The primary objective of pretreatment is to break down the LCB matrix by removing lignin and hemicellulose and de-crystallizing cellulose, thereby enhancing its susceptibility to enzymatic hydrolysis or fermentation. Ideally, the chosen pretreatment method should be both efficient and economically viable. Several factors need to be evaluated to determine the financial feasibility of the selected process. The type of feedstock used is a critical factor, with studies indicating it can account for over 50% of total production costs, although some report a lower contribution of 18–22% (Vasco-Correa and Shah, 2019). A pretreatment method that enhances monomer yield and/or produces highly concentrated treated LCB can significantly improve the overall economics of the process. On the other hand, treating biomass with high monomer yield but low concentration will require large reaction tanks, thereby increasing operating costs. Processes involving high temperatures and pressures (e.g., extrusion, wet oxidation, AFEX, steam explosion,

TABLE 15.1
Comparative Analysis of Different Types of Pretreatment Methods Employed for Lignocellulosic Biomass Treatment

Pretreatment	Effect	Advantages	Disadvantages
Physical pretreatment			
Comminution	Reduces the size and degree of crystallinity	Increased surface area, no production of inhibitory compounds, control of final particle size	Power and energy-intensive, lignin is not solubilized
Microwave	Uniform and rapid heating of large biomass particles, fiber swelling, and fragmentation	Low capital cost, simple operation, and energy efficiency	Substantial energy cost, high investment and operation costs, and limited knowledge of the dielectric properties of biomass
Extrusion	Shortening of fiber, defibrillation, and increased surface area due to high mechanical stress	Low energy requirement, operation at high solids loadings, low production of inhibitory compounds, short operation time	Expensive, more suited for herbaceous biomass, high energy expenditure, and limited effect without the aid of chemical agents
Ultrasonication	Disruption of cavitation bubbles splits the structural polysaccharides and lignin fractions	Short treatment time, high activation energy, and effective mass transfer	Energy intensive
Chemical pretreatment			
Alkaline hydrolysis	Increase in cellulose digestibility and lignin solubilization	Increased accessible surface area and porosity, selective breakdown of lignin structure without degradation of carbohydrates	High capital investment, harsh organic solvents, and the need for a neutralizing step to eliminate lignin and inhibitors
Acid hydrolysis	Hemicellulose and lignin fractionation	An increase in accessible surface area and enzymatic hydrolysis may be avoided if the acid is enough for hydrolysis	Corrosive, hazardous, toxic, requiring expensive corrosion-resistant equipment, and requiring a neutralization step for the removal of acids and inhibitors
Wet oxidation	Delignification, decrystallization, and partial degradation of cellulose	It does not require a dewatering step before treatment	Its nonselective nature may cause significant loss of hemicellulose, considerable expense of catalyst and oxygen, equipment for the high-pressure generation, and production of inhibitors

Physicochemical pretreatment			
Steam explosion	Solubilization of hemicellulose, disruption of the fiber matrix	Lower energy requirement than mechanical comminution, low pollution hazard, and negligible cost for waste stream recycling	Breakdown of xylan fragments, generation of inhibitory byproducts, and incomplete disruption of lignin completely
Liquid hot water	Hydration of cellulosic material, removal of hemicellulose and lignin	Size reduction is not a prerequisite; a corrosion-resistant container is not required, no chemicals or toxic inhibitors are produced, and low-cost neutralization is not required	The average solid load is unsuitable for softwood, and the formation of inhibitors increases as the temperature rises
AFEX	Lignin removal and reduction in cellulose crystallinity	High efficiency and selectivity for altering and solubilizing lignin, an increase in accessible surface area, and higher loadings of solids in the fermentation procedure, as it is a dry-based method	Less effective for softwood, cost of ammonia, environmental concerns, not ideal for high lignin content biomass, compared to dilute acid Pretreatment solubilizes hemicellulose to a lesser extent
Soaking in aqueous ammonia	Lignin removal	Simple, high xylose recovery, minimal sugar degradation, and less inhibitory compounds formation	Low efficiency
Ammonia recycle percolation	Lignin removal	Increased sugar yield, lower ammonia, and water requirement	High energy cost, ineffective for treating high-lignin-containing LCB, the cost of ammonia, and environmental concerns
SCF	Selective removal of lignin	Nontoxic, cheap, noninflammable, green, flexible/versatile solvating power (when CO_2 is used as a solvent)	High set-up cost
Organosolv	Lignin removal and hemicellulose fractionation	Produces low residual lignin substrates that reduce unwanted enzyme adsorption, allowing its recycling and reuse, increasing the accessible surface area, hemicellulose hydrolysis, and convenience restoring and recycling solvents	High capital investment, harsh organic solvents, and inhibitor formation. Pretreatment is necessary in highly restricted environments.

(*Continued*)

TABLE 15.1 (*Continued*)
Comparative Analysis of Different Types of Pretreatment Methods Employed for Lignocellulosic Biomass Treatment

Pretreatment	Effect	Advantages	Disadvantages
Ionic liquids	Decrystallization of cellulose, partial hemicellulose, and lignin removal	Nonflammability, good chemical and thermal stability, recoverable and reusable solvent, solubilization of a large quantity of cellulose at moderate conditions	High cost of ILs, inhibitors formation, strenuous recycling and reuse, lethality to microorganisms and enzymes, poor biodegradability
Carbon dioxide explosion	Disintegration of cellulose and hemicellulose matrix	Green technique, CO_2 is nontoxic and cheap, and increases the digestibility of biomass	For expensive instruments, the lignin structure is not altered and solubilized
Ozonolysis	Hemicellulose solubilization, alteration, and solubilization of lignin structure	The process is carried out at standard temperature and pressure, with no toxic residues and an increase in accessible surface area	Expensive due to a massive amount of ozone requirement, high operational costs
Biological pretreatment	Lignin degradation	No requirement for chemicals, less energy input, mild operating conditions, and environmentally friendly	It is a slow process that requires ample space and careful control of growth conditions. Most ligninolytic fungi solubilize/consume hemicellulose and cellulose in addition to lignin

CDE) require superior construction materials to manufacture the vessels in which these conditions prevail. This will further add to the cost. Land use management, recovery, removal of inhibitory compounds, waste management, steam recycling, chemicals, and so forth will directly impact the economy. The nature and volume of chemicals used (alkali hydrolysis, acid hydrolysis, AFEX, ARP, etc.) must be thoroughly understood and analyzed. Large chemical volumes will need large reaction volumes, and additional expenses must be incurred for disposal or reuse. Handling corrosive chemicals (acid hydrolysis) is risky, poses environmental hazards, and increases operating costs. Dilute or organic acids may counter the high price (da Costa Sousa et al., 2009).

One approach to improve the process economics would be to utilize CO_2 produced during fermentation in pretreatment methods such as CDE and SCF after suitable processing. However, this approach is limited to only a few techniques. Another interesting approach can be universally applied to all pretreatment methods in lignin's recovery and utilization. Lignin valorization can be achieved by the production of bio-oil and by subsequent processing of this unstable, phenolic, acidic oil to obtain (i) valuable chemicals, such as benzene, toluene, and xylene, to name a few, and (ii) hydrocarbons of fuel grade (Kumar et al., 2020). The process of economics is rather complex, as many factors are at play. In practice, no pretreatment can be ideally efficient or economical. After thoroughly analyzing all the aspects to achieve a commercially efficient and economical process, there must be a compromise among the many factors involved.

15.8 CONCLUSION

LCB, in the form of hardwood, softwood, agricultural wastes, and grasses, is a promising energy source for biorefining. Agricultural wastes are of particular interest because they are abundant, and their utilization will also curb pollution. The efficient conversion of LCB to biofuels can help wean the world away from its dependence on fast-depleting petroleum-based fuels and move toward more sustainable biofuels such as ethanol and butanol. However, native LCB is recalcitrant owing to its intrinsic compositional, physicochemical, and structural factors. Pretreatment is a prerequisite for overcoming LCB's recalcitrant nature and enabling efficient bioconversion. It can reduce the crystallinity of biomass and allow easy access to the monomers by hydrolytic enzymes/fermenting culture during bioconversion. Pretreatment can efficiently convert them into fermentable sugars by modifying the physical and chemical properties of the plant cell wall.

The pretreatment technique and the type of lignocellulosic material used will collectively affect the physical and chemical properties of the pretreated biomass. Several physical, chemical, physicochemical, and biological pretreatments are commonly used for LCB pretreatment. All existing techniques have their own benefits and limitations. Commercial-scale pretreatment of LCB faces several challenges, including high energy requirements, high capital and operating costs, and low downstream processing efficiency. Extensive studies are required to address these issues and to exploit LCB as a bio-source at the commercial level efficiently.

Although the primary goal of pretreatment is to fractionate the primary constituents of biomass and release cellulose for enzymatic saccharification, certain undesirable byproducts hinder downstream processes. The inhibiting compounds are mainly composed of organic acids, aromatics, and sugar degradation products. Lignin derivatives inhibit the fermentation of lignocellulosic hydrolysates even at low concentrations and are considered the most hazardous inhibitors. Identifying or conditioning lignocellulosic hydrolysates and slurries is an effective strategy to combat inhibition issues. This is achieved using chemical additives such as polymers, alkali, and other reducing agents.

15.9 ACKNOWLEDGMENTS

This study was supported by the Indian National Academy of Engineering (INAE/121/AKF/22), Gurgaon, India. The opinions, findings, and conclusions expressed in this work are those of the authors and do not necessarily reflect the views of the Indian National Academy of Engineering.

REFERENCES

N.K. Aggarwal, N. Kumar, M. Mittal, Current trends in pretreatment technologies for bioethanol production: Biorefinery concept, in: *Bioethanol Production. Green Chemistry and Sustainable Technology*. Springer, Cham (2022) 27–45. https://doi.org/10.1007/978-3-031-05091-6_3.

D.L. Aguilar, R.M. Rodríguez-Jasso, E. Zanuso, D.J. de Rodríguez, L. Amaya-Delgado, A. Sanchez, H.A. Ruiz, Scale-up and evaluation of hydrothermal pretreatment in isothermal and non-isothermal regimen for bioethanol production using agave bagasse, *Bioresour. Technol.* 263 (2018) 112–119. https://doi.org/10.1016/j.biortech.2018.04.100.

N. Akhtar, K. Gupta, D. Goyal, A. Goyal, Recent advances in pretreatment technologies for efficient hydrolysis of lignocellulosic biomass, *Environ. Prog. Sustain. Energy.* 35 (2016) 489–511. https://doi.org/10.1002/EP.12257.

P. Bajpai, Physical and chemical characteristics of lignocellulosic biomass, *Lignocellul. Biomass Biotechnol.* (2022) 11–24. https://doi.org/10.1016/B978-0-12-821889-1.00001-1.

S. Behera, R. Arora, N. Nandhagopal, S. Kumar, Importance of chemical pretreatment for bioconversion of lignocellulosic biomass, *Renew. Sustain. Energy Rev.* 36 (2014) 91–106. https://doi.org/10.1016/j.rser.2014.04.047.

A.W. Bhutto, K. Qureshi, K. Harijan, R. Abro, T. Abbas, A.A. Bazmi, S. Karim, G. Yu, Insight into progress in pre-treatment of lignocellulosic biomass, *Energy.* 122 (2017) 724–745. https://doi.org/10.1016/j.energy.2017.01.005.

N. Cheng, K. Koda, Y. Tamai, Y. Yamamoto, T.E. Takasuka, Y. Uraki, Optimization of simultaneous saccharification and fermentation conditions with amphipathic lignin derivatives for concentrated bioethanol production, *Bioresour. Technol.* 232 (2017) 126–132. https://doi.org/10.1016/j.biortech.2017.02.018.

H.M. Cho, A.S. Gross, J.W. Chu, Dissecting force interactions in cellulose deconstruction reveals the required solvent versatility for overcoming biomass recalcitrance, *J. Am. Chem. Soc.* 133 (2011) 14033–14041. https://doi.org/10.1021/ja2046155.

S.P.S. Chundawat, R.K. Pal, C. Zhao, T. Campbell, F. Teymouri, J. Videto, C. Nielson, B. Wieferich, L. Sousa, B.E. Dale, V. Balan, S. Chipkar, J. Aguado, E. Burke, R.G. Ong, Ammonia fiber expansion (AFEX) pretreatment of lignocellulosic biomass, *J. Vis. Exp*. 2020 (2020) 1–8. https://doi.org/10.3791/57488.

L. da Costa Sousa, S.P. Chundawat, V. Balan, B.E. Dale, "Cradle-to-grave" assessment of existing lignocellulose pretreatment technologies, *Curr. Opin. Biotechnol*. 20 (2009) 339–347. https://doi.org/10.1016/j.copbio.2009.05.003.

B. Debnath, D. Haldar, M.K. Purkait, Potential and sustainable utilization of tea waste: A review on present status and future trends, *J. Environ. Chem. Eng*. 9 (2021) 106179. https://doi.org/10.1016/j.jece.2021.106179.

W. Den, V.K. Sharma, M. Lee, G. Nadadur, R.S. Varma, Lignocellulosic biomass transformations via greener oxidative pretreatment processes: Access to energy and value-added chemicals, *Front. Chem*. 6 (2018) 1–23. https://doi.org/10.3389/fchem 2018.00141.

A. Devi, A. Singh, S. Bajar, D. Pant, Z.U. Din, Ethanol from lignocellulosic biomass: An in-depth analysis of pre-treatment methods, fermentation approaches and detoxification processes, *J. Environ. Chem. Eng*. 9 (2021) 105798. https://doi.org/10.1016/j.jece.2021.105798.

A.B. Diaz, M. Maria de Souza Moretti, C. Bezerra-Bussoli, C. da Costa Carreira Nunes, A. Blandino, R. da Silva, E. Gomes, Evaluation of microwave-assisted pretreatment of lignocellulosic biomass immersed in alkaline glycerol for fermentable sugars production, *Bioresour. Technol*. 185 (2015) 316–323. https://doi.org/10.1016/j.biortech.2015.02.112.

P. Duarah, D. Haldar, A.K. Patel, C. Di Dong, R.R. Singhania, M.K. Purkait, A review on global perspectives of sustainable development in bioenergy generation, *Bioresour. Technol*. 348 (2022) 126791. https://doi.org/10.1016/j.biortech.2022.126791.

P. Duarah, D. Haldar, M.K. Purkait, Technological advancement in the synthesis and applications of lignin-based nanoparticles derived from agro-industrial waste residues: A review, *Int. J. Biol. Macromol*. 163 (2020) 1828–1843. https://doi.org/10.1016/j.ijbiomac.2020.09.076.

A. Duque, P. Manzanares, M. Ballesteros, Extrusion as a pretreatment for lignocellulosic biomass: Fundamentals and applications, *Renew. Energy*. 114 (2017) 1427–1441. https://doi.org/10.1016/j.renene.2017.06.050.

A. Duque, P. Manzanares, I. Ballesteros, M. Ballesteros, Steam explosion as lignocellulosic biomass pretreatment, in: *Biomass Fractionation Technology for a lignocellulosic Feedstock Based Biorefinery*. (2016) 349–368. https://doi.org/10.1016/B978-0-12-802323-5.00015-3.

M. Ferdeş, M.N. Dincă, G. Moiceanu, B.Ş. Zabava, G. Paraschiv, Microorganisms and enzymes used in the biological pretreatment of the substrate to enhance biogas production: A review, *Sustainability*. 12 (2020). https://doi.org/10.3390/su12177205.

M. Galbe, G. Zacchi, Pretreatment of lignocellulosic materials for efficient bioethanol production, *Adv. Biochem. Eng. Biotechnol*. 108 (2007) 41–65. https://doi.org/10.1007/10_2007_070/COVER/.

A. Gupta, J.P. Verma, Sustainable bio-ethanol production from agro-residues: A review, *Renew. Sustain. Energy Rev*. 41 (2015) 550–567. https://doi.org/10.1016/j.rser.2014.08.032.

D. Haldar, M.K. Purkait, Lignocellulosic conversion into value-added products: A review, *Process Biochem*. 89 (2020) 110–133. https://doi.org/10.1016/j.procbio.2019.10.001.

I.U. Haq, K. Qaisar, A. Nawaz, F. Akram, H. Mukhtar, X. Zohu, Y. Xu, M.W. Mumtaz, U. Rashid, W.A.W.A.K. Ghani, T.S.Y. Choong, Advances in valorization of lignocellulosic biomass towards energy generation, *Catalysts*. 11 (2021) 1–26. https://doi.org/10.3390/catal11030309.

S.S. Hassan, G.A. Williams, A.K. Jaiswal, Emerging technologies for the pretreatment of lignocellulosic biomass, *Bioresour. Technol*. 262 (2018) 310–318. https://doi.org/10.1016/j.biortech.2018.04.099.

T. Hasunuma, A. Kondo, Consolidated bioprocessing and simultaneous saccharification and fermentation of lignocellulose to ethanol with thermotolerant yeast strains, *Process Biochem.* 47 (2012) 1287–1294. https://doi.org/10.1016/j.procbio.2012.05.004.

S. Jayasekara, R. Ratnayake, Microbial cellulases: An overview and applications, *Cellulose.* (2019). https://doi.org/10.5772/intechopen. 84531.

J.M. Jimenez-Gutierrez, R.A.J. Verlinden, P.C. van der Meer, L.A.M. van der Wielen, A.J.J. Straathof, Liquid hot water pretreatment of lignocellulosic biomass at lab and pilot scale, *Processes.* 9 (2021) 1–12. https://doi.org/10.3390/pr9091518.

L.J. Jönsson, C. Martín, Pretreatment of lignocellulose: Formation of inhibitory by-products and strategies for minimizing their effects, *Bioresour. Technol.* 199 (2016) 103–112. https://doi.org/10.1016/j.biortech.2015.10.009.

D. Kim, Physico-chemical conversion of lignocellulose: Inhibitor effects and detoxification strategies: A mini review, *Molecules.* 23 (2018). https://doi.org/10.3390/molecules23020309.

T.H. Kim, Y.Y. Lee, Pretreatment of corn stover by soaking in aqueous ammonia at moderate temperatures, *Appl. Biochem. Biotecnol.* (2007) 81–92. https://doi.org/10.1007/978-1-60327-181-3_8.

N. Kordala, M. Lewandowska, W. Bednarski, Effect of the method for the elimination of inhibitors present in Miscanthus giganteus hydrolysates on ethanol production effectiveness, *Biomass Convers. Biorefinery.* (2021). https://doi.org/10.1007/s13399-020-01255-2.

A. Kumar, Anushree, J. Kumar, T. Bhaskar, Utilization of lignin: A sustainable and eco-friendly approach, *J. Energy Inst.* 93 (2020) 235–271. https://doi.org/10.1016/j.joei.2019.03.005.

B. Kumar, N. Bhardwaj, K. Agrawal, V. Chaturvedi, P. Verma, Current perspective on pretreatment technologies using lignocellulosic biomass: An emerging biorefinery concept, *Fuel Process. Technol.* 199 (2020). https://doi.org/10.1016/j.fuproc.2019.106244.

M. Madadi, A. Abbas, Lignin degradation by fungal pretreatment: A review, *J. Plant Pathol. Microbiol.* 08 (2017). https://doi.org/10.4172/21577471.1000398.

A.R. Mankar, A. Pandey, A. Modak, K.K. Pant, Pretreatment of lignocellulosic biomass: A review on recent advances, *Bioresour. Technol.* 334 (2021) 125235. https://doi.org/10.1016/j.biortech.2021.125235.

J.D. McMillan, Pretreatment of lignocellulosic biomass, in: *Enzymatic Conversion of Biomass for Fuels Production: ACS Symposium Series 566.* (1994) 292–324. https://doi.org/10.1021/BK-1994-0566.CH015.

S. Niju, M. Swathika, M. Balaji, *Pretreatment of Lignocellulosic Sugarcane Leaves and Tops for Bioethanol Production.* INC (2019). https://doi.org/10.1016/B978-0-12-815936-1.00010-1.

M. Nikiema, M.K. Somda, K. Adeoti, D. Traore, Production of efficient microbial complex for organic fraction of municipal organic solid waste pretreatment upstream anaerobic digestion, *Int. J. Environ. Bioremediation Biodegrad.* 5 (2017) 77–85. https://doi.org/10.12691/ijebb-5-3-1.

K. Ninomiya, K. Kamide, K. Takahashi, N. Shimizu, Enhanced enzymatic saccharification of kenaf powder after ultrasonic pretreatment in ionic liquids at room temperature, *Bioresour. Technol.* 103 (2012) 259–265. https://doi.org/10.1016/j.biortech.2011.10.019.

K. Poszytek, M. Ciezkowska, A. Sklodowska, L. Drewniak, Microbial Consortium with High Cellulolytic Activity (MCHCA) for enhanced biogas production, *Front. Microbiol.* 7 (2016) 1–11. https://doi.org/10.3389/fmicb.2016.00324.

M.K. Purkait, S. DasGupta, S. De, Micellar enhanced ultrafiltration of phenolic derivatives from their mixtures, *J. Colloid Interface Sci.* 285 (2005) 395–402. https://doi.org/10.1016/j.jcis.2004.11.036.

S. Rahmati, W. Doherty, D. Dubal, L. Atanda, L. Moghaddam, P. Sonar, V. Hessel, K. Ostrikov, Pretreatment and fermentation of lignocellulosic biomass: Reaction mechanisms and process engineering, *React. Chem. Eng.* 5 (2020) 2017–2047. https://doi.org/10.1039/d0re00241k.

A.A. Salema, F.N. Ani, J. Mouris, R. Hutcheon, Microwave dielectric properties of Malaysian palm oil and agricultural industrial biomass and biochar during pyrolysis process, *Fuel Process. Technol.* 166 (2017) 164–173. https://doi.org/10.1016/j.fuproc.2017.06.006.

F. Taghizadeh, M. Ghaedi, K. Kamali, E. Sharifpour, R. Sahraie, M.K. Purkait, Comparison of nickel and/or zinc selenide nanoparticle loaded on activated carbon as efficient adsorbents for kinetic and equilibrium study of removal of Arsenazo (III) dye, *Powder Technol.* 245 (2013) 217–226. https://doi.org/10.1016/j.powtec.2013.04.020.

M.J. Taherzadeh, K. Karimi, Pretreatment of lignocellulosic wastes to improve ethanol and biogas production: A review, *International Journal of Molecular Sciences.* (2008). https://doi.org/10.3390/ijms9091621.

E. Tomás-Pejó, P. Alvira, M. Ballesteros, M.J. Negro, Pretreatment technologies for lignocellulose-to-bioethanol conversion, *Biofuels.* (2011) 149–176. https://doi.org/10.1016/B978-0-12-385099-7.00007-3.

R. Travaini, J. Martín-Juárez, A. Lorenzo-Hernando, S. Bolado-Rodríguez, Ozonolysis: An advantageous pretreatment for lignocellulosic biomass revisited, *Bioresour. Technol.* 199 (2016) 2–12. https://doi.org/10.1016/j.biortech.2015.08.143.

Ummalyma SB, Sahoo D, Pandey A. Resource recovery through bioremediation of wastewaters and waste carbon by microalgae: a circular bioeconomy approach. *Environmental Science and Pollution Research.* 2021;28(42):58837-58856.

E. van der Pol, R. Bakker, A. van Zeeland, D. Sanchez Garcia, A. Punt, G. Eggink, Analysis of by-product formation and sugar monomerization in sugarcane bagasse pretreated at pilot plant scale: Differences between autohydrolysis, alkaline and acid pretreatment, *Bioresour. Technol.* 181 (2015) 114–123. https://doi.org/10.1016/j.biortech.2015.01.033.

J. Vasco-Correa, A. Shah, Techno-economic bottlenecks of the fungal pretreatment of lignocellulosic biomass, *Fermentation.* 5 (2019). https://doi.org/10.3390/fermentation5020030.

V. Wyman, J. Henríquez, C. Palma, A. Carvajal, Lignocellulosic waste valorisation strategy through enzyme and biogas production, *Bioresour. Technol.* 247 (2018) 402–411. https://doi.org/10.1016/j.biortech.2017.09.055.

H.M. Zabed, S. Akter, J. Yun, G. Zhang, F.N. Awad, X. Qi, J.N. Sahu, Recent advances in biological pretreatment of microalgae and lignocellulosic biomass for biofuel production, *Renew. Sustain. Energy Rev.* 105 (2019) 105–128. https://doi.org/10.1016/j.rser.2019.01.048.

J. Zhang, W. Hou, J. Bao, Reactors for high solid loading pretreatment of lignocellulosic biomass, *Adv. Biochem. Eng. Biotechnol.* 152 (2016) 75–90. https://doi.org/10.1007/10_2015_307/cover/.

C. Zhao, Q. Shao, S.P.S. Chundawat, Recent advances on ammonia-based pretreatments of lignocellulosic biomass, *Bioresour. Technol.* 298 (2020) 122446. https://doi.org/10.1016/j.biortech.2019.122446.

X. Zhuang, W. Wang, Q. Yu, W. Qi, Q. Wang, X. Tan, G. Zhou, Z. Yuan, Liquid hot water pretreatment of lignocellulosic biomass for bioethanol production accompanying with high valuable products, *Bioresour. Technol.* 199 (2016) 68–75. https://doi.org/10.1016/j.biortech.2015.08.051.

16 N-Methyl Morpholine-N-Oxide Pretreatment of Lignocellulosic Biomass for Conversion to Ethanol and Biogas

Na Wu, Shunchang Yang, Spyros Svoronos, and Pratap Pullammanappallil

16.1 INTRODUCTION

Recently, biofuels have received heightened attention amid growing concerns about climate change and energy security. Lignocellulosic biomass is a promising feedstock for biofuel production, as it is abundant and nonedible compared to sugar-based biomass. The abundant supply of lignocellulosic biomass and its low cost not only provide a feasible and sustainable solution to the energy crisis but also offer the potential for environmental and economic benefits. However, to date, biofuels have been commercially produced from sugar-based feedstocks and organic waste. Technologies for producing biofuels from lignocellulosic feedstocks are being developed.

There are two approaches to producing biofuels from bio-renewable resources. One is the sugar platform, where lignocellulosic biomass, specifically cellulose and hemicellulose, is depolymerized to monomeric sugars using various pretreatment techniques, and these sugars are then fermented to produce products such as ethanol, butanol, and other hydrocarbons. The second approach is the syngas platform, in which lignocellulosic biomass is thermally gasified to syngas (a mixture of carbon monoxide and hydrogen), which is then converted to products such as methanol and hydrocarbons. The sugar platform offers many advantages, such as milder operating conditions, higher product specificity and selectivity, and the potential for valuable co-products. Biochemical processes (hydrolysis and fermentation) typically operate at much lower temperatures (often <100°C, sometimes near ambient) and atmospheric pressure compared to the very high temperatures (>700°C) and often elevated pressures required for gasification. This can lead to

 DOI: 10.1201/9781003327608-16

lower capital costs for reactor materials (less need for exotic alloys), simpler reactor designs, and lower energy input for core conversion steps (though pretreatment can be energy-intensive). Operating conditions are generally considered safer. Microbial fermentation pathways can be very specific. By choosing or engineering the right microorganisms, it's possible to produce a high yield of a specific target biofuel (like ethanol or butanol) with fewer undesirable by-products. This contrasts with processes like Fischer–Tropsch synthesis on the syngas platform, which often produce a broader range of hydrocarbon chain lengths, requiring more complex downstream separation and upgrading to meet fuel specifications. Higher selectivity can simplify purification and improve overall process economics for a specific target fuel. The biochemical platform primarily targets the carbohydrate fraction of the biomass (cellulose and hemicellulose). The lignin fraction, which is often separated during pretreatment, can be recovered and utilized as a valuable co-product for materials or chemicals or as a solid fuel (often burned for process heat/power). While the syngas platform utilizes lignin's energy content via gasification, the biochemical route offers the potential to create higher-value streams from lignin beyond burning it, potentially improving overall biorefinery economics. This chapter addresses pretreatment enhancements to the sugar platform to economically increase biofuel yield with minimal environmental impact.

Lignocellulosic biomass contains mainly cellulose, hemicellulose, and lignin. Concentrations of the three components vary across species. Table 16.1 shows the major categories of lignocellulosic biomass. Common agricultural crop residuals, such as corn stover, wheat straw, and rice straw, contain 29–38% of cellulose, 24–32% of hemicellulose, and 16–21% of lignin. The content of these components in agricultural manufacturing residues, such as sugarcane bagasse and banana waste, varies widely. For example, the concentrations of cellulose, hemicellulose, and lignin in sugarcane bagasse are 42%, 25%, and 20%, respectively (Kim and Day, 2011), whereas banana waste contains around 14% of each component (Anwar et al., 2014).

TABLE 16.1
Categories of Lignocellulosic Biomass

Agriculture residues (plants and crop residues, animal residues, manufacturing residues)	Corn stover, corn bobs, wheat straw, rice straw, cattle and swine manure solids, sugarcane bagasse, nut shells, banana waste, cottonseed hairs
Woody biomass (tree and tree residues, wood manufacturing residues)	Hardwood (e.g., birch, willow, poplar, eucalyptus trees), softwood (e.g., pine, spruce).
Grass	Grasses, switchgrass, coastal bermudagrass
Municipal solid waste	Organic portion of solid waste and trash destined for landfills (e.g., sewage sludge, paper, newspaper, cardboard, wastepaper from chemical pulps)

The primary structural materials of plant cell walls of lignocellulosic biomass are cellulose, hemicellulose, and lignin. It is a natural composite material in which each component plays a specific role and interacts closely with the others. Cellulose is the main structural component. It is a long, linear polymer made of glucose units, linked end to end by β-1,4 glycosidic bonds. Many parallel cellulose chains align themselves through extensive hydrogen bonding to form highly ordered, crystalline structures called cellulose microfibrils. These microfibrils are like strong cables providing tensile strength to the plant cell wall. Cellulose provides the fundamental structural framework and strength. Hemicelluloses are branched polymers made up of various sugar units (like xylose, mannose, galactose, arabinose, etc.). They are generally much shorter than cellulose chains and have an amorphous (noncrystalline) structure. Hemicellulose chains coat the surface of the cellulose microfibrils. They interact primarily with cellulose via hydrogen bonds because they are branched and chemically diverse, acting as bridges or tethers between cellulose microfibrils and also connecting to lignin. Lignin is very different from cellulose and hemicellulose. It is a complex, three-dimensional, amorphous polymer made up of phenolic units (derived from phenylpropane alcohols) and is hydrophobic in nature. Lignin acts like glue or cement. It fills the spaces between the cellulose microfibrils and the hemicellulose matrix. Crucially, lignin forms covalent bonds (strong chemical links, primarily ether and ester bonds) with hemicellulose. While direct covalent lignin-cellulose links are thought to be less frequent, lignin effectively encrusts and embeds the cellulose-hemicellulose network. Lignin provides rigidity, stiffness, and compression strength to the cell wall. Its hydrophobic nature prevents excessive water penetration and acts as a barrier protecting the polysaccharides (cellulose and hemicellulose) from enzymatic and microbial degradation. This tightly integrated structure makes lignocellulosic biomass strong and resistant to breakdown, which is essential for the plant but a major challenge when seeking to access its sugars for applications such as biofuel production (Brandt et al., 2013; Potumarthi et al., 2013).

Methods employed to break down the recalcitrant structure of lignocellulosic biomass are referred to as pretreatments. Various pretreatment methods have been developed to facilitate the release of monomeric sugars. However, the pretreatment step is generally considered the most expensive step in the whole process (Zhang, 2011; Potumarthi et al., 2013; Chaturvedi and Verma, 2013). Thus, effective and economical pretreatment techniques are vital in the biofuel conversion process.

16.2 PRETREATMENT OF LIGNOCELLULOSIC BIOMASS

The pretreatment mechanism for lignocellulosic biomass essentially involves disrupting or altering the structure of lignocellulosic materials to increase surface area and porosity, reduce crystallinity, and facilitate chemical or enzyme penetration into cellulose and hemicellulose, accompanied by changes in solubility, depolymerization, and bond-breaking that crosslink the macromolecules.

The pretreatment objectives include the following (Brodeur et al., 2011; Woźniak et al., 2025; Fan et al., 2025; Zhao et al., 2025; Capolupo and Faraco, 2016; Kim and Yoo, 2021; Yang et al., 2018):

1. Preserve cellulose and hemicellulose
2. Being effective on a wide range of lignocellulosic biomass
3. Limit formation of degradation products that affect downstream processes, including inhibiting the growth of fermentative microorganisms
4. Offer high enzymatic hydrolysis and fermentation yields
5. Minimize energy demand
6. Offer cost-effectiveness (inexpensive additives and energy input and possible recycling)
7. Generate value-added coproducts
8. Environmentally friendly (minimize the use of toxic substances)

A fundamental understanding of the mechanisms (both physical and chemical) is essential for selecting a pretreatment method for a given biomass (Mosier et al., 2005). Besides, a comprehensive analysis of the relationships among biomass structure and composition, enzyme digestibility and fermentability, and any associated inhibition and coproducts across the whole process would assist in the overall design, control, and optimization of biofuel production.

Table 16.2 outlines promising pretreatment methods and their effect on cellulose, hemicellulose, and lignin. There are no rigorous boundaries between

TABLE 16.2
Pretreatment Methods and Their Effects

Pretreatment Methods	Cellulose	Hemicellulose	Lignin
Steam explosion	An insignificant amount of cellulose degraded to glucose	Partial hydrolysis and solubilization to mono- and oligosaccharides	Redistribution on fiber surfaces, slightly solubilized
Dilute acid pretreatment	No significant changes	Hydrolyzed, releasing monomeric sugars and soluble oligomers	No significant changes
Alkaline hydrolysis	Partial solubilized under certain conditions	Dissolution under certain conditions	Removal by dissolution or modification
Organosolv process	Hydrolysis to a small extent	Depolymerized by hydrolysis of the glycosidic bonds in hemicelluloses	Hydrolysis of the internal bonds in lignin and also between lignin and hemicellulose
Cellulose solvent-based pretreatments	Dissolved by disrupting the bonds among cellulose	Degradation under certain conditions	No significant delignification

different pretreatments, as some approaches combine methods such as acid-catalyzed steam explosion. Comparing various pretreatment methods is challenging due to the variations in biomass and the configurations of upstream and downstream processes. Nevertheless, an integrated assessment of a biorefinery can be utilized to identify the most suitable pretreatment for a particular feedstock based on the industrial process (Agbor et al., 2011).

Among the above-listed pretreatment methods, solvent-based pretreatment has been shown to achieve greater cellulose accessibility than conventional pretreatments such as acid or alkaline pretreatments (Sathitsuksanoh et al., 2013; Mancini et al., 2016). Substrate accessibility is the bottom line for microbial fermentation of lignocellulosic biomass, meaning that the removal of lignin or hemicellulose has limited benefits, depending on the extent of its effect on substrate accessibility (Sathitsuksanoh et al., 2013). Thus, cellulose solvent-based pretreatments can be promising for different sugar-platform-based microbial conversion processes. In addition, it enables lignocellulosic biomass fractionation to produce value-added compounds by co-utilizing other components, which can be economically attractive.

Lignocellulosic biomass fractionation is a new concept in biorefinery: it uses both carbohydrates and lignin to produce high-value products, unlike conventional ethanol-centric production, which relies on sugars released from carbohydrates (Guragain and Vadlani, 2016). The common cellulose solvents are listed in Table 16.3.

16.3 N-METHYL MORPHOLINE-N-OXIDE

In addition to the above cellulose solvents, N-methylmorpholine-N-oxide (NMMO) can be used to pretreat lignocellulosic biomass with many benefits (Table 16.4). It has been one of the most successful commercial solvents for cellulose (Rabideau and Ismail, 2015). In the NMMO pretreatment method, the NMMO concentration is usually 85%. Most studies are performed at temperatures of 90°C, 110°C, 120°C, and 130°C. Biomass pretreatment with NMMO is a novel and efficient method. It has been found that the regenerated cellulose was three times more reactive than that of untreated cellulose in hydrolysis reactions, due to more β-1,4-glycosidic bonds accessible to acid catalysts as well as the increased amorphous part (Zhao et al., 2007).

16.3.1 What Is NMMO?

NMMO is short for N-methyl morpholine-N-oxide (NMMO). It is an organic compound belonging to the family of aliphatic, cyclic, tertiary amine oxides. Its chemical structure features a morpholine ring (a six-membered ring containing oxygen and nitrogen atoms), with the nitrogen atom bonded to a methyl group (CH_3) and an oxygen atom (forming an N-oxide), both of which are highly polar. Its chemical properties are shown in Table 16.5.

TABLE 16.3
Advantages and Disadvantages of Common Cellulose Solvent-Based Pretreatments

Cellulose Solvent	Description	Mechanism	Advantages	Disadvantages
Ionic liquids	Organic salts having imidazolium or pyridinium cations paired with certain anions (e.g.,., Cl^-, $CF_3SO_3^-$, $CF_3CO_2^-$, $CH_3CO_2^-$, $HCOO^-$, HSO_4^-, $R_2PO_4^-$) (Sathitsuksanoh et al., 2012)	Dissolve cellulose fibers through strong hydrogen bond basicity	High yields of sugar, short processing time, minimum inhibitory product formation, eco-friendly (Li et al., 2010)	Expensive
Concentrated phosphoric acid	Concentrations of H_3PO_4: 85.7% w/w (Mancini et al., 2016), 85% H_3PO_4 (Muranaka et al., 2014), 80% H_3PO_4 mixture with hydrogen peroxide (Wang et al., 2014)	Dissolve and recrystallize cellulose and remove hemicellulose	Flexibility in pretreating different feedstock and size (Wang et al., 2014); yield high sugar fast and low temperature (Zhang et al., 2007); no inhibitory effects for downstream processing (Zhang et al., 2007)	A large amount of usage of phosphoric acid; serious corrosion (expensive materials of construction required)
Concentrated NaOH	Concentration of NaOH: 6–20% w/w (Mancini et al., 2016)	NaOH molecules linked to one anhydroglucose unit to allow for the dissolution of cellulose (Egal et al., 2007)	Operate at ambient pressure and relatively low temperatures (Nieves et al., 2011); low pollution; low cost (Egal et al., 2007)	Inhibitory components can be produced (Nieves et al., 2011); incomplete dissolution for high molecular weight celluloses (Egal et al., 2007)
DMAc/LiCl solution	N, N-dimethylacetamide/lithium chloride, high temperatures (i.e., 150°C) required	Dissolve cellulose by forming strong hydrogen bonds between the hydroxyl protons of cellulose and the Cl^- of the solvent	Generate a complete, preferably direct dissolution of cellulose in non-degrading systems for cellulose analysis, shaping, and chemical modification (Hasani et al., 2013; Zhang et al., 2014)	Retained most of the original crystal structure of cellulose (Wang et al., 2011); high temperature; significantly varying conditions for different biomasses (Hasani et al., 2013)
Sodium carbonate	Na_2CO_3 (4%) with 60 min microwave, 0.5 MNa_2CO_3 at 110°C for 2 hr (Dehghani et al., 2015)	Break the ester bonds between lignin, hemicellulose, and cellulose; enhance the polyionic character of the pretreated lignocelluloses; and promote swelling. (Dehghani et al., 2015)	Inexpensive and environmentally friendly	Inhibition effects of higher concentration due to peeling reactions of carbohydrate end groups (Kaur et al., 2016; Dehghani et al., 2015)

TABLE 16.4
Benefits of the NMMO Pretreatment Method

Operational Benefits	Environmental Benefits	Economic Benefits
1. Rare carbohydrate loss 2. Retains the composition of biomass 3. Flexible in the choice of lignocellulosic biomass 4. No need for chemical neutralization 5. Ambient pressure, relatively moderate conditions (<130°C) 6. High efficiency and yields in enzymatic hydrolysis 7. Potential to be used in a continuous process	1. Human health and ecosystem friendly: nontoxic solvent, no toxic waste produced, fully biodegradable 2. Resources and climate benefits: relatively low energy consumption with moderate operating conditions and high conversion efficiency	High reuse of NMMO (over 98%)

TABLE 16.5
Chemical and Physical Properties of NMMO

Appearance	White Crystalline
Structure	$C_5H_{11}N_2O$
Melting point	180–184°C
Density	1.25 g/cm^3
Saturated vapor pressure	0.35 mm Hg at 25°C, 6.5 mm Hg at 91°C
Molar mass	117.15 g/mol
Water solubility	Unlimited
Crystalline hydrate	a. Monohydrate $C_5H_{11}N_2{\cdot}H_2O$: water content 13.3% (w/w); melting point: 76–78°C b. Di-sesquihydrate (five water molecules per two NMMO molecules) $C_5H_{11}N_2{\cdot}2.5H_2O$: water content 28% (w/w); melting point 39°C

NMMO has been known to be a cellulose solvent since the 1930s (Kulpinski, 2005). Due to the high polarity and weakness of the N—O bond, NMMO has a strong ability to form hydrogen bonds, which is the driving force for cellulose dissolution. It could also be employed as an oxidizing reagent in organic synthesis. This is also due to the energy-rich N—O bond, which can be readily broken and release energy (Rosenau et al., 2001). Besides all these properties, NMMO is stable under normal conditions (Pieterse, 2013), but thermally labile above 100°C (Rosenau et al., 2001, 2002; Ingildeev et al., 2013). The decomposition occurs initially around 100–110°C and becomes more intense at about 130–140°C (Singha, 2012).

There are two crystalline hydrate forms of NMMO (Rosenau et al., 2001). In the monohydrate form of NMMO, one molecule of water is incorporated into the crystal structure and is written as NMMO. H_2O. In the di-sesquihydrate form, NMMO is associated with 2.5 molecules of water, and the formula is NMMO.2.5 H_2O. Anhydrous NMMO cannot be obtained from monohydrate or di-sesquihydrate by simply heating the hydrates above their melting point, as anhydrous NMMO produced in this way is not neat. As mentioned here, NMMO is thermally labile. While heating the monohydrate (melting point ~74°C) or other hydrates will drive off water, NMMO itself undergoes significant thermal decomposition at temperatures well below the melting point of pure anhydrous NMMO (~170°C). Decomposition can become problematic even above 90–120°C, especially under anhydrous conditions. Heating NMMO, particularly to the temperatures required for complete dehydration, leads to various side reactions and degradation products (such as N-methylmorpholine and formaldehyde). Some of these reactions can be autocatalytic and highly exothermic. Because decomposition occurs concurrently with dehydration when hydrates are heated, the resulting anhydrous NMMO is contaminated with these by-products. It is therefore impure or "not neat." Obtaining pure, anhydrous NMMO typically requires methods beyond simple heating, such as azeotropic drying or vacuum sublimation, which remove water under conditions less likely to cause significant thermal decomposition.

16.3.2 How Is It Produced?

NMMO is commercially available in both the monohydrate ($C_5H_{11}NO_2 \cdot H_2O$) and anhydrous forms (Pieterse, 2013). It is produced by the oxidation of N-methylmorpholine with an aqueous solution of hydrogen peroxide (Fink et al., 2001). Hydrogen peroxide oxidizes the nitrogen atom in the N-methylmorpholine molecule. An oxygen atom forms a coordinate covalent bond with the nitrogen atom. The main product formed is N-methyl morpholine-N-oxide. Water (H_2O) is generated as a by-product. CO_2 is used as a catalyst, accelerating the oxidation reaction by forming peroxymonocarbonate (HCO_4), a product of the reaction between bicarbonate and hydrogen peroxide, which is a more potent and selective oxidizing agent for the nitrogen atom in the tertiary amine than hydrogen peroxide. The desired NMMO content in the solution can be achieved by further concentration. Typically, the commercial NMMO usually contains up to 1% by weight of methyl morpholine, up to 0.01% by weight of peroxides calculated as hydrogen peroxide, and up to 0.2% by weight of carboxyl groups (Scholten et al., 1988). Some specific synthesis methods, such as operating in a carbon dioxide atmosphere, could achieve a nitrosamine contamination level below about 10 parts per billion (Zimmerman, 1993).

16.3.3 What Are Its Current Commercial Applications?

As a high-performance cellulose solvent, NMMO is already used for the industrial Lyocell process to produce fiber in bulk quantities (Müssig, 2010). Aqueous N-methylmorpholine-N-oxide solution is also widely used in organic synthesis. For example, it can be used as a co-oxidant with OsO_4 for dihydroxylation of alkenes and oxidation of allylic alcohols; NMMO with ruthenates can oxidize alcohols to aldehydes and ketones as well as sulfides and phosphines to their respective oxides; it could also act as an oxidizing agent under mild conditions (e.g., 60°C) in the conversion of activated halides to aldehydes or ketones and the synthesis of cyclopentenones (Sivik and Edmondson, 2008). NMMO can also be used in biofuel conversion technologies and has shown promising experimental results observed in the pretreatment of both hard and softwoods (Shafiei et al., 2010).

16.4 CELLULOSE DISSOLUTION IN NMMO

The Lyocell process, which uses NMMO as the solvent, is well established for industrial fiber production (Lim et al., 2003; Perepelkin, 2007; Ingildeev et al., 2013; Yoo et al., 2015). Compared to the traditional viscose process, the advantages of the Lyocell process include not only the relatively simple steps, characterized by the direct dissolution of cellulose, but also the higher environmental compatibility of the chemicals involved and their recyclability. On the other hand, the viscose process involves complex derivatization steps (alkalization and xanthation), the handling of toxic chemicals (carbon disulfide), and issues of atmospheric and water pollution. A disadvantage of the Lyocell process in the textile industry is the easy fibrillation of cellulose during spinning due to the higher orientation of Lyocell fibers. In contrast, the viscose process offers greater tunability of spinning conditions (Ingildeev et al., 2013). However, this drawback is not a concern for biofuel production, as cellulose is eventually saccharified into monomeric sugars. In fact, fibrillation, which increases the fiber's surface area, could potentially be advantageous for saccharification by improving enzyme access to the cellulose chains. However, pretreatment steps are usually the dominant factor in determining hydrolysis efficiency.

16.4.1 Interaction of NMMO with Lignocellulosic Biomass

NMMO modifies (opens) the packed crystalline structure of lignocellulosic materials, making them more accessible to cellulolytic enzymes (Rabideau and Ismail, 2015). NMMO dissolves cellulose within the cell wall of lignocellulosic biomass by forming a new, strong hydrogen bond with it while disrupting the intra- and intermolecular hydrogen bonds of cellulose. Specifically, the negatively charged oxygen atom of the N-oxide group forms a hydrogen bond with the hydrogen atom of one of the hydroxyl groups. This process starts in the amorphous region and eventually penetrates the crystalline regions of cellulose. The process does not require the physical removal of lignin and hemicellulose, and it regenerates cellulose on the biomass surface after adding water as an anti-solvent agent. This type of interaction is characteristic of NMMO's role as a solvent for materials rich in hydroxyl groups such as cellulose. It effectively breaks the hydrogen bonds within the cellulose structure and forms new ones with the cellulose chains, allowing them to dissolve.

16.4.2 Effect of Particle Size, Temperature, and Concentration

Particle size is important for a spherical particle's surface/volume ratio and affects pretreatment effectiveness and subsequent steps such as enzyme hydrolysis. Particle size (0.5–16 mm) has been investigated in the bioethanol production process from spruce and birch, which are pretreated with NMMO (Lennartsson et al., 2011). It was found that particle sizes below 2 mm have little effect on the released sugars during enzyme hydrolysis, while particle sizes above 2 mm significantly decrease the released sugars. This has also been observed by other researchers (Aslanzadeh et al., 2014; Teghammar et al., 2010; Li et al., 2010), all of whom used biomass particles below 2 mm.

Temperature has been studied in the interaction between cellulose and N-methylmorpholine-N-oxide (Zhao et al., 2007). NMMO crystal structure collapsed to a liquid-like form between 70°C and 100°C in the cellulose NMMO mixture. Cellulose dissolved in NMMO/H_2O (11% w/w of H_2O) solvents at 100°C as mobile NMMO molecules transformed crystalline cellulose into amorphous cellulose. It was further found that H_2O molecules that hydrogen-bonded to NMMO were replaced by the hydroxyl groups of cellulose when the cellulose-NMMO mixture was heated to 150°C. Varied temperatures (90°C, 110°C, and 130°C) were used to pretreat spruce and oak with NMMO for ethanol fermentation (Shafiei et al., 2010). Almost total conversion of cellulose to ethanol happened at 130°C.

A ternary phase diagram illustrating the composition changes during a process related to producing cellulose fibers, such as the Lyocell process, was presented by Fink et al. (2001). The diagram plots the relative compositions of three components: NMMO, water, and cellulose, with the bottom-left vertex representing 100% NMMO, the bottom-right vertex 100% water, and the top vertex 100% cellulose. A small region is indicated as the dissolution region, where cellulose swells and completely dissolves in the highly concentrated NMMO (13–15% w/w water). The dissolution process is spontaneous when the NMMO-to-water ratio is near or above 1:1 (Rabideau and Ismail, 2015). For fiber formation, ternary solutions of cellulose–NMMO–water are usually formed at elevated temperatures of 90°C to 120°C. The structure of the final fiber depends on each step of the Lyocell process. It was also reported that appropriate solutions have compositions of 8–20% cellulose, 75–80% NMMO, and 5–12% water (Fink et al., 2001). Cellulose crystals can be obtained after cooling and regeneration of the cellulose from the solution. The dissolution, crystallization, and regeneration path has also been studied by Biganska and Navard (2011). In their research, cellulose concentration strongly affects the crystallization velocity and the diffusion coefficient of NMMO. The maximum cellulose concentration suggested is 16% for undissolved cellulose. Water content is another important factor that influences the thermodynamics, structure, and hydrogen bonding in the NMMO–cellulose–water solution (Rabideau and Ismail, 2015). At lower water concentrations, many factors have been found to affect cellulose solubility in NMMO, including the extent to which hydrogen bonding and van der Waals interactions, the root causes of the enthalpy, decrease during cellulose dissolution (Rabideau and Ismail, 2015).

16.4.3 Kinetics

The kinetics of the chemical processes of cellulose dissolution and regeneration in NMMO solution were studied by Tierney (2005). The kinetic parameters (temperature and surface area effects) were derived from rate data obtained by observing the disappearance of cellulose fibers into the solvent and by determining the concentration of cellulose in Lyocell solutions. As mentioned earlier, NMMO has a highly polar N–O group, which results in high water solubility and a tendency to form hydrogen bonds. Both cellulose and water compete to form hydrogen bonds with NMMO; however, because water is preferred, the water content of the mixture must be lower than 17% w/w to dissolve cellulose (Mancini et al., 2016). For the cellulose regeneration to make new cellulose items (like fibers, films, or membranes) using the NMMO method, the cellulose is first dissolved in NMMO. Then this dissolved mixture is transferred to a special liquid bath (usually water-based). This bath is crucial. When the mixture enters the bath, the NMMO solvent begins to leave, and water begins to enter, driven by natural molecular motion (diffusion). Because cellulose doesn't dissolve in water, this swapping of liquids forces the cellulose to turn back into a solid, forming the desired fiber or film shape. This solidification step, driven by liquid exchange, is essential for the NMMO process to work (Biganska and Navard, 2011).

16.5 PRETREATMENT OF BIOMASS AND ITS CONVERSION

The general steps for NMMO pretreatment of lignocellulosic biomass start with evaporating commercial NMMO (50%) to the desired concentration (85%) and then dissolving the biomass in 85% NMMO at high temperatures (usually 120°C/130°C) for several hours. The process is usually carried out in an agitated vessel. The temperature is controlled, and antioxidants are added to prevent the degradation of NMMO and cellulose. Then, the dissolved materials are regenerated by adding boiling water. The regenerated solid is recovered by filtration and washed with water. The NMMO solvent has a high recycle rate and is recycled in an industrial process. The pretreated material is then sent downstream for biofuels production. For ethanol, the subsequent steps are saccharification, fermentation, and product separation. For biogas, the pretreated material is anaerobically digested.

The saccharification yield increases significantly for lignocellulosic materials after NMMO pretreatment, by around 9–11 times compared to untreated biomass (Shafiei et al., 2010; Goshadrou et al., 2013). In many cases, the pretreated cellulose can be completely hydrolyzed (Shafiei et al., 2010; Khodaverdi et al., 2012). This is due to the largely reduced crystallinity and increased enzyme adsorption capacity of cellulose (Khodaverdi et al., 2012). As shown in Table 16.6, with NMMO pretreatment, the ethanol yield improves to 64.6–93.3% of the theoretical ethanol yield. The biogas yield could be improved by 0.43–12 times, depending on the specific biomass and anaerobic digestion design.

In our laboratory, the biochemical methane potential assay of sugarcane bagasse was enhanced by pretreatment with 86% NMMO as the solvent at 130°C and ambient pressure. NMMO pretreatment significantly improved (by 1.5 times) the methane yield. On the other hand, dilute acid pretreatment using phosphoric acid did not improve methane yield. Around 95% of cellulose and 99.5% of hemicellulose were digested in NMMO-pretreated samples, whereas only 68% of cellulose and 50% of hemicellulose were digestible in raw bagasse.

Due to economic concerns arising from its high usage, NMMO is recycled after pretreatment and reused. Usually, the water from the NMMO/water solution obtained after filtration is removed in a rotary evaporator (under vacuum conditions). NMMO is not volatile, so only water is removed. The NMMO/water solution is re-concentrated to 85% and reused. This is also a highlighted advantage of the NMMO pretreatment. The efficiency of recycled NMMO was investigated by Kabir et al. (2014). It was found that the composition of the treated biomass greatly affects the efficiency of recycled NMMO. Experiments have been conducted with barley straw and forest residues. Recycled NMMO maintained similar efficiency in processing barley straw, while its efficiency decreased in the treatment of forest residue. The efficiency loss could be attributed to the accumulation of byproducts from lignin degradation during the pretreatment or to NMMO decomposition. As by-products accumulate, the pretreatment efficiency of recycled NMMO decreases.

The economic effect of recycling NMMO was also evaluated by Teghammar et al. (2014) through a techno-economic analysis of biogas production from forest residues. It was shown that an increase in the recycle rate of NMMO from 99.5 to 99.99% will decrease the production cost greatly from 9.35 €/kg CH_4 to 3.21 €/kg CH_4.

16.6 TECHNO-ECONOMIC ANALYSIS

Techno-economic analysis serves as a tool for benchmarking conceptual process designs, including identifying the process parameters that have the greatest impact on overall economics, production, and costs. Thus, it could be used for comparing

TABLE 16.6
NMMO Pretreatment with Different Lignocellulosic Biomass

Biomass	NMMO (%)	NMMO Usage	Temp (°C)	Time (hr)	Product	Effect of NMMO Pretreatment	Ref.
Corn stalk	Alkali with 50% (w/w) NMMO solution	1 ml/g of biomass	120	7	Ethanol	Ethanol yield increased from 64.6% as compared to 18.8% from untreated biomass.	Cai et al. (2016)
Sugarcane bagasse	86.7 (monohydrate) w/w	5% w/w	130	1	Ethanol	Efficient hydrolysis and 86% of theoretical ethanol yield.	Kuo and Lee (2009)
Spruce and oak	85 w/w	6% w/w	130	2–3	Ethanol	Pretreated oak and spruce resulted in almost total conversion of cellulose to ethanol, with ethanol yields of 85.4% and 89%, respectively.	Shafiei et al. (2010)
Spruce and birch	85 w/w	6% w/w	130	5	Ethanol	Ethanol yields of 128 and 136 mg/g dry wood were obtained in airlift reactors from pretreated spruce and birch, respectively.	Lennartsson et al. (2011)
Rice straw	85 w/w	5% w/w	120	5	Ethanol	Ethanol production yield was improved to 93.3% (from 35.4% for untreated) after treated by NMMO.	Poornejada et al. (2012)
Sugarcane bagasse	85 w/v	5% w/w	130	1	Glucose and ethanol	Enzyme hydrolysis was not affected by the presence of NMMO; the glucose produced was 11.6 g/L, 87.5% of the theoretical yield.	He et al. (2013)

Pinewood	85 w/w	7.5% w/w	120	1–15	Ethanol and biogas	Improved the yields of ethanol up to 86% of the theoretical yield, and the biogas yield up to 222 (mL/g vs.) from pinewood (both chips and powder).	Shafiei et al. (2014)
Waste textile	85 w/w	6% w/w (dry matter)	120	3	Biogas	Doubled the biogas yield.	Jeihanipour et al. (2013)
Cotton linter	85 w/w	5% w/w (dry matter)	120	3	Biogas	Solubilization rates of cellulose increased	Jeihanipour et al. (2011)
Spruce	85 w/w	6% w/w	130	1–15	Biogas	Biogas yields increased by 4–12 times.	Teghammar et al. (2012)
Rice straw	85 w/w	7.5% w/w	130	1–15	Biogas	Biogas yields increased by seven times.	Teghammar et al. (2012)
Triticale straw	85 w/w	7.5% w/w	130	1–15	Biogas	Biogas increased yields by seven times.	Teghammar et al. (2012)
Forest residues	85 w/w	6% w/w	120	12	Biogas	About 141% increase in the methane production.	Aslanzadeh et al., 2014
Manure (cattle and horse)	85 w/w	7.5% w/w	120	15	Biogas	Methane increases by about 50%. Lignin content decreases.	Aslanzadeh et al., 2011
Microalgae (*Nannochloropsis oculata* and *Chlorella vulgaris*)	85 w/w	6% w/w	120	3	Biogas	Methane production was increased by 43% for *N. oculata* and decreased slightly for *C. vulgaris*.	Caporgno et al., 2016
Oil palm empty fruit bunch	85 w/w	6% w/w	120	3	Biogas	Biogas yield increased by 167% compared to untreated OPEFB.	Purwandari et al., 2013
Barley straw and forest residues	85 w/w	6% w/w	90	3–30	Biogas	Resulted in 100% improvement in methane yield.	Kabir et al. (2014)

different pretreatment methods. An NMMO pretreatment step includes evaporation, dissolution, regeneration, filtration, and recirculation of NMMO and wash water (shown in Figure 16.1). The process simulation flowsheet for NMMO pretreatment usually includes an evaporator unit, a flash drum, a pretreatment tank, a solid wash decanter, heat exchangers, and compressors (Shafiei et al., 2011; Shafiei et al., 2014). Units (Figure 16.2) can be optimized for energy-saving considerations such as mechanical vapor recompression evaporators. Compared to other processes (e.g., steam explosion), NMMO-pretreated biomass yields higher biofuel (ethanol/methane) yields due to its higher conversion efficiency. It can also be noted that NMMO is more environmentally friendly than the steam explosion process in a comparative life-cycle assessment using environmental impact categories (Khoshnevisan et al., 2016).

The economic performance of NMMO pretreatment for biofuels' production has been evaluated (Table 16.7) through techno-economic analysis (Shafiei et al., 2011, 2014; Teghammar et al., 2014). Shafiei et al. (2011) investigated the economic effects of key parameters, including plant capacity, feedstock price, and

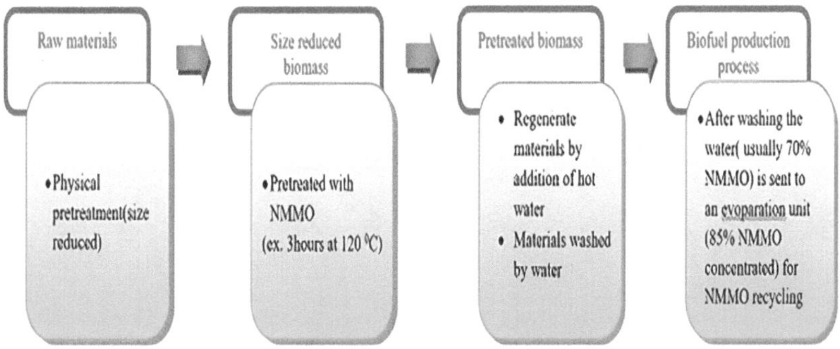

FIGURE 16.1 Process steps for techno-economic studies of biofuels production with NMMO pretreatment.

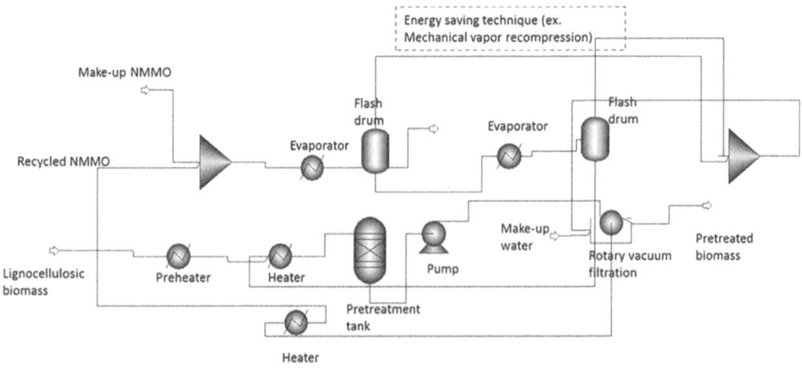

FIGURE 16.2 Unit operations for NMMO pretreatment (process flow diagram).

TABLE 16.7
Recent Techno-Economic Studies of Biofuel Production with NMMO Pretreatment

Biomass	NMMO Pretreatment	NMMO Recovery Rate (%)	Price of NMMO (€/kg)	Biofuels	Main Conclusions	Reference
Spruce wood	85% NMMO, 5 hr, 90°C, 0.05 kg NMMO per kg of biomass	99.9	4	Ethanol and biogas	Lignocellulosic ethanol production with NMMO pretreatment could be economically feasible.	Shafiei et al. (2011)
Forest residues	85% NMMO, 12 hr, 90°C, 0.01 kg NMMO per kg of biomass	99.5	4	Biogas	Biogas produced from forest residues pretreated with NMMO is economically attractive when co-digested with municipal solid waste.	Teghammar et al. (2014)
Pinewood	85% NMMO, 3 h, 120°C, 0.015 kg NMMO per kg of biomass	99.5	4	Ethanol and biogas; biomethane	NMMO pretreatments are slightly more expensive than steam pretreatments during the conversion of pinewood. Producing ethanol is more profitable than producing methane, even though methane has a higher energy yield.	Shafiei et al. (2014)

enzymes, in a novel ethanol production process with NMMO pretreatment. The process includes NMMO concentration by evaporation, pretreatment, filtration and washing, enzymatic hydrolysis, fermentation, ethanol purification, and biogas production, with NMMO and water recycled. The study shows the economic feasibility of the process by estimating the production cost of ethanol to be €0.44 per liter, where high cost is attributed to the price of NMMO, spruce wood feedstock, and enzymes. Similar results were obtained by Teghammar et al. (2014), who conducted a techno-economic study of NMMO pretreatment and biogas production from forest residues. It is also found that the price of NMMO (€4/kg) accounts for 80% of the material cost, the highest share of operating costs. Besides, pretreatment operations such as filtration and evaporation are significant parts of the operation cost. Among all processes for biofuel production, ethanol production with biogas as a by-product, using NMMO pretreatment, has been considered an efficient and economical approach with reduced environmental impacts for converting pinewood (Shafiei et al., 2014; Khoshnevisan et al., 2016). This study considered the profitability of producing ethanol and the environmental benefits of treating waste to generate methane.

The NMMO pretreatment was compared with steam explosion in the production of bioethanol and biomethane from pinewood (Shafiei et al., 2014). NMMO pretreatment cost was higher than the steam explosion cost due to higher material and equipment costs. It was further found that the bioethanol production process is more profitable than the biomethane process; however, biomethane has a lower gasoline-equivalent price. All of the research has shown that biofuels produced by NMMO pretreatment could be economically feasible, although lower material costs would greatly improve the economics.

16.7 CONCLUSION

As a novel and promising method for pretreating biomass to produce biofuels, NMMO has demonstrated high efficiency and economic feasibility, along with notable environmental benefits. However, due to the high price of NMMO and side reactions and degradation that occur during dissolution and recovery, further investigations are needed to improve recycling efficiency and enhance process stability. Also, for the implementation of biofuels technologies, attention should be paid to the entire process, including downstream steps such as product purification and by-product production, which have significant economic and environmental impacts. Overall, NMMO pretreatment shows attractive features both commercially and environmentally for biofuels' production.

REFERENCES

Agbor, V. B., Cicek, N., Sparling, R., Berlin, A. and Levin, D. B. 2011. Biomass pre-treatment: Fundamentals toward application. *Biotech Adv*, 29, 675–685.

Anwar, Z., Gulfraz, M. and Irshad, M. 2014. Agro-industrial lignocellulosic biomass: A key to unlock the future bioenergy: A brief review. *Journal of Radiation Research and Applied Sciences*, 7, 163–173. https://doi.org/10.1016/j.jrras.2014.02.003

Aslanzadeh, S., Berg, A., Taherzadeh, M. J. and Horváth, I. S. 2014. Biogas production from N-Methylmorpholine-N-oxide (NMMO) pretreated forest residues. *Appl Biochem Biotechnol*, 172, 2998 3008. https://doi.org/10.1007/s12010-014-0747-z

Aslanzadeh, S., Taherzadeh, M. J. and Horváth, I. S. 2011. Pretreatment of straw fraction of manure improved biogas production. *BioResources*, 6(4), 5193–5205.

Biganska, O. and Navard, P. 2011. Dissolution, crystallisation, and regeneration of cellulose in N-methylmorpholine N-oxide. MACRO-2004 international conference on polymers for advanced technologies, Dec 2004, Thiruvananthapuram, India. *Society for Polymer Science*, 6, 2004. https://hal-mines-paristech.archives-ouvertes.fr/hal-00579382

Brandt, A., Grasvik, J., Hallett, J. P. and Welton, T. 2013. Deconstruction of lignocellulosic biomass with ionic liquids. *Green Chem*, 15, 550–583.

Brodeur, G., Yau, E., Badal, K., Collier, J., Ramachandran, K. B. and Ramakrishnan, S. 2011. Chemical and physicochemical pretreatment of lignocellulosic biomass: A review. *Enzyme Research*, Article ID 787532. https://doi.org/10.4061/2011/787532

Cai, L.-Y., Ma, Y.-L., Ma, X.-X. and Lv, J.-M. 2016. Improvement of enzymatic hydrolysis and ethanol production from cornstalk by alkali and N-methylmorpholine-N-oxide pretreatments. *Bioresource Technology*, 212, 42–46. http://dx.doi.org/10.1016/j.biortech.2016.04.012

Capolupo, L. and Faraco, V. 2016. Green methods of lignocellulose pretreatment for biorefinery development. *Appl Microbiol Biotechnol*, 100(22), 9451–9467. https://doi.org/10.1007/s00253-016-7884-y

Caporgno, M. P., Olkiewicz, M., Pruvost, J., Lepine, O., Legrand, J., Font, J. and Bengoa, C. 2016. A novel pre-treatment for the methane production from microalgae by using N-methylmorpholine-N-oxide (NMMO). *Bioresource Technology*, 201, 370–373. http://dx.doi.org/10.1016/j.biortech.2015.11.069

Chaturvedi, V. and Verma, P. 2013. An overview of key pretreatment processes employed for bioconversion of lignocellulosic biomass into biofuels and value-added products. *Biotech*, 3, 415–431. https://doi.org/10.1007/s13205-013-0167-8

Dehghani, M., Karimi, K. and Sadeghi, M. 2015. Pretreatment of rice straw for the improvement of biogas production. *Energy Fuels*, 29, 3770–3775. https://doi.org/10.1021/acs.energyfuels.5b00718

Egal, M., Budtova, T. and Navard, P. 2007. Structure of aqueous solutions of microcrystalline cellulose/sodium hydroxide below 0°C and the limit of cellulose dissolution. *Biomacromolecules*, 8, 2282–2287. https://doi.org/10.1021/bm0702399

Fan, J., Lu, Y., An, N., Zhu, W., Li, M., Gao, M., Wang, X., Wu, C. and Wang, Y. 2025. Pretreatment technologies for lignocellulosic biomass: Research progress, mechanisms, and prospects. *BioResources*, 20(2). https://doi.org/10.15376/biores

Fink, H.-P., Weigel, P., Purz, H. J. and Ganster, J. 2001. Structure formation of regenerated cellulose materials from NMMO-solutions. *Prog Polym Sci*, 26, 1473–1524.

Goshadrou, A., Karimi, K. and Taherzadeh, M. J. 2013. Ethanol and biogas production from birch by NMMO pretreatment. *Biomass and Bioenergy*, 49, 95–101. http://dx.doi.org/10.1016/j.biombioe.2012.12.013

Guragain, Y. N. and Vadlani, P. V. 2016. Importance of biomass-specific pretreatment methods for effective and sustainable utilization of renewable resources. In *Biotechnology and Biochemical Engineering, Select Proceedings of ICACE 2015*, Eds: B. D. Prasanna, S. N. Gummadi and P. Vadlani. Springer Nature Link, 207–215.

Hasani, M., Henniges, U., Idström, A., Nordstierna, L., Westman, G., Rosenau, T. and Potthast, A. 2013. Nano-cellulosic materials: The impact of water on their dissolution in DMAc/LiCl. *Carbohydrate Polymers*, 98, 1565–1572. http://dx.doi.org/10.1016/j.carbpol.2013.07.001

He, Y.-C., Xia, D.-Q., Maa, C.-L., Gong, L., Gong, T., Wu, M.-X., Zhang, Y., Tang, Y.-J., Xu, J.-H. and Liu, Y.-Y. 2013. Enzymatic saccharification of sugarcane bagasse by N-methylmorpholine-N-oxide-tolerant cellulase from a newly isolated Galactomyces sp. CCZU11-1. *Bioresource Technology*, 135, 18–22. http://dx.doi.org/10.1016/j.biortech.2012.10.156

Ingildeev, D., Effenberger, F., Bredereck, K. and Hermanutz, F. 2013. Comparison of direct solvents for regenerated cellulosic fibers via the lyocell process and by means of ionic liquids. *J Appl Polym Sci*, 4141–4150. https://doi.org/10.1002/APP.38470

Jeihanipour, A., Aslanzadeh, S., Rajendran, K., Balasubramanian, G. and Taherzadeh, M. J. 2013. High-rate biogas production from waste textiles using a two-stage process. *Renewable Energy*, 52, 128–135. http://dx.doi.org/10.1016/j.renene.2012.10.042

Jeihanipour, A., Niklasson, C. and Taherzadeh, M. J. 2011. Enhancement of solubilization rate of cellulose in anaerobic digestion and its drawbacks. *Process Biochemistry*, 46, 1509–1514. https://doi.org/10.1016/j.procbio.2011.04.003

Kabir, M. M., Niklasson, C., Taherzadeh, M. J. and Horváth, I. S. 2014. Biogas production from lignocelluloses by N-methylmorpholine-N-oxide (NMMO) pretreatment: Effects of recovery and reuse of NMMO. *Bioresource Technology*, 161, 446–450. https://doi.org/10.1016/j.biortech.2014.03.107.

Kaur, K. and Phutela, U. G. 2016. Sodium carbonate pretreatment: An approach towards desilication of paddy straw and enhancement in biogas production. *Paddy Water Environ*, 14, 113–121. https://doi.org/10.1007/s10333-015-0483-1

Khodaverdi, M., Jeihanipour, A., Karimi, K., Taherzadeh, M. J. 2012. Kinetic modeling of rapid enzymatic hydrolysis of crystalline cellulose after pretreatment by NMMO. *J Ind Microbiol Biotechnol*, 39, 429–438. https://doi.org/10.1007/s10295-011-1048-y

Khoshnevisan, B., Shafiei, M., Rajaeifar, M. A. and Tabatabaei, M. 2016. Biogas and bioethanol production from pinewood pre-treated with steam explosion and N-methylmorpholine-N-oxide (NMMO): A comparative life cycle assessment approach. *Energy*, 114, 935–950. https://doi.org/10.1016/j.energy.2016.08.024

Kim, K. H. and Yoo, C. G. 2021. Challenges and perspectives of recent biomass pretreatment solvents. *Front Chem Eng*, 3, 785709. https://doi.org/10.3389/fceng.2021.785709

Kim, M. and Day, D. F. 2011. Composition of sugar cane and sweet sorghum suitable for ethanol production at Louisiana sugar mills. *Journal of Industrial Microbiology and Biotechnology*, 38(7), 803–807. https://doi.org/10.1007/s10295-010-0812-8

Kulpinski, P. 2005. Cellulose nanofibers prepared by the N-methylmorpholine-N-oxide method. *J Appl Polym Sci*, 98, 1855–1859.

Kuo, C.-H. and Lee, C.-K. 2009. Enhanced enzymatic hydrolysis of sugarcane bagasse by N-methylmorpholine-N-oxide pretreatment. *Bioresource Technology*, 100, 866–871. https://doi.org/10.1016/j.biortech.2008.07.001

Lennartsson, P. R., Niklasson, C. and Taherzadeh, M. J. 2011. A pilot study on lignocelluloses to ethanol and fish feed using NMMO pretreatment and cultivation with zygomycetes in an air-lift reactor. *Bioresource Technology*, 102, 4425–4432. https://doi.org/10.1016/j.biortech.2010.12.089

Li, C., Knierim, B., Manisseri, C., Arora, R., Scheller, H. V., Auer, M., Vogel, K. P., Simmons, B. A. and Singh, S. 2010. Comparison of dilute acid and ionic liquid pretreatment of switchgrass: Biomass recalcitrance, delignification and enzymatic saccharification. *Bioresource Technology*, 101, 4900–4906. https://doi.org/10.1016/j.biortech.2009.10.066

Lim, K. Y., Yoon, K. J. and Kim, B. C. 2003. Highly absorbable lyocell fiber spun from celluloses/hydrolyzed starch-g-PAN solution in NMMO monohydrate. *European Polymer Journal*, 39, 2115–2120. https://doi.org/10.1016/S0014-3057(03)00158-7

Mancini, G., Papirio, S., Lens, P. N. L. and Esposito, G. 2016. Solvent pretreatments of lignocellulosic materials to enhance biogas production: A review. *Energy Fuels*, 30, 1892–1903.

Mosier, N., Wyman, C., Dale, B., Elander, R., Lee, Y. Y., Holtzapple, M. and Ladisch, M. 2005. Features of promising technologies for pretreatment of lignocellulosic biomass. *Bioresource Technology*, 96(6), 673–686.

Muranaka, Y., Suzuki, T., Sawanishi, H., Hasegawa, I. and Mae, K. 2014. Effective production of levulinic acid from biomass through pretreatment using phosphoric acid, hydrochloric acid, or ionic liquid. *Industrial & Engineering Chemistry Research*, 53, 11611–11621. https://doi.org/10.1021/ie501811x

Müssig, J. 2010. *Industrial Applications of Natural Fibres: Structure, Properties and Technical Applications*. John Wiley & Sons. https://doi.org/10.1002/9780470660324

Nieves, D. C., Karimi, K. and Horváth, I. S. 2011. Improvement of biogas production from oil palm empty fruit bunches (OPEFB). *Industrial Crops and Products*, 34, 1097–1101. https://doi.org/10.1016/j.indcrop.2011.03.022

Perepelkin, K. 2007. Lyocell fibres based on direct dissolution of cellulose in N-methylmorpholine N-oxide: Development and prospects. *FibreChem*, 39, 163–172.

Pieterse, T. 2013. N-methylmorphine N-oxide. *Synlett*, 24(16), 2175–2176. https://doi.org/10.1055/s-0033-1338973

Poornejada, N., Karimi, K. and Behzad, T. 2013. Improvement of saccharification and ethanol production from rice straw by NMMO and [BMIM][OAc] pretreatments. *Industrial Crops and Products*, 41, 408–413. https://doi.org/10.1016/j.indcrop.2012.04.059

Potumarthi, R., Baadhe, R. R. and Bhattacharya, S. 2013. Fermentable sugars from lignocellulosic biomass: Technical challenges. In *Biofuel Technologies*, Eds: V. K. Gupta and M. G. Tuohy. Springer-Verlag Berlin, 3–27. https://doi.org/10.1007/978-3-642-34519-7_1

Purwandari, F. A., Sanjaya, A. P., Millati, R., Cahyanto, M. N., Horváth, I. S., Niklasson, C. and Taherzadeh, M. J. 2013. Pretreatment of oil palm empty fruit bunch (OPEFB) by N-methylmorpholine-N-oxide (NMMO) for biogas production: Structural changes and digestion improvement. *Bioresource Technology*, 128, 461–466. http://dx.doi.org/10.1016/j.biortech.2012.10.088

Rabideau, B. D. and Ismail, A. E. 2015. Effect of water content in N-methylmorpholine N-oxide/cellulose solutions on thermodynamics, structure, and hydrogen bonding. *J Phys Chem B*, 119, 15014–15022. https://doi.org/10.1021/acs.jpcb.5b07500

Rosenau, T., Potthast, A., Adorjan, I., Hofinger, A., Sixta, H., Firgo, H. and Kosma, P. 2002. Cellulose solutions in N-methylmorpholine-N-oxide (NMMO) – degradation processes and stabilizers. *Cellulose*, 9, 283–291. https://doi.org/10.1023/A:1021127423041

Rosenau, T., Potthast, A., Sixta, H. and Kosma, P. 2001. The chemistry of side reactions and byproduct formation in the system NMMO/cellulose (lyocell process). *Progr Polym Sci*, 26(9), 1763–837.

Sathitsuksanoh, N., George, A. and Zhang, Y. H. P. 2013. New lignocellulose pretreatments using cellulose solvents: A review. *J Chem Technol Biotechnol*, 88, 169–180.

Sathitsuksanoh, N., Zhu, Z. and Zhang, Y. H. P. 2012. Cellulose solvent-based pretreatment for corn stover and avicel: Concentrated phosphoric acid versus ionic liquid [BMIM] Cl. *Cellulose*. https://doi.org/10.1007/s10570-012-9719-z

Scholten, H. and Rindtorff, K. 1988. *Process for Producing Aqueous N-N-N-N-N-N-N-N-Methylmorpholine-N-Oxide Solutions*. United States Patent Number 4,748,241.

Shafiei, M., Karimi, K. and Taherzadeh, M. J. 2010. Pretreatment of spruce and oak by N-methylmorpholine-N-oxide (NMMO) for efficient conversion of their cellulose to ethanol. *Bioresource Technology*, 101, 4914–4918. https://doi.org/10.1016/j.biortech.2009.08.100

Shafiei, M., Karimi, K. and Taherzadeh, M. J. 2011. Techno-economical study of ethanol and biogas from spruce wood by NMMO-pretreatment and rapid fermentation and digestion. *Bioresource Technology*, 102, 7879–7886. https://doi.org/10.1016/j.biortech.2011.05.071

Shafiei, M., Karimi, K., Zilouei, H. and Taherzadeh, M. J. 2014. Economic impact of NMMO pretreatment on ethanol and biogas production from pinewood. *BioMed Research International*, 2014, 13, Article ID 320254. http://dx.doi.org/10.1155/2014/320254

Singha, K. 2012. Importance of the phase diagram in lyocell fiber spinning. *International Journal of Materials Engineering*, 2(3), 10–16. https://doi.org/10.5923/j.ijme.20120203.01

Sivik, M. R. and Edmondson, S. D. 2008. N-methylmorpholine N-oxide. *E-Eros Encyclopedia of Reagents for Organic Synthesis*. https://doi.org/10.1002/047084289X.rm216.pub2

Teghammar, A., Forgács, G., Horváth, I. S. and Taherzadeh, M. J. 2014. Techno-economic study of NMMO pretreatment and biogas production from forest residues. *Applied Energy*, 116, 125–133. http://dx.doi.org/10.1016/j.apenergy.2013.11.053

Teghammar, A., Karimi, K., Horváth, I. S. and Taherzadeh, M. J. 2012. Enhanced biogas production from rice straw, triticale straw and softwood spruce by NMMO pretreatment. *Biomass and Bioenergy*, 36, 116–120. https://doi.org/10.1016/j.biombioe.2011.10.019

Teghammar, A., Yngvesson, J., Lundin, M., Taherzadeh, M. J. and Horváth, I. S. 2010. Pretreatment of paper tube residuals for improved biogas production. *Bioresour Technol*, 101, 1206–1212. https://doi.org/10.1016/j.biortech.2009.09.029

Tierney, J. W. 2005. *Kinetics of Cellulose Dissolution in N-Methyl Morpholine-N-Oxide and Evaporative Processes of Similar Solutions*. Master's Thesis, University of Tennessee. http://trace.tennessee.edu/utk_gradthes/2553

Wang, K., Yang, H. Y., Xu, F. and Sun, R. C. 2011. Structural comparison and enhanced enzymatic hydrolysis of the cellulosic preparation from Populus tomentosa Carr., by different cellulose-soluble solvent systems. *Bioresource Technology*, 102, 4524–4529. https://doi.org/10.1016/j.biortech.2010.12.088

Wang, Q., Wang, Z., Shen, F., Jinguang, H., Sun, F., Lin, L., Yang, G., Zhang, Y. and Deng, S. 2014. Pretreating lignocellulosic biomass by the concentrated phosphoric acid plus hydrogen peroxide (PHP) for enzymatic hydrolysis: Evaluating the pretreatment flexibility on feedstocks and particle sizes. *Bioresource Technology*, 166, 420–428. http://dx.doi.org/10.1016/j.biortech.2014.05.088

Woźniak, A., Kuligowski, K., Świerczek, L. and Cenian, A. 2025. Review of lignocellulosic biomass pretreatment using physical, thermal, and chemical methods for higher yields in bioethanol production. *Sustainability*, 17(1), 287. https://doi.org/10.3390/su17010287

Yang, B., Tao, L. and Wyman, C. E. 2018. Strengths, challenges, and opportunities for hydrothermal pretreatment in lignocellulosic biorefineries. *Biofuels, Bioprod Bioref*, 12, 125–138. https://doi.org/10.1002/bbb.1825

Yoo, M. K., Reza, M. S., Kim, I. M. and Kim, K. J. 2015. Physical properties and fibrillation tendency of regenerated cellulose fiber dry jet-wet spun from high-molecular-weight cotton linter Pulp/NMMO solution. *Fibers Polym*, 16, 1618–1628. https://doi.org/10.1007/s12221-015-5313-y

Zhang, C., Liu, R., Xiang, J., Kang, H., Liu, Z. and Huang, H. 2014. Dissolution mechanism of cellulose in N, N-dimethylacetamide/lithium chloride: Revisiting through molecular interactions. *J Phys Chem B*, 118, 9507–9514. https://doi.org/10.1021/jp506013c

Zhang, Y. H. P. 2011. What is vital (and not vital) to advance economically-competitive biofuels production. *Process Biochemistry*, 46, 2091–2110.

Zhang, Y. H. P., Ding, S. Y., Mielenz, J. R., Cui, J. B., Elander, R. T., Laser, M., Himmel, M. E., McMillan, J. R. and Lynd, L. R. 2007. Fractionating recalcitrant lignocellulose at modest reaction conditions. *Biotechnology and Bioengineering*, 97(2), 214–223.

Zhao, H., Kwak, J. H., Wang, Y., Franz, J. A., White, J. M. and Holladay, J. E. 2007. Interactions between cellulose and N-methylmorpholine-N-oxide. *Carbohydrate Polymers*, 67, 97–103. https://doi.org/10.1016/j.carbpol.2006.04.019

Zhao, Z. T., Ding, J., Pang, J. W., Bao, M. Y., Luo, G., Wang, B. Y., Liu, B. F., Zhang, L. Y., Ren, N. Q. and Yang, S. S. 2025. Pretreatments of lignocellulosic biomass for biohydrogen biorefinery: Recent progress, techno-economic feasibility and prospectives. *Critical Reviews in Environmental Science and Technology*, 1–27. https://doi.org/10.1080/10643389.2025.2484892

Zimmerman, R. L. 1993. *Process for the Preparation of N-Methylmorpholine Oxide*. United States Patent Number 5,216,154.

17 Overview of Biomass Conversion and Process Selection

Bukke Vani, Mamilla Shyam Sunder, and Sundergopal Sridhar

17.1 INTRODUCTION

The formation of fossil fuels (FF) takes millions of years on Earth. The world market depends heavily on FF, such as petroleum crude oils, coal, and natural gas, as sources of thermal energy and other solid, liquid, and gaseous fuels, along with chemicals, as FF reserves are finite and can be depleted as they are consumed. Lignocellulosic biomass is a renewable, natural carbon resource that can be used as a substitute for FF. Biomass can be converted using suitable technologies, but this usually depends on the type and quality of the biomass feedstock, as well as economic and environmental conditions. Various biomass feedstocks are available for conversion into biofuels, chemicals, high-value products, and other power generation applications. Technology selection is also vital in altering feedstock to increase product value by generating biofuels. Many implications involve biomass selection, transport, cost savings, product delivery, and so forth. Further research on biomass can be enabled through international collaboration with various industries and consistent government policy support, leading to the identification of a suitable conversion process that can be commercialized in the market.

1. In developing countries, biomass is used for household cooking, space heating, and lighting. In this scenario, the conversion process of biomass feedstock into energy is between 5% and 15%.
2. In another way of processing biomass-free energy sources, such as tobacco, pig iron, tea, bricks, and tiles, the efficiency of feedstock biomass conversion into useful energy is 15% or lower.
3. The thermal conversion technology of "modern industrial" is expected at 30–60% conversion efficiency.
4. Newly adopted "chemical conversion" technologies, like fuel cells, are capable of converting thermal unit efficiencies.

DOI: 10.1201/9781003327608-17

5. Other upcoming technologies are "biological conversions" techniques such as anaerobic digestion of biomass into biogas production and fermentation of alcohols (Bioenergy 96, 1996).

Biomass is a vast, quiescent renewable energy resource that can be utilized to make biofuels for electricity, transportation, and heating (Lebaka, 2013). The diversity of biomass resources has proved to be an essential component of renewable energy conversations within the framework and is strongly preferred by the European Union, which has been able to transform energy efficiency and environmental protection regulations into strategies for growth. It must be highlighted that biomass is an entirely renewable energy source, as the carbon dioxide (CO_2) emitted during its combustion and use is absorbed by the organic carbon source. To put it another way, plants use CO_2 emitted into the atmosphere as a byproduct of other plants' biodegradation for their metabolic activities and growth. Consequently, using biomass accelerates the release of CO_2 into the atmosphere, where crops will absorb it to produce biomass again (Kaltschmitt, 2013). A detailed illustration of biomass energy technology in a closed-loop cycle is shown in Figure 17.1.

Biomass is any organic material that results either indirectly or directly from photosynthesis. Because of the diversity of materials, applications, and sources, several perspectives on biomass exist. But in the broader sense, biomass is a group

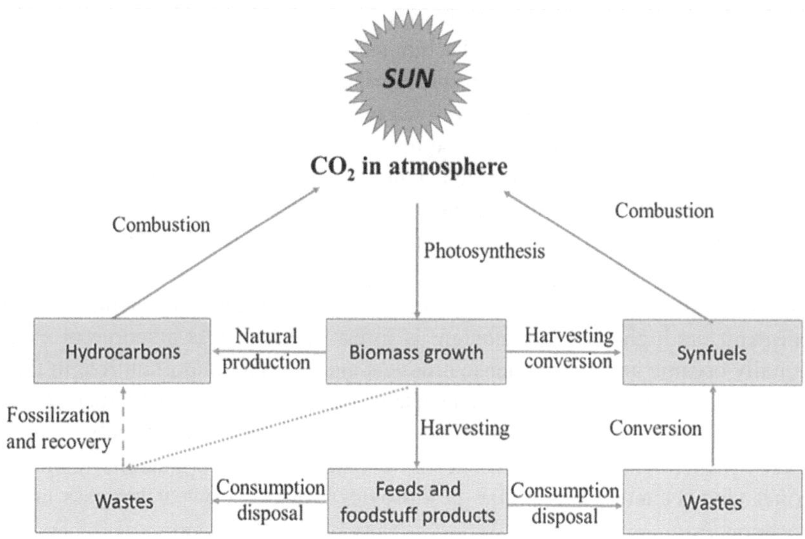

FIGURE 17.1 Illustration of biomass energy technology.

Source: Reproduced from Klass (1998)

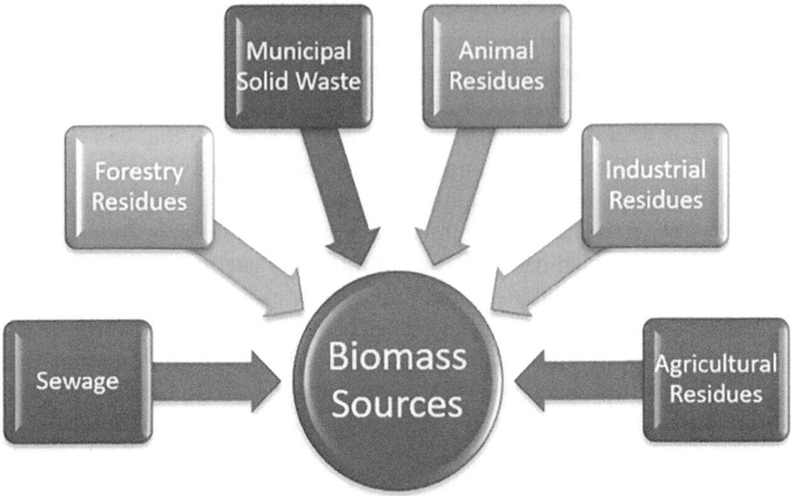

FIGURE 17.2 The major resources of biomass.

of organic value-added products, which includes plant products such as crops, trees, shrubs, and algae, along with other constituents composed of an organic matrix, excluding plastics prepared from hydrocarbons and fossil fuels (McKendry, 2002). The most noteworthy biomasses (depicted in Figure 17.2) include algae, sewage, aquatic crops, forestry, agricultural residues, and animal wastes (from poultry farms), besides solid wastes from the wood-processing sector. Organic matter that can no longer be reused or recycled for its original purpose, such as municipal solid waste (MSW) and garbage released from anthropogenic sources, generally falls under the biomass category (Kaltschmitt, 2013).

It is projected that the carbon content of agricultural biomass is 100 times the world's annual energy usage, indicating the great promise of virgin biomass for energy production. Furthermore, the primary contributor of biomass and the one with the highest carbon content is forest biomass. It is a source of exceptionally organic and energy-dense products and plays an important role in fixing carbon. Additionally, biomass can be used to manufacture synthetic fuels in bulk. Biomass sources with wide variations in energy density, mass density, moisture levels, shape, composition, and intermittent supply must be handled by biomass conversion technologies. Figure 17.3 provides an overview of biomass energy conversion.

There are numerous existing techniques and routes for converting biomass into energy and chemicals. The most frequently used methods are tabulated in Table 17.1: thermo-chemical conversion, biochemical conversion, and physical and chemical conversion.

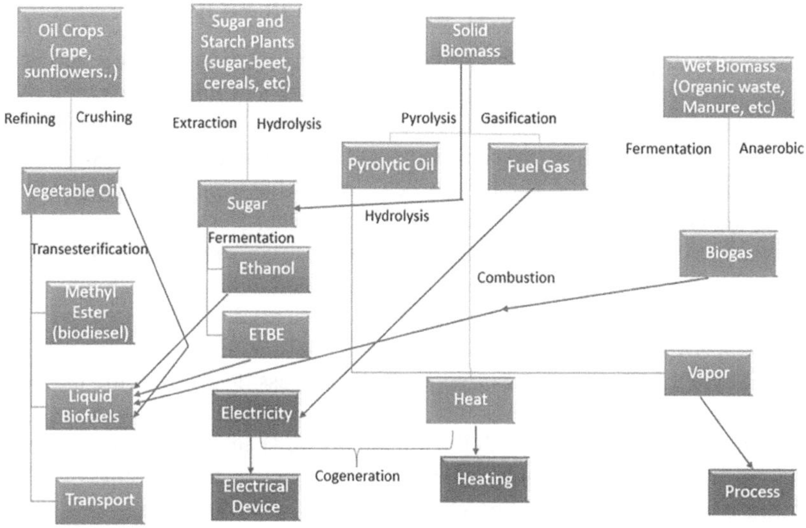

FIGURE 17.3 Overview of biomass energy conversion.

Source: Reproduced from Sumit et al. (2014) with permission

TABLE 17.1
Conversion Technologies and Their Corresponding Products

Conversion Techniques	Methods	Type of Biomass	End Product Use
Thermo-chemical	Combustion	Animal and agricultural wastes, woody residues	Heat and electricity
	Pyrolysis	Agricultural and woody residues	Char, producer gas, and pyrolysis oil
	Gasification	Agricultural and woody residues	Producer gas, char, liquid fuels
	Liquefaction	Woody residues algal biomass	Liquid fuels, biofuel, fertilizer, and syngas
Biochemical	Anaerobic digestion	Sewage and animal wastes	Biogas, liquid fuels, electricity
	Fermentation	Starch, sugars, and agricultural residues	Liquid fuels (bioethanol)
Physicochemical	Esterification/ transesterification	Animal fats, waste, and vegetable oils	Glycerol and liquid fuels

Source: Reproduced from Tursi (2019)

17.2 COMBUSTION TECHNOLOGIES FOR BIOFUELS

Thermochemical conversion of lignocellulosic biomass into biofuels and chemicals can be achieved through combustion, gasification, liquefaction, and pyrolysis. These processes are alternatives and entirely in contrast to the biochemical pathways. In thermochemical conversion, reducing biomass size followed by drying is a preliminary step. The most widely used technologies are gasification and liquefaction, which require further technological improvements.

Nearly 90% of the entire renewable energy derived from biomass is produced by combustion. Numerous feedstocks, such as wood, fallen leaves, tough vegetable hulls, rice bran, and dry animal manure, can be used in combustion processes (Lebaka, 2013).

The type of biomass used throughout the process determines the amount of heat generated, with an average thermal energy output of approximately 20 MJ/kg of feedstock (Nussbaumer, 2003). Equations (17.1) and (17.2) demonstrate that the combustion process is an exothermic reaction in which the biomass is ignited in the presence of air, yielding chemical energy that can be transformed into electrical as well as mechanical energy (Lebaka, 2013). Generation of heat and electricity by combustion is comparable to that of FF-fired power plants, but combustion technologies may cause NOx emissions.

$$\text{Biomass} + O_2 \rightarrow CO_2 + H_2O + \text{Heat} \tag{17.1}$$

The combustion equation can be expressed as follows:

$$CH_{1.44}O_{0.66} + 1.03O_2 \rightarrow CO_2 + 0.72H_2O + \text{Heat} \tag{17.2}$$

Figure 17.4 depicts a typical biomass combustion process. The combustion reaction occurs at temperatures between 800°C and 1,000°C in combustion chambers. The water content of the biomass feedstock, which ought to be less than 50%, is a crucial condition. An average biomass combustion plant produces 20 to 50 MWe, with an associated electrical efficiency of 25% to 30%, using wood and forest waste as fuel. The use of fluidized bed systems, sophisticated gas cleaning, and further innovations of these systems have boosted the amount of electricity produced from biomass. A high moisture level in biomass is not appropriate for this route, and pre-drying may also be necessary in some cases. The combustion ranges from small to large industrial plants, with capacities of 100–3,000 MWe. In coal-fired power plants, where co-combustion of biomass occurs, it is an alternative due to the extraordinary conversion efficiency of the systems.

17.2.1 Grate Technology

Two commonly used boiler designs for burning biomass are fluidized bed combustors and grate-firing devices. Each of these boiler types offers significant fuel

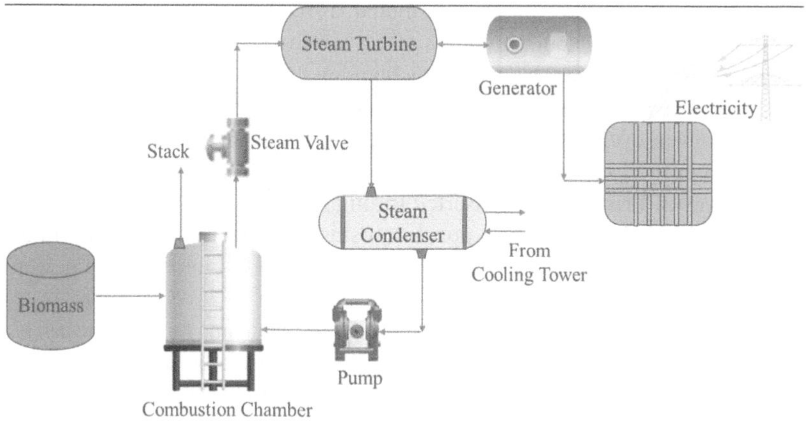

FIGURE 17.4 A typical biomass combustion process.

versatility and can produce energy from biomass in combination. Air-dried biomass with low moisture content should be milled to a particle size below 6 mm and maintained at low moisture levels to facilitate efficient co-firing with coal or natural gas. The use of suspension-fired burners could strongly influence the performance of the boilers.

The working principle and mechanism of the fixed-bed technique are similar to those of the grate technology, which is frequently used to burn biomass feedstock. This method is used when the biomass has irregular particle size, high moisture, and high ash content. This technique evenly distributes the gasoline or fuel mixture over the fuel bed above the grate. The same process, including moisture drying, volatile matter combustion, pyrolysis, and char particle formation, occurs in and above the fuel bed of all grate-fired boilers. Primary air is supplied to the fuel bed through the grate during this phase, aiding heating and accelerating the dehydration of moist fuel via processes such as drying and pyrolysis, thereby achieving char burnout. In addition, the furnaces provided secondary air above the grate to combust the fuel and volatile dust. To reduce NO_2, tertiary air is also supplied to the top furnace via staged combustion.

The various types and commonly used grates are as follows.

Traveling grate: Small packaging boilers are used for biomass firing, whereas large-capacity boilers are used for power and heat generation. In this process, the fuel bed of the boiler unit is continuously stirred on a belt from the fuel inlet to the ash outlet, and the fuel is delivered to the grate by a screw conveyor or stokers for even distribution. The combustion process on the grate is controlled by the bed layer, velocity, and air to achieve complete burnout of the chars. The blends of various biomasses should be evenly distributed, as too high a content can lead to uncontrolled burnout.

Vibrating grate: Vibrating grate technology consists of one or more sections used with various biomass fuels. The sections are independently shaken in cycles that control the stages of the combustion process and prevent the formation of large particles and ash that transfer to the ash conveyor. Primary air is inserted through the grate, while secondary or tertiary air is passed over nozzles positioned directly above the grate. The vibrating grate can be used up to 40 MWe in biomass-fired power plants.

Step grate: The fuel is loaded on one side of the grate and burned; the ash is carried to the ash pit by the grate. It is more controllable and more effective at burning off carbon than a static sloping grate. The complete grate consists of parallel grate sections, which are cooled with water or air. The step grate is high maintenance and requires regular maintenance.

17.2.2 Fluidized Bed Technology

The fluidized bed process is mostly used for the combustion of biomass fuels. There are two types of fluidized bed combustion technologies:

Bubbling fluidized bed technology (BFB): This approach is best suited to small-scale applications, including a variety of biomass fuels with high moisture and ash content and low heating value. A BFB is a furnace or combustion chamber that has a fully refractory-lined bottom and water-cooled walls. The fluidized bed at the bottom of the furnace features nozzles that enhance turbulence-driven mixing of the fuel to create char. Solid particles generally remain in well-stirred beds with a tiny amount of fuel. Then gases move as primary air through a bed of solid materials quickly enough to overcome particle gravitational force. Limestone may be added to the bed to remove or reduce chlorine, sulfur, and coarse bed material, which are withdrawn from the bottom of the bed to avoid ash contamination, that may otherwise cause bed agglomeration. The combustion of primary air is about 30%, and the remaining secondary and tertiary air is injected through air ports above the furnace, depending on the biomass's moisture content. The combustion temperature is normally 800–900°C, with 850°C being the typical bed temperature. Figure 17.5 illustrates a bubbling fluidized bed boiler.

Circulating fluidized bed (CFB): Solid separators separate entrained particulates from the flue gas and recycle them into the lower furnaces, which is how CFB boilers are typically employed in large applications, with fluidizing velocities higher than in BFB. Beyond a certain entrainment velocity, the bed substance gets entrained, and the solids are dispersed all across the furnace. The operation of CFB is fixed over that entrainment velocity. The cyclone recalculates the majority of the

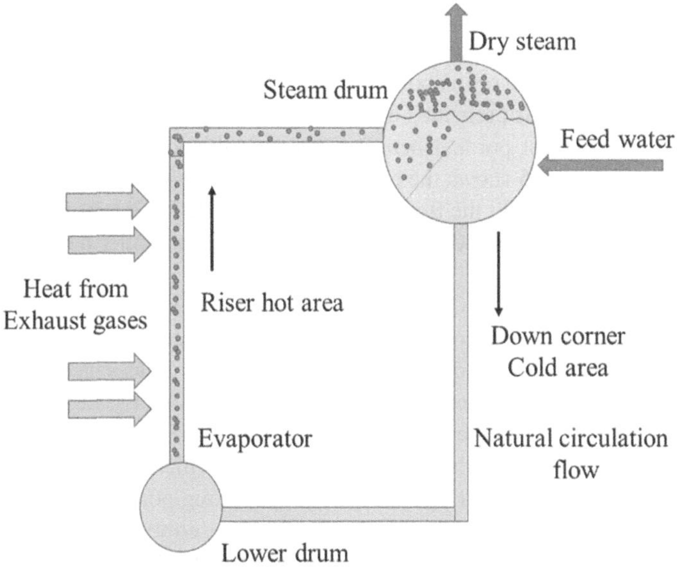

FIGURE 17.5 Evaporation circulation.

Source: Ahmed et al. (2018)

particulates that emerge from the bed, and the boiler's circulating bed substance is employed to regulate temperature. Although sand must be frequently introduced as bed material, and routine maintenance is necessary for the boiler walls, CFB boilers are often expensive. As a result, the costs associated with ash residue are significant.

17.2.3 Boiler Technologies

Boilers convert the energy in hot flue gas from combustion into steam/heat. The main concept, mechanism, and thermodynamics of boilers are similar to those of the steam cycle.

Water and steam boiler: The primary aim of boilers or steam generators is to produce steam at appropriate pressure, temperature, and rate, by transferring heat from the combustion of fuel; the water that has been dried into vapor may be used in diverse applications. The application depends on the steam temperature and pressure for distinct heating, power generation, industrial processes, or a combination. Usually, boilers operate as fire-tube or water-tube boilers, which use a drum at the top; the recirculation of water to convert to steam is called a drum boiler.

The process of a water- and steam-boiler is divided into three main sections: an economizer, an evaporator, and a superheater. The feed water is pumped through the economizer, which heats it to saturated water, and then sent to the evaporator, which contains many downcomer pipes and riser tubes in a closed loop. In addition, these tubes are connected to a header at the bottom of the boiler, which in turn connects to the top of the boiler. Saturated water can enter the drum through the bottom inlet and is preheated by hot combustion gases before being returned to the drum's highest point, where it can be combined with steam to produce electricity. Figure 17.5 shows the evaporation circulating system. The evaporator tubes enclose the walls of the furnace region, and the leftover heat from flue gases is used to preheat combustion air and fumes leaving the boiler before they enter the exhaust gas stream.

Water steam cycle (WSC)**:** In this process, the boiler converts the energy produced by biomass combustion into steam. It is transferred into electrical power in the steam turbine, which is driven by a generator and produces electricity. This is a widely used method for generating electricity from biomass. Figure 17.6 shows the WSC, also known as the Rankin cycle.

The process describes the combustion of fuel, which helps turn water into steam in the boiler, where it is heated above its boiling point using superheaters. The mechanical energy of rotary turbine shafts is used to drive a generator and produce electrical power. The steam exits from turbines and is considered to recirculate into the boiler by condensing through cooling water. The condensed water can be further pumped to the feed tank, which can then be used again as raw material for the boiler to generate steam.

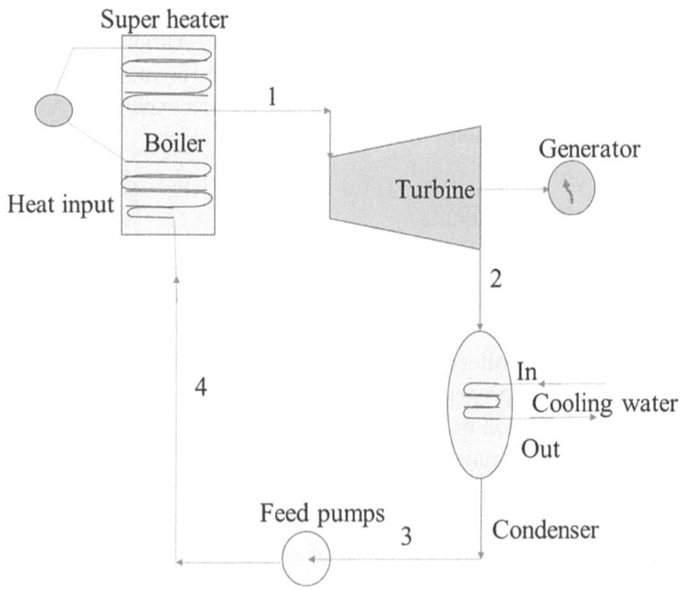

FIGURE 17.6 An overview of the water steam cycle.

Source: Crow and Shippen (2002)

17.3 BIOMASS PYROLYSIS AND ITS CLASSIFICATION FOR BIOFUEL PRODUCTION

Pyrolysis is a thermochemical process in which controlled parameters, such as temperature and pressure, are used to convert raw feedstock into energy products such as bio-oils and gas. These products reduce transport costs by offering convenient combustion characteristics for engines and turbines. Pyrolysis is a method of thermal decomposition of biomass at a certain range of temperatures to produce valuable solids, liquids, and gases. During pyrolysis, biomass is heated in an anaerobic environment, breaking long chains into shorter molecules.

Pyrolysis is the process of partially combusting a type of biomass at about 500°C, in the absence of oxygen, to produce gas, liquid, and solid products, including combustible gas, bio-oil, and charcoal (Lebaka, 2013). The volatile components of the gases that produce biomass can be vaporized at extreme temperatures, and their vapors can then be liquefied. The fuel produced by this method can be stored and later used in a variety of thermal and electric utility applications. The pyrolysis process generates combustible compounds, as well as liquid fuels such as gas and charcoal and numerous other high-value products. The usual process flow diagram for biomass pyrolysis is displayed in Figure 17.7. The benefit of the pyrolysis process is that it converts solid materials into gases and vapors that can be inexpensively transported, stored, and handled. A drawback of the pyrolysis process is that it requires a constant supply of heat, such as fuel, to produce syngas.

According to the choice of biomass feedstock as the raw material for processing from raw material to the final product, the pyrolysis reaction mechanism can be either slow or quick. During pyrolysis, lower temperatures result in a delayed

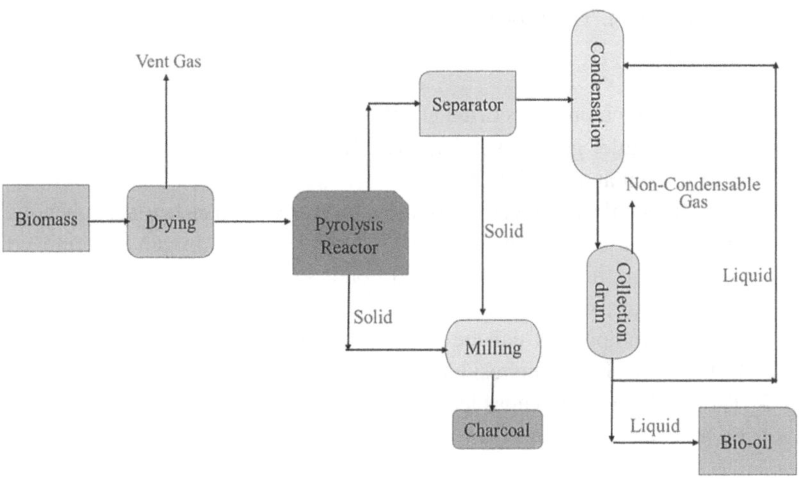

FIGURE 17.7 The pyrolysis of biomass.

reaction that produces biochar, whereas higher temperatures favor the formation of bio-oils. Heating rates in a slow pyrolysis process will be very low, approximately 10–20°C/min, to achieve the process's depolymerization reaction and produce the most solids. Fast pyrolysis generates heat at a pace of up to 200°C/sec to achieve a greater processing temperature, and the residue duration of 2 seconds results in a bio-oil yield of 50–70 wt%. Fast pyrolysis requires biomass with particle sizes less than 1 mm, whereas slow pyrolysis can be performed with particle sizes of 5–50 mm (Chhiti & Kemiha, 2013).

17.3.1 Biomass Pyrolysis Techniques

There are several approaches to the combustion of lignocellulosic biomass, but the conversion of bio-oils, biofuels, and other solid products depends on the available biomass and the reaction conditions used in processing. Many studies by researchers reported that pyrolysis is the best process for producing value-added solids (biochar), liquids (bio-oils), and gases (combustible gases) for day-to-day use. Generally, biomass feedstock or waste is produced by syngas, a mixture of hydrogen, CO, and volatile organic compounds, which can produce a fluid similar to diesel and other products if process conditions are varied accordingly. The physicochemical properties govern the pyrolytic reaction conditions that optimize pyrolysis. Catalytic pyrolysis can produce alcohol from pyrolytic oil. The advantage of this technique is that it captures and combusts methane along with carbon monoxide to produce syngas, which uses energy during the process and produces CO_2 as a greenhouse gas (less potent than methane, offsets FF energy production).

Producing products through this technique requires pathways that include slow pyrolysis, upgradation of syngas, catalytic pyrolysis and hydroprocessing, fast pyrolysis and hydroprocessing, and hydro pyrolysis and hydroprocessing (Dang et al., 2016). The process for the pyrolysis of biomass takes place in the following order:

1. Initially, the biomass is dried at 150°C.
2. Usually, outlet gases like CO, CO_2, N_2, CH_3COOH, and CH_3OH are distilled out at around 275°C.
3. The chemical substances of complex mixtures such as ketones, phenols, aldehydes, esters, ethane, methane, CO, CO_2, and hydrogen are removed by breaking the weakest chemical bonds using an exothermic reaction, which occurs at 300–350°C.
4. Volatile compounds can be removed at 350°C with the formation of CO, C, and H, and the residue remains in the form of charcoal.
5. The production of syngas leads to the formation of residues such as bio-oil and carbonaceous. They are as follows:
    i. The first form of the pyrolysis process is carbonization; in this, solid vegetable coal is recovered at 300–500°C.

ii. Conventional pyrolysis occurs at 500°C and produces 3 fractions in equal proportions (which is slow and takes a longer reaction time).
iii. In fast pyrolysis, the gasification reaction occurs at 500–650°C in a short time and produces a liquid fraction of up to 80wt%, besides generating gas, bio-oil, and coal of 10 to 20%, respectively.
iv. Flash pyrolysis occurs at 650°C in less than 1 second and produces a gaseous fraction with 80% efficiency.

The liquid portion of bio-oil, produced by pyrolysis, can be used as fuel for cogenerators to generate energy.

17.4 GASIFICATION AND LIQUEFACTION METHODS

In this process, biomass can be converted into gaseous and liquid fuels via hydrothermal gasification, which can be applied either in the gaseous phase via supercritical water steam reforming or in the liquid phase via aqueous-phase reforming.

Gasification: Synthesis gas, often called syngas and primarily composed of CO, H_2, and nitrogen, is produced during gasification of solid carbon sources (solid biomass) (Rahimpour et al., 2012). In the petrochemical and refining sectors, syngas can be used as an energy source to generate power or as a raw material for a wide range of products such as ammonia, methanol, and synthetic petrol.

The development of the first gasification devices occurred early in the 20th century. Although there are various forms of treatments and procedures, they share certain commonalities. The predominant method is the fractional oxidation of the solid material at extreme temperatures, resulting in a syngas comprising CO and H_2 in a variety of ratios, accounting for more than 85% of the entire volume, with CO_2 and CH_4 making up the remainder of the gas (Molino et al., 2016). The syngas produced can be further burned to generate heat and power or catalytically converted into liquid fuels, including methanol, ethanol, petrol, diesel, and jet fuels (Brown, 2015). The gasification process is promising because it uses biomass hydrolysates, mixtures of oxygenated hydrocarbons, and converts them into gaseous products. A schematic of the biomass gasification process is shown in Figure 17.8.

This technique is a highly intricate thermochemical procedure performed in an enclosed space at a low air pressure relative to ambient pressure or under air suction. Following gasification, the gas is "cleaned" to simultaneously retrieve trace amounts and remove pollutants. Because it can completely purge contaminants from syngas, gasification is a particularly intriguing technology, especially for compounds that contain significant amounts of heteroatoms or other impurities that are difficult to handle. In fact, using this process, sulfur is routinely recovered in its most basic form; the cleaned gases can be used to produce compounds or energy (Figure 17.9). Depending on the type of biomass and operating conditions, the generated gas is split into various flammable and nonflammable components. The generated gas typically has a calorific value of 4.5–6 MJ/m^3, which is 10–50% of that of natural gas (Akia et al., 2014).

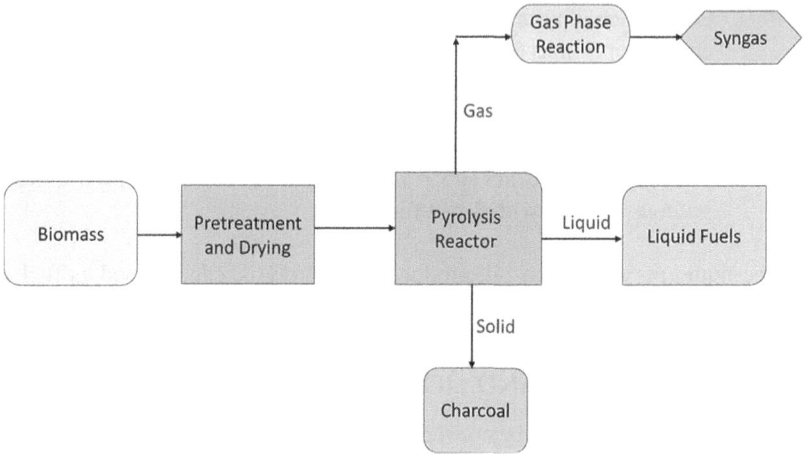

FIGURE 17.8 Biomass gasification.

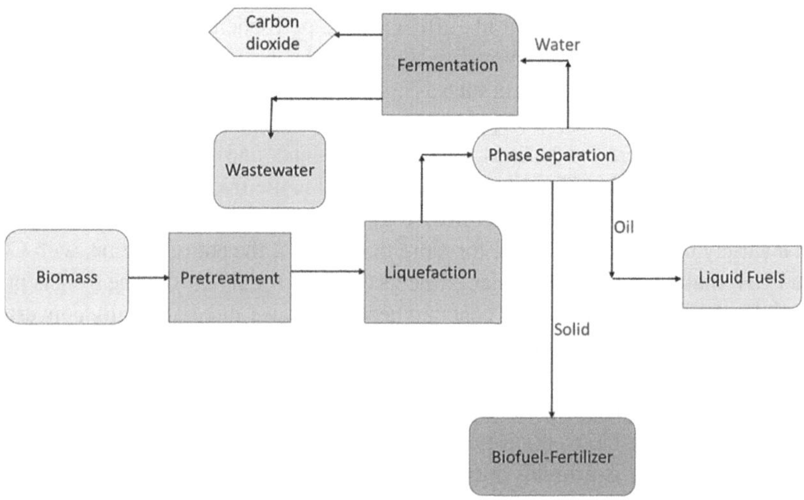

FIGURE 17.9 Process flow diagram of the biomass liquefaction process.

Liquefaction: The conversion of biomass, known as liquefaction, takes place in water at elevated pressures and moderate temperatures of 280–370°C. In addition to other solids, aqueous, and gaseous by-products, a liquid bio-granulate that resembles crude oil is also produced (López Barreiro et al., 2013). Bio-oils can be used as feedstocks to replace petroleum fuels. In addition, phenolics derived from lignin can be hydrogenated to aromatic compounds, while carbohydrates are used in fermentation to produce high-value products. Primarily, the more common method employs lignocellulosic biomass heated to around 350°C and pressed at 150 psi for about 15 min. The spontaneous phase transition occurs in this process, resulting in a gaseous form of CO_2, solid by-products, bio-crude, and a tiny aqueous phase (Rowbotham et al., 2012). The resulting solid-state compound could be used immediately as fertilizer or biofuel. Inside the unit, the aqueous solution could be utilized for water-dependent activities or digesters. Because of its low oxygen content, the resulting bio-crude needs to be refined substantially before it can be used commercially (Yu et al., 2011). Figure 17.9 shows the biomass liquefaction unit in detail.

17.4.1 Oxidation

Each reaction requires a gaseous input to attain the required operating temperature, thereby triggering an endothermic reaction. Any biomass that is to be gasified should first undergo an oxidation reaction to obtain the temperature range required to carry out the endothermic reaction. According to Kaltschmitt (2013), the following reactions occur during the oxidation phase:

Coal combustion:

$$C + O_2 \rightarrow CO_2 \Delta DH = -394 \text{ KJ/mol} \tag{17.3}$$

Partial oxidation:

$$C + Y_2 O_2 \rightarrow CO\Delta H = -111 \text{ KJ/mol} \tag{17.4}$$

Hydrogen combustion:

$$H_2 + ½\, O_2 \; H_2O\Delta H = -242 \text{ KJ/mol} \tag{17.5}$$

The thermal energy required to complete the activity can be obtained from the aforementioned reactions, which are also the primary ones. Complete combustion produces a mixture of CO, CO_2, and H_2O as by-products.

17.4.2 Drying

Sometimes, for a reaction to be effective and produce the highest yields possible, the feedstock must be dehydrated before the reactions can begin. Certain processes employ the moisture present in raw resources, as raw biomass algae can have moisture contents as high as 90%, which can be used to facilitate the transformation into a wide range of products with added value that appear to be beneficial on a global scale. Globally accessible biomass comes in a variety of types and moisture contents ranging from 10% to 90%, which must be removed for enhanced performance in goods. The water present in the feedstock must be eliminated during the drying process at a temperature of 105°C for it to be completed. The heating rate needed for this stage is directly proportional to the moisture content of the raw resources; it is often derived from the oxidation phase that precedes it (Molino et al., 2016).

17.4.3 Pyrolysis

Pyrolysis, which produces ash as a residue and a high-carbon solid fraction known as "char," thermally degrades carbon material derived from biomass under anaerobic conditions. These "tars" are liquid fractions that, at low temperatures, contain intricate, condensable chemical compounds. Pyrolysis gas is a combination of incondensable hydrogen, CO_2, CO, and traces of hydrocarbons, which exist at ambient temperature (Roos, 2010). Higher molecular weight molecule bonds are broken in this stage, resulting in the production of smaller molecules. The endothermic pyrolysis step occurs between 250°C and 700°C.

Biomass:

$$H_2 + CO + CO_2 + CH_4 + H_2O\ (g) = \text{tar} + \text{char} \tag{17.6}$$

As biomass has previously been processed, the term "biomass" in Eq. 17.6 could be replaced by a formula for cellulose ($C_6H_{10}O_6$), the major constituent of the biomass, which accounts for about 55% of the matrix's overall mass. The pyrolysis of cellulose takes place between 600°C and 700°C (Molino et al., 2016). At this phase of the procedure, typically 12.01 kg of carbon is fully oxidized with 22.39 m^3 of O_2, producing 22.26 m^3 of CO and approximately 0.04 GJ of heat.

17.4.4 Reduction

The reduction phases, which occur in gas-phase reactions involving a combination of coal and gas produced during pyrolysis, are converted into products during the gasification process. Interactions between the oxidation and pyrolysis by-products produce the final syngas. Zhang et al. (2013) reported that the reaction in the reduction phases can be demonstrated as follows.

Boudouard reaction:

$$C + O_2 \leftrightarrow 2CO \Delta H = 172\ \text{KJ/mol} \tag{17.7}$$

Character reforms:

$$C + H_2O \leftrightarrow CO + H_2 \Delta H = 131\ \text{KJ/mol} \tag{17.8}$$

Water gas displacement reaction:

$$CO + H_2O \leftrightarrow 2CO \Delta H = -41\ \text{KJ/mol} \tag{17.9}$$

Methanation:

$$C + 2H_2 \leftrightarrow CH_4 \Delta H = -75 \text{ KJ/mol} \quad (17.10)$$

Boudouard reaction and character reforms [Eqs. (17.7) and (17.8)] are endothermic, which favors an increase in temperature; a low temperature [Eqs. (17.9) and (17.10)] favorably fastens exothermic processes. Because the global exothermic contribution is higher than the endothermic impact, the reaction's overall contribution is exothermic, requiring energy throughout the entire phase.

The decrease in temperature, a crucial parameter, governs the composition and properties of syngas and the solid residue. Low levels of solid residues and tar will remain from the process due to the higher oxidation rate of the coal and the maximum operating temperature. Gasification is mostly performed between 800°C and 1,100°C, with only the gasification step using air at 500°C–1,600°C (Shen et al., 2011).

17.5 CONCLUSION

To transform renewable biomass feedstock into biofuels, chemicals, and value-added goods, as well as for energy production and other applications, the selection and implementation of production technologies are crucial. However, the establishment of demand and continuous government initiatives that result in a strong manufacturing policy for any industry are subject to financial and environmental factors.

REFERENCES

Ahmed, S.E.A., Mostafa, E.H., Hesham, A.A., 2018. Modelling and practical studying of heat recovery steam generator (HRSG) drum dynamics and approach point effect on control valves. *Ain Shams Engineering Journal*, 9, 3187–3196.

Akia, M., Yazdani, F., Motaee, E., Han, D., Arandiyan, H., 2014. A review on conversion of biomass to biofuel by nanocatalysts. *Biofuel Research Journal*, 1, 16–25.

Brown, T.R., 2015. A techno-economic review of thermochemical cellulosic biofuel pathways. *Bioresour Technol*, 178, 166–176.

Chhiti, Y., Kemiha, M., 2013. Thermal conversion of biomass, pyrolysis and gasification: A review. *International Journal of Engineering Science*, 2, 75–85.

Crow, I.G., Shippen, K., 2002. Plant engineer's reference book. In Dennis A. Snow (Ed.) *Electricity Generation* (2nd ed). Butterworth-Heinemann, 22-1–22-33. ISBN 9780750644525. https://doi.org/10.1016/B978-075064452-5/50077-8.

Dang, Q., Hu, W., Rover, M., Brown, R.C., Wright, M.M., 2016. Economics of biofuels and bioproducts from an integrated pyrolysis biorefinery. *Biofuels, Bioprod Biorefin*, 10(6), 790–803.

Kaltschmitt, M., 2013. Renewable energy from biomass: Introduction. In M. Kaltschmitt, N.J. Themelis, L.Y. Bronicki, L. Söder and L.A. Vega (Eds.) *Renewable Energy Systems*. Springer, New York.

Klass, D.L., 1998. *Biomass for Renewable Energy, Fuels, and Chemicals*. Academic Press, San Diego, 1–651.Lebaka, V., 2013. Potential bioresources as future sources of biofuels production: An Overview. In V. Gupta and M.G. Tuohy (Eds.) *Biofuel Technology*. Springer, Berlin, 223–258.

López Barreiro, D., Prins, W., Ronsse, F., Brilman, W., 2013. Hydrothermal liquefaction (HTL) of microalgae for biofuel production: State of the art review and future prospects. *Biomass Bioenergy*, 53, 113–127.

McKendry, P., 2002. Energy production from biomass (Part 1): Overview of biomass. *Bioresour Technol*, 83, 37–46

Molino, A., Chianese, S., Musmarra, D., 2016. Biomass gasification technology: The state of the art overview. *J Energy Chem*, 25(1), 10–25.

Noon, C.E., Daly, M.J., Graham, R.L., Zhan, F.B., 1996. *Transportation and Site Location Analysis for Regional Integrated Biomass Assessment (Riba)*. Bioenergy 96-The Seventh National Bioenergy Conference Partnerships to Develop and Apply Biomass Technologies, September 15–20.

Nussbaumer, T., 2003. Combustion and co-combustion of biomass: Fundamentals, technologies, and primary measures for emission reduction. *Energy Fuels*, 17, 1510–1521.

Rahimpour, M.R., Arab Aboosadi, Z., Jahanmiri, A.H., 2012. Synthesis gas production in a novel hydrogen and oxygen perm-selective membranes tri-reformer for methanol production. *J Nat Gas Sci Eng*, 9, 149–159.

Roos, C̄.J., 2010. *Clean Heat and Power Using Biomass Gasification for Industrial and Agricultural Projects*. U.S. Department of Energy.

Rowbotham, J., Dyer, P., Greenwell, H., Theodorou, M., 2012. Thermochemical processing of macroalgae: A late bloomer in the development of third-generation biofuels? *Biofuel*, 3(4), 441–461.

Shen, D.K., Xiao, R., Gu, S., Luo, K.H., 2011. The pyrolytic behavior of cellulose in lignocellulosic biomass: A review. *RSC Adv*, 1(9), 1641–1660.

Sumit, S., Rajendra, M., Amit, S., Pawan, K.G., 2014. Biomass conversion technologies for renewable energy and fuels: A review note. *IOSR Journal of Mechanical and Civil Engineering (IOSR-JMCE)*, 11(2), 28–35.

Tursi A., 2019. A review on biomass: Importance, chemistry, classification, and conversion. *Biofuel Research Journal*, 22, 962–979.

Yu, G., Zhang, Y., Schideman, L., Funk, T., Wang, Z., 2011. Distributions of carbon and nitrogen in the products from hydrothermal liquefaction of low-lipid microalgae. *Energy Environ Sci*, 4(11), 4587–4595.

Zhang, J., Weng, X., Han, Y., Li, W., Gan, Z., Gu, J., 2013. Effect of supercritical water on the stability and activity of alkaline carbonate catalysts in coal gasification. *J Energy Chem*, 22.

18 New Strategies for Conversion of Lignocellulosic Biomass to Biofuels

Mamilla Shyam Sunder

18.1 INTRODUCTION

Lignocellulosic biomass studies have been widely studied, and they have demonstrated new strategies, a feasible technology, and a cost-effective process for value-added products or bioenergy production, with the demand for the products. In the 1920s, the petrochemical industry originated with simple organic chemical reactions such as ethanol and isopropanol from ethylene and propylene of oil refining at an industrial scale. Bioethanol is the most significant volume chemical produced globally by fermentation, and a huge amount of bio-ethylene is currently produced by the dehydration of bioethanol. The feasibility of technology for bio-refineries following the thermochemical or biochemical pathways, or bio-refineries with different complexity, has to be investigated. A techno-economic assessment is used as a standard means, and predefined parameters like production cost and returns rate, which represent techno-economic performance, are evaluated and carried out by determining some common indicators like net present value, payback period, fixed capital cost, total capital cost, breakeven price, and after-tax rate of return. Some studies by researchers argued that biomass conversion to biofuels is strongly influenced by the cost of feedstocks and the technology used (Lange, 2007). For instance, Fischer–Tropsch synthetic crude production is technology dominated, whereas vegetable oil used in biofuel production is significantly influenced by feedstock costs (Parajuli et al., 2015).

The lignocellulosic biomass used in biofuels or bioenergy products results from the type of lignocellulosic material and the method of treatment chosen. Different pretreatment methods are available for producing biofuels and biogas, which show positive effects, but some show adverse effects due to the formation of inhibitors. Alkali pretreatment is generally preferred for biomass containing a higher content of lignin. The pretreatment should be cost-effective, as lignocelluloses may provide lower yield and production rate due to their low accessibility for enzymes and microorganisms. The wide availability of biomass, such as corn

DOI: 10.1201/9781003327608-18

cobs and stalks, can be utilized to convert into bio-hydrogen. Several biofuels can be obtained through lignocellulosic biomass; bio-oil can be produced by fast depolymerization and hydrolysis; fermentation methods can produce bioethanol; and biohydrogen can be produced through thermochemical or biological routes. Biogas and syngas are produced through anaerobic digestion, while gasification produces syngas.

18.2 BIOETHANOL AND BIO-BUTANOL PRODUCTION BY CONSOLIDATED BIO-PROCESSING

Biofuels, namely bioethanol and biobutanol, are the prime biofuels that are renewable and can be produced by the carbohydrate-containing sources of lignocellulosic biomass such as sweet sorghum, sugarcane, corn, pearl millet, and other agricultural residues. Petroleum-derived liquid fuels are the dominant source of fuels, but biofuels proved to be an appropriate option for their substitution (Bhutto et al., 2016). Globally, the transport sector consumes 25% of primary energy annually and is responsible for the related greenhouse gas emissions. Table 18.1 summarizes the techno-economic assessment studies for sugarcane as

TABLE 18.1
Techno-Economic Assessment Studies on Sugarcane Biorefineries Aimed at Biofuel Production

Location	Feedstock/s	Product/s	Capacity (t cane/hr)	Reference
Brazil	Bagasse and trash	EtOH	1,000	Seabra and Macedo (2011)
Colombia	Cane juice	EtOH	146	Sánchez and Cardona (2012)
South Africa	Bagasse and trash	EtOH	300	Mandegari et al. (2017)
Brazil	Cane juice and hemicellulose	EtOH	500	Dias et al. (2013b)
Hungary/USA	Bagasse	EtOH	293	Gubicza et al. (2016)
Brazil	Cane juice, bagasse, and trash	Butanol	500	Pereira et al. (2014)
Brazil	Cane juice	Butanol	500	Mariano et al. (2013)
South Africa	Bagasse and trash	Butanol	300	Farzad et al. (2017b)
Brazil	Cane juice, bagasse, and trash chemicals	Jet fuel	500	Alves et al. (2017)
South Africa	Cane juice, bagasse, and trash	EtOJ/Jet fuel	222	Diederichs et al. (2016)
Brazil	Cane juice, bagasse, and trash	Jet fuel	500	Santos et al. (2017)
South Africa	Bagasse and trash	pH	300	Petersen et al. (2015)

TABLE 18.1 *(Continued)*
Techno-Economic Assessment Studies on Sugarcane Biorefineries Aimed at Biofuel Production

Location	Feedstock/s	Product/s	Capacity (t cane/hr)	Reference
Cuba	Bagasse and trash	EtOH/MeOH	1700	Renó et al. (2014)
Brazil	Cane juice, bagasse, and trash	EtOH/MeOH	500	Albarelli et al. (2015)
South Africa	Bagasse	Pyrolysis products	300	Nsaful et al. (2013)
China/UK	Bagasse	FT/pyrolysis products	667	Michailos et al. (2017)

Source: Mandegari et al. (2017)

feedstock in biorefineries. Day by day, lignocellulosic biomass materials, which are abundantly available biomass resources, are attracting increasing attention as an economical, renewable way to reduce dependency on petroleum resources and minimize energy and material as raw material feedstock cost.

Bioethanol: Ethanol production has dominated the global biofuels industry and has received increasing attention due to its significant environmental benefits. Ethanol fuel can be produced from different types of feedstock biomass containing carbohydrates, such as sugarcane and corn cobs, which produces 110 billion liters of bioethanol in a year (Chum et al., 2014; Baeyens et al., 2015). The United States, Brazil, and other EU members promoted alternative fuel bioethanol in the world (Balan et al., 2013; Chum et al., 2014), and the two commercial bioethanol production plants with a capacity of 40 and 80 ML/year have become operational (Chum et al, 2014; Peplow, 2014), and several other projects are still in progress worldwide (Balan et al., 2013). As the global trend increased toward renewable feedstock, sugarcane bagasse has become more critical; the sugarcane bio-refineries convert sugar syrups, molasses, bagasse, and harvesting residue into biofuel and other bioproducts, as it further converts distillery into ethanol. The production pathway process is the fermentation of sugar to further fuel-grade ethanol, which is blended with gasoline in different ratios for vehicle utilization. Furthermore, it is reported that using 10% bioethanol blends decreases gas emissions and greenhouse effect by 12–20% compared to petroleum-based fuels. The transport sector has been consuming the majority of bioethanol produced worldwide as a fuel, and it is an essential building block for other biofuels and biochemicals. Figure 18.1 shows the possible products from ethanol.

Biobutanol: Butanol is also one of the lignocellulosic biomass-based fuels or renewable products produced by the fermentation process. Due to its superior fuel properties like higher heating values, reduced ignition problems, lower

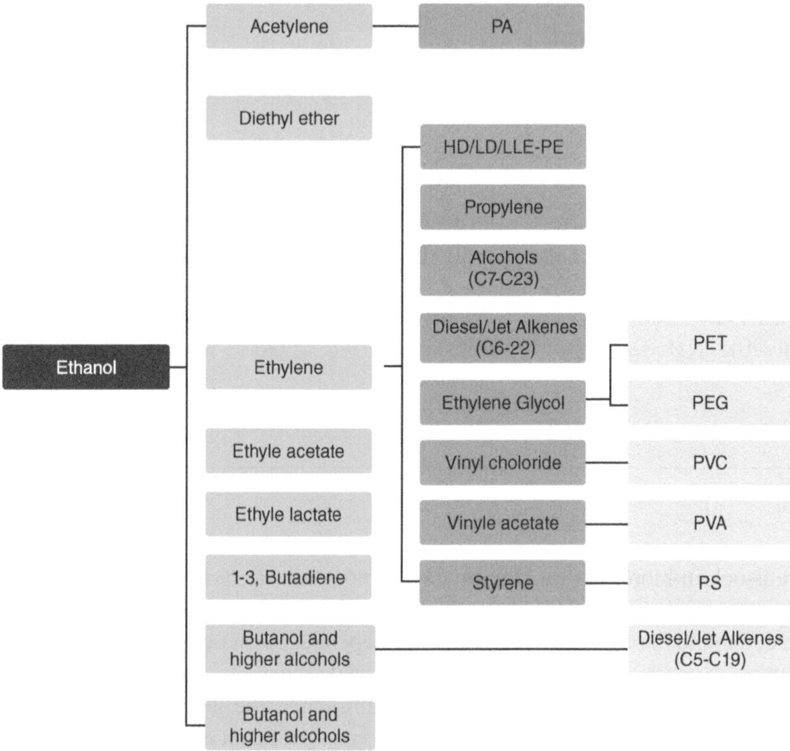

FIGURE 18.1 The possible products from ethanol.

Source: Taylor et al. (2015)

volatility, ease of blending, higher viscosity, easier distribution, and safety of use (Jin et al., 2011), butanol is widely used in blending with petrol. However, ethanol is a well-established biofuel. Butanol can be mixed with gasoline as it has lower polarity (larger hydrocarbon chain). Butanol can be produced by metabolic pathway as fermentation or by chemical synthesis from ethanol (Ndaba et al., 2015).

18.3 BIOCHEMICAL CONVERSIONS OF BIOMASS

Biochemical conversion of biomass produces value-added carbon-based chemicals and products, which are bioproducts like cellulose fiber derivatives, sugars and sugar alcohols, furfural, glycerins, carbonaceous materials, bio-plastics and resins, and other valuable products. The biochemical process to convert biomass by allowing it to decompose with available carbohydrates, which may be converted into biogas and liquid fuels and other types of bioproducts, uses biological agents such as microorganisms like bacteria, yeast, and enzymes (Mahalaxmi and Williford, 2014). However, in the early years, microorganisms were regarded as biochemical "factories" for treating and converting most forms of animal- and human-generated organic waste for ethanol production, which is an ancient ritual.

The biochemical conversion technologies emerged as the studies of microbial engineering encouraged the fermentation technology, both aerobic and anaerobic fermentation, which is used in the production of energy like biogas and fertilizer, and for the use of removal of unwanted products from wastes and waste streams (Cross, 1995). Biochemical conversion of biomass material materials includes the following:

1. Anaerobic digestion includes hydrolysis, acedogenesis, acetogenesis, and methanogenesis.
2. Fermentation process.
3. Physicochemical conversion.

18.3.1 Anaerobic Digestion

The anaerobic digestion process is the microbial digestion of feedstocks. It is a multistep biological process used for proper waste management and generating renewable energy (Zamani, 2015). In anaerobic digestion, organic material is directly converted to a gas, which takes several days to complete, or converted into gas to maintain ideal conditions. The obtained released gas is collectively referred to as biogas. The gas mixture mainly consists of methane and carbon dioxide with small quantities of hydrogen sulfide, heat, and, under a specific condition, hydrogen gas. After the process, the remaining solid digestate is suitable for use as a fertilizer. Anaerobic reactors are generally used to produce methane-rich biogas from human and animal manure and crop residues (Sharma, 2015). They utilize mixed methogenic bacterial culture, allowing digestion to be operated over a wide temperature range up to 60°C. Figure 18.2 shows the anaerobic digestion process.

The anaerobic digestion process is a proven technology, widely used as an ideal process for the waste treatment of 80–90% moisture content. The advantage of anaerobic digestion is that it releases methane gas, a potent greenhouse gas, into the atmosphere and is used directly in ignition gas engines and gas turbines. The overall conversion efficiency can be 21%. The stages for the anaerobic digestion process are as follows (Zamani, 2015):

Hydrolysis: This is the initial phase, in which biomass containing carbohydrates, fats, and proteins is converted into small molecules such as amino acids, simple sugars, and fatty acids (Horan, 2018).

Acidogenesis: The second stage of anaerobic digestion further decomposes the hydrolysis products into ammonia, hydrogen, hydrogen sulfide, carbon dioxide, alcohols, carbonic acids, fatty acids, and other alcohols. As this process is a

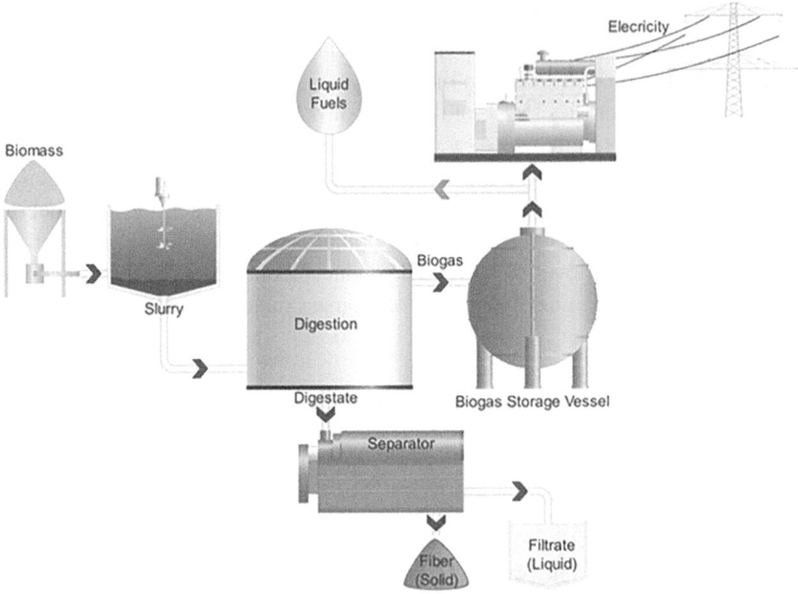

FIGURE 18.2 Biomass anaerobic digestion scheme.

Source: Tursi et al. (2019). DOI:10.18331/BRJ2019.6.2.3

partial decomposition of biomass, a final production of methane, the acetogenesis process, is required.

1. **Acetogenesis:** This process converts the products formed in the acidogenesis phase into acetic acid, carbon dioxide, and hydrogen. Finally, the breakdown process of biomass facilitates the production of methane as a biofuel.
2. **Methanogenesis:** This process is the final stage during which methane is generated from the product of acetogenesis through hydrogenotrophic methanogenesis and acetogenesis methanogenesis, as shown in Equations 18.1 and 18.2.
   i. Hydrogenotrophic methanogenesis:

$$CO_2 + 4H_2 \rightarrow CH_4 + 2H_2O \tag{18.1}$$

   ii. Acetogenetic methanogenesis:

$$CH_3COOH \rightarrow CH_4 + CO_2 \tag{18.2}$$

18.3.2 Fermentation

The fermentation of biomass-derived sugars is necessary to increase the number of commodity chemicals, with advances in metabolic pathway engineering as a cost-effective process. The fermentation of organic materials from biomass or its derived sugars, such as pentoses and hexoses, converts them into ethanol and carbon dioxide under anaerobic conditions using microorganisms as yeast, as shown in Equation 18.3.

$$\text{Sugars} \rightarrow \text{Ethanol} + \text{Carbon dioxide} + \text{By-products} \tag{18.3}$$

Many studies have been carried out and reviewed to determine the challenges involved in achieving commercial viability and productivity yields, as well as other considerations, such as by-product profile and strain robustness, which are involved in the reactions. The microorganisms commonly used for the fermentation process are *Saccharomyces cerevisiae* and *Pichia stipitis*. Theoretically, the product yield process is 51.14 g of ethanol and 48.86 g of carbon dioxide from 100 g of hexoses or pentoses, as given in Equations 18.4 and 18.5. In addition, the by-products produced are glycerol and carboxylic acids. The various factors, such as feedstock, pH, temperature, inoculum, and fermentation time, are the parameters for delivering quality and good yields (Strezov, 2014).

$$C_6H_{12}O_6\,(\text{hexoses}) \rightarrow 2C_2H_5OH + 2CO_2 \tag{18.4}$$

$$3C_5H_{10}O_5\,(\text{pentoses}) \rightarrow 5C_2H_5OH + 5CO_2 \tag{18.5}$$

Fermentation technology enhances ethanol production as a petroleum substitute and fuel, both economically and environmentally beneficial. After the conversion process, ethanol is further distilled and dehydrated to obtain concentrated alcohol, while solid residues are used as fuel in boilers and feed for livestock (Mariod, 2016). Figure 18.3 describes the biomass fermentation process.

18.3.3 Physicochemical Conversion

The production of high-density biofuels from the physicochemical conversion process of biomass by its embedded techniques proved to be the most economical process for products like biodiesel, produced from vegetable oils and animals through esterification and transesterification processes (Fukuda et al., 2001). Figure 18.4 shows the physicochemical conversion process.

Waste cooking and algal oil produce second- and third-generation biofuels and biodiesel. The oil, mainly composed of triglycerides, undergoes the transesterification process that breaks down into constituents such as fatty acids and glycerols, which are converted into methyl or ethyl esters as biodiesel using methyl or

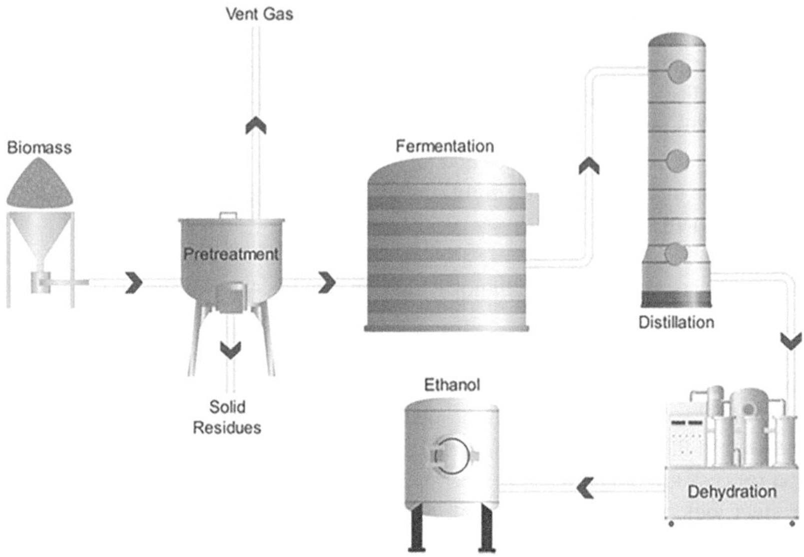

FIGURE 18.3 Biomass fermentation scheme.

Source: Tursi et al. (2019). DOI:10.18331/BRJ2019.6.2.3

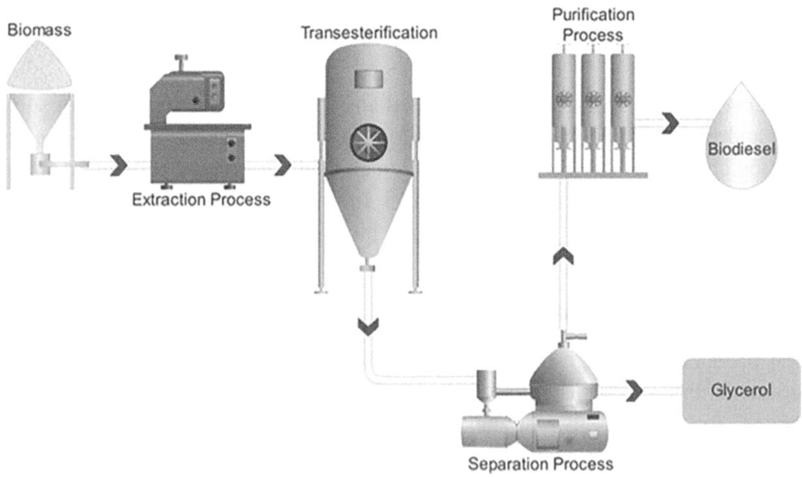

FIGURE 18.4 Biomass physicochemical conversion scheme.

Source: Tursi et al. (2019). DOI:10.18331/BRJ2019.6.2.3

ethyl alcohol in the presence of an alkaline catalyst such as potassium hydroxide or sodium hydroxide, as given in Equation (18.6).

$$\text{Oil} + \text{Short-chain alcohol} \rightarrow \text{Biodiesel} + \text{Glycerol} \tag{18.6}$$

During transesterification, triglycerides occur at low temperatures between 50°C and 70°C at atmospheric pressure. The product obtained is neutralized and purified for glycerol, which is denser than the biodiesel fraction and can be separated by a phase separator (Leung et al., 2010). After glycerol and biodiesel phase separation, the excess alcohol can be removed by distillation and other partial evaporation. Finally, the biodiesel fraction is purified by liquid-liquid extraction to separate or remove catalysts and soaps. The product obtained is dried and stored.

Biodiesel is a biodegradable, nontoxic, and renewable fuel. Its high oxygen content and lubrication properties are unique features, and its close physicochemical parameters ensure efficient biodiesel combustion in diesel engines. Glycerol and glycerine can also be valorized into various value-added products used in the food and pharmaceutical industries (Canakci and Van Gerpen, 1999).

18.4 BIODIESEL AS A RENEWABLE TECHNOLOGY OPTION FROM VARIOUS BIOMASSES

Many plant types available in the world are little known as oil-bearing perennial plants and are a feature of the familiar landscapes of tropical to semiarid climates. However, they are used in traditional culture. Biodiesel, produced from these plant oils, is a viable, renewable fuel for replacing conventional diesel in transportation and other applications, such as electricity generators. Biodiesel is nontoxic and biodegradable and reduces significantly toxic and other emissions when burned as a fuel.

There are many renewable technologies for the biomass raw materials and wind, solar, hydro, and geothermal energy, which are making relatively fast progress (Fridleifsson, 2001) and are commercially competitive as renewable energy sources are often called alternative energy sources. Carbon emissions are primarily from fossil fuels, and about 98% of the pollutants necessitate using renewable and alternative sources to reduce pollutants such as biodiesel. Table 18.2 shows the global renewable energy scenario by 2040. In developed countries, there is a growing trend toward employing modern technologies and efficient bioenergy conversion using a range of biofuels, which are becoming cost competitive with fossil fuel (Puhan, 2005). There are bioethanol and biodiesel, which are biomass-based global liquid transportation fuels that are replacing gasoline and diesel fuel, which offer many benefits of greenhouse gas emission reduction, sustainability, and security of supply (Reijnders, 2006). Biodiesel burns like petroleum diesel, which has better efficiency than gasoline, and has potential for compression-ignition engines and can also be replaced by diesel fuel.

TABLE 18.2
Global Renewable Energy Scenario by 2040

Source	2001	2010	2020	2030	2040
Total consumption (million tons oil equivalent)	10,038	10,549	11,425	12,352	13,310
Biomass	1,080	1,313	1,791	2,483	3,271
Large hydro	22.7	266	309	341	358
Geothermal	43.2	86	186	333	493
Small hydro	9.5	19	49	106	189
Wind	4.7	44	266	542	688
Solar thermal	4.1	15	66	244	480
Photovoltaic	0.2	2	24	221	784
Solar thermal	0.1	0.4	3	16	68
Electricity marine (tidal/wave/ocean)	0.05	0.1	0.4	3	20
Total renewable energy sources	1,365.5	1,745	2,694	4,289	6,351
Renewable energy source contribution (%)	13.6	16.6	3.6	34.7	47.7

Source: Iva Kralova and Johan Sjöblom, 2010.

Biodiesel is nonflammable, renewable, readily available, has higher combustion efficiency, and leads to low formation of sulfur and aromatic content (Ma and Hanna, 1999; Knothe et al., 2006). Biodiesel is mainly produced from biomass, primarily rapeseed, soybean, and palm oils, and is defined as mono-alkyl esters of fatty acids, which are derived from vegetable oils and animal fats. The economic benefits of the biodiesel industry include value added to feedstock, increased income taxes, rural manufacturing jobs, and increased investments in plant and equipment. With expansion in the manufacturing process and improved air quality, biodiesel is exempted from the oil tax. In 2015, the EU accounted for 89% of biodiesel produced worldwide, and the United States became the world's largest single producer, with about 18% of world biodiesel consumption, followed by Germany.

Biodiesel is an alternative diesel obtained by transesterifying triglycerides (Bala, 2005), which is obtained by the extraction of bio-oils from biomass, with methanol. Methanol is preferred due to its low cost and as a base catalyst, which is more effective than an acid catalyst and enzymes (Ma and Hanna, 1999). There are four basic route processes for producing biodiesel from oils and fats. They are base-catalyzed transesterification, conversion of oil into fatty acids and then into biodiesel, and non-catalytic transesterification of oils and fats. Most biodiesel produced today is made via base-catalyzed transesterification due to its high conversion yields, low temperature and pressure requirements, and suitability with simple construction materials (Wang et al., 2007). The base-catalyzed technique for biodiesel production involves mixing alcohol and catalyst, the transesterification reaction, separation, washing of biodiesel, alcohol distillation or removal, glycerine neutralization, and finally, purification of the product. The production of biodiesel can be in batch or a continuous process and is characterized by its diversity, viscosity, cloud or pour points, cetane number, flash point, ash content, distillation range, sulfur content, carbon residue, copper corrosion, acid value, and high heating value.

18.4.1 Bio-Diesel from Coconut and Jatropha

Biomass is an abundant natural raw material. It actively removes carbon dioxide from the atmosphere through photosynthesis and can be converted into biofuels, such as biodiesel for transport systems and other generator applications. Coconut and jatropha are potent biomass sources in the production of biodiesel.

Coconut: *Cocos nucifera*, commonly known as coconut, is grown in many countries and produces 10 million tons of copra (dried coconut flesh). Coconuts provide food, medicine, drink, and shelter, which millions of smallholders rely on to provide their livelihoods. Coconuts as well as their products are an important part of social, cultural, and religious connotations in many parts of the world. Coconut oil is consumed in many countries.

Harvesting coconut plants, rich shells, and residual plants can produce energy. Figure 18.5 shows harvested coconuts and shells. The plant oil produced from

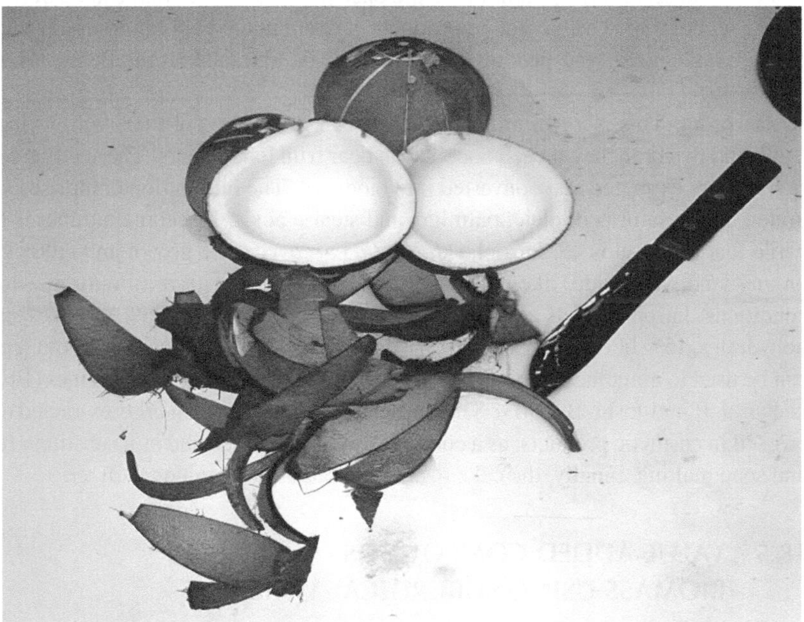

FIGURE 18.5 Harvested coconut and shell.

Source: Frank Rosillo-Calle (2007), Biomass Assessment Handbook

TABLE 18.3
Calculating Potential Oil and Energy Recovery Ratio Rate from Coconut Oil

Statistics	Low	Medium	High
Coconut trees per hectare	151	254	351
Nuts per tree	50	80	120
Flesh per nut (kg; 50% moisture)	0.276	0.34	0.416
Shell per unit (kg)	–	0.2	–
Flesh per hectare (kg; 50% moisture)	2,084	7,004	17,522
Copra per nut (5% moisture)	1146	3852	9637
Recoverable oil per kg copra (kg)	0.3	0.4	0.55
Recoverable oil	344	1541	5300
Recoverable liters of oil/hectare	378	1,693	227.9
Recoverable energy, GJ/hectare	14.8	66.3	227.9

Source: Woods and Hemstock (2003)

coconut can be converted into biodiesel as a diesel substitute. Coconut oil can also may be used directly in diesel engines by modifying fuel supply systems. Table 18.3 describes the potential oil and energy recovery rate that can be derived from coconut. Other value-added products of coconut are copra pulp used as animal feed, charcoal, and producer gas that can be obtained from coconut shells and husks.

Jatropha: This is a perennial shrub that can grow into big trees with a single trunk and two branches at each node. It can bear fruit for 25 years. The seeds are oil rich and are extracted and converted into biodiesel. The oil fraction comprises saturated and unsaturated, oleic, palmitic, and stearic acids. Its cetane number is 51, while that of diesel is 45. Jatropha (*Jatropha curcas*) can be grown and cultivated on any land worldwide, like rocky and fertile land, and with minimum moisture conditions. Jatropha seeds contain 6.2% moisture, 18% protein, 38% fats, 17% carbohydrates, 15% fiber, and 5.3% ash on a dry basis. The oil extracted from the seeds can be used to manufacture biodiesel as an alternative fuel for diesel engines (Bhattacharya, P. and Joshi, B. 2003). The Jatropha beans from which oil is extracted can be used in cosmetic products, as a cooking and lighting fuel, and as a substitute fuel and soap making. Finally, the cake residue is used as an organic fertilizer.

18.5 VALUE-ADDED COMPOUNDS FROM BIOMASS USING SUBCRITICAL WATER

Subcritical water is an essential alternative solvent for extracting value-added compounds from biomass. Studies have reported and proved that subcritical water is a promising alternative solvent for isolating nutrients and photochemicals from natural sources in recent years, and using subcritical water as a solvent results in higher extraction yields and rates than conventional conversion techniques with an organic solvent, which is advantageous. At modest temperatures, ionic and polar species are extracted. Nonpolar compounds can be dissolved and extracted near the critical point at higher temperatures and pressures (Brunner, 2009). Glycosylated phenolics, which are antioxidants, can be converted into aglycones as a side process, which offers numerous advantages, especially in the later stages of the separation process (Ravber et al., 2015a, 2016). Also, use of subcritical water is non-expensive; time-consuming organic solvents can be removed by neutralization, and biomass can be used without prior drying. Supercritical water oxidation is an environmentally acceptable technology that produces clean liquid such as water, clean solid such as salts and metal oxides, and gases such as CO_2 and N_2 (Goto et al., 1998). Therefore, the technology can be classified as a green technology according to sustainable development goals. At high temperatures in a dense, single-phase environment, oxidation reactions are rapid in supercritical water (Marrone, 2013). Due to its precise process conditions and its control, it is possible to extract oil and water-soluble constituents simultaneously.

The bio-constituents, such as proteins, polysaccharides, and glycosides, can be simultaneously hydrolyzed during extraction due to the subcritical water's hydrolytic nature to produce products like amino acids, phenolic aglycones, and sugars. The compounds that are extracted from different materials include essential oils using subcritical water from phenolic compounds, carbohydrates, spices, lipids, and proteins. Studies have reported the simultaneous extraction and hydrolysis of biomolecules, which include hydrolysis of protein to amino acids, lipids to fatty acids, carbohydrates to reducing sugars, phenolic glycosides to phenolic aglycones, and delignification of lignin.

18.5.1 Essential Oils

Subcritical water is an alternate liquid solvent for the extraction of essential oils. By using subcritical water, essential oils can be extracted by extraction process by using coriander seeds (Saim et al., 2008; Pavlić et al., 2015) and oregano (Ayala and Luque de Castro, 2001), which shows that subcritical water extraction is a valuable tool for the isolation of edible essential oils. By the distillation method, higher yields are generally obtained in a shorter extraction time (Saim et al., 2008; Ayala and Luque de Castro et al., 2001). Various process parameters such as temperature and pressure of the reaction or extraction make it possible to manipulate oil composition by subcritical water (Saim et al., .2008).

18.5.2 Protein and Amino Acids

From green microalgae *Chlorella vulgaris*, maximum total carbohydrates and proteins can be obtained by applying the subcritical water extraction process at 277°C for 5 minutes (Awaluddin et al., 2016). By using rice bran, maximum yields of proteins are extracted at 240°C (Hata et al., 2008; Wiboonsirikul et al., 2007); from the peels of *Caryo cathayensis*, maximum protein is yielded at 280°C (Shimanouchi et al., 2014).

Studies have reported that using subcritical water, which is treated with protein, may provide an economical and practical solution for the disposal of protein-rich sources like marine wastes, feathers, and hairs, which are treated as waste (Rogalinski et al., 2005) and can recover amino acids (Esteban et al., 2010; Xian et al., 2008; Yoshida et al., 1999). Continuous hydrolysis of subcritical water from bovine serum albumin produced amino acids (Rogalinski et al., 2005), and at a temperature of 290°C and 65 seconds showed the highest yields of amino acids (Yoshida et al., 1999). Similarly, using subcritical water hydrolysis of fish meat, maximum yields of amino acids were obtained at 270°C.

Production of isoleucine, leucine, and histidine: It was found that the nitrogen and carbon dioxide atmosphere should be used to hydrolyze fish proteins. In contrast, only the air atmosphere might be used (Xian et al., 2008). In the hydrolysis reaction at 250°C with a reaction time of 60 minutes, the supercritical water hydrolysis of hog hair gave the highest amino acid yield, and a large amount of low molecular weight amino acids, such as alanine and glycine, was obtained (Esteban et al., 2010).

18.5.3 Oils and Fatty Acids

Extraction of oil and proteins from soybean flakes and extruded soybean flakes with subcritical water was investigated by Ndlela et al. (Ndlela et al., 2012). It was found that conditions favor both oil and protein extraction from extruded soybean flakes at a temperature of around 150°C and a low solid-to-liquid ratio (1:11.7). From soybean flakes, lower temperature at 66°C and a low solid-to-liquid ratio favored both oil and protein extraction yields.

Studies were conducted by some researchers (Ravber et al., 2015b) on the extraction process with subcritical water for oil and water-soluble compounds like proteins and carbohydrates from sunflower kernels; optimum extraction oil yield was obtained at 130°C at raw material-to-solvent ratio of 1/20 g/mL after 30 minutes; hydrolysis was low. Water-soluble extract was more susceptible to hydrothermal degradation, of which carbohydrates showed the lowest stability. Additionally, hydrolysis of ester and glycoside-bonded antioxidants occurred, which produced oil with much higher antioxidant capacities than oil extracted with Soxhlet extraction method (Ravber et al., 2016).

Simultaneous inactivation of lipase enzyme existing in rice bran was studied by the researchers using the subcritical water technique, and the rice bran oil, which is edible, was obtained by stability by extraction of its oil (Pourali et al., 2009). Also, it was found that subcritical water showed its efficiency toward the extraction process of rice bran in a shorter residence time and also wholly stabilized the extraction oil. As the subcritical water treated oil by time, the lipase enzyme was denatured, and as a result, no increase was observed in total FFA concentration. Using the solvent extraction method of hexane at ambient temperature could not stabilize oil altogether, and results showed that total FFA concentration increased during oil storage (Pourali et al., 2009). Several studies using vegetable oil extraction (Baig et al., 2013; Alenezi et al., 2011; Kocsisova et al., 2006; Milliren et al., 2013; Alenezi et al., 2009) and the thermal stability of fatty acids were reported using subcritical water carried out below 330°C and less than 30 minutes to obtain high yield fatty acids (Shin et al., 2012).

18.5.4 Carbohydrates

For obtaining monosaccharides, oligosaccharides, and other carbohydrate-derived organic compounds, subcritical water showed its use as a medium for the depolymerization of polymeric carbohydrates as cellulose, hemicelluloses, and starch (Milliren et al., 2013). There may be a possibility for further degradation reactions as the formed oligo and monosaccharides can further react with water molecules to form other products until the optimization of the reaction takes place, such as temperature and contact times. Products such as 5-hydroxymethylfurfural (5HMF), 1,3-dihydroxyacetone, pyruvaldehyde, glyceraldehyde, erythrose, and 1,2,4-trihydroxybenzene can occur due to the rearrangement or decomposition of glucose and other monomer sugars. The liquid oil, char, and gases can also be obtained with further temperature and reaction time increase by isomerization, repolymerization, and fragmentation of these small compounds (Sasaki et al., 1998). The formation of chemicals with intact phenolic functional groups and the switch grass conversion at 350°C, 20 MPa pressure, for 60 seconds, indicate lignin hydrolysis. Instead, the fragmentation reaction plays its role during the decomposition reaction of lignin structure (Cheng et al., 2009). The breakdown of the structure bond in lignin by subcritical water under mild conditions results in useful functional products of high value in many industries (Cheng et al., 2009).

Studies done with ultrasound enhanced the use of subcritical water extraction of polysaccharides and have shown maximum yields of polysaccharides (Chao et al. 2013) produced by extraction at 100°C for 53 minutes with a liquid-to-solid ratio of 26 mL/g and a power of 160W ultrasonic electrical power. Subcritical water with ultrasound was superior to other extraction methods due to easy pretreatment and high recovery of polysaccharide yields (Chao et al., 2013). Another study for the separation of sugar alcohol mannitol from olive leaves (Ghoreishi and Shahrestani, 2009) resulted in the highest mannitol yield at 100°C and 5 MPa pressure with subcritical water, which indicates higher extraction yields in contrast to the Soxhlet method using ethanol with lower use of solvent.

18.5.5 Phenolic Compounds: Extracts of Olive Tree Leaves and Peel

It is interesting to have the subcritical water for isolating bioactive phenolic compounds present in biomass and bound to carbohydrates or proteins. Hydrolysis and separation can be performed simultaneously by using water and operating at a specific condition to obtain more active free aglycones. These free phenolic aglycones show much higher antioxidant activities than bonded glycosides (Lindahl et al., 2010). Therefore, the hydrolysis step is more important after the product extraction procedure. Table 18.4 shows the extraction of phenolic compounds with subcritical solvent.

By applying subcritical water to solvents for extraction, many researchers have reported higher yields of phenolic compounds and higher antioxidant activity of extracts (He et al., 2012; Budrat and Shotipruk, 2009; Cheigh et al., 2015; Tunchaiyaphum et al., 2013; Ko et al., 2011; Singh and Saldaña, 2011; Yoswathana et al., 2013; Pavlić et al., 2016; Kumar et al., 2011; Euterpio et al., 2011; García-Marino et al., 2006; Aliakbarian et al., 2012) than those obtained by conventional solvent extraction because simultaneous extraction and hydrolysis of the glyceroids bonded with phenolic compounds into the free aglycones occurred, which increased the total phenolic compound content and antioxidant activity of the extract samples. Further degradation of free aglycones at higher temperatures and long reaction times means that reaction pathways, kinetics, and mechanisms should be studied to optimize the reaction process. The literature corresponds to the systematic studies dealing with the reaction mechanism and kinetics of degradation of standard phenolic glycosides such as hesperidin (Ruen-ngam et al., 2012). See also Ravber et al. (1998, 2016).

The reaction kinetics and the hydrothermal hydrolysis mechanism for conversion of hesperidin (hesperetin-7-O rutinoside) into more valuable compounds such as hesperetin-β-glucoside and aglycones hesperetin have been studied (Ruen-ngam et al., 2012). A temperature of 140°C and pressure of 25 MPa using carbon dioxide resulted in high yields of hesperetin after 3 hr of reaction. Results also show that high temperature, long reaction treatment time, and increasing reaction concentration contribute to higher degradation, and carbon dioxide pressure decreases the degradation process (Ravber et al., 1998).

There are many bioactive compounds, such as antimicrobial and antiviral, which have the capability to extract from biomass available worldwide. Here is one: Olive tree-based waste biomass. Olive tree leaves are generally generated in large amounts as a waste during pruning of trees and harvesting of olives: The valuable phenolic compound being the olive oil (De Leonardis et al., 2008). Many researchers have reported that the olive leaf polyphenols are bioactive compounds, which show antimicrobial, antiviral, anti-inflammatory, antioxidant, and anticarcinogenic properties. They also have active properties such as hypotensive action and atherosclerosis inhibition (De Leonardis et al., 2008). The principal compound contained in olive leaves is oleuropein (OLE); secoiridoids with simple phenols, namely hydroxytyrosol, are present in lower amounts. The molecule of OLE consists of three structural subunits, which are polyphenol hydroxytyrosol (HT), secoiridoid (elenolic acid), and glucose molecule, shown in Figure 18.6. HT is a naturally derived antioxidant, and elenolic acid has strong antiviral properties (Khoufi et al., 2011).

Researchers have investigated the extraction method using subcritical water to recover compounds from olive leaves using temperatures between 80°C and 180°C

TABLE 18.4
Extraction of Phenolic Compounds from Subcritical Water Biomass

Material	Conditions	Cosolvent/Optimal Extraction Conditions, Catalyst
Bitter melon (*Momordica charantia*)	T = 130–200°C; P = 10 MPa; time ≤ 300 min; flow rate = 2–5 mL/min	Main (poly)phenols: Catechin and gallic, gentisic, and chlorogenic acids
Black tea	T = 110–200°C; P = 10 MPa; time = 5–15 min	The yields of myricetin, quercetin, and kaempferol from celery and ginseng leaf plants were maximal at extraction temperatures of 170°C, 170°C, and 200°C, respectively, and they depend on the number of hydroxyl groups included in the chemical structure of the flavonols
Chamomile flowers	T = 65–210°C	Apigenin at 115°C, 4.5 MPa
(*Chamomilla matricaria* L.) Coriandrum	P = 1–9 MPa; time = 5–60 min; T = 100–200°C; P = 3–9 MPa; time = 10–30 min	Total phenols, total flavonoids, and maximal antioxidant activity temperature 200°C, pressure 3 MPa
Fruits of *Terminalia chebula* Retz.	T = 120–220°C, P = 4 MPa; time ≤ 300 min; flow rate = 2–4 mL/min	Gallic and ellagic at 180°C, corilagin at 120°C
Larch wood waste	T = 100–300°C; P = 2–20 MPa; time ≤ 120 min; flow rate = 1–3 mL/min	Highest phenolic content at 300°C; ethanol concentration: 5% and 10% (v/v)
Mango leaves	T = 100°C, P = 4 MPa, Time = 180 min; flow rate =10 g/min	Subcritical water extraction yields more phenolic compounds compared to SC-CO_2 extraction with 20% ethanol
Mango peels	T = 160–220°C, time = 30–120 min, pH: 2–8; citric acid, NaCl	Highest phenolic content at 180°C, extraction time 90 min, solid-to-water ratio 1:40, pH 4
Olive tree	T = 50–200°C, P = 10.34 MPa, time = 20 min	Highest total phenols, 5-HMF, and highest Trolox-equivalent antioxidant capacity at 200°C
Onion skin	T = 100–190°C, P = 9–13.1 MPa, time = 5–30 min	Quercetin at 165°C
Pomegranate (*Punica granatum* L.) seed residue	T = 80–280°C; P = 6 MPa; time = 15–120 min	Total phenolic highest at 220°C, solid-to-solvent ratio 1:40

(Continued)

TABLE 18.4 *(Continued)*
Extraction of Phenolic Compounds from Subcritical Water Biomass

Material	Conditions	Cosolvent/Optimal Extraction Conditions, Catalyst
Potato peel (Red)	T = 100–240°C; P = 6 MPa; time = 30–120 min	Phenolic compounds: Gallic, chlorogenic, caffeic, protocatechuic, syringic, phydroxylbenzoic, ferulic, and coumaric acids, maximal at 180°C and 60 min
Rambutan peels	T = 100–160°C; time 20–60 min; P = 3 MPa	Optimum temperature 160°C, extraction time 20 min, 50% ethanol as cosolvent Ethanol conc.: 5%, 50%, and 95%
Sage (*Salvia*)	T = 120–220°C; time = 10–30 min	Total phenols, the extraction process of Myricetin, Quercetin, and Kaempferol produces maximal yield from celery, extraction temperature of 201.5°C, extraction officinalis L., time 15.8 min, H_2O as extraction solvent
Satureja	T = 79.15–220.5°C; P = 3 MPa; time = 5.9–34.1 min	Total phenols, total flavonoids, and maximal antioxidant activity at temperature 200°C, extraction time, 20.8 min
Seabuckthorn (*Hippophaer-hamnoides*) leaves	T = 100–150°C; $P \leq$ 10 MPa; time 15 min	High flavonoids and phenolic contents at 150°C
Turmeric (*Curcuma ferulic longs* L.)	T= 100–200°C; P = 3 MPa; time 5–120 min	Curcuminoids degradation at 150–200°C to hydroxycinnamic acids as *p*-coumaric acids
Turmeric (*Curcuma longa*)	T = 90–250°C; P = 5 MPa; flow rate = 0.5 mL/min	Highest yield of curcumin at temperature 197°C and pH 1.6, pH 1–7, buffer concentration 25–75 g/L
Winery waste grape seeds	T = 50–150°C; P = 10.34 MPa; time = 30–90 min	Phenolic compounds at 140°C and 11.6 MPa
Winery wastes grape pomace	T = 100–140°C; P = 8–15 MPa; time = 130 min; flow rate =1–3 mL/min	Phenolic compounds at 140°C and 11.6 MPa

Note: Process conditions investigated (temperature, pressure, extraction time, solvent flow rate in case of semicontinuous mode and cosolvents or catalysts used; optimal extraction parameters).
Source: Knez et al. (2018)

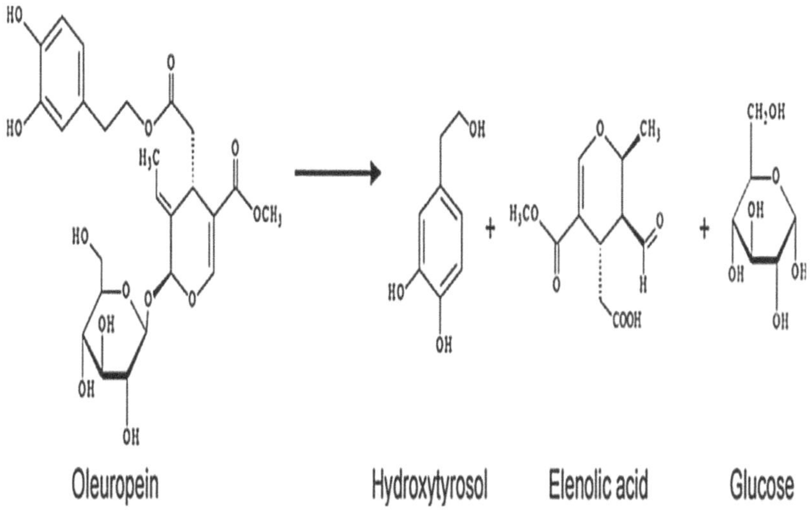

FIGURE 18.6 Hydrolysis of phenolic glycoside oleuropein to its derivatives.

Source: Knez et al. (2018)

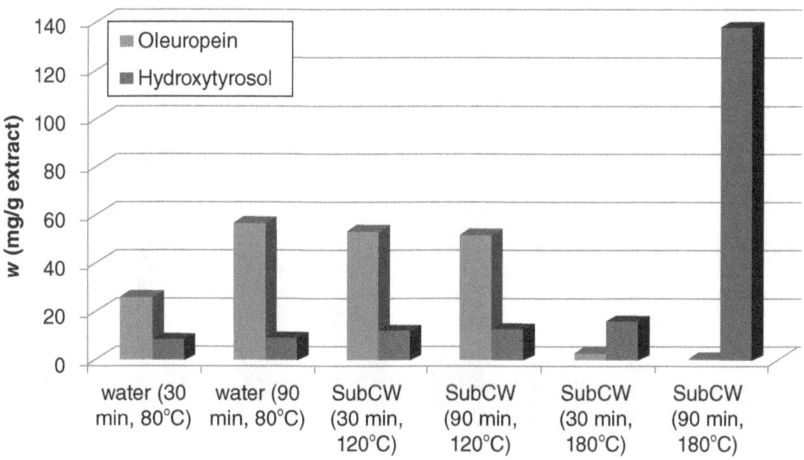

FIGURE 18.7 The phenolic compound extraction from olive oil tree leaves, concentration of oleuropein and its hydrolysate, and hydroxytyrosol in extract.

Source: Knez et al. (2018)

with various residential times (Figures 18.7 and 18.8, respectively). Investigation was also done on the impact of temperature and extract time on product extraction and its hydrolysis by HPLC (Figure 18.9). Subcritical water acts as an environmentally friendly alternative solvent for extracting HT-rich phenolic compounds from olive oil waste. This method allows for the simultaneous extraction of oleuropein (OLE) and its hydrolysis into the powerful antioxidant hydroxytyrosol (HT).

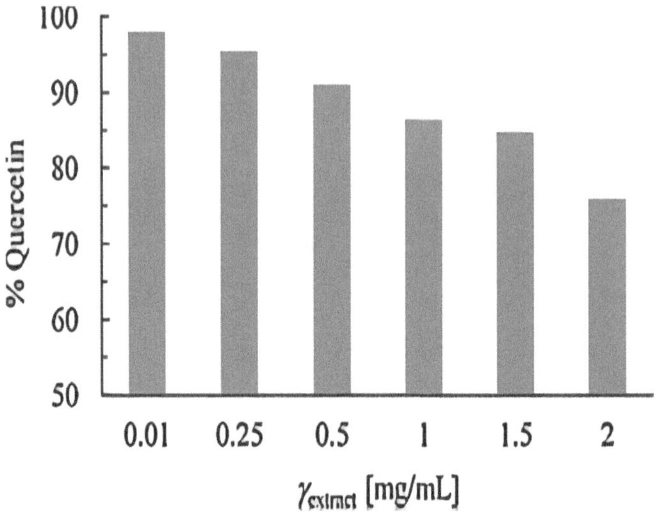

FIGURE 18.8 Extraction of phenolic onion peel extract with subcritical water at $T = 195°C$.

Source: Knez et al. (2018)

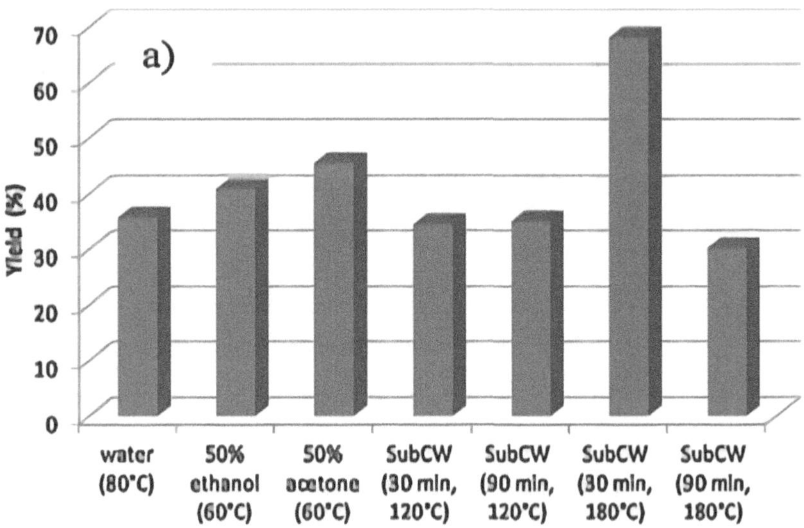

FIGURE 18.9 The phenolic compound extraction from olive oil tree leaves: (a) Yield of extraction of olive tree leaves, (b) concentration of total phenols (TP) in extracts, (c) concentration of tannins (tan) in extracts, and (d) radical scavenging of extracts.

Source: Knez et al. (2018)

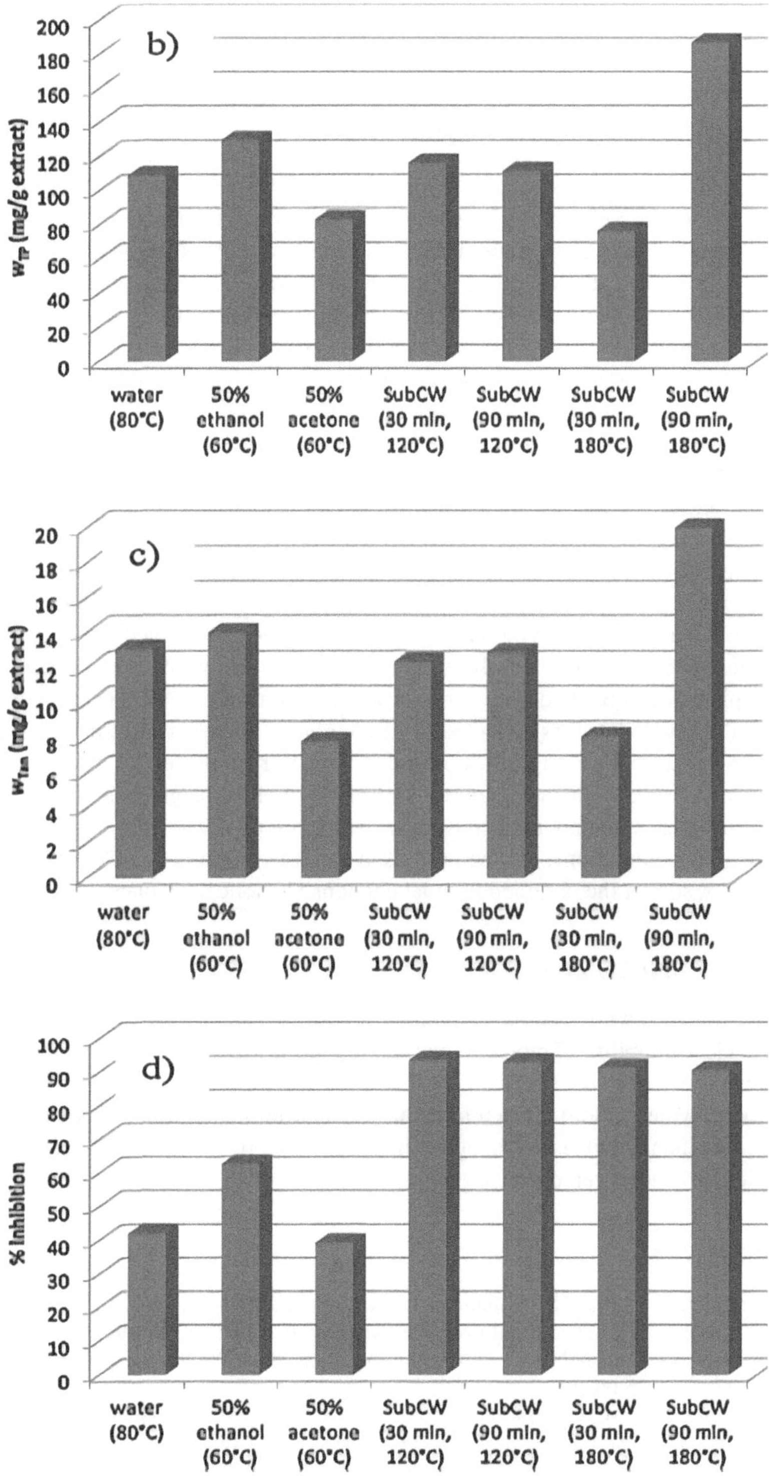

FIGURE 18.9 (Continued)

The hydrolysis of phenolic compound by subcritical water with simultaneous extraction and hydrolysis of natural materials at 140–220°C at optimal conditions give free phenolic compounds. Depending on the research done earlier by hydrolysis of model phenolic glucoside rutin (Ravber et al., 2015a, 2016) and by focusing on the hydrothermal hydrolysis of a natural extract rich in rutin, a natural onion peel extract was obtained by the conventional solvent water extraction at 80°C for 2 hr extraction time with a material-to-solvent ratio 1/20 g/mL. The concentration was determined by hydrolyzing the extract using acid hydrolysis (Škerget et al., 2009) and was quantified with HPLC (Ravber et al., 2015b, 2016). The hydrolysis was performed by dissolving 50 mg of extract in 20 mL of Milli-Q water, and an amount of this extract was treated with HCl and ethanol and refluxed at 90°C for 2 hr to break down quercetin glycosides into their aglycone form. The mixture was diluted and vortexed, and the total quercetin content in the onion peel extract was quantified using HPLC method which served as a reference, indicating complete hydrolysis.

The onion peel extract was hydrolyzed by subcritical water, and the hydrolysis reaction was studied similar to standard rutin. The results were compared, showing that similar data on the onion peel extract were obtained as per the rutin standard (it shows rutin hydrolysis in onion peel extract by subcritical water). The precipitate was obtained with subcritical water concentration by using evaporation. The precipitate was collected by filtering the suspension and washing it with pure water to remove impurities. Both fractions were collected, diluted, and analyzed accordingly. The advantage of hydrolysis of phenolic glucosides using subcritical water is that phenolic aglycones, which are poorly soluble in water under atmospheric conditions, can be easily separated from water-soluble degradation products, so that the obtained product contains phenolic aglycones.

18.6 CONCLUSION

New strategies with feasible technology, a cost-effective conversion process, and the wide availability of biomass material may be utilized to convert biomass into bio-hydrogen (bio-oil obtained by the anaerobic digestion process and further fast depolymerization). Different hydrolysis and fermentation methods can produce bioethanol; biogas and syngas can be produced through anaerobic digestion, while gasification can produce syngas.

REFERENCES

Albarelli, J.Q., Onorati, S., Caliandro, P., Peduzzi, E., Meireles, M.A.A., Marechal, F., Ensinas, A.V., 2015. Multi-objective optimization of a sugarcane biorefinery for integrated ethanol and methanol production. *Energy*. https://doi.org/10.1016/j.energy.2015.06.104

Alenezi, R., Baig, M., Wang, J., Santos, R., Leeke, G.A., 2011. Continuous flow hydrolysis of sunflower oil for biodiesel. *Energy Source*, 32, 460–468.

Alenezi, R., Leeke, G.A., Santos, R.C.D., Khan, A.R., 2009. Hydrolysis kinetics of sunflower oil under subcritical water conditions. *Chem. Eng. Res. Des.*, 87(6), 867–873.

Aliakbarian, B., Fathi, A., Perego, P., Dehghani, F., 2012. Extraction of antioxidants from winery wastes using subcritical water. *J. Supercrit. Fluids*, 65, 18–24.

Alves, C.M., Valk, M., de Jong, S., Bonomi, A., van der Wielen, L.A., Mussatto, S.I., 2017. Techno-economic assessment of biorefinery technologies for aviation biofuels supply chains in Brazil. *Biofuels, Bioprod. Biorefin.*, 11(1), 67–91.

Antonio Tursi, 2019. A review on biomass: Importance, chemistry, classification, and conversion. *Biofuel Research Journal*, 22, 962–979.

Awaluddin, S.A., Thiruvenkadam, S., Izhar, S., Hiroyuki, Y., Danquah, M.K., Harun, R., 2016. Subcritical water technology for enhanced extraction of biochemical compounds from Chlorella vulgaris. *Biomed. Res. Int.*, 2016, 1–10.

Ayala, R.S., Luque de Castro, M.D., 2001. Continuous subcritical water extraction as a useful tool for isolation of edible essential oils. *Food Chem.*, 75, 109–113.

Baeyens, J., Kang, Q., Appels, L., Dewil, R., Lv, Y., Tan, T., 2015. Challenges and opportunities in improving the production of bioethanol. *Prog. Energy Combust. Sci.*, 47, 60–88.

Baig, M.N., Santos, R.C.D., King, J., Pioch, D., Bowra, S., 2013. Evaluation and modelling of continuous flow sub-critical water hydrolysis of biomass derived components; lipids and carbohydrates. *Chem. Eng. Res. Des.*, 91, 2663–2670.

Bala, B.K., 2005. Studies on biodiesels from transformation of vegetable oils for diesel engines. *Energy Edu. Sci. Technol.*, 15, 1–43.

Balan, V., Chiaramonti, D., Kumar, S., 2013. Review of US and EU initiatives toward development, demonstration, and commercialization of lignocellulosic biofuels. *Biofuels, Bioprod. Biorefin.*, 7(6), 732–759.

Bhattacharya, P. and Joshi, B., 2003. Strategies and institutional mechanisms for large scale cultivation of *Jatropha curcas under* agroforestry in the context of the proposed biofuel policy of India. *Indian Institute of Forest Management, ENVIS Bulletin on Grassland Ecosystems and Agroforestry*, 1(2), 58–72. Bhopal, India.

Bhutto, A.W., Qureshi, K., Abro, R., Harijan, K., Zhao, Z., Bazmi, A.A., Abbas, T., Yu, G., 2016. Progress in the production of biomass-to-liquid biofuels to decarbonize the transport sector–prospects and challenges. *RSC Adv.*, 6(38), 32140–32170.

Brunner, G., 2009. Near-critical and supercritical water. Part I. Hydrolytic and hydrothermal processes. *J. Supercrit. Fluids*, 47(3), 373–381.

Budrat, P., Shotipruk, A., 2009. Enhanced recovery of phenolic compounds from bitter melon (Momordica charantia) by subcritical water extraction. *Sep. Purif. Technol.*, 66, 125–129.

Canakci, M., Van Gerpen, J.H., 1999. Biodiesel production via acid catalysis. *Transactions of the ASAE*, 42(5), 1203–1210.

Chao, Z., Ri-Fu, Y., Tai-Qiu, Q., 2013. Ultrasound-enhanced subcritical water extraction of polysaccharides from Lyciumbarbarum L. *Sep. Purif. Technol.*, 120, 141–147.

Cheigh, C.I., Yoo, S.Y., Ko, M.J., Chang, P.S., Chung, M.S., 2015. Extraction characteristics of subcritical water depending on the number of hydroxyl groups in flavonols. *Food Chem.*, 168, 21–26.

Cheng, L., Ye, X.P., He, R., Liu, S., 2009. Investigation of rapid conversion of switchgrass in subcritical water. *Fuel Process. Technol.*, 90, 301–311.

Chum, H.L., Warner, E., Seabra, J.E., Macedo, I.C., 2014. A comparison of commercial ethanol production systems from Brazilian sugarcane and US corn. *Biofuels, Bioprod. Biorefin.*, 8(2), 205–223.

Cross, B. (ed.), 1995. *The World Directory of Renewable Energy Suppliers and Services 1995*. James & James Science, London, United Kingdom.

De Leonardis, A., Aretini, A., Alfano, G., Macciola, V., Ranalli, G., 2008. Isolation of a hydroxytyrosol-rich extract from olive leaves (Olea Europaea L.) and evaluation of its antioxidant properties and bioactivity. *Eur. Food Res. Technol.*, 226, 653–659.

Dias, M.O., Junqueira, T.L., Cavalett, O., Cunha, M.P., Jesus, C.D., Mantelatto, P.E., Rossell, C.E., Maciel Filho, R., Bonomi, A., 2013b. Cogeneration in integrated first and second generation ethanol from sugarcane. *Chem. Eng. Res. Des.*, 91(8), 1411–1417.

Diederichs, G.W., Mandegari, M.A., Farzad, S., Görgens, J.F., 2016. Techno-economic comparison of biojet fuel production from lignocellulose, vegetable oil, and sugar cane juice. *Bioresour. Technol.*, 216, 331–339.

Esteban, M.B., García, A.J., Ramos, P., Márquez, M.C., 2010. Sub-critical water hydrolysis of hog hair for amino acid production. *Bioresour. Technol.*, 101, 2472–2476.

Euterpio, M.A., Cavaliere, C., Capriotti, A.L., Crescenzi, C., 2011. Extending the applicability of pressurized hot water extraction to compounds exhibiting limited water solubility by pH control: Curcumin from the turmeric rhizome. *Anal. Bioanal. Chem.*, 401, 2977–2985.

Farzad, S., Mandegari, M.A., Görgens, J.F., 2017b. Integrated techno-economic and environmental analysis of butadiene production from biomass. *Bioresour. Technol.*, 239, 37–48.

Fridleifsson, I.B., 2001. Geothermal energy for the benefit of the people. *Renew. Sustain Energy Rev.*, 5, 299–312.

Fukuda, H., Kondo, A., Noda, H., 2001. Biodiesel fuel production by transesterification of oils. *J. Biosci. Bioeng.*, 92(5), 405-416.

García-Marino, M., Rivas-Gonzalo, J.C., Ibáñez, E., García-Moreno, C., 2006. Recovery of catechins and proanthocyanidins from winery by-products using subcritical water extraction. *Anal. Chim. Acta*, 563, 44–50.

Ghoreishi, S.M., Shahrestani, R.G., 2009. Subcritical water extraction of mannitol from olive leaves. *J. Food Eng.*, 93, 474–481.

Goto, M., Nada, T., Ogata, A., Kodama, A., Hirose, T., 1998 Supercritical water oxidation for the destruction of municipal excess sludge and alcohol distillery wastewater of molasses. *J. Supercrit. Fluids*, 13, 277–282.

Gubicza, K., Nieves, I.U., Sagues, W.J., Barta, Z., Shanmugam, K.T., Ingram, L.O., 2016. Techno-economic analysis of ethanol production from sugarcane bagasse using a liquefaction plus simultaneous saccharification and co-fermentation process. *Bioresour. Technol.*, 208, 42–48.

Hata, S., Wiboonsirikul, J., Maeda, A., Kimura, Y., Adachi, S., 2008. Extraction of defatted rice bran by subcritical water treatment. *Biochem. Eng. J.*, 40, 44–53.

He, L., Zhang, X., Xu, H., Xu, C., Yuan, F., Knez, Ž., Novak, Z., Gao, Y., 2012. Subcritical water extraction of phenolic compounds from pomegranate (Punica granatum L.) seed residues and investigation into their antioxidant activities with HPLC-ABTS+ assay. *Food Bioprod. Process*, 90(2), 215–223.

Horan, N.J., 2018. Introduction, in: Horan, N., Yaser, A., Wid, N. (eds.), *Anaerobic Digestion Processes. Green Energy and Technology*. Springer, Singapore, pp 1–7.

Jin, C., Yao, M., Liu, H., Chia-Fon, F.L., Ji, J., 2011. Progress in the production and application of n-butanol as a biofuel. *Renew. Sust. Energy Rev.*, 15(8), 4080–4106.

Khoufi, S., Hamza, M., Sayadi, S., 2011. Enzymatic hydrolysis of olive wastewater for hydroxytyrosol enrichment. *Bioresour. Technol.*, 102, 9050–9058.

Knez, Ž., Markočič, E., Leitgeb, M., Primožič, M., Knez Hrnčič, M., Škerget, M., 2014. Industrial applications of supercritical fluids: A review. *Energy*, 77, 235–243. doi.org/10.1016/j.eng.2018.07.003

Knothe, G., Sharp, C.A., Ryan, T.W., 2006. III Exhaust emissions of biodiesel, petrodiesel, neat methyl esters, and alkanes in a new technology engine. *Energy Fuels*, 20, 403–408.

Ko, M.J., Cheigh, C.I., Cho, S.W., Chung, M.S., 2011. Subcritical water extraction of flavonol quercetin from onion skin. *J. Food Eng.*, 102, 327–333.

Kocsisova, T., Juhasz, J., Cvengros, J., 2006. Hydrolysis of fatty acid esters in subcritical water. *Eur. J. Lipid Sci. Technol.*, 108, 652–658.

Kralova, I., Sjöblom, J., 2010. Biofuels–renewable energy sources: A review. *J. Dispers. Sci. Technol.*, 31(3), 409–425. https://doi.org/10.1080/01932690903119674

Kumar, M.S.Y., Dutta, R., Prasad, D., Misra, K., 2011. Subcritical water extraction of antioxidant compounds from Seabuckthorn (Hippophae rhamnoides) leaves for the comparative evaluation of antioxidant activity. *Food Chem.*, 127, 1309–1316.

Lange, J.P., 2007. Lignocellulose conversion: An introduction to chemistry, process and economics. *Biofuels, Bioprod. Biorefin.*, 1(1), 39–48.

Leung, D.Y.C., Wu, X., Leung, M.K.H., 2010. A review on biodiesel production using catalyzed transesterification. *Appl. Energy.*, 87(4), 1083–1095.

Lindahl, S., Ekman, A., Khan, S., Wennerberg, C., Borjesson, P., Sjoberg, P.J.R., Karlsson, E.N., Turner, C., 2010. Exploring the possibility of using a thermostable mutant of β-glucosidase for rapid hydrolysis of quercetin glucosides in hot water. *Green Chem.*, 12, 159–168.

Ma, F., Hanna, M.A., 1999. Biodiesel production: A review. *Bioresource Technology.Bioresources Technol.*, 70, 1–15.

Mahalaxmi, S., Williford, C., 2014. Biochemical conversion of biomass to fuels, in: Chen, W., Suzuki, T., Lackner, M. (eds.), *Handbook of Climate Change Mitigation and Adaptation*. Springer, New York, pp. 1–28.

Mandegari, M.A., Farzad, S., Görgens, J.F., 2017. Economic and environmental assessment of cellulosic ethanol production scenarios annexed to a typical sugar mill. *Bioresour. Technol.*, 224, 314–326.

Mariano, A.P., Dias, M.O., Junqueira, T.L., Cunha, M.P., Bonomi, A., Maciel Filho, R., 2013. Butanol production in a first-generation Brazilian sugarcane biorefinery: Technical aspects and economics of greenfield projects. *Bioresour. Technol.*, 135, 316–323.

Mariod, A.A., 2016. Extraction, purification, and modification of natural polymers, in: Olatunji, O. (ed.), *Natural Polymers*. Springer, Cham, pp. 63–91.

Marrone, P.A., 2013. Supercritical water oxidation – current status of full-scale commercial activity for waste destruction. *J. Supercrit. Fluids*, 79, 283–288.

Michailos, S., Parker, D., Webb, C., 2017. A techno-economic comparison of Fischer–Tropsch and fast pyrolysis as ways of utilizing sugar cane bagasse in transportation fuels production. *Chem. Eng. Res. Des.*, 118, 206–214.

Milliren, A.L., Wissinger, J.C., Gottumukala, V., Schall, C.A., 2013. Kinetics of soybean oil hydrolysis in subcritical water. *Fuel*, 108, 277–281.

Ndaba, B., Chiyanzu, I., Marx, S., 2015. N-Butanol derived from biochemical and chemical routes: A review. *Biotechnol. Rep.*, 8, 1–9.

Ndlela, S.C., Moura, J.M.L.N., Olson, N.K., Johnson, L.A., 2012. Aqueous extraction of oil and protein from soybeans with subcritical water. *J. Am. Oil Chem. Soc.*, 89(6), 1145–1153.

Nsaful, F., Görgens, J.F., Knoetze, J.H., 2013. Comparison of combustion and pyrolysis for energy generation in a sugarcane mill. *Energy Convers. Manage.*, 74, 524–534.

Parajuli, R., Dalgaard, T., Jørgensen, U., Adamsen, A.P.S., Knudsen, M.T., Birkved, M., Gylling, M., Schjørring, J.K., 2015. Biorefining in the prevailing energy and materials crisis: A review of sustainable pathways for biorefinery value chains and sustainability assessment methodologies. *Renew. Sust. Energy Rev.*, 43, 244–263.

Pavlić, B., Vidović, S., Vladić, J., Radosavljević, R., Cindrić, M., Zeković, Z., 2016. Subcritical water extraction of sage (Salvia officinalis L.) by-products-process optimization by response surface methodology. *J. Supercrit. Fluids*, 116, 36–45.

Pavlić, B., Vidović, S., Vladić, J., Radosavljević, R., Zeković, Z., 2015. Isolation of coriander (Coriandrum sativum L.) essential oil by green extractions versus traditional techniques. *J. Supercrit. Fluids*, 99, 23–28.

Peplow, M., 2014. Cellulosic ethanol fights for life. *Nature*, 507(7491), 152.

Pereira, L.G., Dias, M.O.S., Junqueira, T.L., Pavanello, L.G., Chagas, M.F., Cavalett, O., Maciel Filho, R., Bonomi, A., 2014. Butanol production in a sugarcane biorefinery using ethanol as feedstock. Part II: Integration to a second-generation sugarcane distillery. *Chem. Eng. Res. Des.*, 92(8), 1452–1462.

Petersen, A.M., Farzad, S., Görgens, J.F., 2015. Techno-economic assessment of integrating methanol or Fischer–Tropsch synthesis in a South African sugar mill. *Bioresour. Technol.*, 183, 141–152.

Pourali, O., Salak Asghari, F., Yoshida, H., 2009. Simultaneous rice bran oil stabilization and extraction using sub-critical water medium. *J. Food Eng.*, 95(3), 510–516.

Puhan, S., Vedaraman, N., Rambrahaman, B.V., Nagarajan, G., 2005. Mahua (Madhuca indica) seed oil: A source of renewable energy in India. *J. Sci. Ind. Res.*, 64, 890–896.

Ravber, M., Knez, Ž., & Škerget, M., 1998. Degradation of carbohydrates in subcritical water. *J. Agric. Food Chem.*, 46 (12), 4870–4873.

Ravber, M., Knez, Ž., Škerget, M., 2015a. Optimization of hydrolysis of rutin in subcritical water using response surface methodology. *J. Supercrit. Fluids*, 104, 145–152.

Ravber, M., Knez, Ž., Škerget, M., 2015b. Simultaneous extraction of oil- and water-soluble phase from sunflower seeds with subcritical water. *Food Chem.*, 166, 316–323.

Ravber, M., Pečar, D., Goršek, A., Iskra, J., Knez, Ž., Škerget, M., 2016. Hydrothermal degradation of rutin: Identification of degradation products and kinetics study. *J. Agric. Food Chem.*, 64, 9196–9202.

Reijnders, L., 2006. Conditions for the sustainability of biomass based fuel use. *Energy Policy*, 34, 863–876.

Renó, M.L.G., del Olmo, O.A., Palacio, J.C.E., Lora, E.E.S., Venturini, O.J., 2014. Sugarcane biorefineries: Case studies applied to the Brazilian sugar–alcohol industry. *Energy Convers. Manage.*, 86, 981–991.

Rogalinski, T., Herrmann, S., Brunner, G., 2005. Production of amino acids from bovine serum albumin by continuous sub-critical water hydrolysis. *J. Supercrit. Fluids*, 36, 49–58.

Rosillo-Calle, F., de Groot, P., Hemstock, S. L., Woods, J. (eds.), 2007. *The Biomass Assessment Handbook: Bioenergy for a Sustainable Environment*. Earthscan, London & Sterling, VA.

Ruen-ngam, D., Quitain, A.T., Tanaka, M., Sasaki, M., Goto, M., 2012. Reaction kinetics of hydrothermal hydrolysis of hesperidin into more valuable compounds under supercritical carbon dioxide conditions. *J. Supercrit. Fluids*, 66, 215–220.

Saim, N., Osman, R., Yasin, W.A.H.M., Hamid, R.D., 2008. Subcritical water extraction of essential oil from coriander (Coriandrum sativum L.) seeds. *MJAS*, 12, 1–3.

Sánchez, Ó.J., Cardona, C.A., 2012. Conceptual design of cost-effective and environmentally-friendly configurations for fuel ethanol production from sugarcane by knowledge-based process synthesis. *Bioresour. Technol.*, 104, 305–314.

Santos, C.I., Silva, C.C., Mussatto, S.I., Osseweijer, P., van der Wielen, L.A., Posada, J.A., 2017. Integrated 1st and 2nd generation sugarcane bio-refinery for jet fuel production in Brazil: Techno-economic and greenhouse gas emissions assessment. *Renew. Energy*. https://doi.org/10.1016/j.renene.2017.05.011

Sasaki, M., Kabyemela, B., Malaluan, R., Hirose, S., Takeda, N., Adschiri, T., Arai, K., 1998. Cellulose hydrolysis in subcritical and supercritical water. *J. Supercrit. Fluids*, 13(1–3), 261–268.

Seabra, J.E., Macedo, I.C., 2011. Comparative analysis for power generation and ethanol production from sugarcane residual biomass in Brazil. *Energy Policy*, 39(1), 421–428.

Sharma, V.K., 2015. Technology development and innovation for production of next-generation biofuel from lignocellulosic wastes, in: Sharma, A., Kar, S. (eds.), *Energy Sustainability through Green Energy. Green Energy Technology*. Springer, New Delhi, pp. 315–350.

Shimanouchi, T., Ueno, S., Yang, W., Kimura, Y., 2014. Extraction of reducing sugar with anti-oxidative scavengers from peels of Carya cathayensissarg: Use of subcritical water. *Environ. Eng. Res.*, 19(1), 1–5.

Shin, H.Y., Ryu, J.H., Park, S.Y., Bae, S.Y., 2012. Thermal stability of fatty acids in subcritical water. *J. Anal. Appl. Pyrolysis*, 98, 250–253.

Singh, P.P., Saldaña, M.D.A., 2011. Subcritical water extraction of phenolic compounds from potato peel. *Food Res. Int.*, 44, 2452–2458.

Škerget, M., Majhenič, L., Bezjak, M., Knez, Ž., 2009. Antioxidant, radical scavenging and antimicrobial activities of red onion (Allium cepa L.) skin and edible part extracts. *Chem. Biochem. Eng. Q.*, 23, 435–444.

Strezov, V., 2014. Properties of biomass fuels, in: Strezov, V., Evans, T.J. (eds.), *Biomass Processing Technologies*. CRC Press, Boca Raton, pp. 1–32.

Taylor, R., Nattrass, L., Alberts, G., Robson, P., Chudziak, C., Bauen, A., Libelli, I.M., Lotti, G., Prussi, M., Nistri, R., Chiaramonti, D., 2015. *From the Sugar Platform to biofuels and biochemicals: Final report for the European Commission directorate-general energy*. E4tech, London, UK. Report number ENER/C2/423-2012/SI2.673791.

Tunchaiyaphum, S., Eshtiaghi, M.N., Yoswathana, N., 2013. Extraction of bioactive compounds from mango peels using green technology. *Int. J. Chem. Eng. Appl.*, 4, 194–198.

Wang, D., Chen, H., Wang, J., 2007. Biodiesel production by the transesterification of cottonseed oil by solid acid catalysts. *Front. Chem. Eng. China*, 1(1), 101–105.

Wiboonsirikul, J., Hata, S., Tsuno, T., Kimura, Y., Adachi, S., 2007. Production of functional substances from black rice bran by its treatment in subcritical water. *LWT Food Sci. Technol.*, 40, 1732–1740.

Woods, J., Hemstock, S., 2003. *Tuvalu Coconut Oil Bioelectricity Potential*. www.iccept.imperial.ac.uk/research/projects/SOPAC/index.html (accessed 16 February 2006).

Xian, Z., Chao, Z., Liang, Z., Hongbin, C., 2008. Amino acids production from fish proteins hydrolysis in subcritical water. *Chin. J. Chem. Eng.*, 16(3), 456–460.

Yoshida, H., Terashima, M., Takahashi, Y., 1999. Production of organic acids and amino acids from fish meat by sub-critical water hydrolysis. *Biotechnol. Prog.*, 15, 1090–1094.

Yoswathana, N., Eshtiaghi, M.N., 2013. Optimization for subcritical water extraction of phenolic compounds from rambutan peels. *Int. J. Chem. Mol. Nucl. Mater. Metall. Eng.*, 7, 323–327.

Zamani, A., 2015. Introduction to lignocellulose-based products, in: Karimi, K. (ed.), *Lignocellulose-Based Bioproducts*. Springer, Cham, pp. 1–36.

19 Biochemicals from the Bioprocessing of Biomass

Bukke Vani, Mamilla Shyam Sunder, and Sundergopal Sridhar

19.1 INTRODUCTION

The environmental benefits and economic profitability of biochemicals have gained enormous demand during the last decade (Biddy et al., 2016). The formation of fossil fuels (FF) requires millions of years, and their reserves are limited, which will exhaust them in a matter of time. The global energy market is heavily dependent on fossil fuels such as coal, crude oil, and natural gas. However, lignocellulosic biomass has emerged as a promising alternative due to its abundant availability. It is not only a renewable resource but also an economically viable energy source (Mandegari et al., 2017). Biomass plays a crucial role in conversion technologies, enabling the production of value-added products through cost-effective and sustainable methods. Although nonrenewable energy sources continue to be widely used across the globe, they present several drawbacks, including limited availability, environmental harm, and long-term unsustainability (Ahuja et al., 2018).

There are different types of biomass resources available all over the world, like woody plants, agricultural crop residues, grass, vegetable waste, rotten fruits, manures, aquatic plants, and algae. Biomass is also a source of food substitutes for diabetes. In certain conversion technologies, biochemical methods are employed to break down biomass into individual components – primarily monosaccharides and oligosaccharides – which can then be efficiently converted into high-yield, value-added products. The pretreatment of biomass and the hydrolysis step are imperative in generating high-value products or biochemicals by bioprocessing the correct type of biomass. Some essential products that can be produced through the fermentation of biomass are 1,3-propanediol, succinic acid, lactic acid, and xylitol. All over the globe, Asia alone yields 50% of the world's total xylitol, and the rest of the production is by the United States, Australia, and Europe (Gao et al., 2011). Some studies of techno-economic biorefineries for converting sugarcane and its derivatives to biochemicals and biopolymers are reported in Table 19.1.

 DOI: 10.1201/9781003327608-19

TABLE 19.1
Production of Biochemicals/Polymers from Sugarcane

Serial Number	Country	Type of Biomass	End Product	Capacity (t cane/hr)
1	Colombia	Molasses/bagasse	PHB/EtOH	200
2	South Africa	Bagasse and trash	EtOH/butadiene EtOH/lactic acid	300
3	Argentina	Bagasse (hemi fraction)	Furfural/xylitol	–
4	Brazil	Molasses/sucrose	BDO	–

*Source:*Mandegari et al. (2017).

19.1.1 Lactic Acid

Lactic acid can be synthesized using pentoses and hexoses as raw materials through the homo and heterofermentative process, with the implementation of different microorganisms (Gao et al., 2011). The microbial fermentation 1G feedstocks, like carbohydrates, are used for most commercial lactic acid production. However, some plants are available to produce lactic acid even through 2G feedstocks.

The techno-economic studies proved that lactic acid production through the homo fermentative pathway with the utilization of pentoses and hexoses by a sugar mill was an economically attractive option while utilizing the sugarcane bagasse as a raw material (Mandegari et al., 2017). Further, research studies on polylactic acid (PLA) were necessitated to assess various microorganisms and their effects on the economic feasibility of PLA manufacturing. Globally, the increasing demand for biodegradable PLA has led to production, significantly increasing the use of sugarcane bagasse as an eco-friendly, viable substitute to petroleum-derived plastics.

19.1.2 Succinic Acid

Succinic acid (SA) is a valuable biochemical widely used as a pH regulator in the food and beverage industries, as well as an additive in personal care products. With the molecular formula $C_4H_6O_4$, it is a linear, saturated dicarboxylic acid. Succinic acid also serves as a precursor in the production of biopolymers such as polybutylene succinate (PBS) and is used in the manufacturing of polyurethanes, resins, coatings, and plasticizers. It can be synthesized chemically through the catalytic hydrogenation of maleic acid or maleic anhydride in the presence of butane. Alternatively, commercial production of bio-based succinic acid is achieved through microbial fermentation using bacteria or yeast under controlled low pH conditions (Koutinas et al., 2014).

Earlier research investigations, by Sindhu et al. (2016), reported that the sugarcane bagasse hydroxylates showed high conversion rates and higher yields of SA. Meanwhile, ultrasound pretreatment reported that the hydrolysis of sugarcane conversion yielded as high as approximately 79% of SA (Sindhu et al., 2016). Koutinas et al. (2014) and Luo et al. (2010) revealed that glycerol and corn stover can produce SA, and Roger's (2015) studies provide a detailed techno-economic analysis of SA.

19.1.3 Xylitol

Xylitol is an excellent microbial derivative frequently utilized as an artificial sweetener. It is usually called pentitol, and the basic structure of this compound contains five carbons that can be represented as $C_6H_{12}O_5$. Moreover, it is available in white crystals and granular shape, including low carbs that inhibit the demineralization of bone and teeth, as well as respiratory tract infections, tumor growth, and inflammator infections. The first xylitol compound was isolated for the first time from black beech trees in 1890 (Taylor et al., 2015).

It exists in very low quantities in almost all varieties of vegetables such as cauliflower, plums, strawberries, pumpkin, spinach, and natural fruits. Table 19.2

TABLE 19.2
Chemical-Physical Properties of Xylitol

Serial Number	Parameters	Values
1	Chemical formula	$C_5H_{12}O_5$ 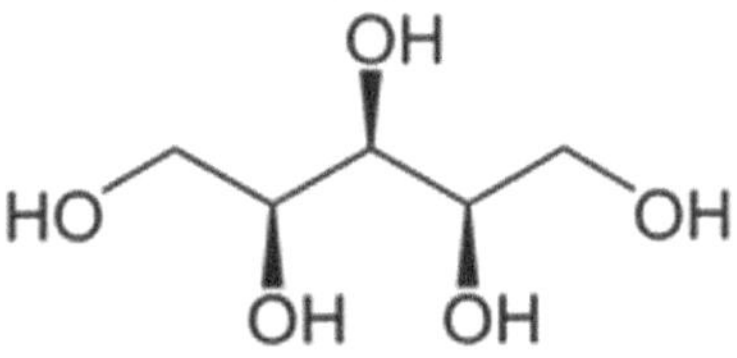
2	Molecular weight of xylitol	152.15
3	Appearance	Crystalline powder 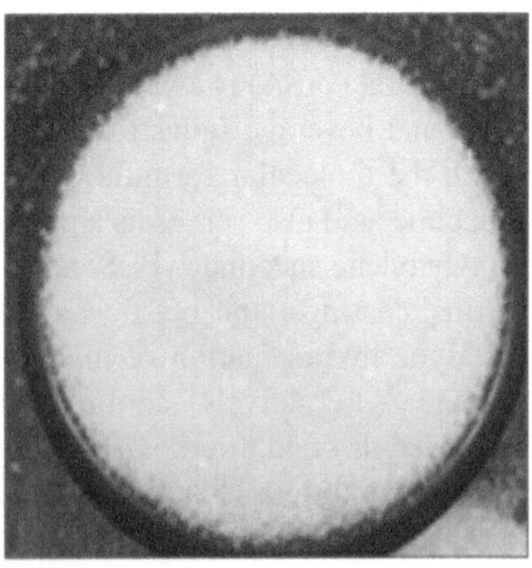

TABLE 19.2 *(Continued)*
Chemical-Physical Properties of Xylitol

Serial Number	Parameters	Values
4	pH	5–7
5	Melting and boiling point	≤ 94.5°C, 216°C
6	Density	1.50 g/L
7	Viscosity (10–60%)	1.23–20.63 cP (centipoise)
8	Caloric value	16.88 J/g

presents the concentrations of xylitol found in various fruits and vegetables. Xylitol has a wide range of applications across multiple industries, particularly in the food, dental (odontological), and pharmaceutical sectors. It is also recommended for medical use, especially in the management of diabetes, as its metabolism occurs independently of insulin, making it beneficial for individuals with insulin resistance. Furthermore, xylitol provides approximately one-third fewer calories than regular sugar, making it a suitable substitute for sucrose in low-calorie products. Table 19.2 describes the physical and chemical characteristics of xylitol in detail.

The major lignocellulosic biomass sources are agricultural, forestry, and agro-industry residues, which are imperishable, sustainable, inexpensive, and viable sources of polysaccharides, which are the primary raw materials for xylitol production (Ahuja et al., 2018). Figure 19.1 illustrates the detailed process of xylitol production using agricultural residue as the main raw material.

Xylans, the most abundant of hemicelluloses, are composed primarily of xylose (~90%) along with gluconic acid, arabinose, acetic acid, and *p*-coumaric acid. Xylose can be extracted from biomass hydrolysis at a specific temperature, and further, xylose can be converted into xylitol by chemical synthesis. Moreover, another way of producing xylitol is by the microbial fermentation of biomass hydroxylate to get the xylitol product (Prabhu et al., 2020; Ur-Rehman et al., 2015).

Table 19.3 presents xylitol production by various microorganisms; Figure 19.2 illustrates xylitol yields from different lignocellulosic sources such as fruits and vegetables (with Figure 19.2a showing xylitol concentration in vegetables and Figure 19.2b that in fruits).

Table 19.4 represents xylitol-based commercial products available in the market, especially in the food industry, along with a concentration of xylitol (%). Xylitol can be used in various concentrations as food products; it mainly depends on end-product use and market demand. Xylitol products developed by famous brands in multiple countries are listed in Table 19.4.

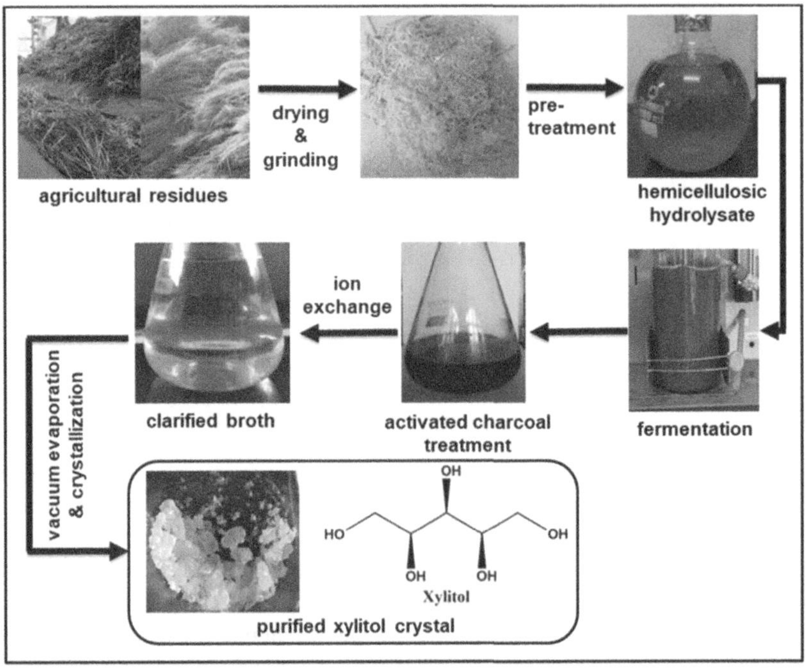

FIGURE 19.1 Xylitol production from lignocellulosic biomass.

Source: Adapted from Ahuja et al. (2018), with permission

TABLE 19.3
Microbial Species Used for Xylitol Manufacturing

Type of Microorganisms	Substrate	Production (g/L)	Reference
Type of bacteria			
Bacillus subtilis	Xylose	Xylose: 213	Cheng et al. (2011)
Cellulomonas cellulans		Xylitol: 1.76 Ethanol: 1.67	Rangaswamy et al. (2002)
Escherichia coli		Xylose: 6.325	Abd Rahman et al. (2020)
Mycobacteriumsmegmatis	D-xylulose	Xylulose: 0.7	Chen et al. (2010)
Type of Fungi			
Aspergillus niger	D-glucose	Biomass: 1.139	Zhao Kang et al. (2016)
Trichoderma reesei	Barely straw	Biomass: 6.1–13.22	Dashtban et al. (2013)
Thermomyceslanuginous	Sugarcane bagasse	Xylose: 4.4 ± 0.13	Zhang et al. (2019)
Type of yeast			
Debaromyces	Xylose	76.6	Sampaio et al. (2004)
Meyerozymaguilliermondii		Xylose: 4.28 ± 1.30	Atzmuller et al. (2020)

TABLE 19.3 *(Continued)*
Microbial Species Used for Xylitol Manufacturing

Type of Microorganisms	Substrate	Production (g/L)	Reference
Saccharomyces cerevisiae	Pretreated corn stover	Ethanol:50.19, xylitol: 45.41	Yang et al. (2020)
Saccharomyces cerevisiae	Wheat stalk	Xylitol: 3.47	Reshamwala et al. (2020)
Pachysolen	Brewer's spent grain	Xylitol: 0.47 ± 0.06	da Silva et al. (2020)
Kluyveromycesmarxianus	Cashew apple bagasse	Xylitol: 6.01	de Albuquerque et al. (2015)
Type of algae and cyanobacteria			
Synechococcus elongates (PCC794)	Xylose	Xylose: 33	Fan et al. (2020)
Chlamydomonas reinhardtii		Xylose: 0.389	Pourmir et al. (2013)

Source: Ahuja et al. (2020).

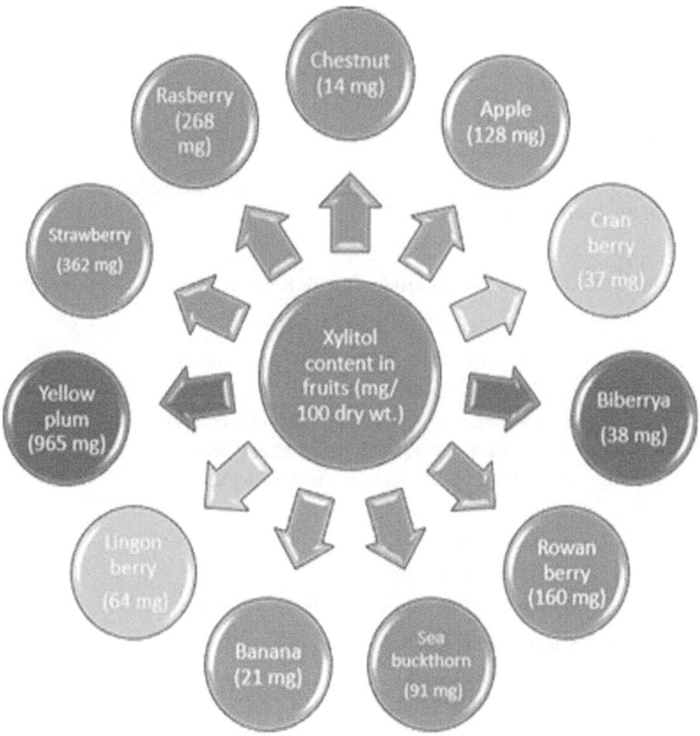

FIGURE 19.2 (a) Xylitol concentration in vegetables and (b) xylitol concentration in fruits.

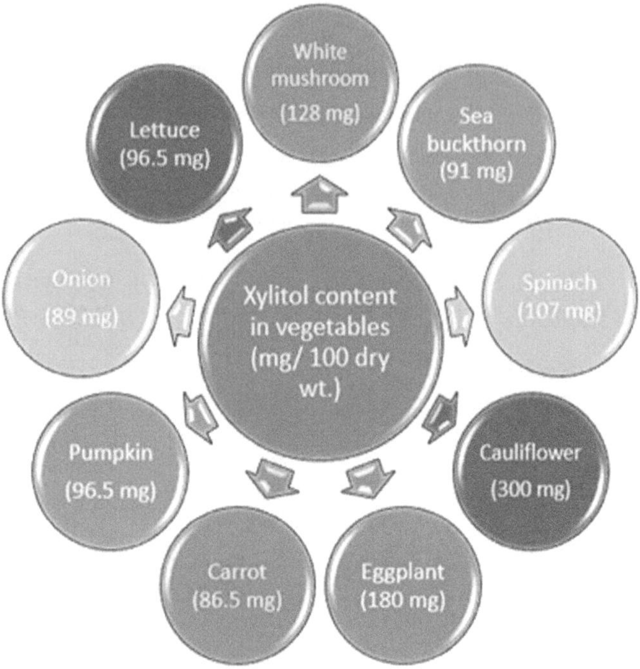

FIGURE 19.2 (Continued)

TABLE 19.4
Xylitol-Based Commercial Products

Country Name	Commercial Products with Brand Name	Concentration (%)
USA	Chewing gum: Trident and Dental Epic	1
	Xylitol-based candies include Ice Chips Candy, Epic Xylitol, Snowflakes, and Xyla.	0.4–2
	Xylitol-containing oral care products include Spry Mouthwash (Xlear), ACT Braces Care (Chattem), TheraMints (3M), and white toothpaste (New Food Solutions).	1–25
	Sweetener: plus Now	1.7
	Beverages: Health Garden	10
Germany	Xylitol-based chewing gum by Hager & Werken	94
	Candies and drops: Hager &Werken	–
Thailand	Chewing gum: Sugar-Free Chewing Gum Lotte	–
	Beverages: Real Bird's Nest by Scotch Real, Thailand	10

TABLE 19.4 *(Continued)*
Xylitol-Based Commercial Products

Country Name	Commercial Products with Brand Name	Concentration (%)
Australia	Beverages: Naturally sweet	6.6
South Africa	Beverages: Yesan-nongsan Co. Ltd.	–
	Sweetener: Alternative Suganon	–
India	Mouthwashes and toothpaste: Bioxtra and Bioxtra-T by Hetero Healthcare Ltd	–
	Sweeteners: Products by Ankur Drugs and Pharma Ltd.	–

Source: Adapted from Ahuja et al. (2020)

19.2 STRAIGHT VEGETABLE OIL/PURE PLANT OIL

Straight vegetable or waste oils are produced from food preparation and other processes, which differ from biodiesel and other conventional diesel. Biodiesel is a renewable fuel derived from fats or vegetable oils, offering the potential to reduce emissions and enhance energy security. Straight vegetable oil (SVO) is another liquid renewable energy source that can be locally produced and contributes to the reduction of greenhouse gas (GHG) emissions.

It contributes to value production in rural areas; it is neither explosive nor flammable and does not release poisonous gases. SVO can also be made from soy, coconut, oil palm, sunflower, cotton, and castor.

SVO/PPO can be extracted by mechanical press and solvent extraction. In a mechanical press, oil seeds are crushed and hard-pressed in a screw press with optional heating either before or during the pressing process. After complete oil is extracted to a maximum level, the residual seed waste can be utilized as animal feed. Meanwhile, solvent extraction is used for oilseed feedstock, in which the amount of oil is in higher concentrations. The process involves the use of solvents, which can be costly due to the high price of both the chemicals and the required equipment. Straight vegetable oil (SVO) or pure plant oil (PPO) can be used as fuel in diesel engines, either directly or after undergoing minor technical modifications. In some cases, these oils can be utilized without any engine alterations. However, their naturally high viscosity poses a challenge, which can be addressed by preheating to ensure smoother combustion. Figure 19.3 illustrates the production pathways and applications of liquid fuels derived from both first- and second-generation feedstocks. Biodiesel, an alternative fuel, can be synthesized from SVO through a chemical process known as transesterification, using methanol as the alcohol and sodium hydroxide as the catalyst.

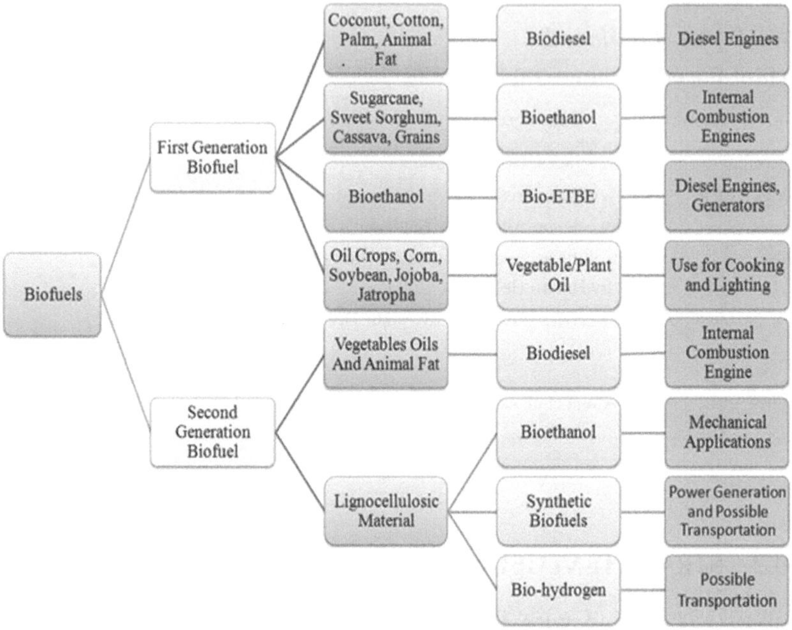

FIGURE 19.3 Production and use of liquid biofuels.

19.3 COOKING-RELATED APPLICATIONS

Biomass feedstocks like straw, bark, husks, shells, pits, sawdust, and seeds are obtained from solid organic by-products of agricultural and silvicultural harvesting with low moisture content. These are suitable for efficient production of briquettes, and biomass densification involves converting complete biomass feedstock into a unique, dense form for generating high-quality fuel. Briquette combustion offers higher efficiency and lower emissions for improved management of household and industrial applications. Briquettes are more straightforward to manage, maintain, and distribute mechanically for residential and commercial procedures.

Cookstoves have been designed specially to operate with ethanol gel and produced with gel stoves that can be reconfigured into many traditional cooking wood burners. It is a clean-burning gel fuel comprising hydrolyzed ethanol mixed with cellulose thickener and water that seems reliable and can be quickly ignited while cooking. This fuel has maximum heating efficiency. Wood fuels and kerosene can be substituted by ethanol gel, which can stabilize the domestic energy market and decrease carbon dioxide emissions, besides reducing indoor air pollution. Gel fuel does not cause respiratory problems, unlike other paraffin, wood, and coal fuel, as it burns with a carbon-free flame and does not produce smoke or smell. Gel tends to last for many days compared to paraffin.

Improved cook stoves for cooking with wood, charcoal, and other forms of biomass are a common source, but the utilization of smokeless, low-cost, and efficient stoves can help to reduce wood fuel demand, indoor air pollution, and deforestation. Improved charcoal kilns and reduced wood consumption should be prioritized alongside enhanced forest management programs and sustainable practices.

19.4 BIOCHAR

New technologies and processes have been developed globally for converting bioenergy and are available commercially today, with the development of research with potential applications of biomass assets. Various biomasses such as compost, manure, organic wastes, agricultural residues, grasses, and other crops subjected to pyrolysis, coupled with the organic matter with maximum carbon source, can be turned into bio-char with half of the original carbon sources. Biochar contains high organic carbon with fine-grained charcoal, which is resistant to decomposition. It can be produced by heating biomass without air or pyrolysis. Figure 19.4 illustrates the production of biochar through low-pressure pyrolysis. Globally, biochar naturally occurs in soils as a result of vegetation fires and certain topsoil management practices. In the Amazon region, researchers have identified biochar-rich dark earth, commonly referred to as "Terra Preta," which exhibits unique properties as an effective soil conditioner. Studies have shown that biochar can reverse soil degradation in many developing countries, promoting sustainable food and fuel production in areas facing severely depleted soils, limited organic resources, restricted access to chemical fertilizers, and water scarcity.

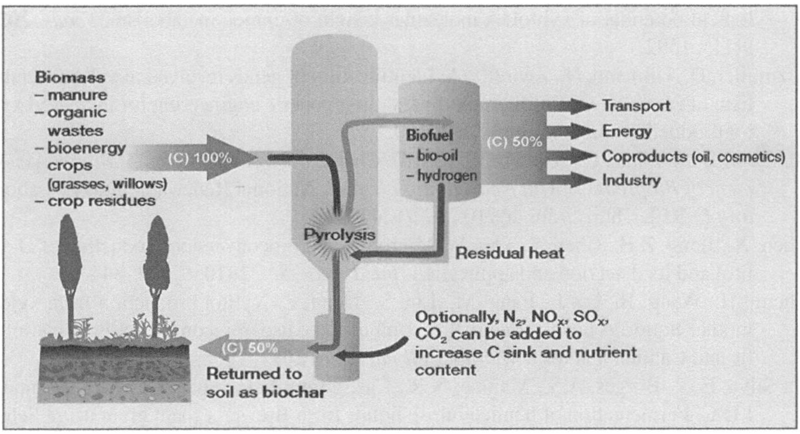

FIGURE 19.4 Production of biochar by low-pressure pyrolysis.

Source: Adapted from Lehmann (2007)

Biochar production with small-scale and low-cost unity can build agriculture, garden, and forest productivity. It can also produce electricity; thermal energy; and eating, drying, and grinding grains with the bioenergy produced.

19.5 CONCLUSION

Varieties of lignocellulosic biomasses are available abundantly globally and can be converted into value-added products. Biomass is a renewable energy source that can serve as an alternative to fossil fuels, especially in response to their depletion, driven by the growing global demand for transportation fuels and other daily energy needs. To contain the depletion and saturation of fossil fuels, alternate processes can be utilized by producing biofuels that can be blended with other commercially available fuels. Biofuels can be made with various biomasses available with eco-friendly and economical technology.

Various lignocellulosic biomass materials – such as wood biomass; agricultural residues (including bagasse, forage crop stalks, and corncobs); grasses; and forest waste – hold significant potential for the production of value-added products such as biochemicals, bio-oils, biochar, and food additives like xylitol in an economically, environmentally, and socially sustainable manner.

REFERENCES

Abd Rahman, N.H., Jahim, J., Abdul Munaim, M.S., Rahman, R.A., Fuzi, S.F.Z., Illias, R. Immobilization of recombinant Escherichia coli on multi-walled carbon nanotubes for xylitol production. *Enzym. Microb. Technol.* **2020**, 135, 109495.

Ahuja, J., Tata, S. V. R. K. (2018). Renewable and non-renewable energy and its impact on environmental quality in south Asian countries. *Int. J. Energy Econ. Policy*, *8*(2), 328–333.

Ahuja, V., Macho, M., Ewe, D., Singh, M., Saha, S., Saurav, K. Biological and pharmacological potential of xylitol: A molecular insight of unique metabolism. *Foods.* **2020**, 9(11), 1592.

Atzmuller, D., Ullmann, N., Zwirzitz, A. Identification of genes involved in xylose metabolism of Meyerozyma guilliermondii and their genetic engineering for increased xylitol production. *Amb. Express.* **2020**, 10, 78.

Biddy, M. J., Scarlata, C., Kinchin, C. (2016). *Chemicals from Biomass: A Market Assessment of Bioproducts with Near-Term Potential.* National Renewable Energy Laboratory (NREL). https://doi.org/10.2172/1244312.

Chen, X., Jiang, Z.H., Chen, S., Qin, W. Microbial and bioconversion production of D-xylitol and its detection and application. *Int. J. Biol. Sci.* **2010**, 6, 834–844.

Cheng, H., Wang, B., Lv, J., Jiang, M., Lin, S., Deng, Z. Xylitol production from xylose mother liquor: A novel strategy that combines the use of recombinant Bacillus subtilis and Candida maltosa. *Microb. Cell Factories* **2011**, 10, 5.

Da Silva, E.G., Borges, A.S., Maione, N.R., Castiglioni, G.L., Suarez, C.A.G., Montano, I.D.C. Fermentation of hemicellulose liquor from Brewer's spent grain using Scheffersomyces stipitis and Pachysolentannophilus for production of 2G ethanol and xylitol. *Biofuels Bioprod. Biorefining.* **2020**, 14, 127–137.

Dashtban, M., Kepka, G., Seiboth, B., Qin, W. Xylitol production by genetically engineered trichoderma reesei strains using Barley Straw as feedstock. *Appl. Biochem. Biotechnol.* **2013**, 169, 554–569.

de Albuquerque, T.L., Gomes, S.D.L., Marques, J.E. Jr., Silva, I.J,Jr., Rocha, M.V.P. Xylitol production from cashew apple bagasse by Kluyveromycesmarxianus CCA510. *Catal. Today* **2015**, 255, 33–40.

Fan, E.S., Lu, K.W., Wen, R.C., Shen, C.R. Photosynthetic reduction of xylose to xylitol using cyanobacteria. *Biotechnol. J.* **2020**, 15, 1900354.

Gao, C., Ma, C., Xu, P. Biotechnological routes based on lactic acid production from biomass. *Biotechnol. Adv.* **2011**, 29(6), 930–939.

Koutinas, A.A., Vlysidis, A., Pleissner, D., Kopsahelis, N., Lopez, G.I., Kookos, I.K., Papanikolaou, S., Kwan, T.L., Carol S.K. Valorization of industrial waste and by-product streams via fermentation for the production of chemicals and biopolymers. *Chem. Soc. Rev.* **2014**, 43(8), 2587–2627.

Lehmann, J. Bioenergy in the black. *Front. Ecol. Environ.* **2007**, 5, 381–387.

Luo, L., van der Voet, E., Huppes, G. Biorefining of lignocellulosic feedstock – technical, economic and environmental considerations. *Bioresour. Technol.* **2010**, 101(13), 5023–5032.

Mandegari, M.A., Farzad, S., Görgens, J.F. Recent trends on techno-economic assessment (TEA) of sugarcane biorefineries. *Biofuel Research Journal* **2017**, 15, 704–712.

Pourmir, A., Noor-Mohammadi, S., Johannes, T.W. Production of xylitol by recombinant microalgae. *J. Biotechnol.* **2013**, 165, 178–183.

Prabhu, A.A., Bosakornranut, E., Amraoui, Y., Agarwal, D., Coulon, F., Vivekanand, V., Thakur, V.K., Kumar, V. Enhanced xylitol production using non-detoxified xylose-rich pre-hydrolysate from sugarcane bagasse by newly isolated Pichia fermentans, **2020**. https://doi.org/10.21203/rs.3.rs-45506/v3

Rangaswamy, S., Agblevor, F. Screening of facultative anaerobic bacteria utilizing D-xylose for xylitol production. *Appl. Microbiol. Biotechnol.* **2002**, 60, 88–93.

Reshamwala, S.M.S., Lali, A.M. Exploiting the NADPH pool for xylitol production using recombinant Saccharomyces cerevisiae. *Biotechnol. Prog.* **2020**, 36, e2972.

Sampaio, F.B.C., Torre, P., Passos, F.V.M.L., Perego, P., Passos, F.J.V., Converti, A. Xylose metabolism in debaryomyces hansenii UFV-170. Effect of the specific oxygen uptake rate. *Biotechnol. Prog.* **2004**, 20, 1641–1650.

Sindhu, R., Gnansounou, E., Binod, P., Pandey, A., Bioconversion of sugarcane crop residue for value-added products – an overview. *Renew. Energy.* **2016**, 98, 203–215.

Taylor, R., Nattrass, L., Alberts, G., Robson, P., Chudziak, C., Bauen, A., Libelli, I.M., Lotti, G., Prussi, M., Nistri, R., Chiaramonti, D., López-Contreras, A.M., Bos, H.L., Eggink, G., Springer, J., Bakker, R. (2015). *From the Sugar Platform to Biofuels and Biochemicals: Final Report for the European Commission Directorate-General for Energy*. The European Commission, Wageningen University & Research (WUR).

Ur-Rehman, S., Mushtaq, Z., Zahoor, T., Jamil, A., Murtaza, M.A. Xylitol: A review on bioproduction, application, health benefits, and related safety issues. *Crit. Rev. Food Sci. Nutr.* **2015**, 55(11), 1514–28.

Yang, B.-X., Xie, C.Y., Xia, Z.Y, Wu, Y.J., Li, B., Tang, Y.Q. The effect of xylose reductase genes on xylitol production by industrial Saccharomyces cerevisiae in fermentation of glucose and xylose. *Process Biochem.* **2020**, 95, 122–130.

Zhang, M., Puri, A.K., Wang, Z., Singh, S., Permaul, K. A unique xylose reductase from Thermomyces lanuginosus: Effect of lignocellulosic substrates and inhibitors and applicability in lignocellulosic bioconversion. *Bioresour. Technol.* **2019**, 281, 374–381.

Zhao Kang, T., Mohammad, S.H., Abd Murad, A.M., Illias, R., Jahim, J.M. Fermentative production of xylitol: A first trial on xylose bifurcation. *Indian J. Sci. Technol.* **2016**, 9, 1–5.

20 Bio-Based Monomers and Bio-Polymers Products from Biomass

Sundergopal Sridhar and Mamilla Shyam Sunder

20.1 INTRODUCTION

Bio-based monomers and biopolymers are considered eco-friendly alternatives to petrochemical polymers due to their composition availability in renewable feedstocks. To understand the concept of the versatile properties of polymers, one must realize that they have occupied a significant niche in commodities. The starch-based polymers, polylactic acid, and polyhydroxyalkanoates, which are biodegradable, have been examined as a solution for the future of our planet (Crank et al., 2004). As only 5% of chemicals are currently produced from renewable feedstocks, and the application of natural substances as a future for the manufacture of polymers is steadily increasing, the world needs to be motivated to stimulate the rational use of biomass as a renewable resource. Nonbiodegradable plastics cause serious ecological problems, and bio-based polymers show biodegradation.

The lignocellulosic biomass showed the conversion into polymers and monomers for novel polymeric materials, which are potentially accessible as they are produced annually in significant amounts in various streams, forests, agriculture, and the paper industry. Lignocellulose comprises three polymers: they are cellulose; hemicelluloses are polysaccharides of hexoses and pentoses; and lignin is a branched polymer of aromatic alcohols. Figure 20.1 shows the production of polymers of monomers. Bio-based polymers are polylactic acid (PLA), polyhydroxyalkonates (PHAs), hyperbranched polymers (HBP), polyilaconic acid (PIA), poly(3-hydroxybutyrate) (PHB), polybutylene succinate (PBS), polyisosorbide terephthalate (PIT), and polyethylene 2,5 furandecarboxylate (PEF); bio-based monomers are butanediol (BDO), butadiene (BD), lactic acid (LA), itaconic acid (IA), succinic acid (SA), diphenolic acid (DPA), and 2,5-furandicarboxylic acid (FDCA).

The production of polymers and monomers from lignocelluloses comprehends the fractionation of lignocelluloses into cellulose, hemicelluloses, and lignin followed by depolymerization into carbohydrates and aromatic monomers and by thermal transformation or catalytic process into chemicals and their conversion

 DOI: 10.1201/9781003327608-20

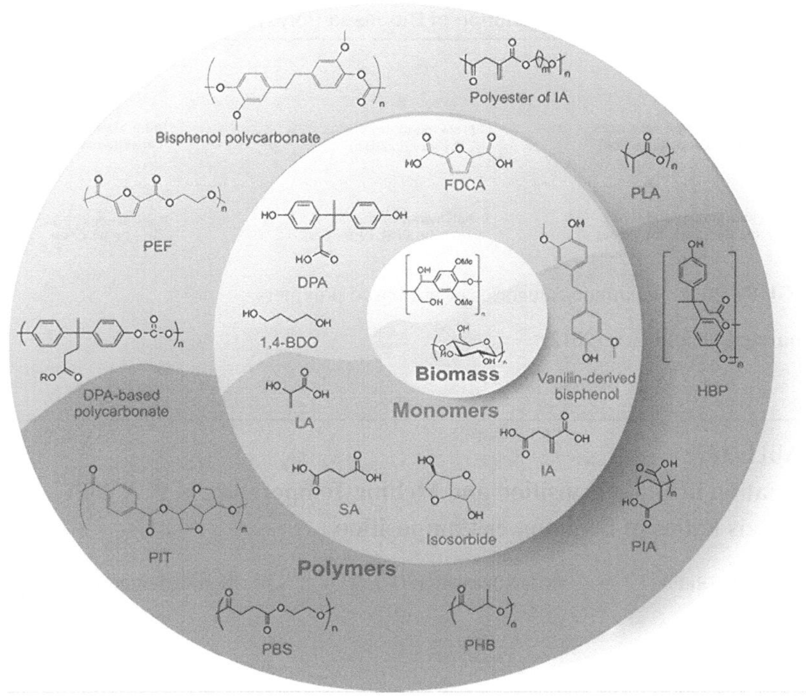

FIGURE 20.1 Production of bio-based polymers and monomers.

Source: **Irina Delidovich et al. (2016)**

into derived alternative monomers and final polymerization of these monomers (Gallezot, 2012; Climent et al. 2011; Kobayashi and Fukuoka, 2013; Delidovich et al., 2014) and potential polymers. Figure 20.2 shows some of the common categories of bio-based polymers.

20.2 POLYLACTIC ACID

Polylactic acid (PLA) has been known since the 18th century and was commercialized in the 1990s. Polylactic acid belongs to the family of aliphatic polyesters, is made of lactic acid, and can be produced from sugars extracted from renewable biomass through microbial fermentation. High-purity lactic acid can be obtained using corn as biomass through an efficient synthetic process and microbial fermentation process. L-lactic acid or D-lactic acid is obtained depending on the strains used. Polylactic acid and polylactic acid copolymers can be obtained depending on the stereochemical nature and nature of monomer L and D, and the final properties of PLA produced depend on the ratio of the L and D forms

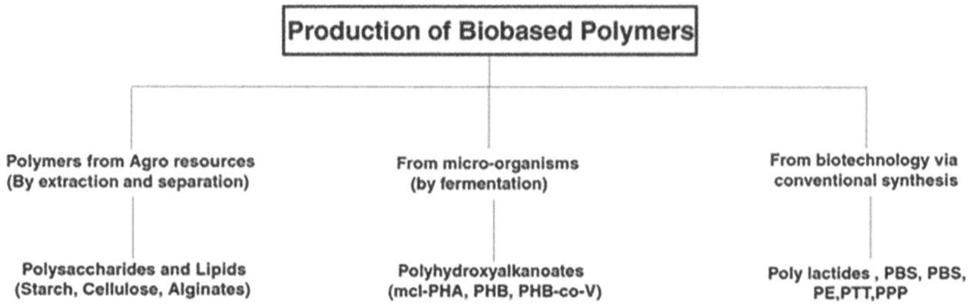

FIGURE 20.2 Common categories of bio-based polymers.

Source: Luc and Eric (2012)

TABLE 20.1
Variation in Glass Transition and Melting Temperature of PLA with Various Ratios of L-Monomer Composition

Copolymer Ratio	Glass Transition (T_g), °C	Melting Temperature (T_m), °C
100:0 (L/DL)-PLA	63	178
95:5 (L/DL)-PLA	59	164
90:10 (L/DL)-PLA	56	150
85:15 (L/DL)-PLA	56	140
80:20 (L/DL)-PLA	56	125

Source: Garlotta (2001)

of lactic acid. Table 20.1 shows the variation in glass transition and melting temperature of PLA with various ratios of L-monomers composition. Polylactic acid can be applied as a bio-based plastic alone or in blend with other polymers and can be reinforced with cellulose fibers in the textiles and packaging industry. It has unique characteristics like glossy appearance, good transparency, and high rigidity. PLA is a thermoplastic polymer that can tolerate various processing conditions and can potentially replace traditional polymers such as PET, PS, and PC (Majid et al., 2010).

Polylactic acid from LA can be produced by direct polycondensation in an azeotropic solution, direct condensation polymerization, and polymerization through lactide formation. Researchers have done many studies on polylactic acid, but they require improving the properties of PLA to suit various applications. Many countries developed commercially available PLA with multiple grades suitable for industrial sectors such as electronics, automobiles, medical devices, and commodity applications. Table 20.2 describes the global supplies of PLA. PLA is used widely daily in food packaging like tableware plates, food trays, water

TABLE 20.2
Global Suppliers of PLA with Country-wise Production Expected by 2030

Company	Brand Names	Country	Planned Capacity (kton/year)
Nature Works	Ingeo®	USA	800–1000
Tate & Lyle	Ingeo®	UK	50–100
Futerro	Futerro®	Belgium	300–400
Purac,	Luminy®,	The Netherlands	200–300
Synbra	Biofoam®	-do-	–
Hycail B.V.	Hycail®	-do-	–
Hisun,	Revode®,	China	2500–3000
Jiangsu	BBCA®	-do-	–
Teijin,	Biofront®,	Japan	200–300
Toyobo	Biomax®	-do-	–

Source: Doug, 2010; Ravenstijn, 2010

bottles, cups, and candy wraps and has heat resistance and mechanical strength. Table 20.3 lists the PLA-based polymer applications in various fields.

20.3 POLYHYDROXY ALKANOATES

Polyhydroxy alkanoates (PHAs) are produced by direct bacterial fermentation of sugars or lipids to store carbon and energy. PHAs are linear polyester families and have the potential to replace hydrocarbon-based polymers that can be produced by microbes with different renewable biomass feedstocks. The production process of PHA involves isolation, fermentation, and purification, followed by blending; 150 PHA monomer constituents of PHAs have been identified (Steinbüchel and Valenti, 1995) to produce a wide range of bio-based polymers.

Three main factors contribute to the production cost of PHAs: the energy required for sterilizing the fermentation equipment, the PHA's yield on the substrate, and the efficiency of the downstream processing. Poly-3-hydroxybutyrate is the first bacterial PHA identified and has received significant attention regarding pathway characterization and industrial-scale production. A techno-economic analysis was performed on a sugarcane biorefinery, evaluating the conversion pathways for sugar, fuel ethanol, PHB, common PHAs, anthocyanins, and electricity. However, slow crystallization, a narrow processing range, and a tendency to "creep" are not attractive for many applications (Reis et al., 2008).

More than 150 different polyhydroxyalkanoates have been identified as useful monomers that can form a large family of polyesters. Poly-3-hydroxybutyrate is

TABLE 20.3
Application of PLA and Their Blends in Various Fields

Polymer	Applications	Reference
PLGA/PGA	Ovine pulmonary valve replacement	Williams et al. (1999); Sodian et al. (1999, 2000); Cheng et al. (2009)
PLA/chitosan, PLA/PLGA, chitosan PLA	Drug carrier/drug release	Jeevitha and Kanchana, (2013); Jayanth and Vinod, (2012); Nagarwal et al. (2010); Chandy et al. (2000); Valantin et al. (2003)
PLGA and copolymers	Degradable sutures	Rajev (2000)
PLA/HA composites	Porous scaffolds for cellular applications	Jung-Ju et al. (2012)
PLA-CaP and PLGA-CaP	Bone fixation devices, plates, pins, screws, and wires, orthopedic applications	Huan et al. (2012)
PDLLA	Coatings on metal implants	Schmidmaier et al. (2001)
PLA/PLGA	Use in cell-based gene therapy for cardiovascular diseases, muscle tissues, bone, and cartilage regeneration, and other treatments of cardiovascular and neurological conditions	Coutu et al. (2009); Kellomäki et al. (2000); Papenburg et al. (2009)
PLA and PLA blends	Electrical appliances, mobile, phone housings, floor mats, and automotive spare parts	Rafael et al., 2010
PLA	Textile applications	Gupta et al., 2007; Avinc and Akbar, 2009

Source: Babu et al. (2013)

a microbial PHA which showed the most excellent potential for industrial-scale production. Many industries produce PHAs as copolymers, such as poly(3-hydroxybutyrate-co-3-hydroxyvalerate), which typically consist of 80–95% (R)-3-hydroxybutyric acid monomers and further 5–20% of secondary comonomer (e.g., 3-hydroxyvalerate) to improve the material properties for various applications.

PHAs can be used in machinery that convert them into injection-molded components, fibers, laminates, films, sheets, and coated articles. These materials are suitable for producing nonwoven fabrics, disposables, hygiene products, synthetic paper, adhesives, paints, waxes, foams, and binders. Food packing applications include cups and closures; disposable items such as spoons, forks, knives, trays, tubs, and hot cup lids; and other products such as cosmetics, housewares, and medical packaging (Philip et al., 2007). PHAs and copolymers are used for making biomedical implant materials. Table 20.4 describes various applications with polymer blends of PHAs.

TABLE 20.4
Application of PHAs and Their Blends in Various Fields

PHA Polymer Type	Applications	Reference
P(3HB), P(3HB-co-3HHX) and blends scaffolds	Nerve regeneration, soft tissue, artificial esophagus, drug delivery, skin regeneration, food additive	Yang et al. (2002); Chen and Qiong (2005); Bayram and Denbas (2008); Tang et al. (2008); Clarinval and Halleux (2005)
mcl-PHA/scl-PHA	Cardiac tissue engineering, drug delivery, cosmetics, drug molecules	Sodian et al. (2000); Wang et al. (2003); de Roo et al. (2002); Zhao et al. (2003); Ruth et al. (2007)
P(4HB)	Heart valve scaffolds, food additive	Clarinval and Halleux (2005); Valappil et al. (2006) P(3HO)
P(3HB-co-4HB)	Drug delivery, scaffolds	Türesin et al. (2001); Williams et al. (1999);
P(3HB-co-3HV)	Heart values, patches to repair gastrointestinal tracts, sutures	Chen et al. (2008); Freier et al. (2002); Kunze et al. (2006); Volova et al. (2003)
PHB, Mirel P103	Commodity applications, shampoo and cosmetic bottles, cups, and food containers	Philip et al. (2007); Amass et al. (1998); Walle et al. (2001)

Source: Babu et al. (2013)

20.4 BUTANEDIOL

Biorefineries are novel and aimed at creating alternatives to many fossil-based products like biomass-based lignocelluloses, creating new sustainable economic growth. 1,4-Butanediol or 2,3-butanediol is a four-carbon primary alcohol produced from readily available, alternative, efficient raw materials and renewable biomass and further has less impact on environment than other fossils. A promising process for producing BDO utilizes a range of lignocellulosic sugars with efficient commercialization potential. Scaling up the catalytic conversion of succinic acid into BDO is a promising strategy.

With 78% total electricity demand, the energy demand can be covered despite low electricity supply. As the current demand of BDO is just under 2 million t/yr, the biorefinery is promising to process 60,000 t/yr of carbon-based biomass for the production of 1,4 butanediol (bio-based). Genomatica, processing BDO, has successfully demonstrated an integrated process utilizing a range of lignocellulosic sugars, which has a potentiality for commercialization, which can meet the demand for these sugars. Alternatively, the purification of BDO requires high pressure stream column.

Application: BDO is a building block used in making plastics, textiles, and automotives. Among other popular applications are shopping bags, packaging, tableware, and industrial and consumer goods molds. BDO is used as PTMEG (polytetramethylene ether glycol) to produce spardex fibers; PBT (polybutylene terephthalate) is used in automotive and cell phones; NMP (N-methyl-2-pyrrolidone) is used in making sports goods; and GBL (gamma-butyrolactone) is used for making PVP polymers, solvents, and in other purposes.

20.4.1 Butadiene

Butadiene is an industrially relevant precursor for the production of polymer, where it is typically polymerized with itself or other monomers to produce synthetic rubber (Langenthal and Schnetger, 2005). 1,3-Butadiene is another monomer whose synthesis from biomass has attracted interest recently, owing to its applications for the production of tires and sealants (Olivera et al., 2016; Langenthal and Schnetger, 2005). Biomass can be converted into butadiene by the formation of tetrahydrofuran (THF); the polymerization method of butadiene with styrene and acrylonitide produces plastic, acrylonitrile butadiene styrene (ABS), which is a polymer of butadiene and styrene (used for the production of automobile types), as butadiene is the chief component used in a broad range of materials. Butadiene plays an essential role in manufacturing automotive parts, sporting

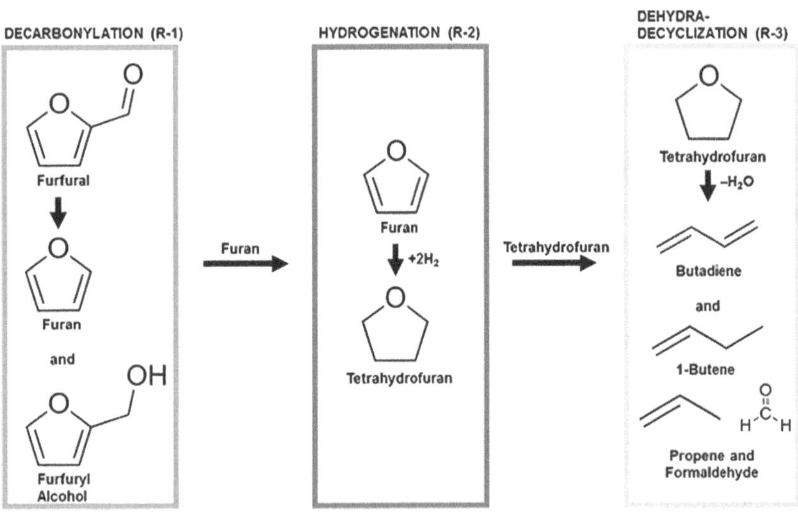

SCHEME 20.1 Process chemistry of three sequential reactors to convert furfural to butadiene.

Source: Kuznetsov et al. (2020)

goods, medical devices, and so forth. Butadiene copolymerizes with acetonitrile from NBR (nitrile butadiene rubber), a resistant rubber used for making scales, hoses, and gloves (Olivera et al., 2016).

Studies on the transition from biomass to butadiene production have been extensively reviewed, focusing on processes that use ethanol or four-carbon alcohols. The renewable biomass is obtained by catalytic conversion of furfural to 1,3-butadiene, which is potential synthetic process for renewable rubber. The process is as follows: decarbonization of the furfural to furan – the hydrogenation of furan to tetrahydrofuran and dehydration of tetrahydrofuran to 1,3-butadiene. Butadiene can be obtained by dehydrogenating n-butene or by naphtha cracking by a by-product of ethylene production. Scheme 20.1 shows the conversion of furfural to butadiene. The first step of conversion of furfural to furan by carbonization can take place in the gas or liquid phase using Pd catalyst, with yields of 98% furan (Sitthisa et al., 2011; Zhang et al., 2011; Jung et al., 1988; Li and Ozer, 2013); Furan with Pd/carbon catalyst gives a quantitative yield of THF and in the final step THF is converted by catalytic dehydra-decyclization to give butadiene. In addition to the present studies for butadiene production, these materials' catalyst characterization and active site structure are required to understand the reaction mechanism in detail.

20.5 CONCLUSION

Bio-based monomers and biopolymers are eco-friendly alternatives to petrochemical polymers when converted with renewable biomass feedstocks due to the availability of cellulose. Hemicelluloses are polysaccharides of the hexoses and pentoses, and further, lignin is a branched polymer of aromatic alcohols.

REFERENCES

Amass W, Amass A, Tighe B (1998) A review of biodegradable polymers: Uses, current developments in the synthesis and characterization of biodegradable polyesters, blends of biodegradable polymers and recent advances in biodegradation studies. *Polymer International* 47:89144.

Avinc A, Akbar K (2009) Overview of poly (lactic acid) fibres. Part I: Production, properties, performance, environmental impact, and end-user applications of poly (lactic acid) fibers. *Fiber Chemistry* 41(6):391–401.

Babu RP, O'Connor K, Seeram R (2013) Current progress on polylactic acid (PLA) and polyhydroxyalkanoates (PHAs) as sustainable alternatives for petroleum-based plastics. *RSC Advances* 3(34):11582–11587.

Bayram C, Denbas EB (2008) Preparation and characterization of triamcinolone acetonide-loaded poly(3-hydroxybutyrate-co-3 hydroxyhexanoate) (PHBHx) microspheres. *J Bioactive and Compatible Polymer* 23:334347.

Chandy T, Das GS, Wilson RF, Rao GHR (2000) Use of plasma glow for surface engineering of biodegradable polymers and their drug release characteristics. *J Biomater Appl* 15(2):127–144.

Chen GQ, Qiong W (2005) The application of polyhydroxyalkanoates as tissue engineering materials. *Biomaterials* 26:65656578.

Chen QZ, Harding SE, Ali NN, Lyon AR, Boccaccini AR (2008) Biomaterials in cardiac tissue engineering: Ten years of research survey. *Materials Sci Eng: Reports* 59:137.

Cheng Y, Deng S, Chen P, Ruan R (2009) Polylactic acid (PLA) synthesis and modifications: A review. *Front Chem China* 4:259264.

Clarinval AM, Halleux J (2005) Classification of biodegradable polymers. In: Smith R (ed) *Biodegradable polymers for industrial applications*. Woodhead, Cambridge.

Climent MJ, Corma A, Iborra S (2011) Converting carbohydrates to bulk and fine chemicals over heterogeneous catalysts. *Green Chem* 13:520–540.

Coutu DL, Yousefi AM, Galipeau J (2009) Three-dimensional porous scaffolds at the crossroads of tissue engineering and cell-based gene therapy. *J Cell Biochem* 108:537–546.

Crank, M, Patel MK, Marscheider-Weidemann F, Schleich J, Hüsing B, Angerer G (2004) *Techno-economic feasibility of large-scale production of bio-based polymers in Europe (PRO-BIP)*. Utrecht University/Fraunhofer Institute; Final Report for European Commission's Institute for Prospective Technological Studies (IPTS).

de Roo G, Kellerhals MB, Ren Q, Witholt B, Kessler B (2002) Production of chiral R-3-R-3-hydroxyalkanoic acids and R-3-hydroxyalkanoic acid methylesters via hydrolytic degradation of polyhydroxyalkanoate synthesized by pseudomonads. *BiotechnolBioeng* 77:717722.

Delidovich I, Leonhard K, Palkovits R (2014) Cellulose and hemicellulose valorisation: An integrated challenge of catalysis and reaction engineering. *Energy Environ Sci* 7:2803–2830.

Doug S (2010) *Bioplastics: Technologies and global markets*. BCC Research Reports PLS050A. www.bccresearch.com/report/bioplastics-technologiesmarkets-pls050a.html

Freier T, Kunze C, Nischan C (2002) In vitro and in vivo degradation studies for development of a biodegradable patch based on poly(3-hydroxybutyrate). *Biomaterials* 23:26492657.

Gallezot P (2012) Conversion of biomass to selected chemical products. *Chem Soc Rev*41:1538–1558.

Garlotta D (2001) A literature review of poly (lactic acid). *J Polyms and the Envir* 9(2):63–84.

Gupta B, Revagade N, Hilborn J (2007) Poly(lactic acid) fiber: An overview. *Prog Polym Sci* 34:455–482.

Huan Z, Joseph GL, Sarit BB (2012) Fabrication aspects of PLA-CaP/PLGA-CaP composites for orthopedic applications: A review. *Acta Biomater* 8(6):1999–2016.

Delidovich I, Hausoul PJC, Deng L, Pfützenreuter R, Rose M, Regina Palkovits (2016) Alternative monomers based on lignocellulose and their use for polymer production. Chem Rev 116:1540–1599.

Jayanth P, Vinod L (2012). Biodegradable nanoparticles for drug and gene delivery to cells and tissue. *Adv Drug Deliv Rev* 64:6171.

Jeevitha D, Kanchana A (2013) Chitosan/PLA nanoparticles as a novel carrier for the delivery of anthraquinone: Synthesis, characterization and in vitro cytotoxicity evaluation. *Colloids Surf B Biointerfaces* 101(1):126–134.

Jung KJ, Gaset A, Molinier J (1988) Furfural decarbonylation catalyzed by charcoal supported palladium: Part II, a continuous process. *Biomass* 16:89–96.

Jung-Ju K, Guang-Zhen J, Hye-Sun Y, Seong-Jun C, Hae-Won K, Ivan BW (2012) Providing osteogenesis conditions to mesenchymal stem cells using bioactive nanocomposite bone scaffolds. *Mater Sci Eng C* 32:25452551.

Kellomäki M, Niiranen H, Puumanen K, Ashammakhi N, Waris T, Törmälä P (2000) Bioabsorbable scaffolds for guided bone regeneration and generation. *Biomaterials* 21(24), 2495–2505.

Kobayashi H, Fukuoka A (2013) Synthesis and utilisation of sugar compounds derived from lignocellulosic biomass. *Green Chem* 15:1740–1763.

Kunze C, Edgar Bernd H, Androsch R (2006) In vitro and in vivo studies on blends of isotactic and atactic poly (3-hydroxybutyrate) for development of a dura substitute material. *Biomaterials* 27:192201.

Kuznetsov A, Kumar G, Ardagh MA, Tsapatsis M, Zhang Q, Dauenhauer PJ (2020) On the economics and process design of renewable butadiene from biomass-derived furfural. ACS Sustain Chem Eng 8(8), 3273–3282.

Langenthal WV, Schnetger J (2005) *Processing of natural and synthetic rubber*. Wiley-VCH.

Li K, Ozer R (2013) Vapor-phase decarbonylation process. *US8* 404:871B2.

Luc A, Eric P (2012) Biodegradable polymers. *In: Environmental silicate nanobiocomposites. Green energy and technology*. Springer, Heidelberg, pp. 13–39.

Majid J, Elmira AT, Muhammad I, Muriel J, St'ephane D (2010) Poly-lactic acid: production, applications, nanocomposites, and release studies. *Comprehensive Rev Food Sci Safety* 9(5):552–571.

Nagarwal RC, Singh PN, Kant S, Maiti P, Pandit JK (2010) Chitosan-coated PLA nanoparticles for ophthalmic delivery: Characterization, in-vitro and in-vivo study in rabbit eye. *J Biomed Nanotechnol* 6:648–656.

Olivera S, Muralidhara HB, Venkatesh K, Gopalakrishna K, Vivek CS (2016) Plating on acrylonitrile-butadiene-styrene (ABS) plastic: A review. *J Mater Sci* 51: 3657–3674.

Papenburg BJ, Liu J, Higuera G, Barradas AMC, Boer J, Blitterswijk VCA, Wessling M, Stamatialis D (2009) Development and analysis of multi-layer scaffolds for tissue engineering. *Biomaterials* 30:62286239.

Philip S, Keshavarz T, Roy I (2007) Polyhydroxyalkanoates: Biodegradable polymers with a range of applications. *J Chemical Tech Biotech* 2(3):233–247.

Rafael A, Loong TL, Susan EM, Selke HT (2010). Poly(lactic acid): Synthesis, structures, properties, processing, and applications. *Chapter* 28:457–467.

Rajev AJ (2000) The manufacturing techniques of various drug-loaded biodegradable poly(lactide-co-glycolide) (PLGA) devices. *Biomaterials* 21:24752490.

Ravenstijn JTJ (2010) *The state-of-the-art on bioplastics: Products, markets, trends and technologies*. Polymedia, Lüdenscheid.

Reis KC, Pereira J, Smith AC, Carvalho CWP, Wellner N, Yakimets I (2008) Characterization of polyhydroxybutyrate-hydroxyvalerate (PHB-HV)/maize starch blend films. *J Food Engg* 89:361369.

Ruth KG, Hartmann R, Egli T, Zinn M, Ren Q (2007) Efficient production of (R)-3 hydroxycarboxylic acids by biotechnological conversion of polyhydroxyalkanoates and their purification. *Biomacromolecules* 8:279–286.

Schmidmaier G, Wildemann A, Stemberger A, Has MR (2001) Biodegradable poly (D, L-lactide) coating of implants for continuous release of growth factors. *J Biomed Mater Res* 58:449455.

Sitthisa S, Pham T, Prasomsri T, Sooknoi T, Mallinson RG, Resasco DE (2011) Conversion of furfural and 2-methylpentanal on Pd/SiO2 and Pd-Cu/SiO2 catalysts. *J Catal* 280:17–27.

Sodian R, Sperling JS, Martin DP, Stock U, Mayer JE Jr, Vacanti JP (1999) Tissue engineering of a trileaflet heart valve—early in vitro experiences with a combined polymer. *Tissue Eng* 5(6):489–494. https://doi.org/:10.1089/ten.1999.5.489

Sodian R, Hoerstrup SP, Sperling JS, Daebritz S, Martin DP, Moran AM, Kim BS, Schoen FJ, Vacanti JP, Mayer JE (2000) Early in vivo experience with tissue-engineered trileaflet heart valves. *Circulation* 102:2229.

Steinbüchel A, Valentin HE (1995) Diversity of bacterial polyhydroxyalkanoic acids. *FEMS Microbiol Lett* 128:219228.
Tang H, Ishii D, Mahara A, Murakami S, Yamaoka T, Sudesh K, Samian R, Fujita M, Maeda M, Iwata T (2008) Scaffolds from electrospun polyhydroxyalkanoate copolymers: fabrication, characterization, bioabsorption and tissue response. *Biomaterials* 29:1307–1317
Türesin F, Gürsel I, Hasirci V (2001) Biodegradable polyhydroxyalkanoate implants for osteomyelitis therapy: In vitro antibiotic release. *J Biomaterials Sci* 12(2):195–207. Polymer Edition.
Valantin MA, Aubron-Olivier C, Ghosn J, Laglenne E, Pauchard M, Schoen H (2003) Polylactic acid implants to correct facial lipoatrophy in HIV-infected patients: Results of the open-label study. *Vega Aids* 17:2471–2477.
ValappilS, Misra S, Boccaccini A, Roy I (2006) Biomedical applications of polyhydroxyalkanoates, an overview of animal testing and in vivo responses. *Expert Rev Med Devices* 3:853868.
Volova T, Shishatskaya E, Sevastianov V, Efremov S, Mogilnaya O (2003) Results of biomedical investigations of PHB and PHB/PHV fibers. *Biochem Eng J* 16:125133.
Walle GAM, de Koning GJM, Weusthuis RA, Eggink G (2001) Properties, modifications and applications of biopolyesters. *Adv BiochemEngBiotechnol* 71:264291.
Wang Z, Itoh Y, Hosaka Y, Kobayashi I, Nakano Y, Maeda I, Umeda F, Yamakawa J, Kawase M, Yagi K (2003) Novel transdermal drug delivery system with polyhydroxyalkanoate and starburst polyamidoamine dendrimer. *J Biosci and Bioengg* 95(5):541–543.
Williams SF, Martin DP, Horowitz DM, Peoples OP (1999) PHA applications: Addressing the price performance issue I. Tissue engineering. *Int J Biol Macromolecules* 25:111121.
Yang F, Li X, Li G, Zhao N, Zhang X (2002) Study on chitosan and PHBHHx used as nerve regeneration conduit material. *J Biomedical Engg* 19:2529.
Zhang W, Zhu Y, Niu S, Li Y (2011) A study of furfural decarbonylation on K-doped Pd/Al2O3 catalysts. *J Mol Catal A: Chem* 335:71–81.
Zhao K, Tian G, Zheng Z, Chen JC, Chen GQ (2003) Production of D-(−)-3 3-hydroxyalkanoic acid by recombinant Escherichia coli. *FEMS Microbiol Lett* 218:5964.

21 Comprehensive Review of Ethanol Fermentation from Lignocellulosic Biomass for the Developing Economies of Tropical Regions

Nivedita Sahu, Mamilla Shyam Sunder, and Sundergopal Sridhar

21.1 INTRODUCTION

The increased exploitation, decreased availability of fossil fuels, and the overwhelming negative impact of petroleum-derived fuels (e.g., about 85% of global CO_2 emissions from global warming) are raising concerns. The second generation of biofuels has been identified as a potential source over the past four decades and is currently the most widely explored in many countries. Ethanol derived from sugarcane or corn juice, a first-generation biofuel, was the best source and tagged as economically viable (Lewis, 1977) in some countries that produced excessive quantities of the respective food crop. For instance, in Brazil, up to 85% of ethanol is blended with petroleum and sold as E85.

21.2 GLOBAL ETHANOL PERSPECTIVE AND PROJECTION

With this development, other countries began exploring various sources for biofuel production, and several reports were published in the late 1970s and early 1980s on crops and wastes (Ladisch et al., 1979; Lewis, 1979). Developments in global ethanol consumption from 2002, with projections up to 2030 for different countries, are shown in Figure 21.1.

DOI: 10.1201/9781003327608-21

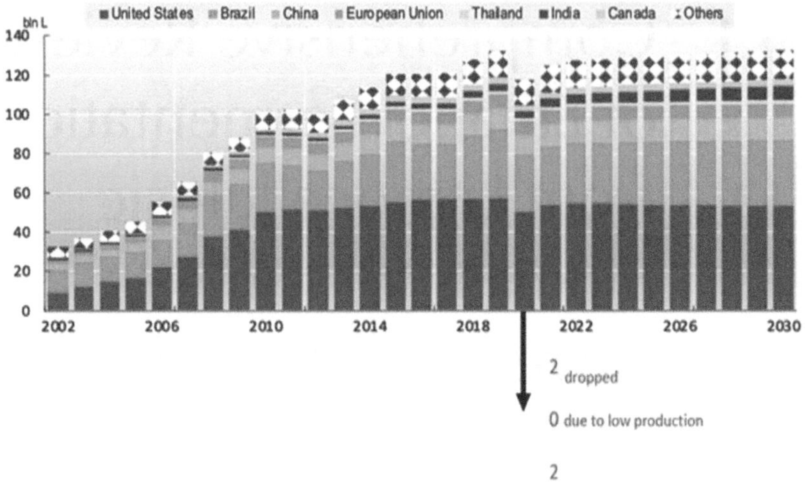

FIGURE 21.1 Global ethanol consumption over the past decades and predicted data up to 2030.

Source: OECD/FAO (2021), "OECD-FAO Agricultural Outlook," OECD Agriculture statistics (database), http://dx.doi.org/10.1787/agr-outl-data-en (modified)

21.2.1 Recent Effect of COVID-19 on Bioethanol

COVID-19 has hit the world, including the biofuel production industries, which have been seriously affected. As a result, ethanol output worldwide dropped drastically in 2020 (Figure 21.1). During the pandemic, even after the lockdown and the slight easing of restrictions, demand for ethanol for hand sanitizers was high. When the pandemic is over and production industries return to normalcy, a rebound is expected. However, worldwide production might not be as strong as before the lockdown period. With an eye toward the future, worldwide ethanol production is expected to increase again, as shown in Figure 21.1.

Soon, concerns emerged about using agricultural land and food crops for biofuel production, sparking the food versus fuel debate, particularly in countries where food crop production was insufficient to meet population needs. Later, the focus shifted to increasing ethanol yields using lignocellulosic biomass, known as second-generation biofuels, rather than using food crops. Xylose fermentation and co-fermentation were also evaluated (Wang et al., 1980). Research efforts were made on multiple product generations through the fermentation of biomass to produce ethanol and other products like acetic acid and butanol to make the process economically viable, competing with food usage (Rosenberg, 1980).

Although there are numerous sources of lignocellulosic biomass worldwide, many factors limit their use for biofuel production and at large scales. Factors such as food demand at the location, cultivation conditions, structural composition, and economic viability determine the selection of the specific biomass for the industrial expansion of the laboratory trials. Figure 21.2 illustrates the distribution of studies (in percentage) carried out globally using different biomasses for bioethanol production. The data represent a comparison of biomass during the research period of 10 years, from 2001 to 2010, and subsequent years from 2011 to 2020. The data labels on the graph bars denote the approximate number of experimental studies conducted on the corresponding biomass in the corresponding periods.

Figure 21.2 reveals that the quantity of research on each lignocellulosic source has increased from the previous decade. This growth fairly represents the interest of researchers and even the government toward second-generation biofuels. However, an inter-biomass comparison shows that wastewater studies were dominant before 2010 and were reduced significantly thereafter, that is, 2011 onward (Figure 21.2). Further, the figure shows that during the previous decade, none of the biomass was studied as extensively as wastewater biomass (56%). The development and increasing demand for innovative wastewater treatment strategies, especially bioremediation coupled with concurrent biofuel generation such as biohydrogen, have progressively supplanted the traditional emphasis on bioethanol production.

21.3 FEEDSTOCK FOR ETHANOL

Sugarcane bagasse in the western continents and rice straw and sorghum stalks in the Asian tropical region have gained significant importance, with almost 75–80% of their respective research studies conducted over the last few years (Figure 21.2). This was followed by wheat straw and corn stover, with sustained research activity (almost 40% of their studies in the previous decade, but more than 60% in the past four years) conducted globally. Developing countries like

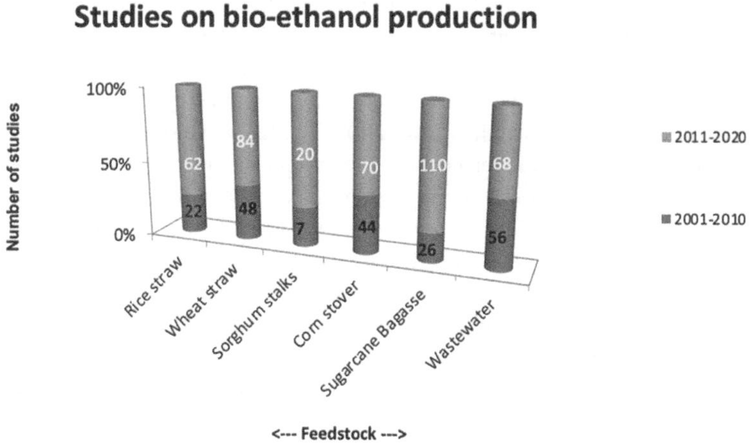

FIGURE 21.2 Investigations into bioethanol production using primary feedstocks.

China and India, whose energy and food demands are increasing exponentially, rely on wheat and rice as primary staple foods. This review provides a deeper insight into the research on renewable energy sources.

The review mainly focuses on sustainable lignocellulosic sources such as sugarcane bagasse, corn stover, and, more importantly, rice straw, wheat straw, and sorghum stalks, which are practically feasible and beneficial for tropical developing countries. The sections mentioned describe a few significant findings for each biomass. Table 21.1 summarizes the latest developments in research studies using sugarcane bagasse, corn stover, rice straw, wheat straw, and sorghum stalks.

21.3.1 Sugarcane Bagasse and Corn Stover

Sugarcane and corn cultivation are most prevalent in the western countries of North and South America; Cuba is known as the world's sugar bowl. Brazil is the world's leading producer of first-generation biofuels. The United States also depends heavily on its corn production for first-generation biofuel generation. These countries are naturally rich in corn stover and sugarcane bagasse and have been actively advancing research facilities for second-generation biofuels since the early 21st century.

During the 1980s and 1990s, preliminary research on sugarcane bagasse was conducted using various pretreatment techniques and wild-type yeast strains. Later, in 2002, Martin Carlos and his team used steam explosion treatment and fermented xylose using a xylose-utilizing recombinant S. cerevisiae TMB 3001 derived from CEN-PK and an industrial strain, *S. cerevisiae* ATCC 96581. The recombinant strain performed better than the industrial strain with an ethanol yield of 0.18 g/g and 0.13 g/g of bagasse, respectively (Martín et al., 2002). Later, in 2007, the same team adapted the recombinant strain to the treated hydrolysate, and an ethanol yield of about 0.38 g/g was achieved (Martín et al., 2007). In a separate study, higher ethanol yields of 0.49 g/g to 0.5 g/g from treated bagasse were obtained by co-culturing *Z. mobilis* with *P. stipitis* (Fu et al., 2009).

Early research on corn stover focused on its availability and feasibility as a bioethanol source. An extensive research study was done by Öhgren and team at the University of Lund, Sweden, from 2005. The team exploited various pretreatment, saccharification, and fermentation techniques. Some key findings highlight a comparison between simultaneous saccharification and fermentation (SSF) and separate hydrolysis and fermentation (SHF). The SSF method yielded approximately 13% higher ethanol than the SHF process (Öhgren et al., 2007a). In a separate SSF process, ethanol yields of about 80.2% were achieved using thermo-active cellulases for saccharification (Öhgren et al., 2007b). A new technique for treating corn stover with Ceriporiopsis subvermispora before fermentation helped remove lignin, producing an ethanol yield of 57.80% (Wan and Li, 2010). Many other studies on sugarcane bagasse report ethanol fermentation using improved pretreatment techniques (Lee et al., 2017; Fockink et al., 2018; Bakare et al., 2019; Espirito Santo et al., 2020; Rahardjo et al., 2021).

TABLE 21.1
Studies on the Various Lignocellulosic Sources

Raw Material	Yeast Strain	Method/Strategy	Ethanol Yield	Reference
Sugarcane bagasse	NA	Xylan removal	74.20%	Li et al. (2014)
Sugarcane bagasse	*K. marxianus*	Thermo-tolerant variant strain	79%	Lin et al. (2013)
Sugarcane bagasse	*Fusariumverticillioides*	Adapted to co-fermentation	0.31 g/g of bagasse	de Almeida et al. (2013)
Sugarcane bagasse	*Escherichia coli* LY 180	Hydrolysate-resistant recombinant strain	0.21 g/g of bagasse	Geddes et al. (2011)
Corn stover	*S. cerevisiae* SyBE005	Ammonia treated	70.1 g/L at 12% loading	Zhu et al. (2014)
Corn stover	*E. coli* KO11	SSF with *Gloeophyllum trabeum*	6.68 g/100g	Vincent et al. (2014)
Corn stover	*E. coli* FBR 5	Hydrothermal treatment	0.49 g/g sugars	Saha et al. (2013)
Corn stover	*S. cerevisiae* ZU-10	Recombinant strain	0.416 g/g	Zhao and Xia (2010)
Rice straw	*S. cerevisiae*	Xylose fermenting and concentrating using NF	76%	Sasaki et al. (2014)
Rice straw	*S. cerevisiae* and *S. stipites*	Optimized co-culturing conditions	99%	Suriyachai et al. (2013)
Rice straw	*Candida tropicalis* ATCC 13803	Hydrolysate-adapted yeast strain	0.48 g/g of sugars	Oberoi et al. (2010)
Wheat straw	*Pichia stipitis*	Aerated co-fermentation	0.41 g/g of sugars	Bellido et al. (2013)
Wheat straw	NA	RSM with Box Behnken Design	70.76%	Zhang et al. (2013)
Wheat straw	*Wickerhamomyces anomalus* and *Scheffersomyces stipites*	Fermentation after integrated storage and pretreatment of moist wheat straw	0.15 g/g of straw, 40% more than dry wheat straw	Passoth et al. (2013)
Wheat straw	*E. coli* FBR 5	SSF with 150 g/L of wheat straw for 120 hr	41.6±0.7 g ethanol/L	Saha et al. (2011)
Sorghum stalk	Mixed cultures	Microwave irradiation	480 g/kg of sugars	Marx et al. (2014)

(*Continued*)

TABLE 21.1 *(Continued)*
Studies on the Various Lignocellulosic Sources

Raw Material	Yeast Strain	Method/Strategy	Ethanol Yield	Reference
Sorghum stalk	*Mucorindicus*	Fungal solid-state fermentation	0.48 g/g of sugars	Molaverdi et al. (2013)
Rice straw	Sugarcane distillery waste isolate *Saccharomyces cerevisiae* NGY10	Fermentation-associated stresses and identification of a robust strain for ethanol production in SHF and SSF.	86.43%	Pandey et al. (2022)
	Saccharomyces cerevisiae DBTIOC S24	In SSF and SHF		(Mishra et al., 2016)
Rice bran (*Oryza sativa*), corn bran (*Zea mays*), sorghum bran (*Sorghum guinense*), and sawdust of *Khayasenegalensis* (red wood), *Terminalia superba* (black wood), *Gmelina arborea* (white wood),	*Saccharomyces cerevisiae* isolated from palm wine (P1)	Yeast isolates from fermented beverages	Cellulose components as 77.78%, 75.55%, 68.59%, 64.83%, 54.82%, and 55.14%, respectively. Ethanol tolerance 14%, and ethanol production ability is 10%	(Bakare et al., 2019)
Rice straw	*Saccharomyces cerevisiae*	Co-fermentation	14 g/L ethanol production	(Lee et al., 2017)

21.3.2 Rice and Wheat Straw

Rice and wheat are the staple foods of more than half of the world's population. They are the most domesticated and widely cultivated food crops in Asian countries. In these countries, sugarcane and corn are not grown in as large a proportion as in Western countries. Due to overpopulation in these countries, available agricultural land has been restricted to staple food crops, neglecting alternative crops. As a result, the researchers have shifted their focus to rice straw, wheat straw, and sorghum stalks for bioethanol production. These biomasses are as competent as sugarcane and corn stover (Rahardjo et al., 2021).

A study conducted by Kadam and his colleagues revealed that rice straw can be exploited as a potential substrate for biofuel production, providing environmental benefits by potentially reducing air pollutants such as VOCs, SOx, NOx, PM10, and silica emissions generated by open-field burning (Kadam et al., 2000). Rice straw was used for ethanol production in a rhomboidal bioreactor to improve fermentation efficiency, which was found helpful in mitigating the disruption caused by the large volumes of CO_2 generated during the process. An ethanol concentration of 57.80 g/L was obtained with an initial rice straw concentration of 200 g/L. The productivity of the fermentation process was 25.43 g/L/hr, and a lower productivity was observed at lower rice straw concentrations (Das et al., 1993).

Dilute-acid-pretreated rice straw was subjected to fermentation using three different organisms, namely *Mucor indicus*, *Rhizopus oryzae*, and *Saccharomyces cerevisiae* (Karimi et al., 2006), aerobically and anaerobically at 38°C with 50 g/L dry mass. The reported ethanol yield for *M. indicus* was 68%, and for *R. oryzae*, it was around 74%, the highest reported.

Wheat straw was used for ethanol production, where, using a wet oxidation process, hemicellulose was preferentially solubilized, resulting in low furfural levels and high ethanol content by Thermoanaerobacter anaerobius (Ahring et al., 1999). Wheat stillage was used to produce hemicellulose sugars in high concentrations by a genetically engineered *Zymomonas mobilis* strain (Davis et al., 2005). A hemicellulose hydrolysate of wheat straw was collected by treating it with lime at a concentration significantly higher than the normal concentration, with prior boiling. Fermentation was performed using *Pichia stipitis NRRL* Y-7124 (Nigam, 2001), which was adapted for several generations.

Saha and coworkers showed that the pretreatment of wheat straw with 0.75% (v/v) sulfuric acid did not produce furfural or HMF (Saha et al., 2005). Fermentation was performed using a recombinant *Escherichia coli* strain FBR5, which produced 19.1 g of ethanol from 78.3 g of wheat straw after 120 hr (Saha et al., 2005). Further experiments by the same research group showed that the recombinant *Escherichia coli* FBR5 strain fermented rice hulls, yielding ethanol at 0.49 g/g (Saha and Cotta, 2007).

21.3.3 Sweet Sorghum

Sweet sorghum is considered a secondary sugar compared to sugarcane, which is primarily used as a food crop and is well explored for biofuel production. An economic study concluded that replacing corn with sweet sorghum juice can significantly reduce bioethanol production costs (Gibbons and Westby, 1989). Sweet sorghum chopped stalks were found to be more beneficial for ethanol production than sorghum juice, and a substantial increase in the removal of leaves from the stalks was observed (Coble et al., 1984). However, microbial contamination was observed as a potential problem for this process.

Mutant yeast strains were developed to confer glucose and ethanol tolerance, enabling an efficient conversion of sugars to ethanol. A conversion efficiency of 93% was achieved in the laboratory, and it was about 89.4% in a large-scale production unit (DeMancilha et al., 1984). Pretreated and non-treated material fermentation was compared using mixed cultures of Fusarium oxysporum F3 and *Saccharomyces cerevisiae* 2541. The untreated biomass could yield only 0.10 g of ethanol per gram of sorghum carbohydrate. In contrast, an ethanol yield of 0.332 g/g was obtained from pretreated sorghum stalk carbohydrates (Christakopoulos et al., 1993). A study on grain sorghum conversion to ethanol yielded 380 liters per ton of grain sorghum (du Preez et al., 1985). Damaged grains were also used for fermentation by *A. niger* and *S. cerevisiae* to produce bioethanol (Suresh et al., 1999).

Squeezing sorghum stalks at high pressure yielded high juice and press-cake concentrations. *Saccharomyces cerevisiae fermented* the juice, producing about 4.8 g of ethanol for 100 g of stalks. In contrast, the press cake fermented with mixed cultures of *Fusarium oxysporum* and *Saccharomyces cerevisiae* yielded about 5.1 g of ethanol per 100 g of stalk (Mamma et al., 1995). Very high gravity (VHG) technology fermented sweet stem sorghum juice and grains for 96 hr under malted and unmalted conditions. Fermentation under VHG conditions produced three times the usual ethanol, although biomass was not fully utilized. Malted fermentation produced 16.8% (v/v) ethanol, whereas under unmalted conditions, only 11% (v/v) ethanol was produced from milled sorghum grain (Bvochora et al., 2000).

Sorghum bagasse containing 200 g/l of total sugar was fermented using immobilized *Saccharomyces cerevisiae.* All the sugars were consumed within 16 hr during fermentation, and the observed ethanol yield was 0.49 g/g (Yu et al., 2007). Various varieties of sorghum plants are now being developed to be biofuel-friendly. There are tall, high-biomass sorghum varieties that are rich in cellulosic content, rather than starchy content. Another variety, brown midrib (bmr) sorghum, has a lower lignin content, making it easier to hydrolyze the stalks.

21.3.4 Woody Biomass

Woody biomass mainly consists of forestry residues, which attained importance owing to their noncompeting nature with food crops and agricultural land. Aspen wood was used for mixed-culture fermentation with S. cerevisiae and P. stipitis, yielding 0.46 g/g of ethanol, equivalent to 94% of the theoretical yield (Delgenes et al., 1998). A variety of woody biomass sources – such as aspen, two Populus hybrids, sweet gum, witch grass, weeping lovegrass, and Sericea lespedeza – were combined with three agricultural residues: corn cobs, corn stover, and wheat straw, to serve as raw materials for lignocellulosic ethanol production (Rahardjo et al., 2021). After pretreatment, a simultaneous saccharification and fermentation process was performed using a mixed culture of *S. cerevisiae* and *B. clausenii* (Wyman et al., 1992). The fermentation process achieved higher final ethanol yields of 80–90% when β-glucosidase was omitted at lower cellulase loadings.

A cellulosic pyrolysate, which was acid hydrolyzed, contained 31.6 g/L glucose. After 24 hr of fermentation with *S. cerevisiae*, ethanol yields of about 0.43 g/g, 0.40 g/g, and 0.39 g/g were obtained from the hydrolysate with initial glucose concentrations of 37.8 g/L, 58.6 g/L, and 95.8 g/L, respectively. The strains were later adapted to the hydrolysate 12 times. The new strain designated as *S. cerevisiae* (R) produced ethanol yields of 0.48 g/g, 0.47 g/g, and 0.44 g/g in the respective hydrolysate media. The adapted strain yielded more ethanol than the parent strain (Yu and Zhang, 2003).

Two strains, one of which is an industrially applied softwood spent sulfite liquor isolate named Tembec T1, and the other a Saccharomyces species (Y-1528) capable of assimilating galactose, were selected to evaluate their fermentation performance and substrate utilization efficiency (Keating et al., 2004). Naturally, they were used for fermenting softwood, softwood spent, and a mixture of lignocellulosic substrates. The natural strain demonstrated superior performance compared to the industrial strain across all substrates. Additionally, strain Y-1528 utilized galactose before glucose and mannose, indicating catabolite repression in galactose metabolism (Keating et al., 2004).

Salix chips were converted to slurries by steam, treated after impregnation with sulfuric acid and sulfur dioxide, and compared with non-impregnated chips. To achieve higher ethanol concentrations, a high dry matter content was maintained during the simultaneous saccharification and fermentation (SSF) process. The highest ethanol yield of about 76% was obtained with SO_2-impregnated Salix chips, which were steamed before fermentation with baker's yeast (Sassner et al., 2006). Most recently, softwood was exploited for bioethanol production using an *S. cerevisiae* XR122N, which produced a yield of about 90% (Hawkins and Doran-Peterson, 2011) of the theoretical yield of 0.51 g/g (Xu et al., 2010). Various other lignocellulosic sources and their respective ethanol yields are summarized in Table 21.2. Table 21.3 summarizes the latest developments in research on ethanol production using key feedstocks such as sugarcane bagasse, corn stover, rice straw, wheat straw, and sorghum stalks; percentages refer to countries' global production shares and rankings during 2018–2020.

21.4 FERMENTATION OF PENTOSES AND CO-FERMENTATION

The lignocellulosic material consists of lignin, cellulose, and hemicellulose. The hemicellulosic part amounts to 25–35% of the material and is broken down to pentose sugars on hydrolysis. The pentose sugars typically obtained are xylose and arabinose, which cannot be efficiently fermented by nonrecombinant strains

TABLE 21.2
Global Production of Primary Feedstock

	Major Feedstock		
Global Production	**Ethanol (%)**	**Ranking**	
The United States	48.2	1	Maize
European Union	4.8	5	Sugarbeet/wheat/maize
Brazil	26.7	2	Sugarcane/maize
China	8.3	3	Maize/cassava
India	2.3	5	Molasses
Canada	1.6	6	Maize/wheat
Indonesia	0.1	20	Molasses
Argentina	1.0	8	Molasses/sugarcane/maize
Thailand	1.4	7	Molasses/cassava/sugarcane
Colombia	0.44	13	Sugarcane
Paraguay	0.42	14	Maize/sugarcane

Source: OECD/FAO (2021), "OECD-FAO Agricultural Outlook," OECD Agriculture Statistics (database), http://dx.doi.org/10.1787/agr-outl-data-en

TABLE 21.3
Various Other Sources for Ethanol Production

Source	Yeast	Ethanol Yield	Reference
Cheese whey powder	*Kluyveromycesmarxianus* NRRL-1195	0.54 g/g	Kargi and Ozmıhcı (2006)
Citrus peel waste	*S. cerevisiae*	24.0–39.60 g/l	Wilkins et al. (2007)
Winter rye	*S. cerevisiae*	66%	Petersson et al. (2007)
Oilseed rape	*S. cerevisiae*	70%	Petersson et al. (2007)
Faba bean	*S. cerevisiae*	52%	Petersson et al. (2007)
Maize silage	NA	82%	Oleskowicz-Popiel et al. (2008)
Agricultural waste	*K. marxianus* 6556	28%	Zhang et al. (2009)
Red sage (*Lantaracamara*)	*Pichia stipitis*	0.32 g/g	Kuhad et al. (2010)
Red sage (*Lantaracamara*)	*S. cerevisiae*	0.48 g/g	Kuhad et al. (2010)
Softwood	*S. cerevisiae* XR122N	90%	Hawkins and Doran-Peterson (2011)
Horticultural waste	*S. cerevisiae*	0.43 g/g	Geng et al. (2012)
Banana waste	*S. cerevisiae*	40%	Santa-Maria et al. (2013)

of *Saccharomyces cerevisiae*. The theoretical yield of ethanol from xylose is about 0.47 g/g (Xu et al., 2010), which makes it a significant contributor to the total ethanol production and yield. Various trials and approaches were made to ferment the pentoses using different fermentation strategies or recombinant yeast strains (Dmytruk et al., 2017; Favaro et al., 2013a, 2013b, 2014; Jansen et al., 2018). Wang and coworkers developed a method for converting D-xylose to ethanol via the intermediary D-xylulose in the early 1980s (Wang et al., 1980). D-xylose reductase and xylitol reductase were the two potential enzymes found in yeast. Although D-xylulose as a substrate could match glucose, ethanol production was slow and inefficient for biomass growth, and its ethanol conversion efficiency was 85% (Wang et al., 1980). Only oxidative fermentation of D-xylose gave ethanol. This study indicated that future scientists should target the hemicellulose part of lignocellulosic biomass by developing xylose-utilizing yeast strains. The pentose-fermenting yeast generally faces two challenges: ethanol tolerance and slow fermentation due to difficulty supplying optimal oxygen levels throughout the reactor (du Preez, 1994; Walker et al., 2020).

Studies were conducted to enhance pentose sugar utilization and overall ethanol yield by recycling the ethanol-containing stream during woody biomass fermentation. This approach also significantly reduced energy consumption during distillation, lowering it from 8 MW to 2 MW (Galbe and Zacchi, 1994). A thermophilic anaerobic bacterial strain, A3, isolated from Icelandic hot springs, was used to ferment wheat straw hydrolysate, and xylose and xylan were successfully converted to ethanol (Ahring et al., 1996). Hardwood-derived hydrolysates were subjected to mixed fermentation for increased ethanol yield. Glucose and xylose were entirely fermented using a respiratory-deficient mutant of *S. diastaticus* co-cultivated with *Pichia stipitis* in continuous culture, but the obtained yield was only 0.25 g/g. However, the monoculture of *Pichia stipitis* yielded 0.37 g ethanol/g of hemicellulosic biomass (Delgenes et al., 1996).

Fermentation was carried out with complete aeration using a respiratory-deficient *S. cerevisiae* CBS 1200 and *P. stipitis* NRRL 11545 in a membrane-associated bioreactor, producing ethanol from a mixture of glucose (35 g/L) and xylose (15 g/L). The overall efficiency achieved was 88% after consuming 100% of the glucose and 60% of the xylose present in the medium (Delgenes et al., 1998). *Candida shehatae* and *Pachysolentannophilus* were identified as potential strains, along with *Pichia stipitis*, for the bioconversion of xylose to ethanol under microaerophilic conditions. It was concluded that controlling oxygen levels was challenging to achieve higher ethanol yields (Szczodrak and Fiedurek, 1996). A feedback-controlled fed-batch method (Nilsson et al., 2001) was used to completely ferment hexose, increasing the productivity by 10 times compared to batch fermentation.

Corn stover contains high concentrations of glucose and xylose in the water-insoluble solid fibers, which can be co-fermented with Saccharomyces cerevisiae TMB3400 to achieve the highest overall yield of 64% within 96 hr (Ohgren et al., 2006). The same strain, TMB3400, co-fermented glucose and xylose in wheat straw, yielding about 75% more ethanol. Xylose consumption increased when adapted using a fed-batch fermentation strategy (Olofsson et al., 2008). A recombinant strain of *S. cerevisiae* 424A was used to study the kinetics and growth pattern during co-fermentation of glucose and xylose in a synthetic medium (Govindaswamy and Vane, 2007).

The synthetic medium containing glucose and xylose was fermented at a total sugar concentration of 60 g/L using *Pichia stipitis CBS* 6054 (Agbogbo et al., 2006). In the co-fermentation, glucose was consumed earlier than xylose. Still, fermentation in the only-glucose medium yielded less ethanol (22.7 g/l) than in the only-xylose medium (24.3 g/l). However, *P. stipitata fermented glucose completely in 96 hr, compared with* xylose (120 hr) (Agbogbo et al., 2006).

Lactobacillus species and *C. shehatae* consumed both glucose and xylose simultaneously, and it was found that this peculiar property was due to carbon catabolite repression (CCR) (Kim et al., 2010). A recent report revealed that a new isolate of the white-rot basidiomycete Trametes versicolor KT9427 co-fermented glucose, xylose, mannose, fructose, and maltose, producing ethanol yields of about 0.45-0.49 g/g. Further, this strain was also found capable of fermenting the untreated lignocellulosic biomass (Okamoto et al., 2014).

21.5 GENETICALLY ENGINEERED STRAINS

A significant breakthrough in genetically engineered strains for bioethanol production was accomplished by Ohta and his team at the University of Florida. They introduced two genes – pyruvate decarboxylase (pdc) and alcohol dehydrogenase II (adhB) – from *Zymomonas mobilis* into an *E. coli* strain, resulting in the development of more than 20 engineered variants (Ohta et al., 1991). These strains could ferment complex nutrients derived from glucose and xylose, yielding ethanol above the theoretical value (Ohta et al., 1991). Later, a novel strain producing ethanol from xylose was developed by transforming the pLOI297 plasmid from the Z. mobilis E. coli strain FBR3. The batch fermentations contained either individual sugars or a mixture of sugars and produced a yield of about 90–91%, better than that of ethanologenic *E. coli* KO11 (Dien et al., 1998). The recombinant strain had the potential to convert pyruvate to ethanol.

Spencer-Martins used defective metabolic mutants and a few genetic engineering tools to identify the key components responsible for sugar transport in yeast and their effects (Spencer-Martins, 1994). A recombinant strain of *Klebsiella oxytoca* was developed and co-cultured with *Saccharomyces pastorianus*, *Kluyveromyces marxianus*, and *Zymomonas mobilis* for simultaneous saccharification and fermentation at different temperatures, aiming to achieve high cellulase activity and enhanced ethanol production. The recombinant strain was found to be ethanol resistant and dominated the co-cultures by the end of the process (Golias et al., 2002).

An engineered *Saccharomyces* strain was developed that contains three xylose-utilizing genes: xylose reductase (XR), xylitol dehydrogenase (XD), and xylulokinase (XK) (Sedlak et al., 2003). They were fused to high-copy glycolytic promoters and placed in the yeast chromosome. They performed a microarray analysis on glucose fermentation and the co-fermentation of glucose and xylose. Another *S. cerevisiae* 259ST parent strain, 259A, was engineered for its resistance to inhibitors and xylose fermentation. The osmotic effects induced ammonium toxicity. However, the growth of the yeast strain and its ability to ferment xylose were mainly affected by the inhibitors, rather than by the overall ethanol yield or the conversion of glucose to ethanol (Helle et al., 2003).

The *Saccharomyces* was transformed with the XylA gene naturally present in the anaerobic fungus Pyromyces sp. for efficient xylose fermentation. The Saccharomyces strain was transformed with the XylA gene derived from the anaerobic fungus Pyromyces sp. (E2; ATCC 76762) to enable efficient xylose fermentation. This minimal genetic modification conferred xylose-fermenting capability, resulting in a high ethanol yield of approximately 0.42 g ethanol per g xylose (Kuyper et al., 2004). A recombinant *Z. mobilis strain* ZM4 (pZB5) was used for the fermentation, which produced 11 g of ethanol after 70 hr from 120 g/L post-fermentation of wheat stillage, which contained 18 g/L xylose, 11.5 g/L arabinose, and 6.5 g/L glucose. However, xylose consumption increased upon the addition of yeast extract and glucose to the hydrolysate, and fermentation was completed within 18 hr. This reflects the significance of co-fermentation, in which glucose concentration was higher than xylose concentration (Davis et al., 2005).

The saccharification by-product, cellobiose, can also inhibit yeast growth. This was overcome by transforming a fungal β-glucosidase gene into *Saccharomyces cerevisiae*. The strain sustained growth in the cellobiose medium. It fermented cellobiose to ethanol, yielding about 0.41 g/g of cellobiose, compared with 0.49 g/g of glucose (van Rooyen et al., 2005). Furthermore, three major *Saccharomyces* recombinant strains were developed and evaluated in comparison to the reference strain CEN. PK113–7D, which cannot ferment xylose. Ethanol production was predominant in the glucose consumption phase, and xylitol and glycerol were predominant in the xylose consumption phase (Zaldivar et al., 2005). Table 21.4 summarizes the various genes responsible for the fermentation of secondary sugars such as xylose and cellobiose.

Recombinants took on a new direction when integrated into a process called consolidated bioprocessing (CBP). It is a technique in which biomass is converted to sugar and, ultimately, to ethanol by one or more organisms in a single reaction vessel, thereby improving the economics of the process. Two genes, cbh1 and cbh2, were transformed from *T. reesei*; cbhB, taken from *Aspergillus niger* and *Phanerochaete chrysosporium*, was used to convert the fourth gene, cbh1–4. The specific activities of all the enzymes were similar to those of the parent strains, even though lower expression levels were observed (Den Haan et al., 2007).

Eight genes were identified by chemogenomics, revealing that their expression confers resistance to high concentrations of glucose, acetic acid, and ethanol (Table 21.5). Another 11 genes were identified as being sensitive to various stresses encountered during interactions during fermentation of lignocellulosic biomass (Pereira et al., 2011). The recombinant *Saccharomyces* strain was able to ferment a mixture of xylose and cellobiose, achieved by transferring genes from a robust industrial *S. cerevisiae* strain (Ha et al., 2013).

TABLE 21.4
Specific Genes Targeted for Following Different Enzymes in Fermentation

Gene of Interest	Parent Strain	Target Strain	Function/Enzyme	Reference
pLOI297 (plasmid)	*Z. mobilis*	*E. coli* FBR3	Xylose utilization	Dien et al. (1998)
bglA	*Aspergillus kawachii*	*S. cerevisiae*	β-Glucosidase	van Rooyen et al. (2005)
bglB	*Candida wickerhamii*	*S. cerevisiae*	β-Glucosidase	van Rooyen et al. (2005)
BGL1	*Saccharomycopsis fibuligera*	*S. cerevisiae*	β-Glucosidase	van Rooyen et al. (2005)
Bgl	*Tichodermaresei*	*S. cerevisiae*	β-Glucosidase	van Rooyen et al. (2005)
XYL1	*Pichia stipitis*	*S. cerevisia* TMB 3001	Xylose reductase	Zaldivar et al. (2005)
XYL2	*Pichia stipitis*	*S. cerevisiae* TMB 3001	Xylitol dehydrogenase	Zaldivar et al. (2005)
XKS1	NA	*S. cerevisiae* TMB 3001	Xylulose kinase	Zaldivar et al. (2005)
XR (XYL1)	*S. cerevisiae* MT8–1/Xyl	*Escherichia coli*	Xylose reductase	Katahira et al. (2006)
XDH (XYL2)	*S. cerevisiae* MT8–1/Xyl	*E. coli*	Xylitol dehydrogenase	Katahira et al. (2006)
XK (XKS1)	*S. cerevisiae* MT8–1/Xyl	*E. coli*	Xylulose kinase	Katahira et al. (2006)
BGL1	*S. cerevisiae* MT8–1/BGL	*E. coli*	β-Glucosidase	Katahira et al. (2006)

TABLE 21.5
Genes Responsible for Resistance to the Organism toward Various Stresses

Stress	Genes Responsible for Tolerance
Ethanol, acetic acid, and glucose	Anp1, Bud31, Hpr1, Pho85, Ppa1, Rpl1B, Vrp1 and Ygl024w
Ethanol, acetic acid, and vanillin	End3, Erg2, Erg24 Gcs1, Rav1 and Tps1
Ethanol, acetic acid, and furfural	Nat3, Ppa1, Rpb4, Prs3 and Vma8

21.6 FERMENTATION INHIBITOR STUDIES

Pretreating lignocellulosic biomass with acids or alkalis offers a significant advantage by effectively removing lignin and facilitating the breakdown of cellulose and hemicellulose into glucose and xylose, respectively. However, these processes have generated a few chemicals that act as inhibitors of yeast fermentation.

They are characterized into three types based on their origin: weak acids, furan derivatives, and phenolic compounds (Palmqvist and Hahn-Hägerdal, 2000a). Three water-soluble inhibitors, furfural, 5-hydroxymethylfurfural (HMF), and acetic acid, have been found to limit the efficient utilization of hydrolysates for ethanol production (Palmqvist et al., 1996).

Many studies have been conducted to either remove or induce resistance to these inhibitors in yeasts. Water recirculation enabled economic efficiency in the bioethanol process and reduced inhibitor effects. The volatile fractions induced no adverse effects on the fermentation. However, the nonvolatile fractions reduced the ethanol yields by inhibiting the fermentation. Softwood was used for its fermentation, and a six-effect evaporation unit was simulated. The experimental data showed that the condensate fractions of intermediate evaporation were most suited for disposal (Larsson et al., 1997).

Comparative studies were conducted on the inhibitory effects of furfural and hydroxymethylfurfural (HMF) during batch and fed-batch fermentations using dilute-acid-pretreated spruce and birch wood, both of which contained high concentrations of furfural and HMF. About 90% furfural and 40–70% HMF conversion were reported in a fed-batch process, leading to complete and efficient yeast fermentation of sugars (Taherzadeh et al., 1999). A research study revealed that fermentation inhibition can be avoided by treating the lignocellulosic hydrolysate with the lignolytic enzyme laccase. It was also observed that pre-fermentation with *T. reesei* could remove nonvolatile inhibitors from the reaction (Palmqvist and Hahn-Hägerdal, 2000b). Other methods, such as extraction with ether or ethyl acetate or treatment with alkali/sulfite, could also reduce the inhibitory effects of furfural and HMF.

Detoxification of dilute-acid-treated hydrolysates was achieved by overliming to pH 10, 11, or 12 (Millati et al., 2002). However, these have shown a significant negative effect on sugar degradation, reducing it by 70% from its initial concentration. Furfural and HMF concentrations were decreased prominently, but the acetic acid concentration remained the same. Methods such as flash evaporation, anion exchange, and chloroform and ethyl acetate extraction revealed at least 35 possible inhibitors in the fermentation of lignocellulosic hydrolysates from hybrid poplar treated with dilute nitric acid (Luo et al., 2002).

Kluyveromyces marxianus was used to analyze the effect of the combination of three different inhibitors, such as furfural, acetic acid, and catechol, using a central composite design (Oliva et al., 2006). They were tested for growth rate, biomass yield, and ethanol yield. However, the furfural concentration affected the specific growth rate, and other factors were affected by the synergistic action of the inhibitors (Oliva et al., 2006). Passing the acid-treated hydrolysates through anion-exchange resin reduced the furan and phenolic concentrations more than other detoxifying agents such as charcoal, laccase, overliming, and neutralized hydrolysate (Chandel et al., 2007).

Adapting xylose-utilizing *Saccharomyces cerevisiae* to a sugarcane bagasse hydrolysate with a high inhibitor content improved ethanol production (Martín et al., 2007). Zeolites, known for their specific adsorption properties, have been successfully used to detoxify hydrolysates (Ranjan et al., 2009). A recent report on metabolic profiling showed that inhibitor-resistant strains were compared with regular strains. It was observed that most amino acids, inositol, and phenethylamine increased in the presence of inhibitors. A higher content of pyrimidines was observed in inhibitor-resistant strains, suggesting that they counteract stress (Ding et al., 2011).

21.7 FACTORS IMPACTING FERMENTATION

The gaseous levels in the fermentation chamber have been a primary factor in altering the final products of fermentation, as mentioned in the previous sections. In 1980, Mudgett conducted an elaborate study to optimize oxygen and carbon dioxide levels at laboratory and industrial scales using mathematical equations and Cooney and Wang correlations (Mudgett, 1980). A response surface methodology experiment was designed to optimize the medium contents for ethanol production using *Clostridium thermocellum* SS19. Filter paper, corn steep liquor, cysteine hydrochloride, magnesium chloride, and ferrous sulfate were identified as the five key factors required for the organism's growth. Among these, magnesium chloride was the least significant factor contributing to the development and fermentation capability of *C. thermocellum*. The optimal concentration combination of all the compounds, with an ethanol yield of 0.41 g/g, was obtained (Balusu et al., 2005).

Aeration is another major factor in yeast's fermentation of sugars into ethanol. Sugar-to-ethanol conversion is an anaerobic process; however, aeration in some fermentation experiments provides additional features. *Fusarium oxysporum* is an xylose-consuming fungus that provides ethanol on aeration instead of xylitol under anaerobic conditions, which is its primary product (Panagiotou et al., 2005). In a separate experiment, micro-aeration has been found to enhance ethanol yields by 100% using an ethanologenic E. coli KO11 (Okuda et al., 2007).

The addition of acetoin, an artificial electron acceptor, to the fermentation culture significantly enhanced xylose consumption, increasing it by approximately 95%. An increase in ethanol production from 0.96 mol/mol to 1.52 mol/mol was observed in a co-culture of glucose and xylose under aerated conditions (Panagiotou et al., 2005). The effects of post-fermentation residual sugars on ethanol production were observed using pervaporation flux through a poly-dimethyl siloxane and selectivity for ethanol. These factors were measured at different temperatures and permeation pressures. At a permeate pressure of 40 mm Hg and a temperature of 60°C, the total flux decreased by 8%, while ethanol selectivity dropped by 15.3% (Aroujalian et al., 2006).

Floc size is an essential factor in yeast cell interactions with the fermentation medium. It was observed that zinc supplementation reduced average floc size, thereby improving ethanol yields (Zhao et al., 2009). One of the significant factors contributing to ethanol fermentation is the initial sugar/raw material present in the medium. Fermentation was performed using various sugar concentrations under different temperature and pH conditions. The optimal parameters were found to be a pH range of 4–5 and a temperature of 30°C. Although fermentation continued at 45°C, it stopped completely at 50°C. The maximum ethanol yield was achieved at a substrate concentration of 40 g/L (Lin et al., 2012).

An industrial strain was used to analyze its performance in ethanol production at a temperature range of 30°C to 47°C. The best results for the industrial strains were obtained at 37°C. At 36 °C, a decoupling between cell growth and glycerol production was observed in a laboratory strain (Amillastre et al., 2012). The presence of salts in water or in hydrolysates might affect fermentation, and Casey and his group demonstrated this using six anion-cation pairs, which showed a high degree of variance in the co-fermentation of glucose and xylose by *S. cerevisiae* (Casey et al., 2013).

A few of the most recent techniques and strategies are now summarized. A novel strategy to overcome product inhibition was developed, where glucose is initially consumed for ethanol production, followed by the introduction of ethanol-tolerant yeast strains during the later stage to ferment xylose and cellobiose in the presence of ethanol. This sequential incubation of *C. shehatae* and *S. cerevisiae* or *B. bruxellensis* has been successful at the laboratory scale, with fermentation (99%) of the total available sugar (Guan et al., 2013). Raman spectroscopy, with real-time monitoring at 785 nm, was used to monitor the fermentation of lignocellulosic biomass (Ewanick et al., 2013). This technique enabled optimization and control of the process on a large scale. The phenotypic microarray analysis was developed to identify yeast species tolerant to fermentation-borne stresses (osmotic, temperature, ethanol, and inhibitors) using growth and metabolic activity as inputs (Wimalasena et al., 2014).

21.8 ETHANOL IN TRADE

Currently, the most popular fuel worldwide is ethanol. In 1925, the automobile industry legend Henry Ford told a *New York Times* reporter that the term "fuel of future" for ethyl alcohol was later widely adopted by the automobile industry (source: Petroleum Service Company *on June 22, 2016, https://petroleumservicecompany.com/blog/henry-fords-fuel-of-the-future-was-ethanol but-we-still-use-gasoline/*). The global ethanol trade is projected to retain a low share of total global production, decreasing from 9% over the base period (2018–2020) to 8% by 2030 (Figure 21.3) (*source: OECD-FAO AGRICULTURAL OUTLOOK 2021–2030 © OECD/FAO 2021*). Brazilian ethanol exports are projected to increase by 0.1%. However, US ethanol exports should decrease over the outlook period due to weak production, and maize-based ethanol is expected to remain a net export. Brazil and the United States are expected to remain the primary exporters of ethanol derived from maize and sugarcane. It is anticipated that both nations' combined export shares will stay around 75%, with the United States acquiring some export shares from Brazil.

According to *OECD/FAO 2021*, while declining demand for transport fuels could lead to reduced ethanol demand in the United States and the European

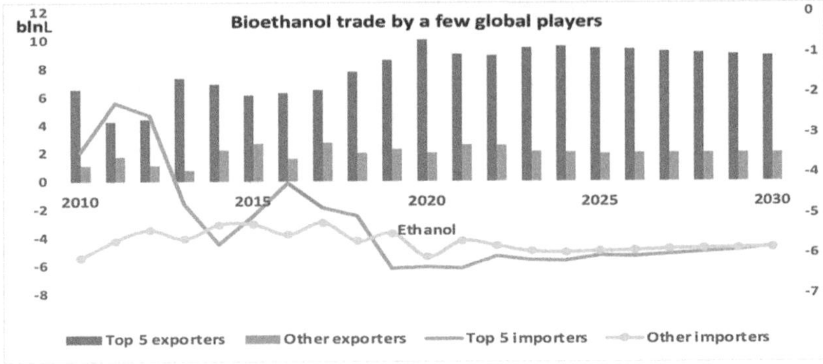

FIGURE 21.3 Classification of biofuels by domestic policies can result in simultaneous exports and imports of biofuels in several countries.

Source: OECD-FAO Agricultural Outlook 2021–2030. © OECD/FAO 2021

Union, strong growth in ethanol trade is expected in Brazil, China, and Thailand. Similar to China, many countries may see a rise in ethanol demand with the introduction of new ethanol mandates (blending regulations). Projections indicate that over the next ten years, developing countries will account for approximately 84% of the total increase in ethanol demand. Despite these advancements, the continuation of sugar export subsidies is likely to hinder the shift toward ethanol production based on sugarcane juice. This will constrain the expansion of blending, and by 2030, the average is expected to be only around E8. Ethanol production is expected to reach nearly seven billion liters in 2030, with the top five lead exporters and importers shown in Figure 21.3.

21.9 INDIA

For instance, India aims to achieve a 10% ethanol blend with petrol by 2022 to reduce reliance on imports. To meet this target, approximately 313 crore liters of ethanol are needed. In line with this goal, the government has begun encouraging sugar mills to shift their focus from sugar production toward increasing ethanol output. To promote biofuels in India, the Union Ministry of New and Renewable Energy (UMoNRE) has formulated a National Policy on Biofuels (NPB) in 2018; it includes a wide range of feedstock from lignocellulosic biomass and garbage waste, such as rural-urban, in line with the "waste-to-wealth" concept for 2G ethanol production. In sway to the consistent under-supply of domestic ethanol from traditional sources, oil PSUs are establishing 12 (second generation) 2G ethanol bio-refineries across 11 states of the country, namely, Punjab, Haryana, Uttar Pradesh, Gujarat, Madhya Pradesh, Maharashtra, Karnataka, Odisha, Bihar, Assam, and Andhra Pradesh, with an approximate expenditure of around Rs. 800–1,000 crore for raising each bio-refinery and an amount of Rs. 10,000 crores for all 12 bio-refineries by the PSUs (*source:* Lahiry Samar 2018. India's ethanol equation, *Energy*, July 2018. Down to Earth, www.downtoearth.org.in/blog/energy/india-s-ethanol-equation-61170). However, by producing 2G ethanol, India can also address a significant environmental issue: crop residue burning, which causes horrific pollution in cities like New Delhi and many others.

21.10 ECONOMIC/COST ANALYSIS

In 1991, a cost analysis model for ethanol production from lignocellulosic biomass was evaluated, highlighting that pretreatment expenses, the capability to ferment pentose sugars, market identification, and marketing strategies to generate by-product credits are key factors influencing the economic viability of producing fermentable sugars from biomass. It was also found that fermentable sugars from enzymatic hydrolysis of cellulose must cost no more than 8.8–11 cents/kg (Ladisch and Svarczkopf, 1991). Ethanol was pursued as a blending material for fossil-derived petroleum, and an economic analysis was performed comparing it with methanol, gasoline, ETBE, MTBE, and isooctane (Wyman, 1994).

A mathematical modelling study was conducted to assess the economic feasibility of an industrial-scale ethanol-producing plant. Producing value-added compounds alongside ethanol could make the process more profitable than a gasoline plant. It was concluded that the optimal plant size is always a trade-off between increasing transportation costs for feedstocks and decreasing plant costs as plant size increases (Kaylen et al., 2000). Furthermore, an economic analysis of feedstock optimization for rice straw revealed that price depends on parameters such as straw moisture, basic and bulk densities, storage conditions, and the optimal number of transport units (Kadam et al., 2000).

Lignocellulosic ethanol production was evaluated for economic and financial viability in the short-, middle-, and long-terms. The study suggests that improvements in pretreatment processes using biotechnology and process combination would increase overall process efficiency to 68% from 35% (Hamelinck et al., 2005). In this study, investments and costs for setting up full-scale plants were also discussed. One of the most recent studies on the economic analysis of using fungi for fermentation revealed that recombinant *S. cerevisiae* provides the best results, as defined by the lowest "Minimum Ethanol Selling Price" (MESP) for the short term. However, when evaluated for the midterm and long term, the analysis showed increased profitability, with possible revenues from by-products used as value-added products and reduced ethanol costs to around $1.98/gallon (Meyer et al., 2013).

21.11 CONCLUSION

The concluding remarks drawn by the authors of this review suggest the following recommendations for researchers in sustainable large-scale production of bioethanol:

1. Selection of effective strains capable of fermenting hexoses and pentoses must be done strategically.

2. Development of a specific culture package, which could consist of single or multiple strains capable of fermenting the hexoses and pentoses present in the hydrolysates.
3. Develop recombinants that can make the fermentation process more selective, that is, produce maximum ethanol with minimal growth of the organism.
4. Development of eco-friendly and cost-effective bioreactors designed for easy maintenance and user-friendliness.

This review focused on process development and encourages researchers, the farmer community, and the government to promote the importance of lignocellulosic biomass and biofuels derived from it.

REFERENCES

Agbogbo, F.K., Coward-Kelly, G., Torry-Smith, M., Wenger, K.S., 2006. Fermentation of glucose/xylose mixtures using Pichia stipitis. *Process Biochem.* 41, 2333–6. doi:10.1016/j.procbio.2006.05.004

Ahring, B.K., Jensen, K., Nielsen, P., Bjerre, A.B., Schmidt, A.S., 1996. Pretreatment of wheat straw and conversion of xylose and xylan to ethanol by thermophilic anaerobic bacteria. *Bioresour. Technol.* 58, 107–13. doi:10.1016/S0960-8524(96)00090-9

Ahring, B.K., Licht, D., Schmidt, A.S., Sommer, P., Thomsen, A.B., 1999. Production of ethanol from wet-oxidised wheat straw by Thermoanaerobacter mathranii. *Bioresour. Technol.* 68, 3–9. doi:10.1016/S0960-8524(98)00077-7

Amillastre, E., Aceves-Lara, C.-A., Uribelarrea, J.-L., Alfenore, S., Guillouet, S.E., 2012. Dynamic model of temperature impact on cell viability and major product formation during fed-batch and continuous ethanolic fermentation in Saccharomyces cerevisiae. *Bioresour. Technol.* 117, 242–50. doi:10.1016/j.biortech.2012.04.013

Aroujalian, A., Belkacemi, K., Davids, S.J., Turcotte, G., Pouliot, Y., 2006. Effect of residual sugars in fermentation broth on pervaporation flux and selectivity for ethanol. *Desalination* 193, 103–8. doi:10.1016/j.desal.2005.06.058

Bakare, V., Abdulsalami, M.S., Onusiriuka, B.C., Appah, J., Benjamin, B., Ndibe, T.O., 2019. Ethanol production from lignocellulosic materials by fermentation process using yeast. *J Appl Sci Environ Manage.* 23(5), 875–88.

Balusu, R., Paduru, R.R., Kuravi, S.K., Seenayya, G., Reddy, G., 2005. Optimization of critical medium components using response surface methodology for ethanol production from cellulosic biomass by Clostridium thermocellum SS19. *Process Biochem.* 40, 3025–30. doi:10.1016/j.procbio.2005.02.003

Bellido, C., González-Benito, G., Coca, M., Lucas, S., García-Cubero, M.T., 2013. Influence of aeration on bioethanol production from ozonized wheat straw hydrolysates using Pichia stipitis. Bioresour. Technol. 133, 51–8. doi:10.1016/j.biortech.2013.01.104

Bvochora, J., Read, J., Zvauya, R., 2000. Application of very high gravity technology to the cofermentation of sweet stem sorghum juice and sorghum grain. *Ind. Crops Prod.* 11, 11–7. doi:10.1016/S0926-6690(99)00029-1

Casey, E., Mosier, N.S., Adamec, J., Stockdale, Z., Ho, N., Sedlak, M., 2013. Effect of salts on the co-fermentation of glucose and xylose by a genetically engineered strain of Saccharomyces cerevisiae. *Biotechnol. Biofuels* 6, 83. doi:10.1186/1754-6834-6-83

Chandel, A.K., Kapoor, R.K., Singh, A., Kuhad, R.C., 2007. Detoxification of sugarcane bagasse hydrolysate improves ethanol production by Candida shehatae NCIM 3501. *Bioresour. Technol.* 98, 1947–50. doi:10.1016/j.biortech.2006.07.047

Christakopoulos, P., Li, L.-W., Kekos, D., Macris, B.J., 1993. Direct conversion of sorghum carbohydrates to ethanol by a mixed microbial culture. *Bioresour. Technol.* 45, 89–92. doi:10.1016/0960-8524(93)90095-S

Coble, C.G., Egg, R.P., Shmulevich, I., 1984. Processing techniques for ethanol production from sweet sorghum. *Biomass* 6, 111–7. doi:10.1016/0144-4565(84)90014-3

Das, D., Gaidhani, N.R., Murari, K., Gupta, P., Sen, 1993. Ethanol production by whole cell immobilization using lignocellulosic materials as solid matrix. *J. Ferment. Bioeng.* 75, 132–7. doi:10.1016/0922-338X(93)90224-V

Davis, L., Jeon, Y.-J., Svenson, C., Rogers, P., Pearce, J., Peiris, P., 2005. Evaluation of wheat stillage for ethanol production by recombinant Zymomonas mobilis. *Biomass and Bioenergy* 29, 49–59. doi:10.1016/j.biombioe.2005.02.006

De Almeida, M.N., Guimarães, V.M., Falkoski, D.L., Visser, E.M., Siqueira, G.A., Milagres, A.M.F., de Rezende, S.T., 2013. Direct ethanol production from glucose, xylose, and sugarcane bagasse by the corn endophytic fungi Fusarium verticillioides and Acremonium zeae. *J. Biotechnol.* 168, 71–7. doi:10.1016/j.jbiotec.2013.07.032

Delgenes, J., Escare, M., Laplace, J., Moletta, R., Navarro, J., 1998. Biological production of industrial chemicals, i.e., xylitol and ethanol, from lignocelluloses by controlled mixed culture systems. *Ind. Crops Prod.* 7, 101–11. doi:10.1016/S0926-6690(97)00038-1

Delgenes, J.P., Laplace, J.M., Moletta, R., Navarro, J.M., 1996. Comparative study of separated fermentations and cofermentation processes to produce ethanol from hardwood-derived hydrolysates. *Biomass and Bioenergy* 11, 353–60. doi:10.1016/0961-9534(96)00019-0

DeMancilha, I.M., Pearson, A.M., Momose, H., Pestka, J.J., 1984. Increasing alcohol yield by selected yeast fermentation of sweet sorghum. II. Isolation and evaluation of mutants and wild types for ethanol production. *Food Chem.* 14, 313–8. doi:10.1016/0308-8146(84)90086-4

Den Haan, R., McBride, J.E., Grange, D.C. La, Lynd, L.R., Van Zyl, W.H., 2007. Functional expression of cellobiohydrolases in Saccharomyces cerevisiae towards one-step conversion of cellulose to ethanol. *Enzyme Microb. Technol.* 40, 1291–9. doi:10.1016/j.enzmictec.2006.09.022

Dien, B.S., Hespell, R.B., Wyckoff, H.A., Bothast, R.J., 1998. Fermentation of hexose and pentose sugars using a novel ethanologenic Escherichia coli strain. *Enzyme Microb. Technol.* 23, 366–71. doi:10.1016/S0141-0229(98)00064-7

Ding, M.-Z., Wang, X., Yang, Y., Yuan, Y.-J., 2011. Comparative metabolic profiling of parental and inhibitor-tolerant yeasts during lignocellulosic ethanol fermentation. *Metabolomics* 8, 232–43. doi:10.1007/s11306-011-0303-6

Dmytruk, K.V., Kurylenko, O.O., Ruchala, J., Abbas, C.A., Sibirny, A.A., 2017. Genetic improvement of conventional and nonconventional yeasts for the production of first and second generation ethanol, in *Biotechnology of yeasts and filamentous fungi*, ed. Sibirny (Cham: Springer). doi:10.1007/978-3-319-588529-2-1.

Du Preez, J.C., 1994. Process parameters and environmental factors affecting d-xylose fermentation by yeasts. *Enzyme Microb. Technol.* 16, 944–56. doi:10.1016/0141-0229(94)90003-5

Du Preez, J.C., de Jong, F., Botes, P.J., Lategan, P.M., 1985. Fermentation alcohol from grain sorghum starch. *Biomass* 8, 101–17. doi:10.1016/0144-4565(85)90021-6

EspiritoSanto, M.C., Fockink, D.H., Pellegrini, V.O.A., Guimaraes, F.E.G., deAzevedo, E.R., Ramos, L.P., et al., 2020. Physical techniques shed light on the differences in sugarcane bagasse structure subjected to steam explosion pretreatments at equivalent combined severity factors. *Ind. Crops Prod.* 158, 113003. doi:10.1016/j.indcrop.2020.113003 [CrossRef] [Google Scholar]

Ewanick, S.M., Thompson, W.J., Marquardt, B.J., Bura, R., 2013. Real-time understanding of lignocellulosic bioethanol fermentation by Raman spectroscopy. *Biotechnol. Biofuels* 6, 28. doi:10.1186/1754-6834-6-28

Favaro, L., Basaglia, M., Casella, S., 2014. Innately robust yeast strains isolated from grape marc have great potential for lignocellulosic ethanol production. *Ann. Microbiol.* 64, 1807–18.

Favaro, L., Basaglia, M., Trento, A., Van Rensburg, E., García-Aparicio, M., Van Zyl, W.H., et al., 2013a. Exploring grape marc as a trove for new thermotolerant and inhibitor-tolerant *Saccharomyces cerevisiae* strains for second-generation bioethanol production. *Biotechnol. Biofuels* 6, 1–14. doi:10.1186/1754-6834-6-168 [PMC free article] [PubMed] [CrossRef] [Google Scholar]

Favaro, L., Basaglia, M., van Zyl, W.H., Casella, S., 2013b. Using an efficient fermenting yeast enhances ethanol production from unfiltered wheat bran hydrolysates. *Appl. Energy* 102, 170–8. doi:10.1016/j.apenergy.2012.05.059 [CrossRef] [Google Scholar]

Fockink, D.H., Sánchez, J.H., Ramos, L.P., 2018. Comprehensive analysis of sugarcane bagasse steam explosion using autocatalysis and dilute acid hydrolysis (H3PO4 and H2SO4) at equivalent combined severity factors. *Ind. Crops Prod.* 123, 563–72. doi:10.1016/j.indcrop.2018.07.017 [CrossRef] [Google Scholar]

Fu, N., Peiris, P., Markham, J., Bavor, J., 2009. A novel co-culture process with Zymomonas mobilis and Pichia stipitis for efficient ethanol production on glucose/xylose mixtures. *Enzyme Microb. Technol.* 45, 210–7. doi:10.1016/j.enzmictec.2009.04.006

Galbe, M., Zacchi, G., 1994. Simulation of ethanol production processes based on the enzymatic hydrolysis of woody biomass. *Comput. Chem. Eng.* 18, S687–91. doi:10.1016/0098-1354(94)80112-6

Geddes, C.C., Mullinnix, M.T., Nieves, I.U., Peterson, J.J., Hoffman, R.W., York, S.W., Yomano, L.P., Miller, E.N., Shanmugam, K.T., Ingram, L.O., 2011. Simplified process for ethanol production from sugarcane bagasse using hydrolysate-resistant Escherichia coli strain MM160. *Bioresour. Technol.* 102, 2702–11. doi:10.1016/j.biortech.2010.10.143

Geng, A., Xin, F., Ip, J., 2012. Ethanol production from horticultural waste treated by a modified organosolv method. *Bioresour. Technol.* 104, 715–21. doi:10.1016/j.biortech.2011.10.076

Gibbons, W.R., Westby, C.A., 1989. Cofermentation of sweet sorghum juice and grain for the production of fuel ethanol and distillers' wet grain. *Biomass* 18, 43–57. doi:10.1016/0144-4565(89)90080-2

Golias, H., Dumsday, G.J., Stanley, G.A., Pamment, N.B., 2002. Evaluation of a recombinant Klebsiella oxytoca strain for ethanol production from cellulose by simultaneous saccharification and fermentation: comparison with native cellobiose-utilising yeast strains and performance in co-culture with thermotolerant yeas. *J. Biotechnol.* 96, 155–68.

Govindaswamy, S., Vane, L.M., 2007. Kinetics of growth and ethanol production on different carbon substrates using genetically engineered xylose-fermenting yeast. *Bioresour. Technol.* 98, 677–85. doi:10.1016/j.biortech.2006.02.012

Guan, D., Li, Y., Shiroma, R., Ike, M., Tokuyasu, K., 2013. Sequential incubation of Candida shehatae and ethanol-tolerant yeast cells for efficient ethanol production from a mixture of glucose, xylose, and cellobiose. *Bioresour. Technol.* 132, 419–22. doi:10.1016/j.biortech.2012.12.040

Ha, S.-J., Kim, S.R., Kim, H., Du, J., Cate, J.H.D., Jin, Y.-S., 2013. Continuous co-fermentation of cellobiose and xylose by engineered Saccharomyces cerevisiae. *Bioresour. Technol.* 149, 525–31. doi:10.1016/j.biortech.2013.09.082

Hamelinck, C.N., Hooijdonk, G. Van, Faaij, A.P., 2005. Ethanol from lignocellulosic biomass: techno-economic performance in short-, middle- and long-term. *Biomass and Bioenergy* 28, 384–410. doi:10.1016/j.biombioe.2004.09.002

Hawkins, G.M., Doran-Peterson, J., 2011. A strain of Saccharomyces cerevisiae evolved for fermentation of lignocellulosic biomass displays improved growth and fermentative ability in high solids concentrations and in the presence of inhibitory compounds. *Biotechnol. Biofuels* 4, 49. doi:10.1186/1754-6834-4-49

Helle, S., Cameron, D., Lam, J., White, B., Duff, S., 2003. Effect of inhibitory compounds found in biomass hydrolysates on growth and xylose fermentation by a genetically engineered strain of S. cerevisiae. *Enzyme Microb. Technol.* 33, 786–92. doi:10.1016/S0141-0229(03)00214-X

Jansen, T., Hoff, J.W., Jolly, N., Van Zyl, W.H., 2018. Mating of natural Saccharomyces cervisiae strains for improved glucose fermentation and lignocellulosic inhibitor tolerance. *Folia Microbiol.* 63, 155–68. doi:10.1007/s12223-017-0546-3.

Kadam, K.L., Forrest, L.H., Jacobson, W.A., 2000. Rice straw as a lignocellulosic resource: collection, processing, transportation, and environmental aspects. *Biomass and Bioenergy* 18, 369–89. doi:10.1016/S0961-9534(00)00005-2.

Kargi, F., Ozmıhcı, S., 2006. Utilization of cheese whey powder (CWP) for ethanol fermentations: effects of operating parameters. *Enzyme Microb. Technol.* 38, 711–8. doi:10.1016/j.enzmictec.2005.11.006

Karimi, K., Emtiazi, G., Taherzadeh, M.J., 2006. Ethanol production from dilute-acid pretreated rice straw by simultaneous saccharification and fermentation with Mucor indicus, Rhizopus oryzae, and Saccharomyces cerevisiae. *Enzyme Microb. Technol.* 40, 138–44. doi:10.1016/j.enzmictec.2005.10.046

Katahira, S., Mizuike, A., Fukuda, H., Kondo, A., 2006. Ethanol fermentation from lignocellulosic hydrolysate by a recombinant xylose- and cellooligosaccharide-assimilating yeast strain. *Appl. Microbiol. Biotechnol.* 72, 1136–43. doi:10.1007/s00253-006-0402-x

Kaylen, M., Van Dyne, D.L., Choi, Y.-S., Blase, M., 2000. Economic feasibility of producing ethanol from lignocellulosic feedstocks. *Bioresour. Technol.* 72, 19–32. doi:10.1016/S0960-8524(99)00091-7

Keating, J.D., Robinson, J., Cotta, M.A., Saddler, J.N., Mansfield, S.D., 2004. An ethanologenic yeast exhibiting unusual metabolism in the fermentation of lignocellulosic hexose sugars. *J. Ind. Microbiol. Biotechnol.* 31, 235–44. doi:10.1007/s10295-004-0145-6

Kim, J.-H., Block, D.E., Mills, D.A., 2010. Simultaneous consumption of pentose and hexose sugars: an optimal microbial phenotype for efficient fermentation of lignocellulosic biomass. *Appl. Microbiol. Biotechnol.* 88, 1077–85. doi:10.1007/s00253-010-2839-1

Kuhad, R.C., Gupta, R., Khasa, Y.P., Singh, A., 2010. Bioethanol production from Lantana camara (red sage): pretreatment, saccharification, and fermentation. *Bioresour. Technol.* 101, 8348–54. doi:10.1016/j.biortech.2010.06.043

Kuyper, M., Winkler, A.A., van Dijken, J.P., Pronk, J.T., 2004. Minimal metabolic engineering of Saccharomyces cerevisiae for efficient anaerobic xylose fermentation: a proof of principle. *FEMS Yeast Res.* 4, 655–64. doi:10.1016/j.femsyr.2004.01.003

Ladisch, M.R., Flickinger, M.C., Tsao, G.T., 1979. Fuels and chemicals from biomass. *Energy* 4, 263–75. doi:10.1016/0360-5442(79)90126-9

Ladisch, M.R., Svarczkopf, J.A., 1991. Ethanol production and the cost of fermentable sugars from biomass. *Bioresour. Technol.* 36, 83–95. doi:10.1016/0960-8524(91)90102-P

Larsson, M., Galbe, M., Zacchi, G., 1997. Recirculation of process water in the production of ethanol from softwood. *Bioresour. Technol.* 60, 143–51. doi:10.1016/S0960-8524(97)00011-4

Lewis, C.W., 1977. Fuels from biomass – energy outlay versus energy returns: a critical appraisal. *Energy* 2, 241–8. doi:10.1016/0360-5442(77)90028-7

Lewis, C.W., 1979. Energy from biomass and wastes. *Energy Policy* 7, 356–7. doi:10.1016/0301-4215(79)90041-7

Li, J., Zhou, P., Liu, H., Wu, K., Xiao, W., Gong, Y., Lin, J., Liu, Z., 2014. Ethanol production from xylan-removed sugarcane bagasse using low loading of commercial cellulase. *Bioresour. Technol.* 163, 390–4. doi:10.1016/j.biortech.2014.04.106

Lin, Y.-S., Lee, W.-C., Duan, K.-J., Lin, Y.-H., 2013. Ethanol production by simultaneous saccharification and fermentation in rotary drum reactor using thermotolerant Kluyveromyces marxianus. *Appl. Energy* 105, 389–94. doi:10.1016/j.apenergy.2012.12.020

Lin, Y.-S., Zhang, W., Li, C., Sakakibara, K., Tanaka, S., Kong, H., 2012. Factors affecting ethanol fermentation using Saccharomyces cerevisiae BY4742. *Biomass and Bioenergy* 47, 395–401. doi:10.1016/j.biombioe.2012.09.019

Luo, C., Brink, D.L., Blanch, H.W., 2002. Identification of potential fermentation inhibitors in conversion of hybrid poplar hydrolyzate to ethanol. *Biomass and Bioenergy* 22, 125–138.

Mamma, D., Christakopoulos, P., Koullas, D., Kekos, D., Macris, B.J., Koukios, E., 1995. An alternative approach to the bioconversion of sweet sorghum carbohydrates to ethanol. *Biomass and Bioenergy* 8, 99–103. doi:10.1016/0961-9534(95)00006-S

Martín, C., Galbe, M., Wahlbom, C.F., Hahn-Hägerdal, B., Jönsson, L.J., 2002. Ethanol production from enzymatic hydrolysates of sugarcane bagasse using recombinant xylose-utilising Saccharomyces cerevisiae. *Enzyme Microb. Technol.* 31, 274–82. doi:10.1016/S0141-0229(02)00112-6

Martín, C., Marcet, M., Almazán, O., Jönsson, L.J., 2007. Adaptation of a recombinant xylose-utilizing Saccharomyces cerevisiae strain to a sugarcane bagasse hydrolysate with high content of fermentation inhibitors. *Bioresour. Technol.* 98, 1767–73. doi:10.1016/j.biortech.2006.07.021

Marx, S., Ndaba, B., Chiyanzu, I., Schabort, C., 2014. Fuel ethanol production from sweet sorghum bagasse using microwave irradiation. *Biomass and Bioenergy* 65, 145–50. doi:10.1016/j.biombioe.2013.11.019

Meyer, P.A., Tews, I.J., Magnuson, J.K., Karagiosis, S.A., Jones, S.B., 2013. Techno-economic analysis of corn stover fungal fermentation to ethanol. *Appl. Energy* 111, 657–68. doi:10.1016/j.apenergy.2013.04.085

Millati, R., Niklasson, C., Taherzadeh, M.J., 2002. Effect of pH, time, and temperature of erliming on detoxification of dilute-acid hydrolyzates for fermentation by Saccharomyces cerevisiae. *Process Biochem.* 38, 515–22.

Mishra, A., Sharma, A.K., Sharma, S., Mathur, A.S., Gupta, R.P., Tuli, D.K., 2016. Lignocellulosic bioethanol production employing newly isolated inhibitor and thermotolerant *Saccharomyces cerevisiae* DBTIOC S24 strain in SSF and SHF. *RSC Adv.* 29, 5–31.

Molaverdi, M., Karimi, K., Khanahmadi, M., Goshadrou, A., 2013. Enhanced sweet sorghum stalk to ethanol by fungus Mucor indicus using solid state fermentation, followed by simultaneous saccharification and fermentation. *Ind. Crops Prod.* 49, 580–5. doi:10.1016/j.indcrop.2013.06.024

Mudgett, R.E., 1980. Controlled gas environments in industrial fermentations. *Enzyme Microb. Technol.* 2, 273–80. doi:10.1016/0141-0229(80)90096-4

Nigam, J.N., 2001. Ethanol production from wheat straw hemicellulose hydrolysate by Pichia stipitis. *J. Biotechnol.* 87, 17–27.

Nilsson, A., Taherzadeh, M.J., Lidén, G., 2001. Use of dynamic step response for control of fed-batch conversion of lignocellulosic hydrolyzates to ethanol. *J. Biotechnol.* 89, 41–53.

Oberoi, H.S., Vadlani, P.V., Brijwani, K., Bhargav, V.K., Patil, R.T., 2010. Enhanced ethanol production via fermentation of rice straw with hydrolysate-adapted Candida tropicalis ATCC 13803. *Process Biochem.* 45, 1299–306. doi:10.1016/j.procbio.2010.04.017

Ohgren, K., Bengtsson, O., Gorwa-Grauslund, M.F., Galbe, M., Hahn-Hägerdal, B., Zacchi, G., 2006. Simultaneous saccharification and co-fermentation of glucose and xylose in steam-pretreated corn stover at high fiber content with Saccharomyces cerevisiae TMB3400. *J. Biotechnol.* 126, 488–98. doi:10.1016/j.jbiotec.2006.05.001

Öhgren, K., Bura, R., Lesnicki, G., Saddler, J., Zacchi, G., 2007a. A comparison between simultaneous saccharification and fermentation and separate hydrolysis and fermentation using steam-pretreated corn stover. *Process Biochem.* 42, 834–9. doi:10.1016/j.procbio.2007.02.003

Öhgren, K., Vehmaanperä, J., Siika-Aho, M., Galbe, M., Viikari, L., Zacchi, G., 2007b. High temperature enzymatic prehydrolysis prior to simultaneous saccharification and fermentation of steam pretreated corn stover for ethanol production. *Enzyme Microb. Technol.* 40, 607–13. doi:10.1016/j.enzmictec.2006.05.014

Ohta, K., Beall, D.S., Mejia, J.P., Shanmugam, K.T., Ingram, L.O., 1991. Genetic improvement of Escherichia coli for ethanol production: chromosomal integration of Zymomonas mobilis genes encoding pyruvate decarboxylase and alcohol dehydrogenase II. *Appl. Environ. Microbiol.* 57, 893–900.

Okamoto, K., Uchii, A., Kanawaku, R., Yanase, H., 2014. Bioconversion of xylose, hexoses, and biomass to ethanol by a new isolate of the white rot basidiomycete Trametes versicolor. *Springerplus* 3, 121. doi:10.1186/2193-1801-3-121

Okuda, N., Ninomiya, K., Takao, M., Katakura, Y., Shioya, S., 2007. Microaeration enhances the productivity of bioethanol from the hydrolysate of waste house wood using ethanologenic Escherichia coli KO11. *J. Biosci. Bioeng.* 103, 350–7. doi:10.1263/jbb.103.350

Oleskowicz-Popiel, P., Lisiecki, P., Holm-Nielsen, J.B., Thomsen, A.B., Thomsen, M.H., 2008. Ethanol production from maize silage as lignocellulosic biomass in anaerobically digested and wet-oxidized manure. *Bioresour. Technol.* 99, 5327–34. doi:10.1016/j.biortech.2007.11.029

Oliva, J.M., Negro, M.J., Sáez, F., Ballesteros, I., Manzanares, P., González, A., Ballesteros, M., 2006. Effects of acetic acid, furfural, and catechol combinations on ethanol fermentation of Kluyveromyces marxianus. *Process Biochem.* 41, 1223–8. doi:10.1016/j.procbio.2005.12.003

Olofsson, K., Rudolf, A., Lid, G., 2008. Designing simultaneous saccharification and fermentation for improved xylose conversion by a recombinant strain of Saccharomyces cerevisiae. 134, 112–20. doi:10.1016/j.jbiotec.2008.01.004

Palmqvist, E., Hahn-Hägerdal, B., 2000a. Fermentation of lignocellulosic hydrolysates. II: inhibitors and mechanisms of inhibition. *Bioresour. Technol.* 74, 25–33. doi:10.1016/S0960-8524(99)00161-3

Palmqvist, E., Hahn-Hägerdal, B., 2000b. Fermentation of lignocellulosic hydrolysates. I: inhibition and detoxification. *Bioresour. Technol.* 74, 17–24. doi:10.1016/S0960-8524(99)00160-1

Palmqvist, E., Hahn-Hägerdal, B., Galbe, M., Zacchi, G., 1996. The effect of water-soluble inhibitors from steam-pretreated willow on enzymatic hydrolysis and ethanol fermentation. *Enzyme Microb. Technol.* 19, 470–6. doi:10.1016/S0141-0229(95)00234-0

Panagiotou, G., Christakopoulos, P., Villas-Boas, S.G., Olsson, L., 2005. Fermentation performance and intracellular metabolite profiling of Fusarium oxysporum cultivated on a glucose – xylose mixture. *Enzyme Microb. Technol.* 36, 100–6. doi:10.1016/j.enzmictec.2004.07.009

Pandey, A.K., Kumar, M., Kumari, S., Gaur, N.A., 2022. Integration of acid pre-treated paddy straw hydrolysate to molasses as a diluent enhances ethanol production using a robust *Saccharomyces cerevisiae* NGY10 strain. *Renewable Energy*. 186, 790–801.

Passoth, V., Tabassum, M.R., Nair, H.A.S., Olstorpe, M., Tiukova, I., Ståhlberg, J., 2013. Enhanced ethanol production from wheat straw by integrated storage and pre-treatment (ISP). *Enzyme Microb. Technol.* 52, 105–10. doi:10.1016/j.enzmictec.2012.11.003

Pereira, F.B., Guimarães, P.M., Gomes, D.G., Mira, N.P., Teixeira, M.C., Sá-Correia, I., Domingues, L., 2011. Identification of candidate genes for yeast engineering to improve bioethanol production in very high gravity and lignocellulosic biomass industrial fermentations. *Biotechnol. Biofuels* 4, 57. doi:10.1186/1754-6834-4-57

Petersson, A., Thomsen, M., Hauggaardnielsen, H., Thomsen, A., 2007. Potential bioethanol and biogas production using lignocellulosic biomass from winter rye, oilseed rape, and faba bean. *Biomass and Bioenergy* 31, 812–9. doi:10.1016/j.biombioe.2007.06.001

Rahardjo, A.H., Azmi, R.M., Muharja, M., Aparamarta, H.W., Widjaja, A., 2021. Pretreatment of tropical lignocellulosic biomass for industrial biofuel production: a review. *IOP Conf. Ser. Mater. Sci. Eng.* 1053, 012097. doi:10.1088/1757–899x/1053/1/012097 [CrossRef] [Google Scholar] [Ref list].

Ranjan, R., Thust, S., Gounaris, C.E., Woo, M., Floudas, C.A., Keitz, M. von, Valentas, K.J., Wei, J., Tsapatsis, M., 2009. Adsorption of fermentation inhibitors from lignocellulosic biomass hydrolyzates for improved ethanol yield and value-added product recovery. *Microporous Mesoporous Mater.* 122, 143–8. doi:10.1016/j.micromeso.2009.02.025

Rosenberg, S.L., 1980. Fermentation of pentose sugars to ethanol and other neutral products by microorganisms. *Enzyme Microb. Technol.* 2, 185–93. doi:10.1016/0141-0229(80)90045-9

Saha, B.C., Cotta, M.A., 2007. Enzymatic saccharification and fermentation of alkaline peroxide pretreated rice hulls to ethanol. *Enzyme Microb. Technol.* 41, 528–32. doi:10.1016/j.enzmictec.2007.04.006

Saha, B.C., Iten, L.B., Cotta, M.A., Wu, Y.V., 2005. Dilute acid pretreatment, enzymatic saccharification and fermentation of wheat straw to ethanol. *Process Biochem.* 40, 3693–700. doi:10.1016/j.procbio.2005.04.006

Saha, B.C., Nichols, N.N., Cotta, M.A., 2011. Ethanol production from wheat straw by recombinant Escherichia coli strain FBR5 at high solid loading. *Bioresour. Technol.* 102, 10892–7. doi:10.1016/j.biortech.2011.09.041

Saha, B.C., Yoshida, T., Cotta, M.A., Sonomoto, K., 2013. Hydrothermal pretreatment and enzymatic saccharification of corn stover for efficient ethanol production. *Ind. Crops Prod.* 44, 367–72. doi:10.1016/j.indcrop.2012.11.025

Santa-Maria, M., Ruiz-Colorado, A.A., Cruz, G., Jeoh, T., 2013. Assessing the feasibility of biofuel production from lignocellulosic banana waste in rural agricultural communities in Peru and Colombia. *BioEnergy Res.* 6, 1000–11. doi:10.1007/s12155-013-9333-4

Sasaki, K., Tsuge, Y., Sasaki, D., Hasunuma, T., Sakamoto, T., Sakihama, Y., Ogino, C., Kondo, A., 2014. Optimized membrane process to increase hemicellulosic ethanol production from pretreated rice straw by recombinant xylose-fermenting Saccharomyces cerevisiae. *Bioresour. Technol.* 169, 380–6. doi:10.1016/j.biortech.2014.06.101

Sassner, P., Galbe, M., Zacchi, G., 2006. Bioethanol production based on simultaneous saccharification and fermentation of steam-pretreated Salix at high dry-matter content. *Enzyme Microb. Technol.* 39, 756–62. doi:10.1016/j.enzmictec.2005.12.010

Sedlak, M., Edenberg, H.J., Ho, N.W., 2003. DNA microarray analysis of the expression of the genes encoding the major enzymes in ethanol production during glucose and xylose co-fermentation by metabolically engineered Saccharomyces yeast. *Enzyme Microb. Technol.* 33, 19–28. doi:10.1016/S0141-0229(03)00067-X

Spencer-Martins, I., 1994. Transport of sugars in yeasts: implications in the fermentation of lignocellulosic materials. *Bioresour. Technol.* 50, 51–7. doi:10.1016/0960-8524(94)90220-8

Suresh, K., Sree, K.N., Rao, V.L., 1999. Utilization of damaged sorghum and rice grains for ethanol production by simultaneous saccharification and fermentation. *Bioresour. Technol.* 68, 301–4. doi:10.1016/S0960-8524(98)00135-7

Suriyachai, N., Weerasaia, K., Laosiripojana, N., Champreda, V., Unrean, P., 2013. Optimized simultaneous saccharification and co-fermentation of rice straw for ethanol production by Saccharomyces cerevisiae and Scheffersomyces stipitis co-culture using design of experiments. *Bioresour. Technol.* 142, 171–8. doi:10.1016/j.biortech.2013.05.003

Szczodrak, J., Fiedurek, J., 1996. Technology for conversion of lignocellulosic biomass to ethanol. *Biomass and Bioenergy* 10, 367–75. doi:10.1016/0961-9534(95)00114-X

Taherzadeh, M.J., Niklasson, C., Lidén, G., 1999. Conversion of dilute-acid hydrolyzates of spruce and birch to ethanol by fed-batch fermentation. *Bioresour. Technol.* 69, 59–66. doi:10.1016/S0960-8524(98)00169-2

Van Rooyen, R., Hahn-Hägerdal, B., La Grange, D.C., van Zyl, W.H., 2005. Construction of cellobiose-growing and fermenting Saccharomyces cerevisiae strains. *J. Biotechnol.* 120, 284–95. doi:10.1016/j.jbiotec.2005.06.013

Vincent, M., Pometto, A.L., van Leeuwen, J.H., 2014. Ethanol production via simultaneous saccharification and fermentation of sodium hydroxide treated corn stover using Phanerochaete chrysosporium and Gloeophyllum trabeum. *Bioresour. Technol.* 158, 1–6. doi:10.1016/j.biortech.2014.01.083

Walker, G.M., Walker, R.S.K., 2018. Enhancing yeast alcoholic fermentations. *Adv. Appl. Microbiol.* 105, 87–129. eds. G.M. Gadd, S. Sariaslani (Cambridge, MA: Academic Press). doi:10.1016/bs.aambs.2018.05.003.

Wan, C., Li, Y., 2010. Microbial pretreatment of corn stover with Ceriporiopsis subvermispora for enzymatic hydrolysis and ethanol production. *Bioresour. Technol.* 101, 6398–403. doi:10.1016/j.biortech.2010.03.070

Wang, P.Y., Shopsis, C., Schneider, H., 1980. Fermentation of a pentose by yeasts. *Biochem. Biophys. Res. Commun.* 94, 248–54. doi:10.1016/S0006-291X(80)80213-0

Wilkins, M.R., Widmer, W.W., Grohmann, K., 2007. Simultaneous saccharification and fermentation of citrus peel waste by Saccharomyces cerevisiae to produce ethanol. *Process Biochem.* 42, 1614–9. doi:10.1016/j.procbio.2007.09.006

Wimalasena, T.T., Greetham, D., Marvin, M.E., Liti, G., Chandelia, Y., Hart, A., Louis, E.J., Phister, T.G., Tucker, G.A., Smart, K.A., 2014. Phenotypic characterisation of

Saccharomyces spp. yeast for tolerance to stresses encountered during fermentation of lignocellulosic residues to produce bioethanol. *Microb. Cell Fact.* 13, 47. doi:10.1186/1475-2859-13-47

Wyman, C.E., 1994. Ethanol from lignocellulosic biomass: technology, economics, and opportunities. *Bioresour. Technol.* 50, 3–15. doi:10.1016/0960-8524(94)90214-3

Wyman, C.E., Spindler, D.D., Grohmann, K., 1992. Simultaneous saccharification and fermentation of several lignocellulosic feedstocks to fuel ethanol. *Biomass and Bioenergy* 3, 301–7. doi:10.1016/0961-9534(92)90001-7

Xu, J., Thomsen, M.H., Thomsen, A.B., 2010. Ethanol production from hydrothermal pretreated corn stover with a loop reactor. *Biomass and Bioenergy* 34, 334–9. doi:10.1016/j.biombioe.2009.11.004

Yu, J., Zhang, X., Tan, T., 2007. An novel immobilization method of Saccharomyces cerevisiae to sorghum bagasse for ethanol production. *J. Biotechnol.* 129, 415–20. doi:10.1016/j.jbiotec.2007.01.039

Yu, Z., Zhang, H., 2003. Ethanol fermentation of acid-hydrolyzed cellulosic pyrolysate with Saccharomyces cerevisiae. *Bioresour. Technol.* 90, 95–100. doi:10.1016/S0960-8524(03)00093-2

Zaldivar, J., Roca, C., Le Foll, C., Hahn-Hägerdal, B., Olsson, L., 2005. Ethanolic fermentation of acid pre-treated starch industry effluents by recombinant Saccharomyces cerevisiae strains. *Bioresour. Technol.* 96, 1670–6. doi:10.1016/j.biortech.2004.12.034

Zhang, M., Shukla, P., Ayyachamy, M., Permaul, K., Singh, S., 2009. Improved bioethanol production through simultaneous saccharification and fermentation of lignocellulosic agricultural wastes by Kluyveromyces marxianus 6556. *World J. Microbiol. Biotechnol.* 26, 1041–6. doi:10.1007/s11274-009-0267-0

Zhang, W., Lin, Y., Zhang, Q., Wang, X., Wu, D., Kong, H., 2013. Optimisation of simultaneous saccharification and fermentation of wheat straw for ethanol production. *Fuel* 112, 331–7. doi:10.1016/j.fuel.2013.05.064

Zhao, J., Xia, L., 2010. Bioconversion of corn stover hydrolysate to ethanol by a recombinant yeast strain. *Fuel Process. Technol.* 91, 1807–11. doi:10.1016/j.fuproc.2010.08.002

Zhao, X.Q., Xue, C., Ge, X.M., Yuan, W.J., Wang, J.Y., Bai, F.W., 2009. Impact of zinc supplementation on the improvement of ethanol tolerance and yield of self-flocculating yeast in continuous ethanol fermentation. *J. Biotechnol.* 139, 55–60. doi:10.1016/j.jbiotec.2008.08.013

Zhu, J.-Q., Qin, L., Li, B.-Z., Yuan, Y.-J., 2014. Simultaneous saccharification and co-fermentation of aqueous ammonia pretreated corn stover with an engineered Saccharomyces cerevisiae SyBE005. *Bioresour. Technol.* 169, 9–18. doi:10.1016/j.biortech.2014.06.085.

22 Physicochemical Strategies for Effective Depolymerization of Lignin

Debosmita Sharmmah, Mihir Acharya, Prasansa Rai, U. Jayakrishnan, Shashi Bhushan, and Siddhartha Moulik

22.1 INTRODUCTION

Lignin is a ubiquitously present phenolic polymer in the biosphere. Lignin is found in ether or ester-linked with hemicellulose/cellulose in lignocellulosic biomass (LCB), which forms the basic component of plants (trees, crops, shrubs, grass, and others). The lignin content in the LCBs can range from 5% to 35%, depending on the type of biomass. The monomeric composition of lignin consists of *p*-coumaryl alcohol, sinapyl alcohol, and coniferyl alcohol (Zhou et al., 2022a). The percentage of monomers also varies with LCB: softwood contains 90–95% coniferyl alcohol, while grass contains all three monomers. These monomers are linked by either carbon-carbon linkages (condensed linkages) or ether linkages, with the latter accounting for more than 56% of the linkages. These monomeric forms form a complex, cross-linked 3D structure consisting of functional groups, including hydroxyl groups (phenolic/aliphatic) and methoxyl groups. These functional groups determine the chemical properties and reactivity of lignin. However, the ratio of these hydroxyl groups varies across lignin sources (Chio et al., 2019).

LCBs are abundantly available as waste biomass from various agro-industrial processes, food and beverage processing industries, paper industries, furniture industries, and other consumer industries. Numerous processes are being applied to convert LCB cellulose and hemicellulose into biochemical and energy applications (Banu et al., 2021). However, lignin is predominantly left as a waste by-product due to its declining market value and low reactivity. Lignin is a significant by-product of the pulping industry. The concept of circular economy pushes the boundaries to close the loop in production by eliminating or reducing wastage (Chio et al., 2019). In line with the concept, converting lignin into value-added products has been an area of intense study. The high carbon-to-oxygen ratio and

DOI: 10.1201/9781003327608-22

aromatic skeleton make lignin a sustainable feedstock for fuel and biochemical production, reducing dependence on fossil fuels and contributing to mitigating climate change (Weng et al., 2021).

One of the primary bottlenecks in realizing the potential of lignin as the feedstock of the future is devising a facile, efficient, and cheap way of depolymerization (cleaving the condensed, β-β, β-1, and β-5 and ether linkage, β-O-4, 5-O-4, and α-O-4) into constituent oligomers or monomers (Ren et al., 2019). The β-aryl ether (β-O-4) linkage accounts for at least 50% of the linkages in hardwood and softwood, making β-O-4 bond cleavage a critical step in depolymerization and downstream conversions (Chio et al., 2019). Strong oxidability/thermal chemistry is necessary to cleave the linkages extensively. However, under strong conditions, repolymerization, char formation, and complex by-product formation occur (Ren et al., 2019). The present chapter provides an in-depth discussion of various aspects of these physical and chemical depolymerization techniques that can be used to valorize lignin derived from LCB.

22.2 DEPOLYMERIZATION OF LIGNIN

22.2.1 Physical Depolymerization

Lignin depolymerization is the physical process of breaking lignin polymers into smaller pieces without chemical interactions. This method creates a structural disruption to lignin without changing its chemical makeup. This treatment mainly depends on physical force to break down lignin.

22.2.1.1 Ultrasound-Assisted Depolymerization

Ultrasound-assisted technology has shown to be a low-cost, more environmentally friendly procedure with improved reaction efficiency (W. Wang et al., 2017). Variations in high- and low-pressure zones are produced as ultrasound waves move through a liquid medium. The swelling of the liquid causes micron-sized bubbles, or acoustic cavitation, to form during the low-pressure period. These bubbles oscillate aggressively in response to changes in acoustic pressure, thereby inducing chemical reactions. Then, these cavities collapse rapidly during the high-pressure phase, producing microjets, shock waves, and localized high temperatures and pressures (5000 K and 200 bar). Due to cavitation induced by ultrasound, reactive species and free radicals are generated in the liquid medium. These substances can then interact with lignin molecules, leading to bond-breaking. These events subject lignin molecules to mechanical pressure, causing them to fragment and depolymerize. Several studies have demonstrated the potential advantages of ultrasonic technology in various processes, including thermal degradation, lignocellulosic biomass hydrolysis, and the cleavage of chemical bonds (B. Liu et al., 2020). Ultrasound vibration can also help biofuel production, decreasing biomass hydrolysis and depolymerization time by 50–80% (Luo et al., 2014).

Organosolv has been used to depolymerize lignin to get phenolic monomers and lignin oil. Ultrasonication power of 90 W, temperature of 250°C, and irradiation time of 6 hr resulted in low molecular weight lignin oil (yield: 56.9%) having phenolic monomers like 2-(1-methylethyl)-phenol and benzene, 1,2,3-trimethoxy-5-methyl, and lesser ether bonds in bio-oil (B. Liu et al., 2020). Ultrasound treatment, along with a catalyst, has been observed to enhance depolymerization performance. Ultrasound-organosolv treatment of lignin in an acidic condition using isopropanol, ultrasound frequency of 30%, and 50% phosphor tungstic acid (PTA/MCM-41) as a catalyst at 310°C for 6 hr yielded 8.63% phenolic monomer product, 86.89% bio-oil, 95.52% liquid fuels, and 98.54% lignin conversion. This outcome showed that lignin depolymerization may be improved by ultrasonic acoustic cavitation, significantly increasing the yield of liquid fuels (Du et al., 2020). Moreover, ultrasonication can be combined with other physical treatments to achieve more effective outcomes. Ashutosh Agarwal and his team used microwave-ultrasound (MW + US) treatment for depolymerization of Kraft lignin and conducted a comparative study with the individual treatments. The result showed that 48.1% of bio-oil (Vanillin, isoeugenol-2, and homovanillic acid) was produced when the Kraft lignin was treated with a combination of both MW + US for 1 hr for autogenous pressure, whereas 42.1% and 25.5% were achieved for MW and US individually (Agarwal et al., 2021).

Lignin can also be pretreated with ultrasonication, thereby increasing the yield percentage. Shorter reaction times, milder reaction conditions, and the absence of harsh chemicals are among the benefits of ultrasound-assisted lignin depolymerization. Increasing lignin conversion and product selectivity through process parameter optimization is a challenge in ultrasonic-assisted lignin depolymerization. Furthermore, the energy efficiency and economic viability of large-scale ultrasonic reactors must be considered for commercial applications. Table 22.1 describes ultrasonication-assisted depolymerization of lignin from different literature (Liang et al., 2024; Abhayasimha et al., 2024; Prabhudesai et al., 2023; Xu et al., 2022; Liu et al., 2022; Schieppati et al., 2022).

22.2.1.2 Microwave-Assisted Depolymerization

Breaking down lignin into smaller molecules under carefully regulated microwave irradiation is known as "microwave-assisted depolymerization." In this technique, lignin undergoes chemical and thermal alterations through rapid, controlled microwave heating. Two essential concepts in microwave heating are dipolar rotation and ionic conductivity. Microwave irradiation produces electromagnetic waves that enter the lignin sample and interact with polar molecules such as lignin's functional groups and water. Extreme oscillation, dipole realignment, and ion migration in the polar liquid are caused by the oscillating electric field generated by molecular waves penetrating the organic molecules. As a result, the material generates friction within itself, which serves as an internal energy source and raises its temperature. The ability of these molecules to absorb microwave energy and convert it into heat causes the lignin matrix to heat rapidly. Localized heating can result in chemical reactions and thermal breakdown (Bundhoo, 2018). The process of depolymerization in microwave-assisted procedures involves the heat-induced breakage of lignin bonds, such as β-O-4, β-5, and β-β linkages, as

TABLE 22.1
Ultrasound-Assisted Depolymerization of Lignin

Lignin Type	Reaction Condition	Major Product	Yield	Reference
Phenoxyphenylethanol (PP-ol) and alkaline lignin	MoS_2/ZnO heterojunction catalysts, 4 hr, ultrasonication, 500°C, 1:1 wt% of TiO_2 nanoparticle and lignin-based biochar (LB) composite	Lignin conversion	95.8%	Liang et al. (2024)
lignin		Lignin-based biochar	96.72%	Abhayasimha et al. (2024)
Pine wood biomass	200–260°C (Pd/ACC), 3 hr/6hr (Pd/ACC); catalysts supported on activated charcoal (ACC), Ni, Pd, Pt, and Ru catalysts	Bio-oil, lignin monomers	20.8%–24.7% 12.5%–17.7%	Prabhudesai et al. (2023)
Lignin	MCM-41 with citrate complex; $LaNiO_3$ perovskite catalyst, 250°C, 6 hr, lignin: catalyst mass = 5:1, with ultrasonic assist	Phenolic monomer, bio-oil	11.46 wt% 68.0 wt%	Xu et al. (2022)
Cornstalk residual lignin	Visible light and WO_3/*g*-C_3N_4/*h*-BN (WCB) photocatalysts, ultra-sonication	Light-oil, phenolic monomer	26% 35%	Liu et al. (2022)
Kraft lignin	NaOH with sodium chloroacetate (SCA) (carboxymethylation), SCA: lignin=1:12 and ultrasound at 20 W and 20 kHz, 30 min	Biodispersing agents	–	Schieppati et al. (2022)

well as aromatic ring opening, thereby speeding up the process and accelerating the production of smaller lignin fragments and soluble products by heating the material quickly and uniformly. Typically, lignin depolymerization facilitated by MW-assisted is divided into two categories: MW-assisted solvolysis at moderate temperatures (<200°C) and MW-assisted pyrolysis at relatively high temperatures (>400°C) (Dhar and Vinu, 2017). Phenolic chemicals, aromatic monomers, oligomers, and volatile gases, including hydrogen, carbon dioxide, and methane, are the by-products of microwave-assisted lignin depolymerization. Several factors, including lignin supply, solvent type, microwave power, and reaction duration, affect the composition and yield of the products.

A recent study used lignin and polypropylene to produce bio-oil via microwave-assisted, fast catalytic co-pyrolysis. At 250°C and a feedstock/catalyst ratio of 2:1, less char/coke was produced, and improved bio-oil and aromatics yields were observed compared with lignin pyrolysis alone (Duan et al., 2017). Dhar and Vinu (2017) used microwave-assisted degradation with organic solvents such as ethylene glycol (EG), dimethyl sulfoxide (DMSO), and dimethyl formamide (DMF) within a temperature range of 100–140°C and a treatment time of 20–80 min; 20% phenolics were obtained in DMF and DMSO at 100°C and 11% in EG at 140°C, containing acetosyringone, guaiacol, syringaldehyde, anisole, and lignin dimers. The lignin extracted from birch sawdust was depolymerized without additional hydrogen in a mixture of water and alcohol (methanol, isopropanol, or ethanol) at 190°C for 3 hr using Pd/C, Pt/C, or Ru/C. The microwave-assisted process produced 65% phenolic monomers (Liu et al., 2021). Table 22.2 summarizes different microwave-assisted depolymerizations of lignin reported

TABLE 22.2
Microwave-Assisted Depolymerization of Lignin

Lignin Type	Reaction Condition	Major Product	Yield	Reference
Alkaline lignin and dealkaline lignin	Formic acid, ethanol	Bio-oil, phenolic monomer	-	Zhou et al. (2022b)
Lignin	10% HBr, 90°C, and 2 hr	Phenolic hydroxyl lignin-based foams	26%	Gao et al. (2021)
Lignin	200–500°C within 8 min under a microwave power of 1,000 W; MoS_2	Liquid products Phenolics	34.1 wt% 32.1 wt%)	Wang et al. (2020)
Bio-enzymatic lignin (BL) organosolv lignin (OL)	CuO, carbon-modified boron nitride (BCN), 30 min under mild conditions (200°C)	Monomers Bio-oil (both BL and OL as substrate)	10 wt% 70 wt%	Cao et al. (2020)
Lignin and waste oil	ZSM-5/MCM-41 as catalyst, SiC microwave absorbent, 400°C, feedstock: catalyst = 10:1	Aromatics Monocyclic aromatic hydrocarbons (MAHs)	50.31% 42.83% –	Zou et al. (2019)
Organosolv lignin	110°C, 7 min, 80 W, $CuSO_4/H_2O_2$	Vanillin, vanillic acid, 4 4-hydroxybenzaldehyde	–	Dai et al. (2018)
Organosolv lignin	100W, 160°C, 30 min, H_2SO_4/HCl/H_3PO_4	Char Levoglucosenone	47.9% 21%	Tayier et al. (2018)

in the literature (Zhou et al., 2022b; Gao et al., 2021; Wang et al., 2020; Cao et al., 2020; Zou et al., 2019; Dai et al., 2018; Tayier et al., 2018).

22.2.2 Thermal Depolymerization

Thermal and other physical treatments are often used because high temperatures are a common and efficient way to break chemical interactions. Hydrothermal liquefaction (HTL), gasification, combustion, and pyrolysis are examples of thermal depolymerization. As an important method for the thermal depolymerization of lignin, pyrolysis – high-speed/flash pyrolysis – and HTL have received much interest in comparison to combustion and gasification under extremely high temperatures (Zhou et al., 2022a). These procedures for lignin's heat treatment are performed in the presence or absence of additional catalysts (Chio et al., 2019).

22.2.2.1 Hydrothermal Liquefaction of Lignin

Under high pressure and temperature in the presence of water, lignin undergoes a thermochemical process called hydrothermal liquefaction, which transforms it into biocrude oil and other valuable products. Because HTL can effectively depolymerize lignin and generate a high-energy-density liquid bio-oil, it has attracted interest as a potential lignin valorization technique. Because water has a high ionic product (*K*w, or the concentration of [H_3O^+] & [OH^-] ions by self-dissociation) and low viscosity, it may function as an acid-base catalytic system. In the presence of water as the solvent, hydrothermal liquefaction of lignin typically occurs at temperatures between 250°C and 400°C and pressures between 10 MPa and 25 MPa (Kumar et al., 2017). Compared to many other biomass conversion methods, HTL is helpful because of its comparatively low oxygen concentration and consistency of the liquids (Lui et al., 2020). Methane, carbon dioxide, hydrogen, other gases, and solid residues (char) are produced during the hydrothermal liquefaction of lignin.

Other products derived from this process include biocrude oil and an aqueous phase, depending on optimization of the efficiency and selectivity of the hydrothermal liquefaction. The emeraldine liquefaction of lignin can be improved by using catalysts, such as solid acids/bases, metal oxides, and transition metals, which can alter product distributions, enhance bio-oil production, and promote lignin depolymerization. Concerns regarding hydrothermal lignin liquefaction include catalyst deactivation, product separation, reactor design, and techno-economic viability. The primary objectives of the research include improving product quality and yield, creating effective catalysts, and optimizing process conditions.

Previous reviews have shown that, using the hydrothermal liquefaction/carbonization process, lignin can be broken down to yield bio-oil (a low-oxygen liquid) and phenolics such as syringol, vanillin, guaiacol, trimers, and oligomers (Cao et al., 2018). Corn straw lignin was hydrothermally liquefied with different catalysts [nano ferrite + inorganic base catalyst ($CoFe_2O_4$), $ZnFe_2O_4$] at different temperatures. At 220°C, this yielded benzofuran, 2,3-dihydro-2-methoxy-4-vinylphenol, and vanillin at 31.42%, 17.64%, and 10.82%, respectively, and 34.2% heavy oil at 180°C (Chen et al., 2021). When Kraft lignin, a Ni-Al/MCM-41 catalyst, and different solvents (water, methanol, and ethanol) were used during hydrothermal liquefaction at 280°C, bio-oil was produced as the product. However, the yield varied with the solvent; with water, 44.3 wt% bio-oil was obtained, whereas with methanol and ethanol, the yields were 48.1 wt.% and 56.2 wt%, respectively (Feng et al., 2021). Table 22.3 describes the use of various factors in the HTL of lignin from different literature sources.

22.2.2.2 Pyrolysis of Lignin

Pyrolysis is the process of breaking down lignin by heat at high temperatures in the absence of oxygen. Lignin is broken down but does not fully transform into carbon dioxide due to the lack of oxygen. In the process, liquids and gases, including solid char, bio-oil, and gases, are produced. Because pyrolysis can transform lignin into valuable compounds, including high levels of aromatic monomers, it is indicated that pyrolysis may have the potential to convert lignin and biomass into other value-added biomaterials (Bridgwater, 2012). The normal temperature range for lignin pyrolysis in an oxygen-free atmosphere is 300–600°C. This temperature range helps break ester bonds, including α-O-4 and β-O-4, two of the most common bonds in lignin (Chio et al., 2019). The temperature of 400°C is critical during the pyrolysis process, because at this range (secondary pyrolysis), lignin undergoes structural alteration, which causes the release of free radicals. These radicals help break the C—C bonds present, producing oligomers and monomers (Li and Takkellapati, 2018). The concentration of products can be affected by temperature: lower temperatures favor bio-oil synthesis, while higher temperatures favor gas formation. Adding catalysts can affect the yield of the bio-oil produced from lignin pyrolysis and improve its quality. Various catalysts, such as metal oxides, supported metals, and zeolites, can improve lignin depolymerization and desired product yield. The mechanistic outlook for depolymerization via pyrolysis is shown in Figure 22.1. The earlier studies used low-sulfonated Kraft lignin and were treated by Zn- or Mo-loaded HZSM-5 catalyst, in CH_4 and CH_4-D (breakdown of CH_4 (CH4-D)) atmospheres during pyrolysis.

The result showed a more significant methylation of alkyl moieties and a 33% increase in the overall output of benzene, toluene, and xylenes, as well as a by-product, pyrolytic oil (Farooq et al., 2022). These produced bio-oils are now an important research topic for the energy industry. So, these by-products have commercial, economic, and biological values. However, the presence of oxygen-sensitive functional groups in lignin poses a challenge for lignin pyrolysis, as they may lead to unwanted side reactions and degrade the quality of the bio-oil. So, more studies are being conducted to optimize the process using a catalyst or a reactor to increase overall efficiency. Zhipeng Wu and coworkers (2019) used raw lignin (RL) and base-catalysis (SEBC) pretreated lignin (SL) and heated them simultaneously at 20°C/min, 60°C/min, 80°C/min, and 100°C/min up to 720°C. From this, they obtained a temperature range of 200–500°C.

TABLE 22.3
Hydrothermal Liquefaction of Lignin

Lignin type	Reaction conditions	Major product	Yield	Reference
Alkali lignin	Cu/HBC (catalytic process of mesoporous homologous biochar), 0.05 g Cu/HBC, 18 mL water, 0.2 g alkali lignin, 280°C, 6 hr,	Monophenol bio-oil	5.01 ±0.76 mg/g 57.98% ± 1.76%	Zhang et al. (2023)
Alkali lignin	Bimetallic catalyst Ni-Co/AC (activated bio-char carbon), catalyst quantity (5–20 wt%), 260 to 300°C, 15 min, Ni-Co/AC with ethanol, water, methanol	Benzene, phenol, vanillin, bio-oil	1.1–2.1% 8.6–18.2% 32.1–36.2% 72.0 wt%	Biswas et al. (2021)
Aqueous waste	356°C, 37 min, 19 mL/g (HTL-AW/biocrude), hydrogen to carbon effective (H/Ceff) ratio of 1.07	Energy, N-heterocyclic compounds, n-hexadecanoic acid	80% 10.15% 22.23%	B. Li et al. (2021)
Oak wood	Nano-spike Ni catalysts (10–50 wt%), 330°C, and 10 min	Bio-crude	36.63%	de Caprariis et al. (2020)
Pinewood sawdust	300°C for 30 min, ethanol/water co-solvent without any catalyst and with Na_2CO_3 and NaOH catalysts, separately; pure water without any catalyst and with Na_2CO_3 and NaOH catalysts, separately.	Bio-crude oil, solid residue Bio-crude oil, solid residue	81.94–67.87% 3.29–12.61% 21.54–55.51% 32.48–76.72%	Hu et al. (2020)
Corncob lignin	290°C with a retention time of 0 min	Heavy oil, phenol, vanillin, 2-methoxyphenol, 4-ethylphenol, 4-ethyl-2-methoxy-phenol, 2,6-dimethoxy-phenol, 1, 3-dimethylbenzene, p-xylene	10.2% 15.5% – 34.6% 17.6% 10.2% – –	Yang et al. (2015)
Lignin	Methanol, 200°C, 30 min residence time	Phenols and aromatic ethers	85%	Singh et al. (2014)

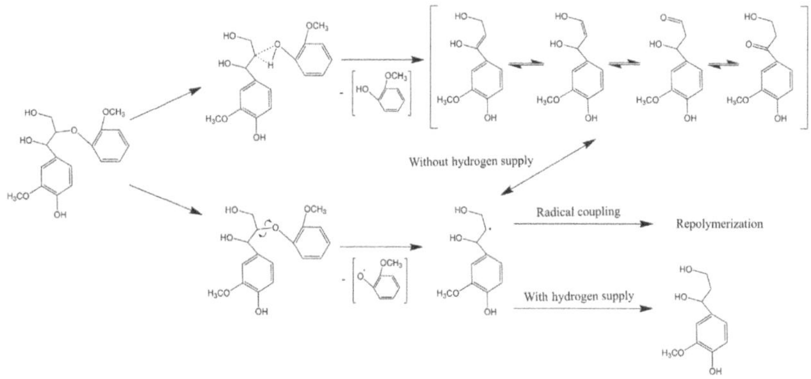

FIGURE 22.1 Breakage of β-O-4 linkages by pyrolysis: a compensatory mechanism.

Source: Reproduced with permission from Elsevier (Chio et al., 2019)

In the experiment, they used 10% wt NaOH at 1.5 MPa. They obtained phenol as the primary product when pretreated lignin (SL) was used, whereas raw lignin yielded 2-methoxy-4-ethylphenol as the main product. When lignin from Japanese cedar wood was used, diphenoxybenzene (an aprotic solvent) was used during pyrolysis, keeping the temperature range between 270°C and 380°C. At 270°C, the yield was relatively low, but as the temperature increased, oligomer yield increased to more than 80 wt% (Wang et al., 2022). Table 22.4 describes different investigations into lignin depolymerization by pyrolysis (Li et al., 2023; Dong et al., 2022; Zhang et al., 2021; L. Xu et al., 2021; Hoang et al., 2021; Wang et al., 2019; Huang et al., 2018).

22.2.3 Chemical Depolymerization

This depolymerization process is a chemical-dependent method for breaking the complex structure of lignin polymers into more useful products, which also have different value-added prospects. Additionally, the chemical way is more manageable and less energy-consuming than thermal depolymerization and yields more environmentally friendly energy resources (Zhou et al., 2022a)

We use various acids and bases for chemical treatment, along with oxidative and reductive catalysts (as discussed in the subsequent sections).

22.2.3.1 Acid-Based Depolymerization

Acid hydrolysis is a chemical degradation technique that cleaves ether bonds and alters lignin structure, breaking it down into smaller molecules. This process uses acid to break through the lignin's β-O-4 bonds. Due to its firm acidity and capacity to successfully dissolve ether bonds, sulfuric acid (H_2SO_4) is frequently used for the acid hydrolysis of lignin (H. Wang et al., 2019). Organic acids, such

TABLE 22.4
Pyrolysis of Lignin

Lignin Type	Reaction Condition	Major Product	Yield	Reference
Alkali lignin	650°C, niobium-doped HZSM-5 catalyst (H[Nb]ZSM-5) and only HZSM-5 catalyst	Monoaromatic hydrocarbons, aliphatic hydrocarbons, phenol	43.4–35.5% 20.8–3.2% 2.8–24.9%	Z.M. Li et al. (2023)
Lignin	3% ammonium borate, 650°C	Diphenols	80%	Dong et al. (2022)
Hydrotreatment of alkaline lignin	850°C	Olefins, benzene, toluene, char, guaiacol, cresol, phenol, 4-ethyl-2-methoxy-, vanillin, etc.	3.1 wt% 4.8 wt% 36.46 wt% – –	Zhang et al. (2021)
Lignin to PF resins of 1:1	Phenol-formaldehyde (PF) resins, HZSM-5–3 zeolite (Si/Al ratio of 80) catalyst, 650°C	Aromatic amines	32.2%	L. Xu et al. (2021)
Clean wood	250 and 600°C	Bio-oil	60–75 wt%	Hoang et al. (2021)
Kraft lignin	Sodium formate (SF), calcium formate (CF), nickel formate (NF) 200–420°C	Carbon residue, monophenols, 3-methylcatechol, 4-methylcatechol, hydrocarbons (toluene and o-cymene)	52.1wt–47.3wt% 53.77% 16.81% 5.53% 10.12%	Wang et al. (2019)
Rice husks	500°C, the feeding rate is 20 g/min, and the superficial gas velocity is 0.340 m/s	Bio-oil (acetic acid, furfural, phenol, and phenol derivatives)	30.4%	Huang et al. (2018)

as formic and acetic acids, and other acids, such as hydrochloric, formic, and peracetic, can be used as catalysts for cleaving ether bonds (Roy et al., 2022). Phenolic compounds are produced during hydrolysis when the acids supply H_3O^+ to break the ether linkages. Acid hydrolysis generally occurs under high-pressure, high-temperature conditions to accelerate lignin breakdown. After combining the lignin source with the preferred acid solution, the process is heated to around 120°C and 200°C. Although higher temperatures could speed up reactions, they are also prone to undesired reactions and, as a result, degrade the quality of the intended products (Ren et al., 2019). Oxonium ions are formed when the H^+ ion of the acid reacts with the ether bonds in the lignin polymer. Smaller lignin fragments are released as those ions get hydrolyzed, breaking down the ether linkages. Furthermore, the pH levels allow the lignin to become soluble in the media, making the reaction viable (Gasson et al., 2012). Figure 22.2 describes the impact of the acid-catalyzed reaction on lignin structure.

In a 1:1 water/ethanol solvent solution, sulfuric acid has been used as the catalyst for the reaction, generating roughly 70% of the polymer breakdown (Mahmood et al., 2015). The study conducted by de Carvalho and Colodette (2017) used lignin from sugarcane bagasse, eucalyptus, and sugarcane straw. It was

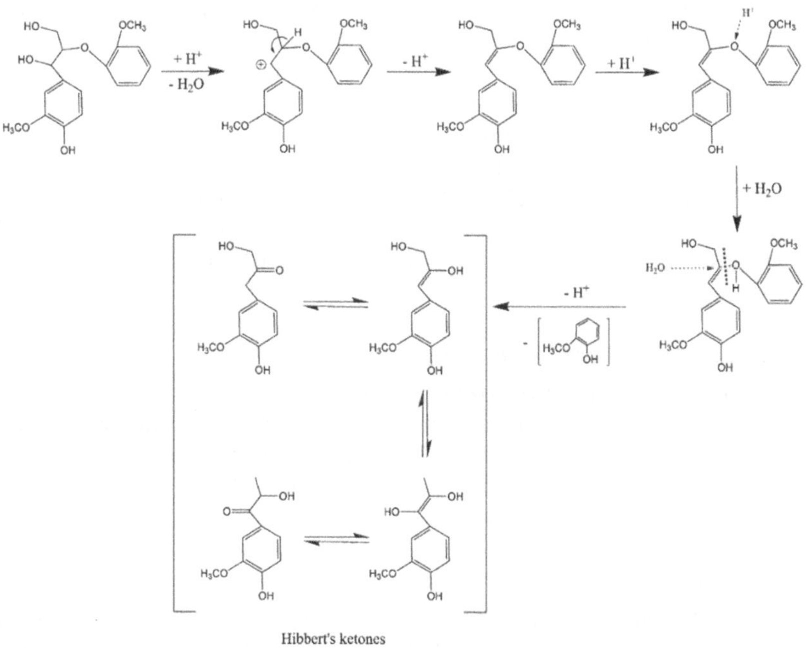

FIGURE 22.2 Acid catalyst-induced hydrolysis of β-O-4 linkages: A compensatory mechanism.

Source: Reproduced with permission from Elsevier (Chio et al., 2019)

hydrolyzed with 6.15 mol/L H_2SO_4 at 121°C for 90 min, which turned lignin into its monomeric form. The experiment done with organosolv lignin and H_2SO_4 at 300°C for 1 hr having H-Y zeolite (SiO_2/ Al_2O_3= 10) showed 92.5% lignin conversion having aromatic monomer 1.02% and phenolic compound 6.02% (4-ethylguaicol 1.37%, 4-ethylphenol 1.23%, guaiacol 1.23%, vanillin 0.22%, phenol 0.68%, Syringol 1.09%) (Wanmolee et al., 2016). Burcu Güvenatam processed the soda lignin by triflating Lewis acidic metals (aluminum, copper, and nickel) in an ethanol-water combination at 400°C for 4 hr under a pressure of 375–400 bars. The reaction also broke the α–O–4, β–O–4 (C—O—C) ether linkage bridge by alkylation. It resulted in the following compounds: aliphatic hydrocarbons (paraffin and olefins), aromatic hydrocarbons (highly alkylated non-oxygenated mono-aromatics, primarily alkylbenzenes as well as mono-aromatic oxygenates, primarily phenolics), condensation products (primarily naphthalene), and saturated oxygenates (ketones and carboxylic acids) (Güvenatam et al., 2016)

The acid-mediated hydrolysis of lignin yields many kinds of low-molecular-weight fragments, including ketones, aromatic, volatile aldehydes, phenolic compounds, and carboxylic acids, as breakdown products. The composition and quantity of these compounds can be affected by lignin supply, acid content, and reaction conditions, among other variables (X. Liu et al., 2020). To stop the acid-catalyzed reactions upon completion of the depolymerization step, the acid-treated lignin mixture must be neutralized. Generally, a base is added to neutralize the solution. The depolymerized lignin can be retrieved from the resultant mixture by solvent extraction, precipitation, or filtering. A significantly longer reaction time, a higher temperature, and greater pressure are required for this method to work. Also, it yields hazardous waste products that are very harmful to the environment, raising reaction costs considerably due to storage and removal requirements (Roy et al., 2022). Table 22.5 contains the breakdown of the lignin depolymerization using acid (Žula et al., 2023; Asawaworarit et al., 2019; Du et al., 2019; Nandiwale et al., 2019; J. Wang et al., 2017; Deepa and Dhepe, 2015; Gasson et al., 2012).

22.2.3.2 Alkali-Based Depolymerization

Lignin can also be depolymerized by base hydrolysis, which involves treating lignin with alkali. This approach treats lignin at high temperatures, generally between 150°C and 250°C, with alkaline solutions that include strong bases, usually potassium hydroxide (KOH) or sodium hydroxide (NaOH). By severing ether bonds and dissolving ester connections, base hydrolysis breaks down the structure of lignin and produces shorter lignin pieces and soluble compounds (Thring, 1995). According to the individual settings and expected outcomes, the base concentration and reaction period might fluctuate (Zhou et al., 2022a), but high pressure and temperatures above 300°C are typically used. The β-O-4 bond, the most prevalent link in lignin, begins to cleave at 270°C. Phenolic monomers are formed when cations from the base aid in producing cation conjugates, facilitating a six-membered transition on the β-O-4 bond (Roberts et al., 2011). Alkaline

TABLE 22.5
Acid-Based Lignin Depolymerization

Lignin Type	Reaction Condition	Major Product	Yield	Reference
Benzyl phenyl ether (BPE)	Solvent (methanol, ethanol, γ-valerolactone, water), catalyst loading (0.5–1.5 wt% of H_2SO_4), 160–200°C	Alkoxylated and hydroxyl group-bearing products	–	Žula et al. (2023)
Bagasse organosolv fractionalized lignin	Standardized acids (i.e., H_2SO_4, H_3PO_4, and HCl) and heterogeneous carboniferous solid acids; 350°C for 3 hr using methyl isobutyl ketoneas solvent	Phenolic products like 4-ethylphenol and guaiacol; vanillin and ethyl guaiacol	Total phenolic yield 32.8%	Asawaworarit et al. (2019)
Bulrush lignin (BL)	Phosphotungstic acid catalyst (0.25 g), H_2O_2 (3 mL), and ethanol/water (v/v, 30 mL/30 mL), 250°C for 6 hr	Biochar, monomer EL-soluble, monomer tetrahydrofuran (THF) soluble	44.41 wt% 17.24 wt% 30.39 wt%	Du et al. (2019)
Corn stover lignin (organosolv)	Acetic acid, Zr-KIT-5 (Si/Zr = 20) catalyst, 250°C for 60 min	Extractable ethyl acetate, 12 phenolic monomers (like phenyl acetate, guaiacol, phenyl-b-d-glucoside, ethyl guaiacol, 2-ethylphenol)	~43 wt% 28 wt%	Nandiwale et al. (2019)
Microwave-assisted black liquor lignin	Formic acid, 160°C for 30 min	Bio-oil 1 (mainly aromatic monomers) Bio-oil 2 (mainly aromatic oligomers)	9.69% 54.39%	Q. Wang et al. (2017)
Bagasse lignin	Zeolite HHSZ-100, SiO_2-Al_2O_3 catalyst, water-methanol (1:5 v/v), 250°C, 30 min, RPM 1,000 (not more than 1,200)	Vanillin, methyl vanillate, Syringol, homovanillic acid, and vinyl guaiacol	59%	Deepa and Dhepe (2015)
Wheat straw lignin	10 wt% formic acid, 77–81wt%, ethanol at 360°C, 25 MPa pressure	Methoxyphenols, catechols, phenols	2.0–2.9 wt% 1.7–1.5 wt% 1.5–2.0 wt%	Gasson et al. (2012)

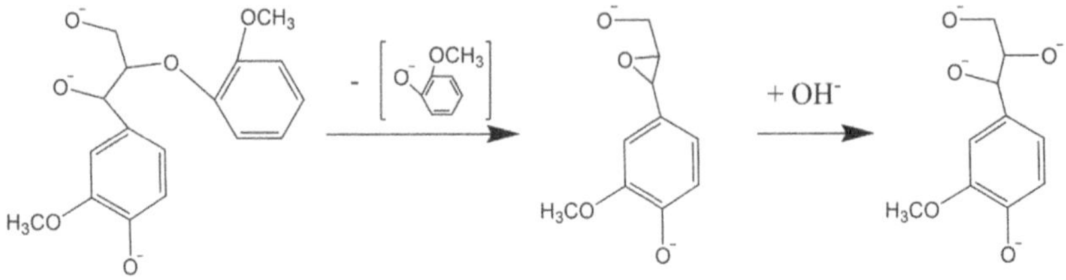

FIGURE 22.3 Alkaline catalyst-induced hydrolysis of β-O-4 linkages: A compensatory mechanism.

Source: Reproduced with permission from Elsevier (Chio et al., 2019).

hydrolysis is a nucleophilic process where hydroxide ions (OH^-) attack the interactions between esters in the lignin polymer. As a result, the lignin structure breaks apart into smaller units, and the bonds are cleaved. However, strong bases are corrosive and may harm the ecosystem, so their transportation and disposal should be done carefully. Figure 22.3 demonstrates how a base catalyst functions to break the lignin.

Hanna Paananen et al. (2021) used Kraft lignin obtained from softwood and phenol mixtures treated with NaOH, and they hydroxymethylated it at a high temperature (above 100°C). As a product, they obtained oxidized lignin molecules and used phenol-formaldehyde resins to replace phenols. However, lignin from two different sources, agricultural (hemp) and forestry (softwood), was treated with base-catalysis (NaOH) at 1,300–1,900 psi pressure and 300–330°C temperature in a bioreactor. The product they obtained contained 10% monomers (propanoic acid, phenol, o-cresol, m-cresol, guaiacol, catechol, 1,2-dimethoxybenzene, 2-ethylphenol, 6-methylguaiacol, 5-methylguaiacol, 4-methylguaiacol, 3,4-dimethoxytoluene, Syringol, 2-methoxyresorcinol, 4-ethylguaiacol, 3-methylcathecol, 1,2,3-trimethoxybenzene, 2-methoxyethyl phenol, vanillin, 1,2,3-trimethoxy-5-methylbenzene, 4,5-dimethylcathecol, BHT, 4,5-dimethoxy-2-methylphenol, acetovanillon, syringaldehyde, acetosyringone), a mixture containing up to 60% dimers and trimers and 30% char (Lavoie et al., 2011). Moreover, softwood Kraft lignin was treated with 7.50 wt% lignin by 3.75 wt% NaOH solution at a pressure of 250 bar and temperature of 320°C for 10 minutes; the extracted lignin segments were vacuum dried at 40°C. They found numerous products that could substitute for phenol and phenolic resins (50–70 wt%). They found products in monomeric-rich (BCD-oil) and oligomeric (BCD-oligomers), such as lignin phenol-formaldehyde (LPF) (Solt et al., 2018). Table 22.6 describes base-mediated lignin depolymerization from the available literature (K. Li et al.,

TABLE 22.6
Alkali-Based Lignin Depolymerization

Lignin Source	Reaction Condition	Major Product	Yield	Reference
Soda-P1000 OS-Alcell KraftIndulin AT OS-spruce OS-wheat straw	NaOH catalyst in hot compressed water	Char Lignin oil Monomer Monomer in lignin oil Residue	1–2%(w/w) 20–30% (w/w) 11–13% (w/w) 42–55% (w/w) 43–70% (w/w)	Purushothaman et al. (2023)
Kraft lignin	NaOH (1.67 and 2.50 wt%), 513–573 K, 0.055–1.000 L vol, flow rate of mass (10–20 kg/hr)	Phenolic oligomers	–	Bernhardt et al. (2021)
Alkaline lignin	Base 5–9 min, 300°C, 61.0–80.0% lignin	Phenols: Guaiacol and Syringol	5.5–6.9 wt% –	Kudo et al. (2021)
Kraft lignin from black liquor retentate (BLR)	170–210°C, 2% NaOH, 10 min	Monomers and dimers	–	K. Li et al. (2021)
Klason lignin from coconut coir	NaOH, 200–250°C, 1 hr, 1,000 RPM	Aromatic products	64%	Chaudhary and Dhepe (2019)
Pine Kraft lignin (Indulin AT)	NaOH/lignin ≡1(w/w), 5 wt% lignin solids, 170–250°C	Low-molecular-weight phenolics	–	Abdelaziz et al. (2018)
Lignin	Lignin: NaX = 1:1 *wt/wt*, EtOH: H_2O (1:2 *v/v*), lignin: catalyst mass = 1:1; 250°C, 1 hr, 1000 RPM	Phenyl	5%	Chaudhary and Dhepe (2017)
		Diethylterephthalate	0.6 wt%	
		Homovanillic acid	0.3 wt%	
		Hexadecane	0.5 wt%	
		2,4-Ditertbutylphenol	0.5 wt%	
		Acetoguaiacone	4.1 wt%	
		Vanillin	3.6 wt%	
		2,6-Dimethoxy phenol	0.4 wt%	
		4-Hydroxybenzyl alcohol	1.4 wt%	
		Resorcinol	0.8 wt%	
		2-Methoxy-4-methylphenol	3.7 wt%	
		Guaiacol	1 wt%	
		Pyrocatechol	0.3 wt%	
		Eugenol	0.4 wt%	
		1,2,4- trimethoxybenzene	0.03 wt%	
		3,4- dimethoxyphenol	0.02 wt%	
		4-hydroxy-3- methoxy-benzyl alcohol	0.3 wt%	
		Acetoguaiacone	4.1 wt%	
		Dimethyl polysiloxane	95%	
		Guaiacol	1 wt%	
		Pyrocatechol	0.3 wt%	

2021; Chaudhary and Dhepe, 2019; Abdelaziz et al., 2018; Chaudhary and Dhepe, 2017).

22.2.4 Oxidative Depolymerization

This process involves oxidizing agents such as oxygen, ozone, hydrogen peroxide, or other oxidants (Crestini et al., 2006). They are used for lignin's oxidative depolymerization process to break its polymer down into smaller chunks, as depicted in Figure 22.4. It is feasible to substitute acid- or base-catalyzed methods for lignin conversion into monomers under less harsh conditions (Stärk et al., 2010). The C—O and C—C bonds in its polymeric structure must be cleaved to commercialize lignin. In such processes, catalysts are commonly used to reduce energy consumption, reaction time, temperature, and pressure and to simultaneously increase product yields and selectivity (Abdelaziz et al., 2022). For the depolymerization process, various oxidants are used, for example, permanganate, nitrobenzene, copper oxide, hydrogen peroxide, chlorine, and hypochlorite. By preserving the aromatic nature, the oxidative degradation method selectively cleaves the ether bonds. Hydrogen peroxide (H_2O_2) is an oxidizing agent that can break down lignin polymer chains into smaller pieces by cleaving lignin bonds through oxidation. It can react with the phenolic and non-phenolic components in lignin, breaking the long polymer chains. Depolymerization of lignin using H_2O_2 usually occurs under mild reaction conditions such as near-neutral pH and ambient or slightly elevated temperature. To improve the efficiency and selectivity of the process, enzyme catalysts or transition-metal ions (such as Fe2+ or Cu2+) are typically used. Strong oxidants can effectively break the bonds between aromatic moieties in lignin.

As taken from previous studies, when O_2/$NaNO_2$/DDQ/NHPI for oxidation and Ni-Mo sulfide catalyst were used for hydration to break the bonds of the lignin from birch wood, as per the concept of two-step oxidation-hydrogenation, 32% of phenol monomers in the by-product were accomplished (Zhang et al., 2017). Kerstin Stärk (Stärk et al., 2010) used beech lignin and depolarized it in the presence of an ionic liquid. $Mn(NO_3)_2$ in 1-ethyl-3-methylimidazolium

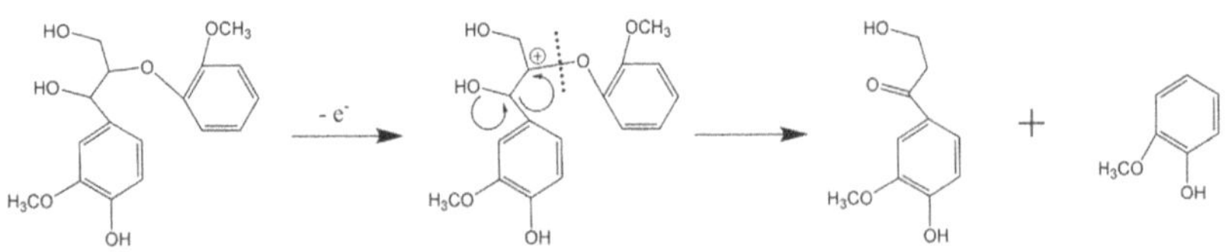

FIGURE 22.4 The dissociation process of β-O-4 links with the oxidant agent. It depicts one of the various products. The oxidation level might alter the actual products.

Source: Reproduced with permission from Elsevier (Chio et al., 2019)

trifluoromethanesulfonate [EMIM][CF_3SO_3] was used as the batch reactor system at 100°C, 84 × 10^5 Pa air for 24 hr (multi-parallel way of working); 66.3% lignin (11 g) was converted to give a solution of phenols, unsaturated propylaromatics, and aromatic aldehydes such as syringaldehyde and 2,6-dimethoxy-1,4-benzoquinone (DMBQ) (having 11.5 wt% yield). On the other hand, as lignin was converted into aromatic components, cerium-oxide-supported palladium nanoparticles (Pd/CeO_2) and CH_3OH solvent were used at 185°C, 1 bar O_2 for 24 hr to yield 2-phenoxy-1-phenylethanol, phenol, acetophenone (breaking of β-O-4 bond), and benzoic acid and methyl benzoate (breaking of C_α-C_β bond, catalyzed by CeO_2). Under mild temperatures, such as 458 K, it can also be converted into guaiacol and 4-hydroxylbenzaldehyde (Deng et al., 2015).

To hasten lignin oxidation, oxidative depolymerization steps are often carried out at high pressure and temperature. The specific procedure and desired product determine the choice of oxidizing agent and reaction conditions (Zhang et al., 2017). Table 22.7 shows the experimental parameters for lignin depolymerization using oxidative catalysts from the literature (Song et al., 2019; Hdidou et al., 2018; Jennings et al., 2017).

22.2.5 Reductive Depolymerization

Reducing agents can simplify the process of breaking the lignin bonds by reductive reactions. Examples of these agents include hydrogen gas and metal catalysts like nickel and palladium.

22.2.5.1 Metal-Catalyzed Depolymerization

Lignin may be broken down into smaller pieces by using metallic catalysts. These catalysts can be noble metals such as ruthenium and platinum or transition metals such as nickel, palladium, and iron. The depolymerization of lignin by metallic catalysts is summarized in Figure 22.5. Because of their tendency to activate oxygen and promote redox reactions, transition metals – especially those with fluctuating oxidation states – are frequently used as catalysts for lignin depolymerization. Noble metals tend to be more valuable but can also be effective catalysts in their own right. Depolymerization processes usually take place at mild-to-moderate temperatures and pressures, depending on the specific catalysts and reaction mechanisms. The solvent and the reaction surroundings also influence the method. Metal-catalyzed depolymerization can occur via a variety of mechanisms, including oxidative cleavage, hydrodeoxygenation, hydrogenolysis, and reductive reactions. Different product variations and characteristics could result from these paths. The activation energy for depolymerization was significantly reduced by the addition of metallic catalysts, enabling moderate reaction conditions. The C—O and C—C cleavages of lignin remained the focus of metal-catalyzed reactions when hydrogen sources such as ethanol or water were present. Accessible metal sites were created on the outer surface by nickel or other

TABLE 22.7
Oxidative Lignin Depolymerization

Lignin Type	Reaction Condition	Major Product	Yield	Reference
Softwood LignoBoost Kraft lignin (LB)	Zirconia-supported vanadium, copper catalysts (VCu*x*:*y*Zr) with alkaline water at 150°C under an O_2 pressure of 5 bar for 10 min	Vanillin Monomer	59% 9 wt%	Abdelaziz et al. (2023)
Kraft lignin	$NaOH/H_2O$ and Pd-PVP/TiO_2 and Pd/TiO_2cata-lysts having 150°C, 20 bar, 5 g lignin/L, 1–10 wt% metal	Vanillic acid Vanillin	1–2% 1.5–2.5%	Y. Xu et al. (2021)
Organosolv lignin (hardwood) Kraft lignin Organosolv lignin (softwood)	$NaOH/H_2O$, Au/TiO_2 and Pt/TiO_2 catalysts, 150°C, 20 bar air pressure, concentration of NaOH: 10 g/L, 1 hr, 5 g lignin/L,0.1 wt% metal	Vanillin	1.7–5.1%	Almada et al. (2021)
Organosolv lignin	CH_3CH_2OH; Ce-Cu/MFI nanosheets catalysts, 150°C, 10 bar, 24 hr	Diethyl maleate Aromatics C3-C5 esters	18.1% 5.1% 6.2%	L. Li et al. (2020)
Organosolv lignin	Au/CeO_2 20 wt% catalyst, O_2, CH_3OH, 453 K, 10 bar, 4 g lignin/L	Vanillin Methyl vanillate Methylene syringate	10.5 wt% 6.8 wt% 3.4 wt%	Song et al. (2019)
Organosolv lignin	Co_3O_4, Fe_2O_3, and CoFeO heterogenous catalyst, 10%O_2/N_2, 150–200°C, 1–2 bar, 2–4 hr, 1.66 g lignin/L, 20–40 wt% catalyst	Aromatic molecules (syringaldehyde and Vanillin)	19.6% (H_2O, 150°C) 16.6% (H_2O + CH_3OH, 200°C)	Hdidou et al. (2018)
Lignin	Hydrogen peroxide/2-adamantanone/SnO_2 for the ketones' Baeyer-Villiger oxidation	Ester	81%	Jennings et al. (2017)

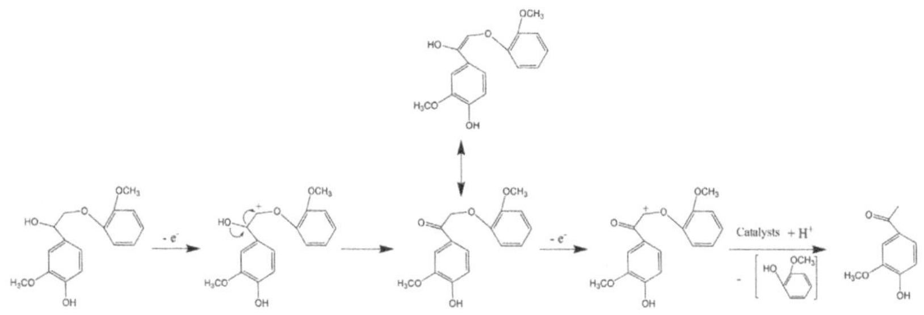

FIGURE 22.5 Metal-catalyzed cleavage of β-O-4 linkages: A compensatory mechanism.

Source: Reproduced with permission from Elsevier (Chio et al., 2019)

solid catalysts, facilitating the chemical reaction during depolymerization. This approach showed considerable potential for process selectivity, along with the minimization of the required reaction temperature (Wang et al., 2013).

Hi-Ming Su, Jack Twilton, and their team (2022) analyzed an alternative energy source and decided to work with 4-hydroxybenzoic acid, vanillic acid, and syringic acid, which are derived from hardwood lignin. They treated the system electrochemically using Ni/DPEPhos as a catalyst, $NiCl_2$/phenanthroline/PdC12/phosphine as a cocatalyst, and Zn as a chemical reductant; this yielded the by-product biphenyl-4,4′-dicarboxylic acid (BPDA), which they used as a plasticizer.

Metal-catalyzed depolymerization looks promising, but there are still limitations with catalyst selectivity, stability, and recyclability. Reaction conditions also need to be optimized to maximize product yields while reducing side reactions.

22.2.5.2 Hydrogenolysis Depolymerization

In hydrogenolysis lignin depolymerization, lignin linkages are usually broken by hydrogen gas (H_2) and an appropriate catalyst (Dou et al., 2022). This technique has attracted interest because it has the potential to produce high-quality, low-oxygen lignin-derived compounds and can operate under very moderate conditions compared to other depolymerization processes. Known catalysts for lignin depolymerization in hydrogenolysis are transition metals, including ruthenium (Ru), nickel (Ni), palladium (Pd), platinum (Pt), and nickel (Ni). These catalysts promote the hydrogenation of lignin bonds by cleaving and fragmenting lignin into smaller fragments (Xiao et al., 2017). Hydrogenolysis reactions usually occur in the presence of hydrogen gas over a range of pressures (1–50 bar) and temperatures (100–300°C). The catalyst loading, reaction time, and solvent selection can also impact the process's efficiency and selectivity. Hydrogen gas combines with ether, carbonyl, and carboxyl bonds in the lignin polymer to cause hydrogenation and subsequent breakdown of bonds. Normally, the end products have the potential to yield useful compounds and intermediates that can be used to make fuels, polymers, resins, and specialized chemicals, which can serve as alternatives to fossil fuels, helping create renewable and sustainable options. Catalyst deactivation, product selectivity, and the need for effective lignin pretreatment techniques to improve accessibility and reactivity are among the challenges in hydrogenolysis lignin depolymerization. Additionally, optimization is needed to maximize overall process efficiency and economic feasibility when implementing hydrogenolysis into biorefinery processes. The development of effective catalysts, understanding of reaction processes, and optimization of process conditions remain the main areas of research for scalable, affordable depolymerization of lignin by hydrogenolysis. Table 22.8 provides an overview of reductive lignin depolymerization results (Dou et al., 2021, 2022; H. Li et al., 2020; T. Li et al., 2020; Xiao et al., 2017; Q. Wang et al., 2017; Kloekhorst et al., 2015).

22.2.6 Ionic Liquid-Assisted Depolymerization

Salts with a melting point below 100°C are usually referred to as ionic liquids. Being a "designer solvent and/or catalyst" (Zhu et al., 2018) implies that it has adaptable characteristics that can be transformed by modifying the amounts of anions and cations present in the salt and having a low melting point, minimal vapor pressure, among other features, which make it easy to change the salt into a high concentration ionic liquid while providing a favorable condition for electrochemical reactions (Chio et al., 2019). Ionic liquids (ILs) offer unique qualities, such as good thermal stability and flexible chemical structures, making them an interesting choice as catalysts in depolymerization (Huddleston et al., 2001). Unlike other solvents, ILs have significant potential for dissolving a variety of biomasses, thereby boosting the management of natural resources (Hossain and Aldous, 2012). Some ILs have inherent catalytic activity that may promote base- or acid-catalyzed processes that lead to lignin depolymerization. Specific products can be formed by selectively cleaving lignin linkages with ILs containing basic or acidic functional groups (Zhu et al., 2018). Lignin depolymerization processes aided by ILs often occur at mild temperatures and pressures, minimizing environmental impacts and energy consumption. Different ILs and reaction conditions employ different methods for lignin depolymerization. While basic ILs can break activated lignin bonds in a nucleophilic way, in the absence of H+, acidic ILs may protonate lignin functional groups, making it possible for the bond to break.

Zhang-Min Li et al. (2020) used herbaceous lignin to produce methyl *p*-hydroxycinnamate (MPC), where they added M-DES $ChCl[FeCl_3]_2$ as a catalyst and ChCl: $FeCl_3$ (1:2) as ionic solvent under a mild temperature of 160°C for 8 hr. They used 50 mg lignin and 0.1–0.5 mmol M-DES catalyst with 5–15 mL methanol, stirred at 500 rpm in an oil bath to maintain a temperature of 120–200°C; they obtained methyl phydroxycinnamate (MPC) with a yield of 105.8 mg/g (74.1%) as a byproduct. On the other hand, when methanol/choline chloride (MeOHChCl) was used as an ionic solvent and $Cu(OAc)_2$/1,10-phenanthroline as a catalyst for alkali lignin at 0.4–3.0 MPa O_2, 60°C for 3 hr,

TABLE 22.8
Reductive Lignin Depolymerization

Lignin Type	Reaction Condition	Major Product	Yield	Reference
Native poplar lignin	Pd-PdO/TiO_2 catalyst, 180°C, self-hydrogen transfer hydrogenolysis (STH)	Monomers	40 *wt%*	Dou et al. (2022)
Kraft lignin	$ZnCoO_x$ nanoplate catalyst/1, 4-dioxane and methanol, 2 MPa H_2, 300°C for 24 hr	Monomers and dimers	71% wt%	Dou et al. (2021)
Lignin	La^{3+}-doped Ni/MgO catalyst, hydrogenolysis, 270°C for 4 hr	4-Ethyl phenol Biochar	7.17% wt% 11.04% wt%	H. Li et al. (2020)
Lignin	Ru nanoparticles (Ru/NCM-10) supported N_2-doped carbon, >700°C, hydrogenolysis	Aromatic monomers	40.7% wt%	T. Li et al. (2020)
Enzymatic mild acidolysis lignins (EMALs)	Nanostructured MoO_x/CNT, under H_2 atmosphere MeOH/EtOH/PrOH/ethylene glycol solvent	Lignin oil Monomers	29–67 wt% 14–33 wt%	Xiao et al. (2017)
Kraft lignin	$S_2O_8^{2-}$-KNO_3/TiO_2; co-catalyst, Ru/C, 320°C for 6 hr	Monomeric and dimeric degradation products	60–93%	J. Wang et al. (2017)
Alcell® lignin	Ru/C catalyst, formic acid, 673 K, 4 hr, IPA/FA solvent/ethanol/FA solvent/methanol/FA solvent	Lignin oil Aromatics Alkylphenolics Catechols Guaiacols Alkanes	71.2–63.4 wt% 10–10.6 wt% 6-19.2 wt% 8.7 wt% 1.3 wt% 5.2 wt%	Kloekhorst et al. (2015)

46.09% and 40.64% acetovanillone and acetic acid, respectively, were obtained; as by-products, vanillic acid, vanillin, 2-methoxy-4-vinylphenol, 2-methoxyphenol, dihydroconiferyl alcohol, among others, were also obtained (Hdidou et al., 2018). While double enzymatic lignin (DEL) was extracted from *Eucalyptus*, after it was allowed to react with ChCl:lactic acid (1:10) ionic solvent at 60–140°C for 6 hr, the C—O and C—C bonds in the lignin were broken, which separated the aryl ether linkage (β-O-4), which is one of the main chains in lignin nanoparticle, having less aliphatic hydroxyl groups and higher phenolic hydroxyl. With an increase in temperature, 8.0 g/kg lignin converted into 2.5 g/kg guaiacol, 0.31 g/kg guaiacylacetone, 1.0 g/kg vanillin, 0.6 g/kg syringaldehyde, and 0.08 g/kg acetovanillone (Shen et al., 2020).

Despite its promise, IL-assisted lignin depolymerization faces some difficulties, including high cost, potential toxicity, and the recovery and recycling of ILs. Reusing or recycling ILs is crucial, as their high cost significantly limits commercial lignin depolymerization. Reaction product evaluation and industrial chemical purification are among the requirements for separating products from ILs (Zakzeski et al., 2010). The main goal is to create affordable ILs, enhance IL recovery techniques, and provide insight into how IL-based activities affect the environment. Table 22.9 provides details of some ionic-liquid-based lignin depolymerization results (Cox and Ekerdt, 2012; Pinkert et al., 2011; Stärk et al., 2010).

22.3 CONCLUSION: CHALLENGES AND FUTURE PERSPECTIVE

The chapter delves extensively into a vital part of lignin valorization, that is, depolymerization, by implementing physical, chemical, and thermal conditions. The monomers or oligomers can be further used downstream for biochemical and energy applications. Lignin is biosynthesized by random coupling of its monolignols, giving it a 3D structure that is resistant to biological/chemical degradation. The heterogeneity of lignin structure across different feedstocks and isolation methods makes it difficult to formulate depolymerization pathways (H. Wang et al., 2019). Special care must be taken during the design of the biomass fractionation to prevent recondensation of the reactive lignin stream. The interplay of these factors determines the necessary condition and the extent of cleavage that can be attained on the native inter-unit ether linkage in the lignin matrix (Brienza et al., 2023). Hence, a combination of factors, like biomass fractionation, lignin's native structure, targeted end product, energy consumption, scale-up probability, environmental impact, economic valuation, conversion efficiency, and downstream processing, dictates the method to be adopted (Chio et al., 2019).

Selecting the appropriate depolymerization method for specific reactions and end products tailored to a particular application is necessary to efficiently utilize lignin for value addition (Zhou et al., 2022a). At the same time, tailored/novel catalysts to depolymerize lignin and generate specific end products are required to enhance the output of the valorization process. Nanotechnology can significantly alter the efficacy of lignin depolymerization. These targeted conversions

TABLE 22.9
Ionic Liquid-Assisted Lignin Depolymerization

Lignin Type	Reaction Condition	Major Product	Yield	Reference
Lignin	1-Ethyl-3-methylimidazolium acetate ([C_2mim][OAc]), TiO_2/AgCl nanoparticles, 120°C	Vanillin Guaiacol	3 g/kg 1 g/kg	Pena et al. (2024)
Alkaline lignin	Lactic acid and choline chloride (deep eutectic solvent thermal degradation), 180°C and 9 hr	Aromatic monomers Vanillin butyrovanillone	12.56% 0.67% 0.64%	P. Li et al. (2023)
Lignin model compound with 2-phenoxy-aceto-phenone and 2-(2-methoxy-phenoxy)-1-phenyl-ethanone with methoxyl group	1-Octyl-3-methylimidazolium acetate [OMIm][OAc] solvent; O_2, H_2O, 373 K	Phenol Benzoic acid	96–98% 85–86%	Yang et al. (2017)
Lignin	HCl as the catalyst; 120°C, 8 hr, and lignin-to-IL mass ratio of 1:10 with BnMIMCl (IL) and BnMIMTFA (IL)	Vanillic acid, acetovanillone, isovanillin, 1-(4-hydroxy-3-methoxyphenyl)-ethanone, acetophenone	75.45% [BnMIMCl (IL)] about 60% [BnMIMTFA (IL)]	Xue and Yan, (2014)
Oak wood lignin	1-Methyl-3-ethyl-imi-dazoliumacetate with acidic ionic liquid 1-H-3-methylimidazolium chloride under mild conditions, 110–150°C	Alkyl-aryl ether Linkage cleavage	–	Cox and Ekerdt, (2012)
Wood lignin	dry N2, with both ILs 1-butyl-3-methylimidazolium acesulfamate ([BMIM]Ace) and 1-ethyl-3 methylimidazolium acesulfamate ([EMIM]Ace); 473 K, 2hr, 10Kpa pressure	Monomers, dimers	–	Pinkert et al. (2011)
Beech lignin	Mn $(NO_3)_2$ in 1-ethyl-3-methylimidazolium trifluoromethanesulfonate [EMIM][CF3SO3]; 24 hr at 100°C, 84 × 10^5 Pa air	Syringaldehyde, 2,6-Dimethoxy-1,4-benzoquinone (DMBQ).	66.3% (11.5 wt% DMBQ)	Stärk et al. (2010)

can significantly reduce the downstream processing costs of the derived product. An approach for a continuous depolymerization system can alleviate degradation efficiency, facilitate catalyst reclamation, and improve the industrial perspective of the lignin biorefinery (Nandiwale et al., 2020).

REFERENCES

Abdelaziz, O.Y., Clemmensen, I., Meier, S., Bjelić, S., Hulteberg, C.P., Riisager, A., 2023. Oxidative depolymerization of kraft lignin to aromatics over bimetallic V – Cu/ZrO2 catalysts. *Top. Catal.* 66, 1369–1380. https://doi.org/10.1007/s11244-023-01826-3

Abdelaziz, O.Y., Clemmensen, I., Meier, S., Costa, C.A.E., Rodrigues, A.E., Hulteberg, C.P., Riisager, A., 2022. On the oxidative valorization of lignin to high-value chemicals: A critical review of opportunities and challenges. *ChemSusChem* 15, e202201232. https://doi.org/10.1002/cssc.202201232

Abdelaziz, O.Y., Li, K., Tunå, P., Hulteberg, C.P., 2018. Continuous catalytic depolymerisation and conversion of industrial kraft lignin into low-molecular-weight aromatics. *Biomass Convers. Biorefinery* 8, 455–470. https://doi.org/10.1007/s13399-017-0294-2

Abhayasimha, K.C., Rao, C.S., Nair, V., 2024. Combination of ensemble machine learning models in photocatalytic studies using nano TiO2 – lignin based biochar. *Chemosphere* 352, 141326. https://doi.org/10.1016/J.Chemosphere.2024.141326

Agarwal, A., Jo, Y.T., Park, J.H., 2021. Hybrid microwave-ultrasound assisted catalyst-free depolymerization of kraft lignin to bio-oil. *Ind. Crops Prod.* 162, 113300. https://doi.org/10.1016/j.indcrop.2021.113300

Almada, C.C., Kazachenko, A., Fongarland, P., Perez, D.D.S., Kuznetsov, B.N., Djakovitch, L., 2021. Supported-metal catalysts in upgrading lignin to aromatics by oxidative depolymerization. *Catalysts* 11. https://doi.org/10.3390/catal11040467

Asawaworarit, P., Daorattanachai, P., Laosiripojana, W., Sakdaronnarong, C., Shotipruk, A., Laosiripojana, N., 2019. Catalytic depolymerization of organosolv lignin from bagasse by carbonaceous solid acids derived from hydrothermal of lignocellulosic compounds. *Chem. Eng. J.* 356, 461–471. https://doi.org/10.1016/j.cej.2018.09.048

Banu, R.J., Sugitha, S., Kavitha, S., Kannah, Y.R., Merrylin, J., Kumar, G., 2021. Lignocellulosic biomass pretreatment for enhanced bioenergy recovery: Effect of lignocelluloses recalcitrance and enhancement strategies. *Front. Energy Res.* 9, 646057. https://doi.org/10.3389/fenrg.2021.646057

Bernhardt, J.J., Rößiger, B., Hahn, T., Pufky-Heinrich, D., 2021. Kinetic modeling of the continuous hydrothermal base-catalyzed depolymerization of pine wood-based kraft lignin in pilot scale. *Ind. Crops Prod.* 159, 113119. https://doi.org/10.1016/J.INDCROP.2020.113119

Biswas, B., Kumar, A., Kaur, R., Krishna, B.B., Bhaskar, T., 2021. Catalytic hydrothermal liquefaction of alkali lignin over activated bio-char supported bimetallic catalyst. *Bioresour. Technol.* 337, 125439. https://doi.org/10.1016/j.biortech.2021.125439

Bridgwater, A.V., 2012. Review of fast pyrolysis of biomass and product upgrading. *Biomass and Bioenergy* 38, 68–94. https://doi.org/10.1016/j.biombioe.2011.01.048

Brienza, F., Cannella, D., Montesdeoca, D., Cybulska, I., Debecker, D.P., 2023. A guide to lignin valorization in biorefineries: Traditional, recent, and forthcoming approaches to convert raw lignocellulose into valuable materials and chemicals. *RSC Sustain.* 2, 37. https://doi.org/10.1039/d3su00140g

Bundhoo, Z.M.A., 2018. Microwave-assisted conversion of biomass and waste materials to biofuels. *Renew. Sustain. Energy Rev.* 82, 1149–1177. https://doi.org/10.1016/j.rser.2017.09.066

Cao, L., Yu, I.K.M., Liu, Y., Ruan, X., Tsang, D.C.W., Hunt, A.J., Ok, Y.S., Song, H., Zhang, S., 2018. Lignin valorization for the production of renewable chemicals: State-of-the-art review and future prospects. *Bioresour. Technol.* 269, 465–475. https://doi.org/10.1016/j.biortech.2018.08.065

Cao, Y., Chen, S.S., Tsang, D.C.W., Clark, J.H., Budarin, V.L., Hu, C., Wu, K.C.W., Zhang, S., 2020. Microwave-assisted depolymerization of various types of waste lignins over two-dimensional CuO/BCN catalysts. *Green Chem.* 22, 725–736. https://doi.org/10.1039/c9gc03553b

Chaudhary, R., Dhepe, P.L., 2017. Solid base catalyzed depolymerization of lignin into low molecular weight products. *Green Chem.* 19, 778–788. https://doi.org/10.1039/c6gc02701f

Chaudhary, R., Dhepe, P.L., 2019. Depolymerization of lignin using a solid base catalyst. *Energy and Fuels* 33, 4369–4377. https://doi.org/10.1021/acs.energyfuels.9b00621

Chen, Y., Duan, P., Dong, L., Zhu, C., Jin, L., Tian, F., 2021. The study of hydrothermal liquefaction of corn straw with nano ferrite + inorganic base catalyst system at low temperature. *Bioresour. Technol.* 333, 125185. https://doi.org/10.1016/j.biortech.2021.125185

Chio, C., Sain, M., Qin, W., 2019. Lignin utilization: A review of lignin depolymerization from various aspects. *Renew. Sustain. Energy Rev.* 107, 232–249. https://doi.org/10.1016/j.rser.2019.03.008

Cox, B.J., Ekerdt, J.G., 2012. Depolymerization of oak wood lignin under mild conditions using the acidic ionic liquid 1-H-3-methylimidazolium chloride as both solvent and catalyst. *Bioresour. Technol.* 118, 584–588. https://doi.org/10.1016/j.biortech.2012.05.012

Crestini, C., Caponi, M.C., Argyropoulos, D.S., Saladino, R., 2006. Immobilized methyltrioxo rhenium (MTO)/H2O2 systems for the oxidation of lignin and lignin model compounds. *Bioorganic Med. Chem.* 14, 5292–5302. https://doi.org/10.1016/j.bmc.2006.03.046

Dai, J., Styles, G.N., Patti, A.F., Saito, K., 2018. CuSO4/H2O2-catalyzed lignin depolymerization under the irradiation of microwaves. *ACS Omega* 3, 10433–10441. https://doi.org/10.1021/acsomega.8b01978

De Caprariis, B., Bracciale, M.P., Bavasso, I., Chen, G., Damizia, M., Genova, V., Marra, F., Paglia, L., Pulci, G., Scarsella, M., Tai, L., De Filippis, P., 2020. Unsupported Ni metal catalyst in hydrothermal liquefaction of oak wood: Effect of catalyst surface modification. *Sci. Total Environ.* 709, 136215. https://doi.org/10.1016/j.scitotenv.2019.136215

de Carvalho, D.M., Colodette, J.L., 2017. Comparative study of acid hydrolysis of lignin and polysaccharides in biomasses. *BioResources.* 12(4), 6907–6923.

Deepa, A.K., Dhepe, P.L., 2015. Lignin depolymerization into aromatic monomers over solid acid catalysts. *ACS Catal.* 5, 365–379. https://doi.org/10.1021/cs501371q

Deng, W., Zhang, H., Wu, X., Li, R., Zhang, Q., Wang, Y., 2015. Oxidative conversion of lignin and lignin model compounds catalyzed by CeO2-supported Pd nanoparticles. *Green Chem.* 17, 5009–5018. https://doi.org/10.1039/c5gc01473e

Dhar, P., Vinu, R., 2017. Understanding lignin depolymerization to phenols via microwave-assisted solvolysis process. *J. Environ. Chem. Eng.* 5, 4759–4768. https://doi.org/10.1016/j.jece.2017.08.031

Dong, Z., Yang, H., Liu, Z., Chen, P., Chen, Y., Wang, X., Chen, H., Wang, S., 2022. Pyrolysis of boron-crosslinked lignin: Influence on lignin softening and product properties. *Bioresour. Technol.* 355, 127218. https://doi.org/10.1016/J.BIORTECH.2022.127218

Dou, X., Li, W., Zhu, C., 2021. Catalytic hydrotreatment of kraft lignin into liquid fuels over porous ZnCoOx nanoplates. *Fuel* 283, 118801. https://doi.org/10.1016/j.fuel.2020.118801

Dou, Z., Zhang, Z., Wang, M., 2022. Self-hydrogen transfer hydrogenolysis of native lignin over Pd-PdO/TiO2. *Appl. Catal. B Environ.* 301, 120767. https://doi.org/10.1016/J.APCATB.2021.120767

Du, B., Chen, C., Sun, Y., Yang, M., Yu, M., Liu, B., Wang, X., Zhou, J., 2020. Efficient and controllable ultrasound-assisted depolymerization of organosolv lignin catalyzed to liquid fuels by MCM-41 supported phosphotungstic acid. *RSC Adv.* 10, 31479–31494. https://doi.org/10.1039/d0ra05069e

Du, B., Liu, B., Yang, Y., Wang, X., Zhou, J., 2019. A phosphotungstic acid catalyst for depolymerization in bulrush lignin. *Catalysts* 9. https://doi.org/10.3390/catal9050399

Duan, D., Wang, Y., Dai, L., Ruan, R., Zhao, Y., Fan, L., Tayier, M., Liu, Y., 2017. Ex-situ catalytic co-pyrolysis of lignin and polypropylene to upgrade bio-oil quality by microwave heating. *Bioresour. Technol.* 241, 207–213. https://doi.org/10.1016/j.biortech.2017.04.104

Farooq, A., Shiung Lam, S., Hoon Rhee, G., Lee, J., Ali Khan, M., Jeon, B.H., Park, Y.K., 2022. Technical benefits of using methane as a pyrolysis medium for catalytic pyrolysis of kraft lignin. *Bioresour. Technol.* 353, 127131. https://doi.org/10.1016/J.BIORTECH.2022.127131

Feng, L., Li, X., Wang, Z., Liu, B., 2021. Catalytic hydrothermal liquefaction of lignin for production of aromatic hydrocarbons over metal-supported mesoporous catalyst. *Bioresour. Technol.* 323, 124569. https://doi.org/10.1016/j.biortech.2020.124569

Gao, C., Li, M., Zhu, C., Hu, Y., Shen, T., Li, M., Ji, X., Lyu, G., Zhuang, W., 2021. One-pot depolymerization, demethylation, and phenolation of lignin catalyzed by HBr under microwave irradiation for phenolic foam preparation. *Compos. Part B Eng.* 205, 108530. https://doi.org/10.1016/j.compositesb.2020.108530

Gasson, J.R., Forchheim, D., Sutter, T., Hornung, U., Kruse, A., Barth, T., 2012. Modeling the lignin degradation kinetics in an ethanol/formic acid solvolysis approach. Part 1. Kinetic model development. *Ind. Eng. Chem. Res.* 51, 10595–10606. https://doi.org/10.1021/ie301487v

Güvenatam, B., Heeres, E.H.J., Pidko, E.A., Hensen, E.J.M., 2016. Lewis acid-catalyzed depolymerization of soda lignin in supercritical ethanol/water mixtures. *Catal. Today* 269, 9–20. https://doi.org/10.1016/j.cattod.2015.08.039

Hdidou, L., Khallouk, K., Solhy, A., Manoun, B., Oukarroum, A., Barakat, A., 2018. Synthesis of CoFeO mixed oxides via an alginate gelation process as efficient heterogeneous catalysts for lignin depolymerization in water. *Catal. Sci. Technol.* 8, 5445–5453. https://doi.org/10.1039/c8cy00576a

Hoang, A.T., Ong, H.C., Fattah, I.M.R., Chong, C.T., Cheng, C.K., Sakthivel, R., Ok, Y.S., 2021. Progress on the lignocellulosic biomass pyrolysis for biofuel production toward environmental sustainability. *Fuel Process. Technol.* 223, 106997. https://doi.org/10.1016/j.fuproc.2021.106997

Hossain, M.M., Aldous, L., 2012. Ionic liquids for lignin processing: Dissolution, isolation, and conversion. *Aust. J. Chem.* 65, 1465–1477. https://doi.org/10.1071/CH12324

Hu, Y., Gu, Z., Li, W., Xu, C.C., 2020. Alkali-catalyzed liquefaction of pinewood sawdust in ethanol/water co-solvents. *Biomass and Bioenergy* 134, 105485. https://doi.org/10.1016/j.biombioe.2020.105485

Huang, A.N., Hsu, C.P., Hou, B.R., Kuo, H.P., 2018. Production and separation of rice husk pyrolysis bio-oils from a fractional distillation column connected fluidized bed reactor. *Powder Technol.* 323, 588–593. https://doi.org/10.1016/j.powtec.2016.03.052

Huddleston, J.G., Visser, A.E., Reichert, W.M., Willauer, H.D., Broker, G.A., Rogers, R.D., 2001. Characterization and comparison of hydrophilic and hydrophobic room temperature ionic liquids incorporating the imidazolium cation. *Green Chem.* 3, 156–164. https://doi.org/10.1039/b103275p

Jennings, J.A., Parkin, S., Munson, E., Delaney, S.P., Calahan, J.L., Isaacs, M., Hong, K., Crocker, M., 2017. Regioselective Baeyer-Villiger oxidation of lignin model compounds with tin beta zeolite catalyst and hydrogen peroxide. *RSC Adv.* 7, 25987–25997. https://doi.org/10.1039/c7ra03830e

Kishimoto, T., Kadla, J.F., Chang, H.M., Jameel, H., 2003. The reactions of lignin model compounds with hydrogen peroxide at low pH. *Holzforschung* 57, 52–58. https://doi.org/10.1515/HF.2003.008

Kloekhorst, A., Shen, Y., Yie, Y., Fang, M., Heeres, H.J., 2015. Catalytic hydrodeoxygenation and hydrocracking of Alcell® lignin in alcohol/formic acid mixtures using a Ru/C catalyst. *Biomass and Bioenergy* 80, 147–161. https://doi.org/10.1016/j.biombioe.2015.04.039

Kudo, S., Honda, E., Nishioka, S., Hayashi, J., 2021. Formation of p-p-p-unsubstituted phenols in base-catalyzed lignin depolymerization. *MATEC Web Conf.* 333, 05006. https://doi.org/10.1051/matecconf/202133305006

Kumar, G., Shobana, S., Chen, W.H., Bach, Q.V., Kim, S.H., Atabani, A.E., Chang, J.S., 2017. A review of thermochemical conversion of microalgal biomass for biofuels: Chemistry and processes. *Green Chem.* 19, 44–67. https://doi.org/10.1039/c6gc01937d

Lavoie, J.M., Baré, W., Bilodeau, M., 2011. Depolymerization of steam-treated lignin for the production of green chemicals. *Bioresour. Technol.* 102, 4917–4920. https://doi.org/10.1016/j.biortech.2011.01.010

Li, B., Liu, Y., Yang, T., Feng, B., Kai, X., Wang, S., Li, R., 2021. Aqueous phase reforming of biocrude derived from lignocellulose hydrothermal liquefaction: Conditions optimization and mechanism study. *Renew. Energy* 175, 98–107. https://doi.org/10.1016/j.renene.2021.04.127

Li, H., Zheng, X., Zhang, H., Li, X., Long, J., 2020. Selective cleavage of ester linkages in lignin catalyzed by La-doped Ni/MgO. ACS sustain. *Chem. Eng.* 8, 15685–15695. https://doi.org/10.1021/acssuschemeng.0c05360

Li, K., Prothmann, J., Sandahl, M., Blomberg, S., Turner, C., Hulteberg, C., 2021. Investigating lignin-derived monomers and oligomers in low-molecular-weight fractions separated from depolymerized black liquor retentate by membrane filtration. *Molecules* 26. https://doi.org/10.3390/molecules26102887

Li, L., Kong, J., Zhang, H., Liu, S., Zeng, Q., Zhang, Y., Ma, H., He, H., Long, J., Li, X., 2020. Selective aerobic oxidative cleavage of lignin C[sbnd]C bonds over novel hierarchical Ce-Cu/MFI nanosheets. *Appl. Catal. B Environ.* 279, 119343. https://doi.org/10.1016/j.apcatb.2020.119343

Li, P., Jiang, Z., Yang, C., Ren, J., Jiang, B., Wu, W., 2023. Degradation of Alkaline lignin in the lactic acid-choline chloride system under mild conditions. *J. Renew. Mater.* 11, 2233–2248. https://doi.org/10.32604/jrm.2023.025279

Li, T., Lin, H., Ouyang, X., Qiu, X., Wan, Z., Ruan, T., 2020. Impact of nitrogen species and content on the catalytic activity to C – O bond cleavage of lignin over N-doped carbon-supported Ru-based catalyst. *Fuel* 278, 118324. https://doi.org/10.1016/j.fuel.2020.118324

Li, T., Takkellapati, S., 2018. The current and emerging sources of technical lignins and their applications. *Biofuels, Bioprod. Biorefining* 12, 756–787. https://doi.org/10.1002/bbb.1913

Li, Z.M., Long, J.X., Zeng, Q., Wu, Y.H., Cao, M.L., Liu, S.J., Li, X.H., 2020. Production of methyl p-hydroxycinnamate by selective tailoring of herbaceous lignin using metal-based deep eutectic solvents (DES) as catalyst. *Ind. Eng. Chem. Res.* 59, 17328–17337. https://doi.org/10.1021/acs.iecr.0c01307

Li, Z.M., Zhang, H., Yang, D., Hu, Z., Wang, F., Zhang, Z., 2023. Efficient conversion of lignin to aromatics via catalytic fast pyrolysis over niobium-doped HZSM-5. *Molecules* 28. https://doi.org/10.3390/molecules28104245

Liang, J., Han, J., Zhou, M., Fakayode, O.A., Yagoub, A.E.A., Li, H., Ren, M., Kong, F., Zhou, C., 2024. Ultrasonic-enhanced photocatalysis through piezoelectric and cavitation effects for lignin depolymerization. *Int. J. Biol. Macromol.* 264, 130526. https://doi.org/10.1016/J.IJBIOMAC.2024.130526

Liu, B., Du, B., Sun, Y., Zhu, M., Yang, Y., Wang, X., Zhou, J., 2020. Ultrasound acoustic cavitation enhances depolymerization of organosolv lignin to phenolic monomers and low molecular weight lignin bio-oils. *Fuel Process. Technol.* 203, 106387. https://doi.org/10.1016/j.fuproc.2020.106387

Liu, C., Liu, B., Wang, X., Xie, Z., Tong, L., Kong, X., Fan, Y., Xiao, R., 2022. Tandem strategy of photocatalytic preoxidation-ultrasonic cavitation depolymerization for lignin valorization. *Bioresour. Technol.* 363, 127880. https://doi.org/10.1016/J.BIORTECH.2022.127880

Liu, X., Bouxin, F.P., Fan, J., Budarin, V.L., Hu, C., Clark, J.H., 2020. Recent advances in the catalytic depolymerization of lignin towards phenolic chemicals: A review. *ChemSusChem* 13, 4296–4317. https://doi.org/10.1002/cssc.202001213

Liu, X., Bouxin, F.P., Fan, J., Budarin, V.L., Hu, C., Clark, J.H., 2021. Microwave-assisted catalytic depolymerization of lignin from birch sawdust to produce phenolic monomers utilizing a hydrogen-free strategy. *J. Hazard. Mater.* 402, 123490. https://doi.org/10.1016/j.jhazmat.2020.123490

Lui, M.Y., Chan, B., Yuen, A.K.L., Masters, A.F., Maschmeyer, T., 2020. Hydrothermal liquefaction of α-O-4 aryl ether linkages in lignin. *ChemSusChem* 13, 2002–2006. https://doi.org/10.1002/cssc.201903263

Luo, J., Fang, Z., Smith, R.L., 2014. Ultrasound-enhanced conversion of biomass to biofuels. *Prog. Energy Combust. Sci.* 41, 56–93. https://doi.org/10.1016/j.pecs.2013.11.001

Mahmood, N., Yuan, Z., Schmidt, J., Xu, C.C., 2015. Hydrolytic depolymerization of hydrolysis lignin: Effects of catalysts and solvents. *Bioresour. Technol.* 190, 416–419. https://doi.org/10.1016/j.biortech.2015.04.074

Nandiwale, K.Y., Danby, A.M., Ramanathan, A., Chaudhari, R.V., Motagamwala, A.H., Dumesic, J.A., Subramaniam, B., 2020. Enhanced acid-catalyzed lignin depolymerization in a continuous reactor with stable activity. *ACS Sustain. Chem. Eng.* 8, 4096–4106. https://doi.org/10.1021/acssuschemeng.9b06556

Nandiwale, K.Y., Danby, A.M., Ramanathan, A., Chaudhari, R.V., Subramaniam, B., 2019. Dual function Lewis acid catalyzed depolymerization of industrial corn stover lignin into stable monomeric phenols. *ACS Sustain. Chem. Eng.* 7, 1362–1371. https://doi.org/10.1021/acssuschemeng.8b05077

Paananen, H., Alvila, L., Pakkanen, T.T., 2021. Hydroxymethylation of softwood kraft lignin and phenol with paraformaldehyde. *Sustain. Chem. Pharm.* 20, 100376. https://doi.org/10.1016/j.scp.2021.100376

Pena, C.A., Rodil, E., Rodríguez, H., 2024. Capacity of aqueous solutions of the ionic liquid 1-ethyl-3-methylimidazolium acetate to partially depolymerize lignin at ambient temperature and pressure. *J. Agric. Food Chem.* 72, 1136–1145. https://doi.org/10.1021/acs.jafc.3c04047

Pinkert, A., Goeke, D.F., Marsh, K.N., Pang, S., 2011. Extracting wood lignin without dissolving or degrading cellulose: Investigations on the use of food additive-derived ionic liquids. *Green Chem.* 13, 3124–3136. https://doi.org/10.1039/c1gc15671c

Prabhudesai, V.S., Saravanakumar, K., Gurrala, L., Vinu, R., 2023. Ultrasound-assisted low-temperature catalytic lignin-first depolymerization of pine wood biomass to selectively produce propyl guaiacol. *Sustain. Energy Fuels* 7, 2117–2129. https://doi.org/10.1039/d2se01796b

Purushothaman, R.K.P., van Erven, G., van Es, D.S., Rohrbach, L., Frissen, A.E., van Haveren, J., Gosselink, R.J.A., 2023. New insights into the base-catalyzed depolymerization of technical lignins: A systematic comparison. *RSC Adv.* 13, 4898–4909. https://doi.org/10.1039/d2ra06998a

Ren, T., Qi, W., Su, R., He, Z., 2019. Promising techniques for depolymerization of lignin into value-added chemicals. *ChemCatChem* 11, 639–654. https://doi.org/10.1002/cctc.201801428

Roberts, V.M., Stein, V., Reiner, T., Lemonidou, A., Li, X., Lercher, J.A., 2011. Towards quantitative catalytic lignin depolymerization. *Chem. – A Eur.* J. 17, 5939–5948. https://doi.org/10.1002/chem.201002438

Roy, R., Rahman, M.S., Amit, T.A., Jadhav, B., 2022. Recent advances in lignin depolymerization techniques: A comparative overview of traditional and greener approaches. *Biomass* 2, 130–154. https://doi.org/10.3390/biomass2030009

Schieppati, D., Dreux, A., Gao, W., Fatehi, P., Boffito, D.C., 2022. Ultrasound-assisted carboxymethylation of lignoforce kraft lignin to produce biodispersants. *J. Clean. Prod.* 366, 132776. https://doi.org/10.1016/J.JCLEPRO.2022.132776

Shen, X.J., Chen, T., Wang, H.M., Mei, Q., Yue, F., Sun, S., Wen, J.L., Yuan, T.Q., Sun, R.C., 2020. Structural and morphological transformations of lignin macromolecules during bio-based deep eutectic solvent (DES) pretreatment. *ACS Sustain. Chem. Eng.* 8, 2130–2137. https://doi.org/10.1021/acssuschemeng.9b05106

Singh, R., Prakash, A., Dhiman, S.K., Balagurumurthy, B., Arora, A.K., Puri, S.K., Bhaskar, T., 2014. Hydrothermal conversion of lignin to substituted phenols and aromatic ethers. *Bioresour. Technol.* 165, 319–322. https://doi.org/10.1016/j.biortech.2014.02.076

Solt, P., Rößiger, B., Konnerth, J., van Herwijnen, H.W.G., 2018. Lignin phenol formaldehyde resoles using base-catalysed depolymerized kraft lignin. *Polymers (Basel)* 10, 1–11. https://doi.org/10.3390/polym10101162

Song, W.L., Dong, Q., Hong, L., Tian, Z.Q., Tang, L.N., Hao, W., Zhang, H., 2019. Activating molecular oxygen with Au/CeO2 for the conversion of lignin model compounds and organosolv lignin. *RSC Adv.* 9, 31070–31077. https://doi.org/10.1039/c9ra04838c

Stärk, K., Taccardi, N., Bösmann, A., Wasserscheid, P., 2010. Oxidative depolymerization of lignin in ionic liquids. *ChemSusChem* 3, 719–723. https://doi.org/10.1002/cssc.200900242

Su, Z.M., Twilton, J., Hoyt, C.B., Wang, F., Stanley, L., Mayes, H.B., Kang, K., Weix, D.J., Beckham, G.T., Stahl, S.S., 2022. Ni- and Ni/Pd-catalyzed reductive coupling of lignin-derived aromatics to access biobased plasticizers. *ACS Cent. Sci.* https://doi.org/10.1021/acscentsci.2c01324

Tayier, M., Duan, D., Zhao, Y., Ruan, R., Wang, Y., Liu, Y., 2018. Depolymerization of lignin. *BioResources* 13, 412–424.

Thring, R.W., 1995. Alkaline degradation of Alcell lignin. *Biomass and Bioenergy* 7, 125–130.

Wang, H., Pu, Y., Ragauskas, A., Yang, B., 2019. From lignin to valuable products – strategies, challenges, and prospects. *Bioresour. Technol.* 271, 449–461. https://doi.org/10.1016/j.biortech.2018.09.072

Wang, H., Tucker, M., Ji, Y., 2013. Recent development in chemical depolymerization of lignin: A review. *J. Appl. Chem.* 2013, 1–9. https://doi.org/10.1155/2013/838645

Wang, J., Li, W., Wang, H., Ma, Q., Li, S., Chang, H.M., Jameel, H., 2017. Liquefaction of kraft lignin by hydrocracking with simultaneous use of a novel dual acid-base catalyst and a hydrogenation catalyst. *Bioresour. Technol.* 243, 100–106. https://doi.org/10.1016/j.biortech.2017.06.024

Wang, J., Minai, E., Kawamoto, H., 2022. Stable Oligomer Formation from Lignin by Pyrolysis of Softwood in an Aprotic Solvent with a Hydrogen Donor. ChemistryOpen 11. https://doi.org/10.1002/open.202200104

Wang, Q., Guan, S., Shen, D., 2017. Experimental and kinetic study on lignin depolymerization in water/formic acid system. *Int. J. Mol. Sci.* 18. https://doi.org/10.3390/ijms18102082

Wang, W., Ma, Z., Zhao, X., Liu, S., Cai, L., Shi, S.Q., Ni, Y., 2020. Effect of various microwave absorbents on the microwave-assisted lignin depolymerization process. *ACS Sustain. Chem. Eng.* 8, 16086–16090. https://doi.org/10.1021/acssuschemeng.0c04658

Wang, W., Wang, M., Huang, J., Zhao, X., Su, Y., Wang, Y., Li, X., 2019. Formate-assisted analytical pyrolysis of kraft lignin to phenols. *Bioresour. Technol.* 278, 464–467. https://doi.org/10.1016/j.biortech.2019.01.078

Wang, W., Wu, X., Chantapakul, T., Wang, D., Zhang, S., Ma, X., Ding, T., Ye, X., Liu, D., 2017. Acoustic cavitation assisted extraction of pectin from waste grapefruit peels: A green two-stage approach and its general mechanism. *Food Res. Int.* 102, 101–110. https://doi.org/10.1016/j.foodres.2017.09.087

Wanmolee, W., Daorattanachai, P., Laosiripojana, N., 2016. Depolymerization of organosolv lignin to valuable chemicals over homogeneous and heterogeneous acid catalysts. *Energy Procedia* 100, 173–177. https://doi.org/10.1016/j.egypro.2016.10.161

Weng, C., Peng, X., Han, Y., 2021. Depolymerization and conversion of lignin to value-added bioproducts by microbial and enzymatic catalysis. *Biotechnol. Biofuels* 14, 84. https://doi.org/10.1186/s13068-021-01934-w

Wu, Z., Zhu, X., Guo, H., Jiang, Y., Gu, X., 2019. A kinetic study of lignin pyrolysis over base catalyst during steam exploded depolymerization. *Catal. Today* 226–234. https://doi.org/10.1016/j.cattod.2018.04.044

Xiao, L.P., Wang, S., Li, H., Li, Z., Shi, Z.J., Xiao, L., Sun, R.C., Fang, Y., Song, G., 2017. Catalytic hydrogenolysis of lignins into phenolic compounds over carbon nanotube supported molybdenum oxide. *ACS Catal.* 7, 7535–7542. https://doi.org/10.1021/acscatal.7b02563

Xu, J., Yang, Y., Liu, B., Kong, Y., Du, B., Guo, Y., Zhou, J., Wang, X., 2022. Ultrasonic assisted enhanced catalytic effect of perovskite to promote depolymerization of lignin. *Int. J. Biol. Macromol.* 218, 431–438. https://doi.org/10.1016/J.IJBIOMAC.2022.07.120

Xu, L., He, Z., Zhang, H., Wu, S., Dong, C., Fang, Z., 2021. Production of aromatic amines via catalytic co-pyrolysis of lignin and phenol-formaldehyde resins with ammonia over commercial HZSM-5 zeolites. *Bioresour. Technol.* 320, 124252. https://doi.org/10.1016/j.biortech.2020.124252

Xu, Y., Burel, L., Goc, F., Fongarland, P., Philippe, R., Aubert, G., Aymonier, C., Rataboul, F., Djakovitch, L., 2021. Investigating (Pseudo)-heterogeneous Pd-Catalysts for kraft lignin depolymerization under mild aqueous basic conditions. *Catalysts* 11, 1311. https://doi.org/10.3390/catal11111311

Xue, L., Yan, L., 2014. Effect of hydrothermal carbonization reaction parameters on. *Environ. Prog. Sustain. Energy* 33, 676–680. https://doi.org/10.1002/ep

Yang, S., Yuan, T., Li, M., Sun, R., 2015. Hydrothermal degradation of lignin: Products analysis for phenol formaldehyde adhesive synthesis. *Int. J. Biol. Macromol.* 72, 54–62. https://doi.org/10.1016/j.ijbiomac.2014.07.048

Yang, Y., Fan, H., Meng, Q., Zhang, Z., Yang, G., Han, B., 2017. Ionic liquid [OMIm][OAc] directly inducing oxidation cleavage of the β-O-4 bond of lignin model compounds. *Chem. Commun.* 53, 8850–8853. https://doi.org/10.1039/c7cc04209d

Zakzeski, J., Bruijnincx, P.C.A., Jongerius, A.L., Weckhuysen, B.M., 2010. The catalytic valorization of lignin for the production of renewable chemicals. *Chem. Rev.* 110, 3552–3599. https://doi.org/10.1021/cr900354u

Zhang, C., Li, H., Lu, J., Zhang, X., Macarthur, K.E., Heggen, M., Wang, F., 2017. Promoting lignin depolymerization and restraining the condensation via an oxidation-hydrogenation strategy. *ACS Catal.* 7, 3419–3429. https://doi.org/10.1021/acscatal.7b00148

Zhang, J., Ge, Y., Li, Z., 2023. Catalytic hydrothermal liquefaction of alkali lignin for monophenols production over homologous biochar-supported copper catalysts in water. *Int. J. Biol. Macromol.* 253, 126656. https://doi.org/10.1016/J.IJBIOMAC.2023.126656

Zhang, L., Choi, C., Machida, H., Huo, Z., Norinaga, K., 2021. Catalytic hydrotreatment of alkaline lignin and its consequent influences on fast pyrolysis. *Carbon Resour. Convers.* 4, 219–229. https://doi.org/10.1016/j.crcon.2021.09.001

Zhou, N., Thilakarathna, W.P.D.W., He, Q.S., Rupasinghe, H.P.V., 2022a. A review: Depolymerization of lignin to generate high-value bio-products: Opportunities, challenges, and prospects. *Front. Energy Res.* 9, 758744. https://doi.org/10.3389/fenrg.2021.758744

Zhou, N., Yang, J., Lu, X., Xin, Z., Xu, C., He, Q., 2022b. Microwave-assisted depolymerization of lignin and a biphasic extraction method for the recovery of bio-oil and phenolic monomers. *J. Anal. Appl. Pyrolysis* 161, 105403. https://doi.org/10.1016/J.JAAP.2021.105403

Zhu, X., Peng, C., Chen, H., Chen, Q., Zhao, Z.K., Zheng, Q., Xie, H., 2018. Opportunities of ionic liquids for lignin utilization from biorefinery. *ChemistrySelect* 3, 7945–7962. https://doi.org/10.1002/slct.201801393

Zou, R., Wang, Y., Jiang, L., Yu, Z., Zhao, Y., Wu, Q., Dai, L., Ke, L., Liu, Y., Ruan, R., 2019. Microwave-assisted co-pyrolysis of lignin and waste oil catalyzed by hierarchical ZSM-5/MCM-41 catalyst to produce aromatic hydrocarbons. *Bioresour. Technol.* 289, 121609. https://doi.org/10.1016/j.biortech.2019.121609

Žula, M., Jasiukaitytė-Grojzdek, E., Grilc, M., Likozar, B., 2023. Understanding acid-catalysed lignin depolymerisation process by model aromatic compound reaction kinetics. *Chem. Eng. J.* 455. https://doi.org/10.1016/j.cej.2022.140912

23 Valorization of Lignin Derived from Lignocellulosic Biomass for Biochemical Production and Energy Applications

Mihir Acharya, Debosmita Sharmmah, Prasansa Rai, U. Jayakrishnan, Shashi Bhushan, and Siddhartha Moulik

23.1 INTRODUCTION

Lignocellulosic biomass is a cornerstone in the continuously evolving landscape of sustainable technologies. Lignocellulosic biomass is considered a carbon-neutral, renewable, and edible bioresource, as plants play a vital role in life on Earth. These are constituted mainly by varying lignin, cellulose, and hemicellulose proportions. Meanwhile, copious amounts of this biomass are available as waste or by-products of several agro-industrial and forestry processes. Hence, managing these residues also raises concern, as the traditional disposal route has been reported to impact environmental quality significantly. Recent investigations suggest that stubble-burning in surrounding paddy fields contributed 30–35% of Delhi-NCR's (India) air pollution during October–November 2021, lowering the air quality index to 401 (Govardhan et al., 2023). Hence, sustainable and cost-effective utilization of these biomasses has been in demand for decades, demonstrating immense valorization potential. Cellulose and hemicellulose are abundant sources of carbohydrates that can be converted into a wide range of value-added products, leaving behind lignin. Several technological interventions and process intensification have enabled continued improvement in separating cellulose/hemicellulose from biomass and in converting them into platform chemicals, biopolymers, methane, hydrogen, ethanol, lipids, biodiesel, and other products. However, lignin derived from biomass remains underutilized (Banu et al., 2021). Currently,

 DOI: 10.1201/9781003327608-23

lignin waste is used as a combustion fuel to meet the establishments' internal energy requirements. Several countries have published mandates to increase the use of second-generation biofuels, such as ethanol, as blends with petroleum (Wang et al., 2019). India has also published its roadmap to implement a 20% ethanol-petroleum blend to meet global emission standards and attain fuel independence (NITI Aayog, 2021). This increasing demand would produce more lignin than can be combusted. Further improvement in lignin utilization is required to make the lignocellulosic-biomass-based biorefinery system cost-competitive (Wang et al., 2019).

Lignin is the second-most-abundant naturally occurring polymer, after cellulose, accounting for 15–30% of biomass dry weight. Lignin acts as a cross-linker between cellulose and hemicellulose, binding the lignocellulosic matrix and strengthening the plant cell wall (Chio et al., 2019). It is a three-dimensional heteropolymer with high chain branching, intra- and inter-chain coupling, and an amorphous structure, showing variability across plant species and extraction techniques. Lignin is formed by the radical condensation of three monolignols (hydroxycinnamyl alcohols) of coniferyl alcohol, *p*-coumaryl alcohol, and syringyl alcohol. In the polymer, these monolignols form phenylpropanoid units of guaiacyl, *p*-hydroxyphenyl, and syringyl. The monomers are linked through chemical bonds of phenylcoumaran (β-5), dibenzodioxocin (5–5), resinol (β-β), biphenyl ether (5-O-4), and aryl ether (β-O-4) (Weng et al., 2021). The high frequency of ether linkages leads to the predominance of non-phenolic units over aromatic units in the lignin. Hence, lignin becomes resistant to low-redox-potential oxidoreductases such as peroxidases. The structural bulkiness and chemical linkages make the lignin polymer impervious to biological action and require harsher thermal/chemical action to induce structural changes (Ruiz-Dueñas and Martínez, 2009).

The growing acceptance of waste as wealth rather than an object of repugnance promotes the exploration of novel ways to utilize every component of waste material (Jayakrishnan et al., 2021). Lignin is now being identified as a promising feedstock due to its bulky carbonaceous aromatic skeleton, availability of functional groups, higher carbon-to-oxygen ratio, and high antioxidant capacity (Weng et al., 2021). However, most studies on the valorization of lignin lag behind in the commercial arena due to its recalcitrant nature, highly reactive depolymerized fractions, and low yields and quality of the end product (Wang et al., 2019). The efficient disruption of lignocellulosic biomass (LCB) and the extraction/separation of the released lignin polymers/oligomers are prerequisites for any downstream lignin valorization process. Designing and implementing a cost-effective, environmentally friendly, and high-yielding depolymerization method with simplified process control are essential to convert lignin further. The depolymerized lignin can be converted simultaneously or subsequently into simple phenols, nutraceuticals, hydrocarbons, polymers, cosmetics, drugs, bio-oil, syngas, and so forth. The subsequent sections of this chapter describe lignin separation from biomass, the different techniques used for depolymerization, the various valorization products of lignin and their production routes, and future perspectives on lignin biorefinery.

23.2 SEPARATION AND PURIFICATION OF LIGNIN

The primordial and crucial task in lignin biorefinery is the maximum delignification of LCB, followed by purification with a less condensed structure. Specific reactive components in lignin can be covalently linked to hemicellulose, requiring stronger conditions to separate the components. Hence, delignification involves rupture of these covalent linkages and partial depolymerization of lignin into oligomers that facilitate further solubilization from biomass into the bulk. The high reactivity of these smaller fractions can form new C—C bonds, leading to repolymerization and the formation of different intermediates with varying properties. Therefore, the structure of lignin separated is influenced by the feedstock used, the extraction route adopted, and the extent of extraction (Wang et al., 2019).

The biorefinery approach has been extensively investigated for delignification to convert LCBs into a wide variety of bio-based products, including methane, ethanol, hydrogen, biodiesel, nanocellulose, and others. Separating cellulose from other components was the primary focus, leaving lignin as a substantial and neglected by-product. Several biomass pretreatment or fractionation strategies have been developed and explored to enhance cellulose recovery while simultaneously releasing abundant lignin (Wang et al., 2019). These pretreatment techniques are optimal strategies for lignin biorefineries. The substrate influences the selection of pretreatment techniques and the desired outcomes, as LCBs vary in composition and structure. The biomass pretreatment techniques employed to date can be broadly classified into thermal, mechanical, chemical, and biological methods, with respective advantages and disadvantages (Banu et al., 2021).

Several thermal techniques have been employed to solubilize LCB, including autoclave, hot-air oven, water bath, microwave, and steam explosion (Veluchamy and Kalamdhad, 2017). As the temperature rises, hydrogen bonds and other linkages increase and break down, decreasing viscosity and increasing solubility (Banu et al., 2021). Each thermal technique varies in the delignification process depending on how temperature affects the substrate. In microwave treatment, a hot spot forms across the biomass due to the induced oscillatory motion of polar molecules, thereby generating the heating effect. Meanwhile, the conductive and convective heat transfer from hot air, pressurized steam, and heated water imparts thermal degradation (Haldar and Purkait, 2021; Veluchamy and Kalamdhad, 2017). High energy consumption, high-pressure requirements, and possible inhibitor formation impacting downstream applications place limitations on thermal pretreatment (Banu et al., 2021).

Mechanical pretreatment involves disrupting LCB polymers into oligomers or smaller fragments, altering the crystallinity of lignin/cellulose/hemicelluloses, and providing a higher surface area that renders LCB more amenable to downstream processes (Veluchamy and Kalamdhad, 2017). Elementary mechanical processes like grinding, chipping, extrusion, and milling (ball milling, roll milling, etc.) involve cutting, tearing, breaking, compression, and shearing. However, these are suitable for particle size reduction and can significantly influence subsequent applications beyond delignification (Arce and Kratky, 2022). Advanced processes using mechanical/physical interactions with the lignocellulosic backbone have been developed, with immense applications such as ultrasonication, hydrodynamic cavitation techniques, electrodialysis, and high-pressure homogenization. In these processes, mechanical implosion, shear, breaking, and so forth are highly localized, providing significant energy to break molecular bonds (Bimestre et al., 2022). These advanced mechanical treatment methods are more efficient than conventional ones, with little harmful by-product generation, but consume high energy and are expensive (Veluchamy and Kalamdhad, 2017).

Among all delignification strategies, chemical pretreatment has proven highly efficient at achieving greater lignin and hemicellulose removal. The type of chemical pretreatment also varies with the solvent used, including alkaline, acid, oxidative reagents, ammonia, and supercritical fluid. The specificity and accuracy of these processes are provided by the breakage and rearrangement of intermolecular ester linkages between lignin and hemicellulose, which leads to the leakage of components and the solubilization of intact biomass (Baruah et al., 2018). The conventional chemical treatment requires a high solvent-to-biomass ratio, resulting in several intermediates (such as furfural) that affect further applications and produce relatively toxic effluent. Hence, greener approaches such as ionic liquids, deep eutectic solvents, and organosolv were investigated. These methods are environmentally friendly, provide good delignification under mild conditions, and facilitate easy recovery/separation. However, the high cost of these green solvents still raises the issue of real-world implementation (Bharadwaj et al., 2023).

Leveraging a biological system's capacity to degrade lignin and other components is biological pretreatment. Biological pretreatment employs fungi/bacteria as whole-cell systems or enzymes to restructure LCB (Baruah et al., 2018). The primary enzymes involved in delignification are laccase, versatile peroxidase, manganese peroxidase, and lignin peroxidase. Enzymes are used in crude, pure, or cocktail form, with cocktails shown to provide better degradation of LCB. Enzymatic actions are specific and require longer incubation times to elicit higher hydrolysis (Zabed et al., 2019). The activity and specificity of these enzymes have been modulated using modified surface immobilization, mutagenesis, chemical modification, bioprospecting, and other methods (Bhushan et al., 2023). The mechanism of whole-cell pretreatment can occur in the attached or suspended form. In the attached form, the cell binds to the LCB surface through receptor-ligand binding (like carbohydrate binding motifs), adsorption onto the surface, and extracellular polysaccharide production. In suspended form, the microenvironment between substrate-bacteria/fungi and bulk diffusion plays a vital role. In both cases, the lignin backbone is disrupted by enzymes and other biomolecules secreted (Bhushan et al., 2023). Bioprospecting, metabolic interventions, genetic engineering, and so forth can modify whole-cell pretreatment to enhance hydrolytic activity against LCBs. Meanwhile, bacteria/fungi can continuously produce enzymes during growth, whereas enzymatic pretreatment requires optimized dosing (enzyme-to-substrate ratio) for optimal outcomes (Zabed et al., 2019). Biological pretreatment is environmentally friendly, has reduced energy consumption, and avoids inhibitor formation. However, the process becomes costly and time-consuming, requiring stricter process conditions for optimal performance (Veluchamy and Kalamdhad, 2017).

Acidification is one of the processes used to recover lignin from black liquor. The process was employed by Jablonský and the team, who precipitated lignin by adjusting the pH of black liquor to 2, 3, or 4. It was then filtered using a vacuum filtration unit. The recovered lignin was washed with hot water to remove the impurities (if any) (Jablonský and Haz, 2016). Likewise, soda lignin was isolated by acidification using three different inorganic acids (HCl, H_2SO_4 and H_3PO_4) at different concentrations. The precipitated lignin was centrifuged at 3,500 rpm for 12 minutes, and the pellet was washed with water several times for further characterization (Domínguez-Robles et al., 2016). Similarly, alkali-extracted lignin from steam-exploded stalk was recovered by gradient acid precipitation using HCl solution (Wang and Chen, 2013).

Aside from this, lignin is also purified using ionic liquids (ILs) such as 1-butyl-3-methylimidazolium methyl sulfate and 1-ethyl-3-methylimidazolium acetate (Radotić and Mićić, 2016; Szalaty and Klapiszewski, 2020). Lignin can be extracted from soda pulping with a 5% NaOH solution, known as soda lignin. The dried, impure lignin was then fractionated using ILs based on the 1-buthyl-3-methylimidazolium ([Bmim]) cation combined with various anions: chloride ([Bmim]Cl), dimethylphosphate ([Bmim] Me_2PO_4), acetate ([Bmim]OAc), and tosylate ([Bmim]OTs) at a 1:20 ratio. After 6 hr of incubation under an inert atmosphere, the mixture was added to an acetone-water mixture (1:1) and centrifuged at 5,500 rpm for 15 minutes. The precipitated lignin was washed and vacuum-dried. The highest yield of lignin (more than 60%) was observed for [Bmim] Me_2PO_4 and [Bmim] OAc (Lauberts et al., 2017). Similarly, Mohtar et al. (2015) extracted lignin-rich IL solution from oil palm biomass (OPB) and purged the solution with CO_2 gas at 60°C for 30 minutes. The solution was kept still overnight, and the precipitate formed was segregated by filtration and vacuum dried overnight at 50°C. The lignin extracted from *Eucalyptus urophylla* by microwave-assisted ionic liquid approach was recovered by adding the residual lignin (from the extraction process) drop-wise to acidified water (pH 2), precipitating it, and then washing the precipitated lignin with water several times (Sun et al., 2019).

Nitsos et al. (2016) recovered lignin from the black liquor by precipitating lignin in water. To reduce the solubility of lignin, the pretreated lignin was diluted with cold washing liquid and cold deionized water in a ratio of 1:3. Then, using a vacuum filter, the precipitated lignin was separated, after which the purified lignin was washed with deionized water, air dried, and stored for further use. Natural biomass resources (wheat straw, flax fiber, pine straw, and Alfalfa fiber) were used for lignin extraction. After delignification, the spent liquor was heated at 105°C. The lignin from the liquor was then precipitated by adding distilled water, filtered in a Buchner funnel, and washed with distilled water (Watkins et al., 2015).

23.3 DEPOLYMERIZATION OF LIGNIN DERIVED FROM LIGNOCELLULOSIC BIOMASS

Several depolymerization approaches based on physical methods such as ultrasound, microwave, pyrolysis, and hydrothermal techniques, and chemical methods such as acid/base-catalyzed and ionic liquid-mediated, have shown varying capacities to break down lignin into its monomeric forms, which can be subsequently converted to different products (Ren et al., 2019). However, these methods use harsh conditions, which can cause over-condensation; produce toxic by-products that increase environmental concerns; become energy-intensive; and raise the possibility of repolymerization, monomer degradation, and other issues (Chio et al., 2019). Biological depolymerization is an environmentally benign method, enabling fast depolymerization at milder conditions, with reduced polymerization, over-condensation, degradation, and toxic-by-product formation (Weng et al., 2021)

23.4 BIOLOGICAL DEPOLYMERIZATION OF LIGNIN

Biological depolymerization of lignin employs bacteria, fungi, or enzymes secreted by them for its degradation. Hence, it is also referred to as "enzymatic combustion," in which the oxidizing capabilities of ligninolytic enzymes, such as hydrogen peroxidase, laccases, and DyP peroxidases, from fungi or bacteria are used to oxidize aromatic units of lignin (Khan and Ahring, 2019). Figure 23.1 depicts the basic working model of biological lignin degradation.

23.4.1 Lignin Degradation by Fungi

Lignin-degrading fungi, particularly white rot, brown rot, and soft rot fungi, break down lignin polymer chains into smaller fragments, a process known as lignin depolymerization. The ligninolytic enzymes found in these fungi are diverse and catalyze the oxidation and cleavage of lignin bonds, thereby depolymerizing lignin.

Many studies reported that white rot fungi and brown rot fungi are important in lignin depolymerization. *Phanerochaete chrysosporium*, a white-rot *Basidiomycete*, is an extensively studied fungus for lignin degradation. In a study by Khatami et al. (2019), ultra-high-resolution mass spectrometry showed that the ligninolytic enzymes from the fungus introduced oxidation into the aromatic rings of lignin. This led to the opening of the ring, which in turn produced aliphatic

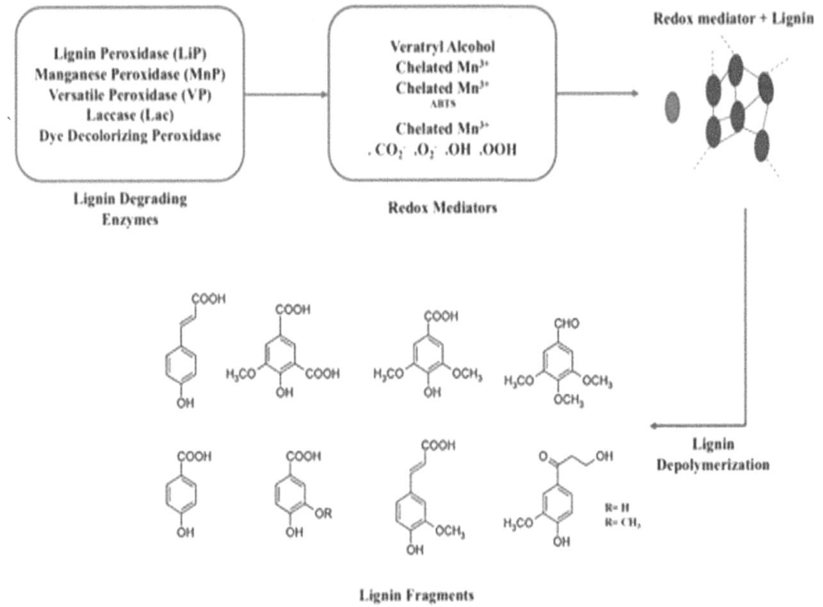

FIGURE 23.1 Microbial lignin degradation model.

Source: Reproduced with permission from Elsevier (Khan and Ahring, 2019)

compounds. The fungus has a good number of oxidative enzymes that may be involved in lignin depolymerization. Among all, lignin peroxidase (LiP) enzyme is the most studied. It brings about the C (alpha)—C (beta) cleavage of the propyl side chain of lignin and aromatic cleavage of non-phenolic lignin compounds.

On the other hand, manganese peroxidase (MnP) enzyme, in the presence of H_2O_2 and oxalate, oxidizes manganese II (Mn^{2+}) to manganese III (Mn^{3+}). *Trametes villosa* is another white fungus that secretes a high-redox-potential laccase that, at 50/μg in the presence of 2.5% 1-hydroxybenzotriazole (HBT), depolymerizes and removes lignin (Gutiérrez et al., 2012). *Gloeophyllum trabeum* is a brown rot fungus that can break the inter-monomeric side chain of lignin non-selectively, and its fermentation can result in 16% of lignin loss in spruce wood (Yelle et al., 2008). *Postia placenta* follows the Fenton reaction, wherein the aryl glycerol β aryl ether linkage of lignin is cleaved at its aromatic four positions to produce phenyl glycerol when an electrophilic hydroxyl radical is added (Yelle et al., 2011). Furthermore, soft rot fungi can also degrade lignin by attacking the syringyl units of lignin. *Ascomycetes* and *Deuteromycetes* are the soft rot fungi that can degrade hardwoods. Apart from this, *Aspergillus niger* and *Penicillium chrysogenum* are another group of soft-rot fungi that degrade pine and sycamore wood (Weng et al., 2021).

23.4.2 Lignin Degradation by Bacteria

Due to poor adaptability to diverse temperatures, pH, and anoxic conditions, the application of fungi for lignin degradation is limited in industries. Hence, bacteria come into the picture. Numerous bacteria, including those in the phyla Actinobacteria, Proteobacteria, Firmicutes, and Bacteroidetes, are known to decompose lignin. These bacteria are found in various environments, including soil, freshwater, and marine environments and the gastrointestinal systems of animals. These bacteria possess a range of enzymes that catalyze the oxidation and cleavage of lignin bonds, ultimately leading to lignin depolymerization.

In the experiment by Zhu et al. (2017), aerobic bacteria, *Bacillus ligniniphilus* L1, degraded 38.9% of lignin within seven days of incubation. SEM showed that the particle size of the lignin treated with the strain was reduced in the 30–300 µm range. The decolorization of lignin was due to the activities of MnP and laccase. Proteins such as peroxiredoxin, cytochrome oxidase, and ferredoxin were upregulated during lignin degradation, suggesting their roles. *Bacillus amyloliquefaciens* degrades lignin of tobacco straw by 22.26% and 11.70% (Mei et al., 2020). A thermotolerant lignin-degrading bacterium, *Aneurinibacillus* sp. LD3, could degrade lignin by 61.28%, which was more effective and better than *Bacillus* sp. The bacterium also has higher ligninolytic activities (Wu et al., 2022). *Streptomyces viridosporus* and *Streptomyces setonii* can oxidize ^{14}C labeled lignocellulose to $^{14}CO_2$ and besides, they also efficiently metabolize varieties of single-ring aromatic compounds (Sutherland et al., 1981). In addition to aerobic bacteria, a few anaerobic bacteria can degrade lignin. The anaerobic pathway for degradation employs demethylation and aromatic ring cleavage. Table 23.1 describes examples of different bacteria involved in lignin depolymerization, taken from the literature (Khan et al., 2022; An et al., 2022; Liu et al., 2021; Lin et al., 2019; He et al., 2017).

23.4.3 Lignin Degradation by Enzymes

Enzymes are biological catalysts that enhance the degradation process of lignin without changing its properties after reaction. Enzymes that are naturally occurring or artificially modified are used in lignin depolymerization to break down lignin polymer chains into smaller pieces. Lignin may be depolymerized enzymatically, providing environmental benefits, gentle reaction conditions, and selectivity. Lignin undergoes enzymatic depolymerization in moderate reaction conditions, such as near-neutral pH and mild temperature. Mediators and cofactors can be added to the system to enhance enzyme activity during lignin breakdown.

Enzymes are normally obtained from fungi and bacteria to carry out lignin degradation. Ligninolytic enzymes, such as heme peroxidases (lignin peroxidase, manganese peroxidase, and versatile peroxidase, multifunctional peroxidases) and phenol oxidases (laccases, different oxidases), have shown a considerable

TABLE 23.1
Lignin Degradation by Bacteria

Bacteria	Lignin Type	Reaction Condition	Lignin Degradation	Reference
Erwinia billingiae QL-Z3	Lignin	LiP, MnP, and Lac enzymes, which were isolated from fermentation (supernatant) having activities 367.50 U/L, 839.50 U/L, and 219.00 U/L, respectively, by orthogonal optimization.	Lignin degradation rate was 25.24% using 1.5 g/L lignin as the only carbon source	Zhao et al. (2024)
*Bacillus amyloliquefaciens*MN-13,	Alkaline lignin	Collaborative effects of glucose and sodium carboxymethyl cellulose to lignin breakdown, where lignin was used as the only carbon source in AL-MSM media by using glycolysis, TCA cycle, and central carbon metabolism.	–	Li et al. (2024)
Bacillus altitudinis SL7	Alkaline lignin	Bacteria show metabolization and transformation of lignin's functional group at 40°C and pH 8.0; lignin load 3 g/L, degradation time 5 days, by extracellular laccase enzyme.	Lignin degradation by 44%; vanillin, 2-methoxyphenol, 3-methylphenol, oxalic acid, and ferulic acid	Khan et al. (2022)
Arthrobacter sp.AXJ-M1 *and Serratia* sp.AXJ-M	Lignin in paper-making black liquor	The extracted thermo-alkali-stable endoglucanase (*bcsZ*) gene was most active at 70°C, pH 9 in presence of Mn^{2+}, Ca^{2+}, Mg^{2+}, and Tween-20	Lignin degradation by 30% and increased up to 70%	An et al. (2022)
Azotobacter AC-1	Straw lignin	360 hr, 60°C, using bacterial component *Tepidimicrobium*, *Haloplasma*, *norank-f-Limnochordaceae*, *Ruminiclostridium*, *Rhodothermus*	Degradation of lignin by 20.12% at 60°C	Liu et al. (2021)
Pseudomonas putida A514	Alkali lignin	DypB (B subfamily dye-decolorizing peroxidases), Mn^{2+} independent lignin depolymerizes and cleaves the ring structure in the presence of O_2 via central and peripheral pathways to form aromatic compounds.	Degradation of lignin by 27%	Lin et al. (2019)
Rhodococcusopacus PD630 and *Rhodococcusjostii* RHA1 VanA (wild and engineered, respectively)	Alkali-treated straw lignin	The linkage is oxidized to aromatic intermediates via the β-ketoadipate pathway, which converts aromatic-derived carbon into TCA cycle intermediates and produces lipids via lipid biosynthetic pathways.	Degradation of lignin by 31.60% (dry weight), palmitic acid (35.8%), oleic acid (47.9%), and other fatty acids, vanillin, 3-hydroxy-4-methoxy-benzaldehyde	He et al. (2017)

amount of lignin degradation capability and thus have attracted the attention of researchers. These enzymes catalyze oxidative processes that result in lignin depolymerization by cleaving lignin bonds (Weng et al., 2021)

Lignin peroxidase: Lignin peroxidase is a ligninolytic enzyme produced by certain fungi, such as white rot fungi, which catalyzes the depolymerization of lignin by oxidizing lignin substrates. Oxidative reactions targeting certain bonds, such as aryl-ether and aryl-aryl couplings, inside lignin polymer chains are catalyzed by lignin peroxidase. It produces highly reactive intermediates that attack lignin substrates, breaking down chemical bonds and forming smaller fragments. Examples of these intermediates include peroxyl and free radicals. Neutral to slightly acidic pH and moderate temperatures are typical reaction conditions for lignin depolymerization by lignin peroxidase. The one oxidation and two reduction phases that make up LiP's catalytic cycle are described in Figure 23.2.

Lignin peroxidase catalyzes the oxidation of lignin substrates by transferring electrons from the substrate to a heme cofactor within the enzyme active site (ferric enzyme ([LiP]-Fe(III)) native form) in the presence of hydrogen peroxide (H_2O_2) or other peroxidase substrates and forms a compound I oxo-ferryl intermediate [Fe(IV)]. This process generates highly reactive intermediates, such as radical species, when compound I reduces to compound II by taking one electron in, and as it goes to the resting native ferric state, it attacks lignin polymer chains,

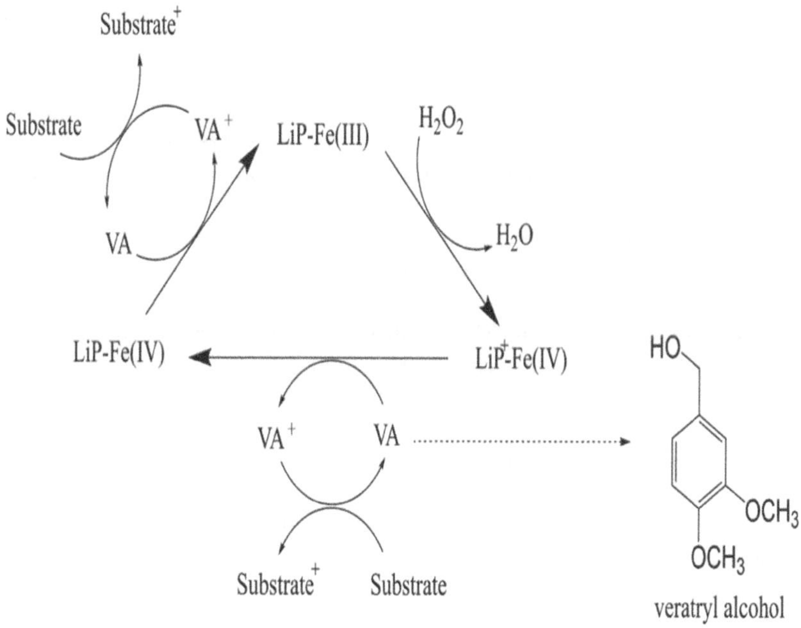

FIGURE 23.2 The process of breakdown of lignin mediated by LiP.

Source: Reproduced with permission from Elsevier (Chio et al., 2019)

leading to the cleavage of chemical bonds and the production of smaller lignin fragments (Datta et al., 2017). LiP degradation of lignin follows one oxidation and two reduction steps. At first, compound I oxo-ferryl intermediate [Fe(IV)] is formed by the two-electron oxidation of native (LiP)-FeIII enzyme by H_2O_2. It is followed by the reduction of compound I to form compound II (LiP-Fe IV) by a non-phenolic aromatic reducing substrate A. Compound II is reverted to the native enzyme by gaining one more electron (Datta et al., 2017). Fan et al. (2019) determined the optimal conditions for lignin degradation using the Michaelis-Menten Model. The maximum μ_a (max) was determined using a one-factor-at-a-time design and an orthogonal array. The maximum μ_a, the maximum lignin oxidative degradation, was achieved with the combination of optimal parameters. Lignin peroxidase, manganese peroxidase, and laccase together have a greater influence on degradation than the individual enzymes (Zhang et al., 2022).

Laccase: Laccases, blue multi-copper phenoloxidases, can oxidize a wide range of phenolic and non-phenolic substrates by taking electrons from oxygen (Datta et al., 2017). Laccase transfers electrons from the substrate to an active site on the enzyme that contains copper, catalyzing the oxidation of lignin substrates. The lignin polymer chains are attacked by extremely reactive intermediates (phenoxyl free radical) produced by oxidized phenolic compounds in this process, such as radical species, which, being very unstable, react and cleave chemical bonds, producing smaller lignin fragments (Chio et al., 2019). By a two-step process, laccase catalyzes the oxidation of lignin substrates. A radical intermediate is created when laccase oxidizes a substrate molecule in the first stage by removing an electron. The second process involves additional oxidation or polymerization of the radical intermediate, leading to the breakage of lignin linkages and the formation of smaller lignin fragments. Normally, *B. licheniformis*, *B. pumilus*, *B. subtilis*, *Streptomyces cyaneus*, *Thermus thermophilus*, and so forth are the bacterial sources of this enzyme. Figure 23.3 demonstrates the action of laccase in lignin depolymerization.

Manganese peroxidase: Just like lignin peroxidase, manganese peroxidase (glycoproteins) also catalyzes target-specific bonds within lignin polymer chains. It utilizes manganese ions as a mediator and hydrogen peroxide (H_2O_2) as an oxidant. MnP oxidizes Mn^{2+} to Mn^{3+}, which uses free radicals and uses the oxidation energy for the cleavage of chemical bonds and the formation of smaller lignin fragments. Figure 23.4 shows the enzymatic activity of manganese peroxidase.

MnP oxidizes Mn^{2+} to Mn^{3+} in the presence of H_2O_2 as mentioned, which, in turn, converts lignin phenolic compounds to phenoxy radicals (Weng et al., 2021). Arantes et al. (2007) reported that the –OH radical is an important participant in Azure B degradation. Further, the pretreatment of Azure B with low molecular weight fraction Fe-reducing activity ($LMWF_{FeRA}$), ferric iron, and hydrogen peroxide, followed by the addition of high molecular weight fraction of MnP ($HMWF_{MnP}$) and high molecular weight fraction of Lac ($HMWF_{Lac}$), had significant Azure degradation (approximately 40%). Versatile peroxidase, on the other hand, was extracted from a white rot fungus, *P. vitreus PF18*, and expressed in *E. coli*. They found that the recombinant rVP1 not only exhibited

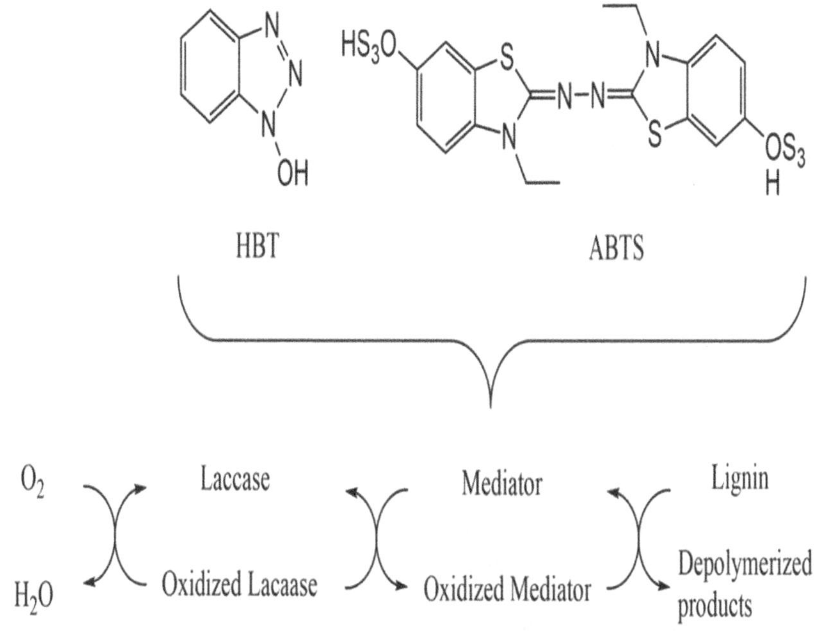

FIGURE 23.3 The process of breakdown of lignin mediated by laccase.

Source: Reproduced with permission from Elsevier Chio et al. (2019)

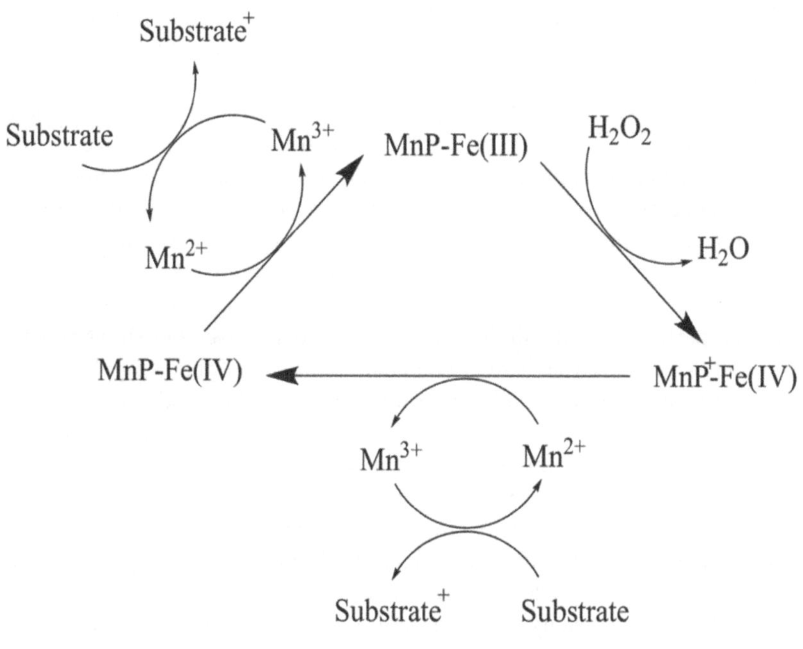

FIGURE 23.4 The process of breakdown of lignin mediated by manganese peroxidise (Chio et al., 2019).

Source: Reproduced with permission from Elsevier (Chio et al., 2019)

Mn-dependent activity but also oxidized low or high-redox-potential substrates. The rVP1 also resulted in the increment in the G/S ratio (5.4 fold), which in turn led to the lignin condensation (Liu et al., 2019). Besides these three dye-decolorizing peroxidases (DyP) and the biphenyl bond cleavage enzyme, versatile peroxidase (VP) can also be used for delignification (Kumar and Chandra, 2020). Unlike other lignin depolymerization technologies, biological depolymerization of lignin is cost-effective and specific, although there are a few limitations such as low yield and poor productivity.

23.5 DERIVING BIOCHEMICAL AND ENERGY APPLICATIONS FROM DEPOLYMERIZED LIGNIN

23.5.1 Energy Conversion from Lignin

Battery: Lignin has been recognized as a promising precursor for the production of active carbon-based materials for energy storage devices. However, their limited electrical conductivity has been a significant barrier to their direct use as electrode materials in energy storage and conversion devices. As a result, researchers have been exploring different synthetic methods and structural transformation strategies to improve their conductivity, electrochemical performance, and mechanical properties (Wu et al., 2020). Converting lignin into battery-active carbon materials via high-temperature pyrolysis with chemical activation agents such as KOH, K_2CO_3, and $ZnCO_3$ results in the formation of active carbon suitable for battery applications (Wu et al., 2020; Zhu et al., 2020). This process imparts advanced properties to the carbon derivative, including a hierarchical nanomicro-pore system, high conductivity, and mechanical robustness, thereby enhancing fast kinetics, stability, and charge storage capacity. Like graphite, lignin-derived carbons have been extensively studied for use in various energy storage applications, such as metal ion and redox flow batteries. Unlike graphite, the polymeric nature of lignin enables tailored modifications, such as surface functionalization and molecular grafting, before carbonization and heteroatom doping, yielding carbon materials with diverse morphologies and improved functional properties. This flexibility enables lignin derivatives to exhibit beneficial properties across different battery components, making lignin a highly attractive precursor material for carbon-based battery materials. In a study, the importance of pore structure, high surface area, and network was highlighted by producing fine porous carbon nanofibers (CNFs) via electrospinning a blend of lignin and polylactic acid (PLA), followed by carbonization at 900°C. These lignin/PLA-based CNFs exhibited a surface area of 670 m^2/g, enhancing ion transport and cycling stability as a lithium-ion battery (LIB) anode, achieving a capacity of 611 mA h/g after 500 cycles, nearly double the theoretical capacity of graphite. Despite the higher capacity of lignin-derived carbons compared to graphite, they still show low initial Coulombic efficiency (CE), and the use of organic polymer blends and chemical activation agents at high temperatures may compromise environmental benefits. Furthermore, the growing demand for high-energy-density batteries, especially for electric mobility applications, cannot be met solely with lignin-derived carbon materials.

Jet fuel: Due to its abundance, inedible characteristics, and cost-effectiveness, lignocellulose (comprising cellulose, hemicellulose, and lignin) is the most viable biomass source for the production of transportation fuels (Cheng and Brewer, 2017). Lignocellulose is used to produce cost-effective fuels, while more expensive feedstocks such as oils, terpenes, and sugars are typically reserved for high-value fine chemicals. Lignin, being the second most abundant component in lignocellulose, is primarily used for fuel production. However, biomass-derived fuels cannot entirely replace traditional fuels because they lack aromatic and cycloalkane hydrocarbons, which are crucial for jet turbine fuels. To ensure that quality and performance standards are met, a blend of biomass-derived fuels and conventional fuels is necessary for alternative jet fuels. Given lignin's abundance in aromatic benzene ring structures, it can be used to create 100% biomass-derived jet fuel. This biofuel offers a more affordable option, helps mitigate supply disruptions, and reduces the environmental impact of aviation emissions. The cost of lignin-derived jet fuel ranges from USD 1,300 to USD 6,400 per ton when blended with fossil jet fuel at concentrations of 1–50% (Amezcua-Allieri and Aburto, 2018).

Lignin-based carbon fibers for electronic double-layer capacitors (EDLC): Lignin has been combined with support polymers such as polyvinyl alcohol (PVA) and polyethylene glycol (PEG) to facilitate the electrospinning of supercapacitor electrodes. Ago et al. (2016) achieved the production of high-surface-area free-standing electrospun mats using lignin/PVA solutions. By incorporating a low PVA content (25%), they created flexible, free-standing carbon networks with a high surface area of 2,000 m^2/g. These free-standing fibers, when used as electrodes, exhibited outstanding specific double-layer capacitance and maintained 83% capacity over 1,500 cycles. This exceptional performance was attributed to the microphase separation between lignin and PVA, resulting in a wide pore distribution in the mesopore range of the carbon fibers.

Lignin-based activated carbon fibers (ACFs) were produced using a range of electrospinning methods and diverse lignin varieties (You et al., 2015). These ACFs were evaluated as electrodes for EDLCs and internal tandem EDLCs (IT-EDLCs). A significant discovery highlighted in their study was the reduction in thermostabilization time for lignin-based carbon fibers to just 3 hr by incorporating hexamethylenetetramine (hexamine) into a solvent mixture of acetic acid/carbon tetrachloride (8/2). You et al. (2016a) created electrodes for *use* in EDLCs using polyethylene glycol (PEG) and soda lignin (SL) through dry electrospinning. These fibers had a smaller diameter than PEG fibers produced by dry and melt spinning methods. The fibers underwent thermostabilization at a high heating rate but for a short duration.

Additionally, the ACFs/SL electrodes exhibited an impedance of 4.5 Ω and a specific capacitance of 55.6 F/g, which were higher than those of the PEG-ACFs electrodes. To develop EDLCs with a broad potential window and high energy density, thick ACFs made from polyethylene glycol lignin (PEGL) were introduced as electrodes for IT-EDLCs (You et al., 2016b). These electrodes were internally laminated and connected in series, parallel, and a series/parallel combination. The findings showed that the combined connections were more effective than a single cell. In IT-EDLCs, the potential window was expanded through a series connection, while capacitance was enhanced through a parallel connection.

Lignin as a photosensitizer of dye-sensitized solar cells (DSSC): Solar cells are devices that convert sunlight into electrical energy. Lignin and ligno-phenols, when combined with conducting polymers (CP), have been explored for developing alternative photosensitizers for dye-sensitized solar cells (DSSCs) and polymer solar cells (PSCs) (Fonseca et al., 2017). Water-soluble poly(3,4-ethylenedioxythiophene) lignosulfonate (PEDOT/LS) and poly(3,4-ethylenedioxythiophene) alkali lignin (PEDOT/AL) composites have been investigated for hole transport in PSCs. Studies have shown that the presence of phenolic hydroxyl groups from lignin enhances the power conversion efficiency of PSCs (Aoyagi and Funaoka, 2004). In photovoltaic applications, polystyrene sulfonic acid (PSS) is commonly used as a dopant for PEDOT. Wu et al. (2016) synthesized grafted sulfonated-acetone-formaldehyde lignin (GSL) as a dopant and dispersant for PEDOT. Compared with PEDOT/PSS, PEDOT/GLS exhibited higher efficiency. This improvement was attributed to the smaller particle size and better dispersion of PEDOT/GSL, which can enhance charge transport and improve the electrical conductivity of PSCs.

Before use in DSSCs, lignin must undergo chemical modifications to function as a photosensitizer. Aoyagi and Funaoka (2006) explored the use of certain lignophenols derived from modified lignins as photosensitizers. They observed that p-cresol, catechol, resorcinol, and pyrogallol exhibited strong interactions with the titanium dioxide (TiO_2) surface. These ligno-phenols demonstrated greater stability than lignin due to the positioning of benzyl groups, which are blocked by -OH groups. The efficiency of these DSSCs was 0.11%. DSSCs were developed using lignophenols directly synthesized on the mesoporous TiO_2 electrode. The light-to-electricity conversion in a sandwich-type cell reached 3.61%, whereas in a single TiO_2 cell, it was 0.81%. The molecular weight and chemical structure of the lignophenols influenced these outcomes.

23.5.2 Biochemicals from Lignin

Lignin as a source of aromatic compounds: One fascinating aspect of lignin is its ability to be broken down into various building blocks. By reducing these building blocks, essential substances such as benzene, toluene, xylene, and phenol can be produced. This process highlights the versatility and potential of lignin as a valuable resource for producing important chemical compounds with a wide range of applications. 4-Ethylphenol and guaiacol (phenolic yield of 32.8%) were synthesized from lignin extracted from sugarcane bagasse using methyl isobutyl ketone and lignin-derived carbonaceous solid acids (Asawaworarit et al., 2019). Benzene, toluene, and xylene (BTX) are widely utilized in various applications, making them highly valuable in the chemical industry. The potential of lignin-based BTX is significant, as it closely resembles petroleum-derived BTX, making it a viable substitute. With BTX accounting for 60% of all aromatics and 24% of the global petrochemical market, lignin-based BTX offers a promising opportunity for sustainable, environmentally friendly chemical production. Fast pyrolysis of lignin under a hydrogen atmosphere and a temperature of 850°C resulted in the aromatic hydrocarbon products such as benzene and toluene (4.8 wt%) (Zhang et al., 2021)

Phenol plays a crucial role in the production of plastics and various materials, particularly in the manufacturing of phenol-formaldehyde resins, polyurethane foams, and polyurethanes for the automobile industry. Currently, the market value of phenol ranges from approximately USD 1,000 to USD 2,000 per metric ton. With an annual production of 8 million tons in 2012, phenol is of significant importance in the chemical industry. One key advantage of producing phenol from lignin is its independence from fluctuating oil prices, providing a more stable market value. As a renewable source, lignin offers a sustainable and reliable alternative for phenol production, contributing to a more consistent market outlook. Phenolic resins with superior bonding strength for plywood exterior applications, lower formaldehyde emissions, and faster cure kinetics can be obtained by partial replacement with demethylated lignin (Argyropoulos et al., 2023).

Carbon fibers from lignin: Carbon fibers (CFs) are prominent as they are fibers that contain mainly carbon (>90 wt%) with outstanding mechanical properties due to their high strength-to-weight ratio. This makes them ideal as the load-bearing component in lightweight composites used in the aerospace and automotive industries, as well as for constructing wind turbine blades, premium sporting goods, and so forth. In 2018, the global output of carbon fibers was 108,000 tons, and the growth rate was at double digits (~12.5%) for the ninth consecutive year. Kraft lignin has been used for various biomedical applications via different processes (Argyropoulos et al., 2023). Similarly, continuous processing of hardwood Kraft lignin in carbon nanotubes was demonstrated in a tubular furnace with ferrocene and thiophene as catalysts. The carbon fiber exhibited superior electrical conductivity (1.19×10^5 S/m) and tensile strength (1.33 GPa) compared to other carbon materials derived from biomass (Liu et al., 2022).

Lignin as a macromolecule: Unmodified lignin lacks the necessary properties to be utilized as a standalone material; however, it can be effectively blended with other synthetic or bio-based polymers to enhance its functionality. When combined with polymers such as polyethylene, polystyrene, polypropylene, or natural rubber, lignin is a valuable UV-degradation stabilizer or a thermo-oxidation stabilizer. By incorporating lignin into these polymer blends, its stabilizing properties can be harnessed to improve the overall performance and durability of the resulting composite materials, showcasing the versatility and potential of lignin to enhance the properties of various polymer products (Zhou et al., 2022).

For example, lignin reinforcement (3/5%) in polyhydroxybutyrate produced from volatile fatty acids and activated sludge as the inoculum showed better thermal properties than the pristine polymer (Naresh Kumar et al., 2021).

Adsorbents from lignin: Lignin's ability to adsorb heavy metal ions has sparked interest in its potential as an adsorbent for wastewater purification. Phenolic hydroxyl groups play a key role in lignin sorption. Studies have investigated lignin's adsorption capabilities against various heavy metals, including chromium, cadmium, lead, zinc, nickel, mercury, and cobalt. This research highlights lignin's effectiveness in removing these contaminants from wastewater, showcasing its promise as a sustainable solution for water treatment processes (Argyropoulos et al., 2023). In a recent study, methylene blue removal showed 14 times higher removal (127.91 mg/g) using lignin nanoparticle synthesized using hydrotrope method (*p*-toluenesulfonic) compared to lignin powder (20.74 mg/g) (Pourbaba et al., 2024)

23.6 CONCLUSION: CHALLENGES AND FUTURE PERSPECTIVES

Lignin has been mostly viewed as a recalcitrant macromolecule that impedes the effective conversion of biomass into products and fuels. However, lignin's recognition as a natural polymer for its ubiquitous availability, chemical versatility, antioxidant capacity, reinforcing ability, biocompatibility, and abundant carbon reserve has opened opportunities in diverse sectors. Understanding this potential has led to divergent attempts to isolate lignin from biomass, purify the extracted lignin, depolymerize it, and valorize it. The chapter extensively delves into crucial lignin valorization processes, namely, lignin isolation, purification, depolymerization, and value-added products. Tailoring depolymerization for prospective applications and required properties remains a challenging endeavor in lignin biorefineries. However, concerted efforts have faced several challenges that are being addressed to project a large-scale application of lignin biorefinery.

A large body of literature on biomass delignification exists, with varying efficiencies and economic considerations. However, in these techniques, the fate of lignin is neglected, with emphasis on the hemicellulose/cellulose fraction. For developing and ratifying cost-effective lignin, biorefinery techniques are critical for improving lignin valorization (Zhou et al., 2022). The solid-to-liquid (solvent) ratio needs to be considered when developing or modifying the lignin extraction process, as this could significantly affect the economics of upscaling (Zhou et al., 2022). An approach for a continuous depolymerization system can potentially alleviate degradation efficiency, enable possible catalyst reclamation, and improve the industrial perspective of the lignin biorefinery (Nandiwale et al., 2020). Lignin's unique structural and functional properties have enabled numerous applications, including the reinforcement of biopolymer blends/composites, slow-release fertilizers, and more. The investigations have yet to reveal large-scale feasibility due to aspects related to tailoring properties and modifying the process in a scale-up scenario. Further investigation on this application should take into account the effects of chemical modifications on lignin before blend formation, combination with other materials in binary/ternary systems, lignin with varying particle size, and the combination of biopolymer and lignin from different sources (Lu et al., 2022; Mariana et al., 2021).

The origin/source of biomass induces a certain degree of variability in the physicochemical properties of lignin. This variability increases the challenges and economic design of the strategy to ensure the required lignin recovery and characteristics, ensuring a constant process flow for biorefinery products (Brienza et al., 2023). This requires a concerted technical and economic analysis to understand and curate every conversion process in lignin biorefinery and the life cycle of lignin-derived products. The complex nature of lignin from LCB results in a multitude of product streams, which complicates separation and purification and alters the economic calculation of the process (Zhou et al., 2022). Bioengineering plant feedstock to control lignin monomer composition and functionality relevant to the production of high-value intermediates is a prospective research area to explore in the future. Strategizing the development of a lignin biorefinery with respect to functional derivatives with market applications is crucial to the process's viability. In addition, expanding the boundary conditions of protocols from the lab to a larger scale is necessary to assess process scalability, maximize revenue, and identify checkpoints to focus on further improving the process (Zhou et al., 2022). Finally, extended actions in the front of deciphering newer functional intermediates derived from lignin depolymerization and their application in various niches of human life should be concomitant with other attempts in lignin biorefinery.

REFERENCES

Ago, M., Borghei, M., Haataja, J.S., Rojas, O.J., 2016. Mesoporous carbon soft-templated from lignin nanofiber networks: Microphase separation boosts supercapacitance in conductive electrodes. *RSC Adv.* 6, 85802–85810. https://doi.org/10.1039/c6ra17536h

Amezcua-Allieri, M.A., Aburto, J., 2018. Conversion of lignin to heat and power, chemicals or fuels into the transition energy strategy, in: *Lignin – Trends and Applications*. InTech. https://doi.org/10.5772/intechopen.71211

An, X., Zong, Z., Zhang, Q., Li, Z., Zhong, M., Long, H., Cai, C., Tan, X., 2022. Novel thermo-alkali-stable cellulase-producing Serratia sp. AXJ-M cooperates with Arthrobacter sp. AXJ-M1 to improve the degradation of cellulose in papermaking black liquor. *J. Hazard. Mater.* 421, 126811. https://doi.org/10.1016/j.jhazmat.2021.126811

Aoyagi, M., Funaoka, M., 2004. A new polymeric photosensitizer for dye-sensitized solar cell with porous TiO2 from forest carbon resources. *J. Photochem. Photobiol. A Chem.* 164, 53–60. https://doi.org/10.1016/j.jphotochem.2004.01.025

Aoyagi, M., Funaoka, M., 2006. A photochemical cell with a nano-porous TiO2 electrode sensitized by lignophenol under visible light irradiation. *J. Photochem. Photobiol. A Chem.* 181, 114–119. https://doi.org/10.1016/j.jphotochem.2005.11.012

Arantes, V., Maria, A., Milagres, F., 2007. The synergistic action of ligninolytic enzymes (MnP and Laccase) and Fe 3 + -reducing activity from white-rot fungi for degradation of Azure B. *Enzyme Microb. Technol.* 42, 17–22. https://doi.org/10.1016/j.enzmictec.2007.07.017

Arce, C., Kratky, L., 2022. Mechanical pretreatment of lignocellulosic biomass toward enzymatic/fermentative valorization. *iScience* 25, 104610. https://doi.org/10.1016/j.isci.2022.104610

Argyropoulos, D.D.S., Crestini, C., Dahlstrand, C., Furusjö, E., Gioia, C., Jedvert, K., Henriksson, G., Hulteberg, C., Lawoko, M., Pierrou, C., Samec, J.S.M., Subbotina, E., Wallmo, H., Wimby, M., 2023. Kraft lignin: A valuable, sustainable resource, opportunities and challenges. *Chem Sus Chem* 16, e202300492. https://doi.org/https://doi.org/10.1002/cssc.202300492

Asawaworarit, P., Daorattanachai, P., Laosiripojana, W., Sakdaronnarong, C., Shotipruk, A., Laosiripojana, N., 2019. Catalytic depolymerization of organosolv lignin from bagasse by carbonaceous solid acids derived from hydrothermal of lignocellulosic compounds. *Chem. Eng. J.* 356, 461–471. https://doi.org/10.1016/j.cej.2018.09.048

Banu, R.J., Sugitha, S., Kavitha, S., Kannah, Y.R., Merrylin, J., Kumar, G., 2021. Lignocellulosic biomass pretreatment for enhanced bioenergy recovery: Effect of lignocelluloses recalcitrance and enhancement strategies. *Front. Energy Res.* 9, 646057. https://doi.org/10.3389/fenrg.2021.646057

Baruah, J., Nath, B.K., Sharma, R., Kumar, S., Deka, R.C., Baruah, D.C., Kalita, E., 2018. Recent trends in the pretreatment of lignocellulosic biomass for value-added products. *Front. Energy Res.* 6, 141. https://doi.org/10.3389/fenrg.2018.00141

Bharadwaj, A.V.S.L.S., Dev, S., Zhuang, J., Wang, Y., Yoo, C.G., Jeon, B.H., Aggarwal, S., Park, S.H., Kim, T.H., 2023. Review of chemical pretreatment of lignocellulosic biomass using low-liquid and low-chemical catalysts for effective bioconversion. *Bioresour. Technol.* 368, 128339. https://doi.org/10.1016/j.biortech.2022.128339

Bhushan, S., Jayakrishnan, U., Shree, B., Bhatt, P., Eshkabilov, S., Simsek, H., 2023. Biological pretreatment for algal biomass feedstock for biofuel production. *J. Environ. Chem. Eng.* 11, 109870. https://doi.org/10.1016/j.jece.2023.109870

Bimestre, T.A., Júnior, J.A.M., Canettieri, E.V., Tuna, C.E., 2022. Hydrodynamic cavitation for lignocellulosic biomass pretreatment: A review of recent developments and future perspectives. *Bioresour. Bioprocess.* 9, 7. https://doi.org/10.1186/s40643-022-00499-2

Brienza, F., Cannella, D., Montesdeoca, D., Cybulska, I., Debecker, D.P., 2023. A guide to lignin valorization in biorefineries: Traditional, recent, and forthcoming approaches to convert raw lignocellulose into valuable materials and chemicals. *RSC Sustain.* 2, 37. https://doi.org/10.1039/d3su00140g

Cheng, F., Brewer, C.E., 2017. Producing jet fuel from biomass lignin: Potential pathways to alkylbenzenes and cycloalkanes. *Renew. Sustain. Energy Rev.* https://doi.org/10.1016/j.rser.2017.01.030

Chio, C., Sain, M., Qin, W., 2019. Lignin utilization: A review of lignin depolymerization from various aspects. *Renew. Sustain. Energy Rev.* 107, 232–249. https://doi.org/10.1016/j.rser.2019.03.008

Datta, R., Kelkar, A., Baraniya, D., Molaei, A., Moulick, A., Meena, R.S., Formanek, P., 2017. Enzymatic degradation of lignin in soil: A review. *Sustain.* 9. https://doi.org/10.3390/su9071163

Domínguez-Robles, J., Espinosa, E., Savy, D., Rosal, A., 2016. Selective lignin precipitation using mineral acids. *BioResources* 11, 7061–7077.

Fan, Y., Zhang, Z., Wang, F., Li, J., Hu, K., Du, Z., 2019. Lignin degradation in corn stover catalyzed by lignin peroxidase from Aspergillus oryzae broth : Effects of conditions on the kinetics. *Renew. Energy* 130, 32–40. https://doi.org/10.1016/j.renene.2018.06.037

Fonseca, S.M., Moreira, T., Parola, A.J., Pinheiro, C., Laia, C.A.T., 2017. PEDOT electrodeposition on oriented mesoporous silica templates for electrochromic devices. *Sol. Energy Mater. Sol. Cells* 159, 94–101. https://doi.org/10.1016/j.solmat.2016.09.002

Govardhan, G., Ambulkar, R., Kulkarni, S., Vishnoi, A., Yadav, P., Choudhury, B.A., Khare, M., Ghude, S.D., 2023. Stubble-burning activities in north-western India in 2021: Contribution to air pollution in Delhi. *Heliyon* 9, e16939. https://doi.org/10.1016/j.heliyon.2023.e16939

Gutiérrez, A., Rencoret, J., Cadena, E.M., Rico, A., Barth, D., del Río, J.C., Martínez, Á.T., 2012. Demonstration of laccase-based removal of lignin from wood and non-wood plant feedstocks. *Bioresour. Technol.* 119, 114–122. https://doi.org/10.1016/j.biortech.2012.05.112

Haldar, D., Purkait, M.K., 2021. A review on the environment-friendly emerging techniques for pretreatment of lignocellulosic biomass: Mechanistic insight and advancements. *Chemosphere* 264, 128523. https://doi.org/10.1016/j.chemosphere.2020.128523

He, Y., Li, X., Ben, H., Xue, X., Yang, B., 2017. Lipid production from dilute alkali corn stover lignin by Rhodococcus strains. *ACS Sustain. Chem. Eng.* 5, 2302–2311. https://doi.org/10.1021/acssuschemeng.6b02627

Jablonský, M., Haz, A., 2016. Characterization of lignins precipitated with nitric and hydrochloric acid. *Int. J. Recent. Sci. Res.* 7, 9177–9180.

Jayakrishnan, U., Deka, D., Das, G., 2021. Waste as feedstock for polyhydroxyalkanoate production from activated sludge: Implications of aerobic dynamic feeding and acidogenic fermentation. *J. Environ. Chem. Eng.* 9, 105550. https://doi.org/10.1016/j.jece.2021.105550

Khan, M.U., Ahring, B.K., 2019. Lignin degradation under anaerobic digestion: Influence of lignin modifications-a review. *Biomass and Bioenergy* 128. https://doi.org/10.1016/j.biombioe.2019.105325

Khan, S.I., Zarin, A., Ahmed, S., Hasan, F., Belduz, A.O., Çanakçi, S., Khan, S., Badshah, M., Farman, M., Shah, A.A., 2022. Degradation of lignin by Bacillus altitudinis SL7 isolated from pulp and paper mill effluent. *Water Sci. Technol.* 85, 420–432. https://doi.org/10.2166/wst.2021.610

Khatami, S., Deng, Y., Tien, M., Hatcher, P.G., 2019. Formation of water-soluble organic matter through fungal degradation of lignin. *Org. Geochem.* 135, 64–70. https://doi.org/10.1016/j.orggeochem.2019.06.004

Kumar, A., Chandra, R., 2020. Ligninolytic enzymes and its mechanisms for degradation of lignocellulosic waste in environment. *Heliyon* 6, e03170. https://doi.org/10.1016/j.heliyon.2020.e03170

Lauberts, M., Sevastyanova, O., Ponomarenko, J., Dizhbite, T., Dobele, G., Volperts, A., Lauberte, L., Telysheva, G., 2017. Fractionation of technical lignin with ionic liquids as a method for improving purity and antioxidant activity. *Ind. Crops Prod.* 95, 512–520. https://doi.org/10.1016/j.indcrop.2016.11.004

Li, X., Li, Z., Li, M., Li, J., Wang, Q., Wang, S., Li, S., Li, H., 2024. Transcriptomic and metabolomic analysis reveals the influence of carbohydrates on lignin degradation mediated by Bacillus amyloliquefaciens. *Front. Microbiol.* 15, 1–12. https://doi.org/10.3389/fmicb.2024.1224855

Lin, L., Wang, X., Cao, L., Xu, M., 2019. Lignin catabolic pathways reveal unique characteristics of dye-decolorizing peroxidases in Pseudomonas putida. *Environ. Microbiol.* 21, 1847–1863. https://doi.org/10.1111/1462-2920.14593

Liu, F., Wang, Q., Zhai, G., Xiang, H., Zhou, J., Jia, C., Zhu, L., Wu, Q., Zhu, M., 2022. Continuously processing waste lignin into high-value carbon nanotube fibers. *Nat. Commun.* 13, 5755. https://doi.org/10.1038/s41467-022-33496-2

Liu, H., Zhang, L., Sun, Y., Xu, G., Wang, W., Piao, R., Cui, Z., Zhao, H., 2021. Degradation of lignocelluloses in straw using AC-1, a thermophilic composite microbial system. *PeerJ* 9, 1–13. https://doi.org/10.7717/peerj.12364

Liu, J., Zhang, S., Shi, Q., Wang, L., Kong, W., Yu, H., Ma, F., 2019. Highly efficient oxidation of synthetic and natural lignin-related compounds by Physisporinus vitreus versatile peroxidase. *Int. Biodeterior. Biodegrad.* 136, 41–48. https://doi.org/10.1016/j.ibiod.2018.10.009

Lu, J., Cheng, M., Zhao, C., Li, B., Peng, H., Zhang, Y., Shao, Q., Hassan, M., 2022. Application of lignin in preparation of slow-release fertilizer: Current status and future perspectives. *Ind. Crops Prod.* 176, 114267. https://doi.org/10.1016/j.indcrop.2021.114267

Mariana, M., Alfatah, T., Abdul Khalil, H.P.S., Yahya, E.B., Olaiya, N.G., Nuryawan, A., Mistar, E.M., Abdullah, C.K., Abdulmadjid, S.N., Ismail, H., 2021. A current advancement on the role of lignin as sustainable reinforcement material in biopolymeric blends. *J. Mater. Res. Technol.* 15, 2287–2316. https://doi.org/10.1016/j.jmrt.2021.08.139

Mei, J., Shen, X., Gang, L., Xu, H., Wu, F., Sheng, L., 2020. A novel lignin degradation, bacteria-Bacillus amyloliquefaciens SL-7, used to degrade straw lignin efficiently. *Bioresour. Technol.* 310, 123445. https://doi.org/10.1016/j.biortech.2020.123445

Mohtar, S.S., Tengku Malim Busu, T.N.Z., Md Noor, A.M., Shaari, N., Yusoff, N.A., Bustam Khalil, M.A., Abdul Mutalib, M.I., Mat, H.B., 2015. Extraction and characterization of lignin from oil palm biomass via ionic liquid dissolution and non-toxic aluminium potassium sulfate dodecahydrate precipitation processes. *Bioresour. Technol.* 192, 212–218. https://doi.org/10.1016/j.biortech.2015.05.029

Nandiwale, K.Y., Danby, A.M., Ramanathan, A., Chaudhari, R.V., Motagamwala, A.H., Dumesic, J.A., Subramaniam, B., 2020. Enhanced acid-catalyzed lignin depolymerization in a continuous reactor with stable activity. *ACS Sustain. Chem. Eng.* 8, 4096–4106. https://doi.org/10.1021/acssuschemeng.9b06556

Naresh Kumar, A., Kim, G.-B., Muhorakeye, A., Varjani, S., Kim, S.H., 2021. Biopolymer production using volatile fatty acids as resource: Effect of feast-famine strategy and lignin reinforcement. *Bioresour. Technol.* 326, 124736. https://doi.org/10.1016/j.biortech.2021.124736

Nitsos, C., Stoklosa, R., Karnaouri, A., Vörös, D., Lange, H., Hodge, D., Crestini, C., Rova, U., Christakopoulos, P., 2016. Isolation and characterization of organosolv and alkaline lignins from hardwood and softwood biomass. *ACS Sustain. Chem. Eng.* 4, 5181–5193. https://doi.org/10.1021/acssuschemeng.6b01205

Pourbaba, R., Abdulkhani, A., Rashidi, A., Ashori, A., 2024. Lignin nanoparticles as a highly efficient adsorbent for the removal of methylene blue from aqueous media. *Sci. Rep.* 14, 9039. https://doi.org/10.1038/s41598-024-59612-4

Radotić, K., Mićić, M., 2016. Methods for extraction and purification of lignin and cellulose from plant tissues, in: Micic, M. (Ed.), *Sample Preparation Techniques for Soil, Plant, and Animal Samples: Springer Protocols Handbooks*. Humana Press, New York, pp. 365–376. https://doi.org/10.1007/978-1-4939-3185-9.

Ren, T., Qi, W., Su, R., He, Z., 2019. Promising techniques for depolymerization of lignin into value-added chemicals. *Chem Cat Chem* 11, 639–654. https://doi.org/10.1002/cctc.201801428

Ruiz-Dueñas, F.J., Martínez, Á.T., 2009. Review microbial degradation of lignin: How a bulky recalcitrant polymer is efficiently recycled in nature, and how we can take advantage of this. *Microb. Biotechnol.* 2, 164–177. https://doi.org/10.1111/j.1751-7915.2008.00078.x

Sarwal, R., Kumar, S., Mehta, A., Varadan, A., Kumar Singh, S., Ramakumar, S.S.V., Mathai, R., 2021. *Road Map for Ethanol Blending in India 2020–25: Report of the Expert Committee*. NITI Aayog, India, pp. 1–67.

Sun, Y., Liu, X., Wang, T., Xue, B., Sun, R., 2019. Green process for extraction of lignin by the microwave-assisted ionic liquid approach: Toward biomass biorefinery and lignin characterization. *ACS Sustain. Chem. Eng.* 7, 13062–13072. https://doi.org/10.1021/acssuschemeng.9b02166

Sutherland, J.B., Crawford, D.L., Pometto, A.L., 1981. Catabolism of substituted benzoic acids by Streptomyces species. *Appl. Environ. Microbiol.* 41, 442–448. https://doi.org/10.1128/aem.41.2.442-448.1981

Szalaty, T.J., Klapiszewski, Ł., Jesionowski, T., 2020. Recent developments in modification of lignin using ionic liquids for the fabrication of advanced materials – A review. *J. Mol. Liq.* 301, 112417. https://doi.org/https://doi.org/10.1016/j.molliq.2019.112417

Veluchamy, C., Kalamdhad, A.S., 2017. Influence of pretreatment techniques on anaerobic digestion of pulp and paper mill sludge: A review. *Bioresour. Technol.* 245, 1206–1219. https://doi.org/10.1016/j.biortech.2017.08.179

Wang, G., Chen, H., 2013. Fractionation of alkali-extracted lignin from steam-exploded stalk by gradient acid precipitation. *Sep. Purif. Technol.* 105, 98–105. https://doi.org/10.1016/j.seppur.2012.12.009

Wang, H., Pu, Y., Ragauskas, A., Yang, B., 2019. From lignin to valuable products: Strategies, challenges, and prospects. *Bioresour. Technol.* 271, 449–461. https://doi.org/10.1016/j.biortech.2018.09.072

Watkins, D., Hosur, M., Tcherbi-Narteh, A., Jeelani, S., 2015. Extraction and characterization of lignin from different biomass resources *J. Mater. Res. Technol.* 4, 26–32.

Weng, C., Peng, X., Han, Y., 2021. Depolymerization and conversion of lignin to value-added bioproducts by microbial and enzymatic catalysis. *Biotechnol. Biofuels* 14, 84. https://doi.org/10.1186/s13068-021-01934-w

Wu, X., Amanze, C., Wang, J., Yu, Z., Shen, L., Wu, X., Li, J., Yu, R., Liu, Y., Zeng, W., 2022. Isolation and characterization of a novel thermotolerant alkali lignin-degrading bacterium Aneurinibacillus sp. LD3 and its application in food waste composting. *Chemosphere* 307, 135859.

Wu, X., Jiang, J., Wang, C., Liu, J., Pu, Y., Ragauskas, A., Li, S., Yang, B., 2020. Lignin-derived electrochemical energy materials and systems. *Biofuels, Bioprod. Biorefining*. https://doi.org/10.1002/bbb.2083

Wu, Y., Wang, J., Qiu, X., Yang, R., Lou, H., Bao, X., Li, Y., 2016. Highly efficient inverted perovskite solar cells with sulfonated lignin doped PEDOT as hole extract layer. *ACS Appl. Mater. Interfaces* 8, 12377–12383. https://doi.org/10.1021/acsami.6b00084

Yelle, D.J., Ralph, J., Lu, F., Hammel, K.E., 2008. Evidence for cleavage of lignin by a brown rot basidiomycete. *Environ. Microbiol.* 10, 1844–1849. https://doi.org/10.1111/j.1462-2920.2008.01605.x

Yelle, D.J., Wei, D., Ralph, J., Hammel, K.E., 2011. Multidimensional NMR analysis reveals truncated lignin structures in wood decayed by the brown rot basidiomycete Postia placenta. *Environ. Microbiol.* 13, 1091–1100. https://doi.org/10.1111/j.1462-2920.2010.02417.x

You, X., Duan, J., Koda, K., Yamada, T., Uraki, Y., 2016a. Preparation of electric double layer capacitors (EDLCs) from two types of electrospun lignin fibers. *Holzforschung* 70, 661–671. https://doi.org/10.1515/hf-2015-0175

You, X., Koda, K., Yamada, T., Uraki, Y., 2015. Preparation of electrode for electric double-layer capacitor from electrospun lignin fibers. *Holzforschung* 69, 1097–1106. https://doi.org/10.1515/hf-2014-0262

You, X., Koda, K., Yamada, T., Uraki, Y., 2016b. Preparation of high-performance internal tandem electric double-layer capacitors (IT-EDLCs) from melt-spun lignin fibers. *J. Wood Chem. Technol.* 36, 418–431. https://doi.org/10.1080/02773813.2016.1212893

Zabed, H.M., Akter, S., Yun, J., Zhang, G., Awad, F.N., Qi, X., Sahu, J.N., 2019. Recent advances in biological pretreatment of microalgae and lignocellulosic biomass for biofuel production. *Renew. Sustain. Energy Rev.* 105, 105–128. https://doi.org/10.1016/j.rser.2019.01.048

Zhang, L., Choi, C., Machida, H., Huo, Z., Norinaga, K., 2021. Catalytic hydrotreatment of alkaline lignin and its consequent influences on fast pyrolysis. *Carbon Resour. Convers.* 4, 219–229. https://doi.org/10.1016/j.crcon.2021.09.001

Zhang, S., Dong, Z., Shi, J., Yang, C., Fang, Y., Chen, G., Chen, H., Tian, C., 2022, Enzymatic hydrolysis of corn stover lignin by laccase, lignin peroxidase, and manganese peroxidase. *Bioresour. Technol.* 361, 127699.

Zhao, S., Deng, D., Wan, T., Feng, J., Deng, L., Tian, Q., Wang, J., Aiman, U.E., Mukhaddi, B., Hu, X., Chen, S., Qiu, L., Huang, L., Wei, Y., 2024. Lignin bioconversion based on genome mining for ligninolytic genes in Erwinia billingiae QL-Z3. *Biotechnol. Biofuels Bioprod.* 17, 1–18. https://doi.org/10.1186/s13068-024-02470-z

Zhou, N., Thilakarathna, W.P.D.W., He, Q.S., Rupasinghe, H.P.V., 2022. A review: Depolymerization of lignin to generate high-value bio-products: Opportunities, challenges, and prospects. *Front. Energy Res.* 9, 758744. https://doi.org/10.3389/fenrg.2021.758744

Zhu, D., Zhang, P., Xie, C., Zhang, W., Sun, J., Qian, W.J., Yang, B., 2017. Biodegradation of alkaline lignin by Bacillus ligniniphilus L1. *Biotechnol. Biofuels* 10, 1–14. https://doi.org/10.1186/s13068-017-0735-y

Zhu, J., Yan, C., Zhang, Xin, Yang, C., Jiang, M., Zhang, Xiangwu, 2020. A sustainable platform of lignin: From bioresources to materials and their applications in rechargeable batteries and supercapacitors. *Prog. Energy Combust. Sci.* https://doi.org/10.1016/j.pecs.2019.100788

24 Membrane Bioreactors for Industrial and Domestic Wastewater Treatment

Sajja Srinivas Chandrasekhar,
Sugali Chandra Sekhar, Bukke Vani,
Nazia Shaik, and Sundergopal Sridhar

24.1 INTRODUCTION

The world is facing a global crisis of water scarcity and contamination. Population growth and urbanization, rapid industrialization, and expanding and intensifying food production put pressure on water resources and increase the unregulated or illegal discharge of contaminated water within and beyond national borders (Li et al., 2016). Therefore, interest in wastewater treatment is increasing, driven by the growing focus on water conservation. In addition, urbanization is creating a demand for more compact wastewater treatment plants. Activated sludge treatment is often used for municipal and domestic wastewater purification and achieves high organic matter removal efficiency. However, activated sludge treatments are susceptible to external disturbances of physical and/or chemical nature, which often result in high suspended solids and turbidity in the effluent, reducing the amount of active biomass in the bioreactor. Currently, recycling and reuse of wastewater have become economically and environmentally viable processes, driven by restrictive wastewater discharge parameters, the imposition of charges for water collection and effluent discharge, and reduced availability of water quality resources. This being the case, the most promising technologies for wastewater treatment are reuse membrane separation systems and the combination of these systems with other technologies (Jin et al., 2014; Yi et al., 2011).

24.2 MEMBRANE

In membrane processes, the membrane acts as a semipermeable barrier, a thin layer that separates permeate and reject components from the feed sample. It acts

DOI: 10.1201/9781003327608-24

as a filtration and separation process driven by pressure applied to the thin layer's surface, according to Ho and Sirkar (1992).

24.2.1 Classification of the Membrane Processes

Based on pore size and pressure-driven forces, membranes are classified into four types: microfiltration (MF), ultrafiltration (UF), nanofiltration (NF), and reverse osmosis (RO). NF and UF are low-pressure-driven processes to clarify and separate suspended and colloidal particles from the selected solution. NF is a moderate-pressure-driven process used for water and wastewater treatment and other applications. RO requires higher pressure than other membrane processes and is widely used for water filtration and other applications.

24.2.2 Conventional Activated Sludge Process

It mainly consists of two steps. The first step involves treating the wastewater in an aeration tank using activated sludge. After treatment, the treated water and sludge are separated in the sedimentation tank or secondary clarifier. Further, activated sludge can be collected in a sedimentation tank, and the lighter fraction is carried out with the treated effluent.

24.3 PROCESS FOR THE MEMBRANE BIOREACTOR

A membrane bioreactor combines biological action with a separation process to degrade pollutants and impurities in selected wastewater and produce high-quality treated water for reuse in various applications (Santasmasas et al., 2014). The membrane bioreactor (MBR) is a key step in wastewater treatment for contaminant separation, a promising and advanced solution (Peinemann and Nunes, 2010; Norman et al., 2008). Membrane bioreactors provide efficient separation and allow high organic loading with a compact system footprint. MBRs are divided into submerged/internal and side-stream/external configurations, depending on the way the membrane module is coupled. In a submerged membrane bioreactor (SMBR), the modules are immersed in the bioreactor, and filtration is driven by vacuum pressure. The filtration tank is often separated from the bioreactor tank, with the mixed liquor circulated between them. In a side-stream membrane bioreactor (SSMBR), the membrane modules are coupled to the bioreactor by an external sludge recirculation loop to create cross-flow velocity.

24.3.1 Types of Membrane Bioreactor

MBRs are classified into two configurations: submerged membrane bioreactor (SMBR) and side-stream membrane bioreactor (SSMBR).

24.3.1.1 Submerged/Immersed

In the submerged/immersed membrane bioreactor, the membrane is directly immersed in the bioreactor. The membranes are configured either horizontally

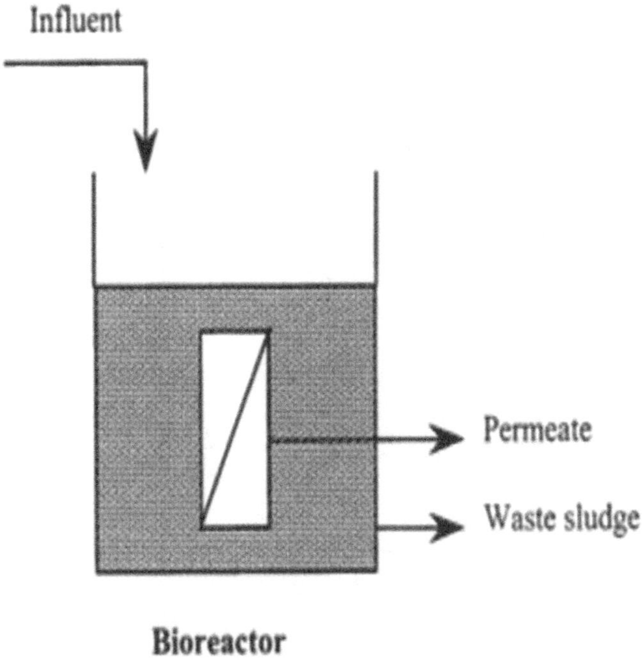

FIGURE 24.1 Submerged membrane bioreactor.

or vertically. The membrane component involves significantly more membrane area per unit volume than the membrane component involved in the (side-stream) external MBR configuration (Al-Shammari et al., 2015) (Figure 24.1).

24.3.1.2 Side Stream/External

In this MBR configuration, the membrane is located outside the reactor. The tubular membranes control the membrane flow at a well-defined flow velocity (Figure 24.2).

24.4 ADVANTAGES OF THE MBR PROCESS

MBR has many advantages over the activated sludge process (ASP). It includes higher biomass concentration; a smaller footprint; less sludge production; decoupled sludge (SRT) and hydraulic retention time; and highly improved, consistent effluent quality. Moreover, the membrane bioreactor is commonly considered an innovative wastewater treatment technology and reclamation with high water filtration flux and recovery. The membrane bioreactor is simple and easy to operate. The advantages of MBRs with conventional ASP include a small footprint and reduced sludge production. The submerged MBR requires only half the area of a conventional activated sludge process and sludge production. A membrane bioreactor is an advanced technology for alleviating membrane fouling and improving

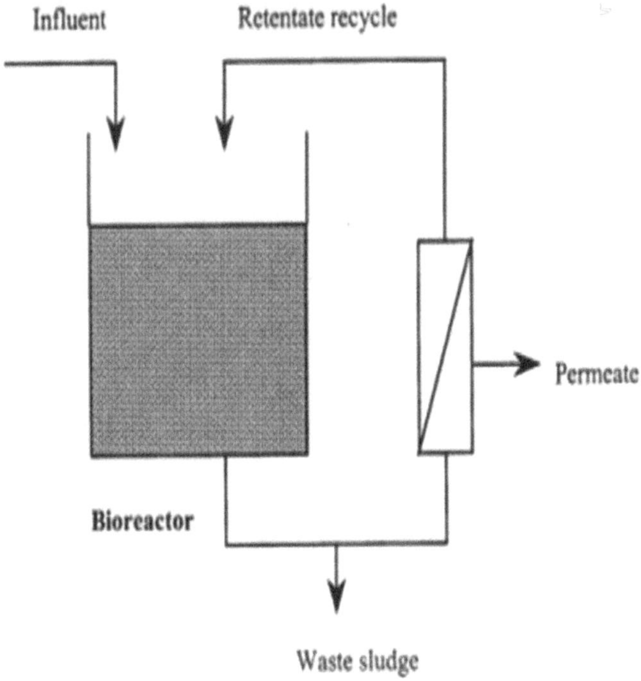

FIGURE 24.2 Side-stream membrane bioreactor.

wastewater treatment efficiency, with good performance and a promising future in applications (Al-Asheh et al., 2021). Challenges facing membrane-based technologies for water reuse applications, including institutional barriers, financial constraints, and public awareness, are identified as areas requiring further research and development to improve the production of reusable water and reduce freshwater consumption.

24.5 CHARACTERISTIC PARAMETERS OF THE WASTEWATER AND ANALYTICAL METHODS AS PER STANDARDS

The characteristics of wastewater are determined as per the American Public Health Association (APHA) and the pollution control board (PCB) standards. Turbidity is purely an appearance of the optical property of a sample measured with the help of a turbidity meter. The turbidity of wastewater is measured with Formazin Attenuation Units (FAU). The pH and conductivity of the sample are measured using a digital pH and EC meter, and buffer solutions are used to maintain the required pH and EC. Total suspended solids are determined using a simple weighing balance method, and total suspended solids are measured by an HM digital TDS meter with a range of 0–5,000 ppm. The closed titrimetric method analyzed chemical oxygen demand after 2 hr of incubation.

24.6 APPLICATION OF MBR FOR TREATMENT OF INDUSTRIAL AND DOMESTIC WASTEWATERS

24.6.1 Industrial Wastewater (Laundry Wastewater) Treatment

The laundry industry generates large quantities of wastewater among all the industries with a lot of detergents, fats, dyes, excess surfactants, solvents, plasticizers, emulsifiers, even pathogens, and other chemicals, which cause a rapid pollution load on the environment, which in turn increases chemical oxygen demand and biological oxygen demand and interrupts the balance of aquatic and ecological ecosystem (Giagnorio et al., 2017; Manouchehri and Kargari, 2017; Mozia et al., 2017). Wastewater recovery and reuse are important and necessary to meet industrial and public water demands, treating wastewater generated by the industrial sector. Most reports state that various techniques, such as coagulation, electrocoagulation, flotation, adsorption, chemical oxidation, and membrane filtration, followed by biological treatment, are primarily used instead of conventional methods. Numerous studies have reported on the implementation of membrane technology for laundry wastewater treatment, mostly in combination with other processes. Most studies focused on the reuse of water without considering treatment economics and environmental aspects, but membrane technology has been adopted for wastewater treatment due to its high separation efficiency and economic and environmental advantages (APHA, 2000, 2005). Membrane processes are pressure-driven membrane techniques that are considered the best solutions for water reuse (Szwast and Polak, 2018).

Efficient removal of impurities was observed as follows: 93% of total suspended solids (TSS); 74% for chemical oxygen demand; and 22% for total phosphorus (TP), by combining coagulation with an MF system (Kim et al., 2014; Shang et al., 2015). A 55–65% decrease in COD and complete removal of turbidity have been reported using a combined coagulation and MF process. Sumisha et al. (2015) achieved more than 90% turbidity and more than 80% COD removal using the UF membrane process alone for laundry wastewater treatment. Pollutant removal efficiency was improved by applying adsorption after coagulation treatment of laundry wastewater, along with membrane filtration such as ultrafiltration (UF) and reverse osmosis. The results showed that a single coagulation step was ineffective for removing surfactant. The treatment was analyzed with chemical oxygen demand and biological oxygen demand to get higher-quality treated wastewater for reuse in the laundry industry (Sostar-Turk et al., 2005). The results from the membrane bioreactor process show good-quality treated water for reuse. The reuse of laundry wastewater to meet the water demands of the rinsing processes was studied by Hoinkis and Panten (2008).

Treatment of laundry wastewater using clay oil can be used as a resource in urban areas to meet daily needs (Misra & Sivongxay, 2009). The NF process produces high-quality permeate water free of microbes and suspended solids, with a chemical oxygen demand of 48 mg (Guilbaud et al., 2010), for the recycling of laundry wastewater. Laundry wastewater treatment using microfiltration and recovered water shows that the process is reliable for use in washing machines, toilets, irrigation, and so forth (Manouchehri &Kargari, 2017). Commercial laundry wastewater was treated in two-stage bioreactors; the treated wastewater met discharge standards and was of good quality (Bering et al., 2018).

24.6.2 Domestic Wastewater (Kitchen Wastewater) Treatment

Domestic wastewater typically has high concentrations of suspended and dissolved solids, turbidity, chemical oxygen demand, biological oxygen demand, and other pollutants. The membrane bioreactors consist of a cell growth reactor and a membrane filtration device combined into a single unit process. The membrane unit can be placed externally, as in side-stream operation, or submerged in the reactor. In the externally mounted membrane system, the side-stream membrane bioreactor operates independently. The effluent enters the bioreactor as input, is further degraded by microorganisms, and is filtered by a membrane filtration unit operated on a pressure-driven pump. The membrane permeate is the treated product, and the retentate is continuously returned to the bioreactor. In the submerged membrane bioreactor, the modules are immersed in the bioreactor, and filtration is driven by vacuum pressure. The filtration tank is often separated from the bioreactor tank, with the mixed liquor circulated between them.

Significant reductions in turbidity and COD were observed with the HF-UF membrane.

In the aerobic mode of SMBR, after 21 days of the experimental study, a sharp drop in turbidity from 71 FAU in the feed to 6 FAU in the permeate was observed, resulting in 92% turbidity removal efficiency. Similarly, a 97% reduction in COD was observed, from 3,967 ppm to 120 ppm. Decreases in TDS from 1,382 ppm to 1,000 ppm and in TSS from 450 ppm to 120 ppm were observed by Chandrasekhar et al. (2017). The treatment method with MBRs resulted in effective removal of organics, TSS, surfactants, and micropollutants from different wastewater streams. The process of MBRs has achieved constant removal rates of 90–95% for COD, 80–99% for NH4-N, and 70–99% for total phosphorus (Hai et al., 2018; Song et al., 2018), as concluded by Alturki et al. (2010).

24.6.3 Procedure for Membrane Cleaning

Cleaning in place (CIP) is necessary to clean the membrane module, prevent membrane fouling, and improve flux and water recovery. Cleaning can remove organic, inorganic, suspended, and dissolved particles; pathogens; and scale from the membrane surface and pores. The membrane's cleaning procedure includes the use of citric acid, NaOH, EDTA, and SLS as chemical and chelating reagents; a 1% citric acid solution is recirculated throughout the membrane module for 20 minutes to remove inorganic and organic contaminants, followed by a water wash for 20 minutes. After the acid wash, the membrane is cleaned with an alkali solution containing 0.5% EDTA and 1% NaOH for 20 minutes to remove salts formed on the membrane surface, followed by a water wash for 10 minutes. After the membrane cleaning process, it is stored in 0.1% SMBS solution for the membrane durability span (Chandrasekhar et al., 2020, 2021, 2022).

24.6.4 Results and Discussion

Experimental results are shown in Tables 24.1 and 24.2. The pH, conductivity, turbidity, TDS, COD, and color values decrease from feed to permeate in both laundry and kitchen wastewater systems (Figures 24.3 and 24.4). This indicates that separation is occurring and the MBR is working well.

TABLE 24.1
Characteristic Parameters of Laundry Wastewater: Feed and Permeate Values

Serial Number	Parameters	Feed	Permeate	Percentage Removal
1	pH	8.5	7.25	15
2	Conductivity (mS/cm)	2.98	0.45	85
3	Turbidity (FAU)	350	5	98.5
4	Total dissolved solids, TDS (ppm)	1,907	288	85
5	Chemical oxygen demand (COD) (mg/L)	2,800	120	96
6	Color (Pt-Co)	120	8	93

TABLE 24.2
Characteristic Parameters of Kitchen Wastewater: Feed and Permeate Values

Serial Number	Parameters	Feed	Permeate	Percentage Removal
1	pH	8.20	7.10	13.41
2	Conductivity (mS/cm)	2.00	0.65	67.5
3	Turbidity (FAU)	165	4	97.57
4	Total dissolved solids, TDS (ppm)	2,065	416	79.89
5	Chemical oxygen demand (COD) (mg/L)	3,010	115	96.17
6	Color (Pt-Co)	110	5	95.45

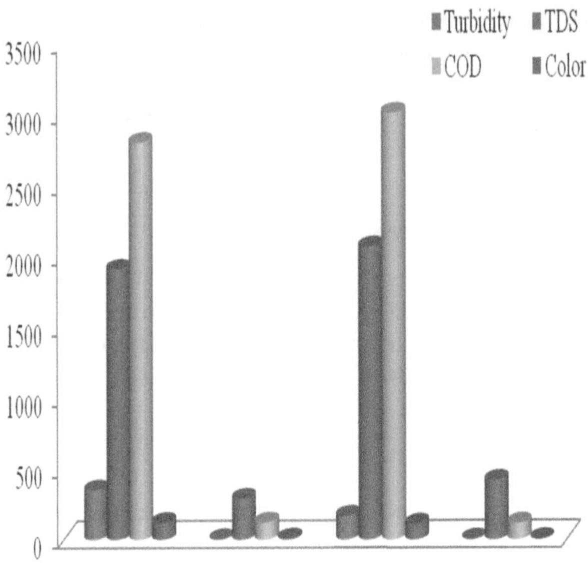

FIGURE 24.3 Characteristic parameters of laundry and domestic wastewater.

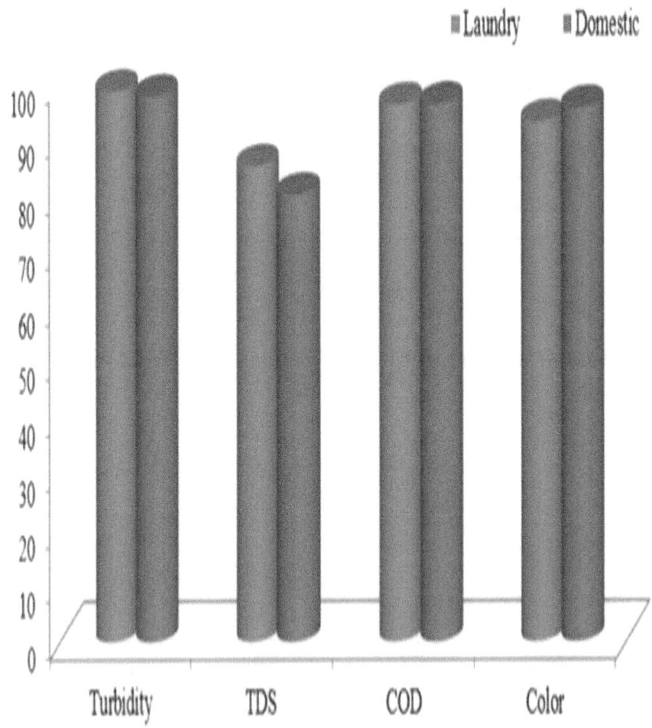

FIGURE 24.4 Percentage removal of impurities in laundry and domestic wastewater.

24.6.5 Summary on Membrane Bioreactor

MBR is a membrane separation process for the efficient separation performance of membrane bio-solids, with high concentration, which can be retained within the bioreactor, enabling operation in high organic loading and compacting the equipment. MBRs are divided into submerged/internal and side-stream/external configurations, depending on how the membrane is coupled. In the submerged membrane bioreactor, the modules are immersed in the bioreactor, with filtration driven by vacuum pressure. The filtration tank is often separated from the bioreactor tank, with the mixed liquor circulated between them. In a side-stream membrane bioreactor, the membrane modules are coupled to the bioreactor by an external sludge recirculation loop to create cross-flow velocity. MBR has many advantages over the conventional activated sludge process, including a higher biomass concentration; a smaller footprint; less sludge production; a decoupled sludge and hydraulic retention time process; and highly improved, consistent effluent quality. Moreover, MBR is commonly considered an innovative wastewater treatment and reclamation technology with high water filtration efficiency (simple and easy to operate). The MBR process leads to a small footprint and reduced sludge production. Submerged MBRs require only half the land area of a traditional ASP and produce less sludge. To maintain long-term membrane performance and manage membrane fouling, filtration is typically performed in cycles that include relaxation or backwash (physical cleaning methods), maintenance, and intensive chemical cleaning. To extend membrane life, modules can be stored in an SMBS solution to prevent pore blockage. The obtained permeate water meets APHA and PCB standards, and reclaimed water quality can be reused in different applications. MBR is an excellent technology, alleviating membrane fouling and improving wastewater treatment efficiency, with good performance and a bright future in applications. Challenges are institutional blocks, financial allocation, and public awareness. It needs further research and development to reduce freshwater consumption.

24.7 CONCLUSION

The basic concepts of MBRs and case studies of their application for industrial (laundry) and domestic (kitchen) wastewater treatment are discussed. In laundry wastewater, COD and TDS decreased by 96% and 85%, respectively. From the kitchen wastewater, the COD levels and TDS values decreased by 96% and 80%, respectively. Reduction in COD and TDS values indicates better treatment efficiency. Membrane fouling is addressed through effective cleaning.

24.8 ACKNOWLEDGMENT

The authors are thankful to the Membrane Separations Laboratory, Department of Process Engineering and Technology Transfer, CSIR Indian Institute of Chemical Technology (IICT), Hyderabad, and AcSIR, Ghaziabad, Uttar Pradesh, India.

REFERENCES

Al-Asheh, S., Bagheri, M., & Aidan, A. 2021. Membrane bioreactor for wastewater treatment: A review. *Case Studies in Chemical and Environmental Engineering*,4, 100109.

Al-Shammari, S.B., Sameer, B.H., Al-Saffar, A., Salman, M., & Al-Sairafi, A. 2015. Treatment of dairy wastewater effluent using submerged membrane microfiltration system. *Journal of Environmental Science and Engineering*,4, 107–118.

Alturki, A.A., Tadkaew, N., McDonald, J.A., Khan, S.J., Price, W.E., & Nghiem, L.D. 2010. Combining MBR and NF/RO membrane filtration for the removal of trace organics in indirect potable water reuse applications. *J. Membr. Sci.*, 365, 206–215.

APHA (American Public Health Association). 2000. *Standard Methods for Examination of Water and Wastewater*, 21st edition. Washington, DC.

Bering,S., Mazur, J., Tarnowski, K., Janus, M., Mozia, S., & Morawski, A.W. 2018. The application of moving bed bio-reactor (MBBR) in commercial laundry wastewater treatment. *Sci. Total Environ.*, 627, 1638–1643.

Chandrasekhar, S.S., Chandra Sekhar, S., Kalyani, S., & Sridhar, S. 2022. Performance assessment of a side-stream membrane bioreactor for the treatment of kitchen wastewater. *Biochemical Engineering Journal*, 180, 108366.

Chandrasekhar, S.S., Sahu, N., & Sridhar, S. 2017.Processing of dairy industrial effluent and kitchen wastewater by integration of microbial action with membrane processes. *Membrane Technology*, 493–514.

Chandrasekhar, S.S., Sahu, N., & Sridhar, S. 2021. Treatment of textile industrial wastewater using hydrophilized polyamide nanofiltration membrane for water recovery and reuse. *Journal of Water Pollutionand Purification Research*, 8(3).

Chandrasekhar, S.S., Vaishnavi, D., Sahu, N., & Sridhar, S. 2020. Design of an integrated membrane bioreactor process for effective and environmentally safe treatment of highly complex coffee industrial effluent. *Journal of Water Process Engineering*, 37, 101436.

Federation, W.E., & Association, A.P.H. 2005. *Standard Methods for the Examination of Water and Wastewater*. American Public Health Association (APHA), Washington, DC, USA.

Giagnorio, M., Amelio, A., Grüttner, H., & Tiraferri, A. 2017. Environmental impacts of detergents and benefits of their recovery in the laundering industry. *J. Clean. Prod.*, 154, 593–601.

Guilbaud, J., Masse Andres, Y., Combe, F., & Jaouen, P. 2010. Laundry water recycling in ship by direct nanofiltration with tubular membranes. *Resour. Conserv. Recy.*, 55, 148–154.

Hai, F.I., Yamamoto, K., & Lee, C.-H. 2018. *Membrane Biological Reactors: Theory, Modeling, Design, Management and Applications to Wastewater Reuse*, 2nd edition. IWA Publishing, London, UK. ISBN 978-1-78040-916-0.

Ho, W.S.W., & Sirkar, K.K. 1992. *Membrane Handbook*. Van Nostrand, New York, p. 393.

Hoinkis, J., & Panten, V. 2008. Wastewater recycling in laundries-from pilot to large-scale plant. *Chem Eng Process.*, 47, 1159–1164.

Jin, L., Zhang, G., & Tian, H. 2014. Current state of sewage treatment in China. *Water Research*, 66, 85–98.

Kim, H.-C., Shang, X., Huang, J.H., & Dempsey, B.A. 2014. Treating laundry wastewater: Cationic polymers for removal of contaminants and decreased fouling in microfiltration. *J. Membr. Sci.*, 456, 167–174.

Li, K., Wang, J., Liu, J., Wei, Y., & Chen, M. 2016. Advanced treatment of municipal wastewater by nanofiltration: Operational optimization and membrane fouling analysis. *Journal of Environmental Sciences*, 43, 106–117.

Manouchehri, M., & Kargari, A. 2017. Water recovery from laundry wastewater by the cross-flow microfiltration process: A strategy for water recycling in residential buildings. *J. Clean. Prod.*, 168, 227–238.

Misra, K.R., & Sivongxay, A. 2009. Reuse of laundry greywater as affected by its interaction with saturated soil. *J. Hydrol.*, 366, 5561.

Mozia, S., Janus, M., Brożek, P., Bering, S., Tarnowski, K., Mazur, J., & Morawski, A.W. 2017. Possibilities of application of advanced oxidation – membrane separation system for treatment and reuse of laundry wastewater. *Desalin. Water Treat.*, 64, 218–222.

Norman, N.L., Anthony, G.F., Winston Ho, W.S., & Takeshi, M. 2008. *Advanced Membrane Technology and Applications*. Wiley-AIChE, p. 1016. ISBN: 978-0-471-73167-2.

Peinemann, K.V., & Nunes, S.P. 2010. *Membranes for Water Treatment*. John Wiley and Sons, Membrane Technology, p. 4.

Santasmasas, C., Rovira, M., Clarens, F., & Valderrama, C. 2014. Wastewater treatment by MBR pilot plant: Flat sheet and hollow fiber case studies. *Desalination and Water Treatment*,51(10–12), 2423–2430.

Shang, X., Kim, H.-C., Huang, J.H., & Dempsey, B.A. 2015. Coagulation strategies to decrease fouling and increase critical flux and contaminant removal in microfiltration of laundry wastewater. *Sep. Purif. Technol.*, 147, 44–50.

Song, X., Luo, W., Hai, F.I., Price, W.E., Guo, W., Ngo, H.H., & Nghiem, L.D. 2018. Resource recovery from wastewater by anaerobic membrane bioreactors: Opportunities and challenges. *Bioresour. Technol.*, 270, 669–677.

Sostar-Turk, S., Petrinic, I., & Simonic, M. 2005. Laundry wastewater treatment using coagulation and membrane filtration. *Resour. Conserv. Recy.*, 44, 185–196.

Sumisha, A., Arthanareeswaran, G., Thuyavan, Y.L., Ismail, A.F., & Chakraborty, S. 2015. Application of equisetum hyemale in constructed wetland: Influence of wastewater dilution and contact time. *Ecotox. Environ. Saf.*, 121, 174–179.

Szwast, M., & Polak, D. 2018. Nowemembrany do filtracji ścieków z pralniprzemysłowych. *Przem. Chem.*, 97, 439–441.

Yi, L., Jiao, W., Chen, X., & Chen, W. 2011. An overview of reclaimed water reuse in China. *Journal of Environmental Sciences*, 23(10), 1585–1593.

25 Membranes in Biorefineries

Sundergopal Sridhar

25.1 INTRODUCTION

Over the last few decades, the adverse environmental effects of fossil fuels (coal and petroleum) have contributed to global warming, rising sea levels, and the depletion of resources needed to meet the world's energy demands. Alternatives to coal or petroleum should reduce greenhouse gas emissions and be produced from renewable, sustainable feedstocks. Bioethanol can be used as a neat fuel or blended with gasoline in cars and automobiles. Bioethanol is used as a fuel for transportation. The fermentation process primarily produces sugar. Ethanol is a colorless, odorless liquid that undergoes combustion, providing energy with carbon dioxide and water as byproducts. Bioethanol is relatively less toxic, safe, and biodegradable. Bioethanol is one of the most widely used alternative automotive fuels worldwide (Bowen et al., 2005). The production of chemicals and biofuels, such as ethanol, from processing biomass waste containing cellulose, lignin, and hemicellulose is a promising alternative route for generating renewable energy with greater efficiency than its sustainable counterparts (Chandel et al., 2007). In this process, biomass is pretreated with acids to separate lignin and reduce the size of the feedstock, thereby facilitating the production of sugars through hydrolysis and bioethanol by fermentation. Hydrolysis breaks down cellulose and hemicellulose into sugars, which are then fermented. Figure 25.1 illustrates the overall process for the conversion of lignocellulosic biomass to bioethanol, which includes mechanical unit operations for shredding, crushing, and sieving of the biomass, followed by pretreatment using dilute acid or alkali, saccharification of cellulose to produce glucose, fermentation of glucose to bioethanol, and finally distillation to separate water and concentrate bioethanol to the desired purity.

25.1.1 Sources Used to Produce Bioethanol

First-generation process plants include sugarcane, corn, wheat, and sweet sorghum, among others, while second-generation plants comprise *miscanthus*, *eucalyptus*, and so forth. Biomass conversion should be cost-competitive with rapid and efficient separation of fermented product from the biological media (Moiser et al., 2005; Bowen et al., 2005). Ethanol is a green liquid fuel that, upon combustion, produces CO_2 and H_2O but does not emit any harmful gases such as SO_2

 DOI: 10.1201/9781003327608-25

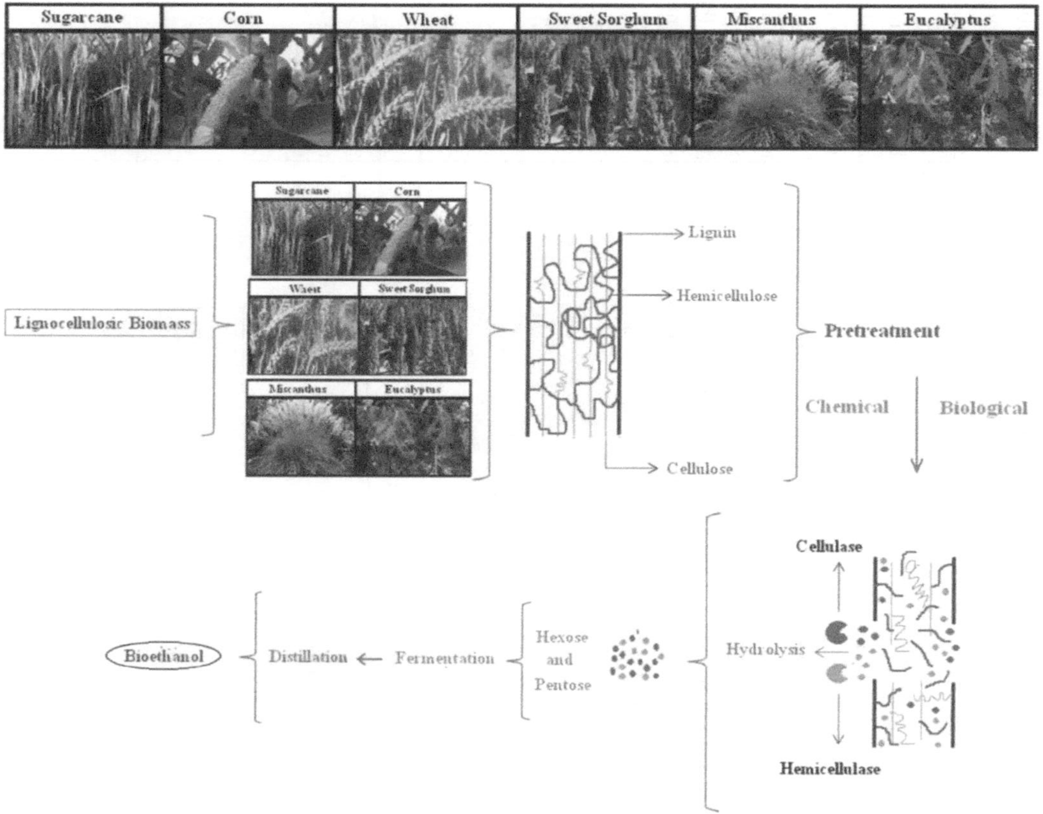

FIGURE 25.1 Overview of the process for conversion of lignocellulosic biomass to bioethanol.

and NO_2 In Brazil, ethanol is used as a neat fuel, i.e., 95% ethanol + 5% water, directly to run vehicles (Wyman, 1994; Wyman and Hinman, 1990).

Pretreatment processes: Pretreatment is one of the most crucial steps for recovering lignin-based biomass from cellulosic feedstocks. Pretreatment breaks down the lignin barrier, enabling recovery of cellulose, which is then enzymatically hydrolyzed to fermentable sugars. Over the past few decades, several pretreatment processes have been developed to generate cost-effective fermentable sugars from lignocellulosic matter containing cellulose and hemicellulose (Yang et al., 2008; Zahid Anwar et al., 2014). In this context, several reports are available on pretreatment technologies, suitable for various raw material feedstocks that conserve hemicellulose fragments, yield maximum fermentable sugars, minimize carbohydrate loss to prevent inhibitor formation from product degradation, and require minimal energy input. Chemical or biological methods can be used to hydrolyze lignocellulosic biomass (Yang et al., 2008, 2011; Asgher et al., 2013; Hamzeh et al., 2013). Pretreatment of biomass is energy-intensive, and the price of enzymes used in saccharification is also substantial, posing challenges that need to be decisively addressed. Figure 25.2 shows a magnified view of the mechanical unit operations involved in fragmenting lignocellulosic biomass into a processable form for pretreatment.

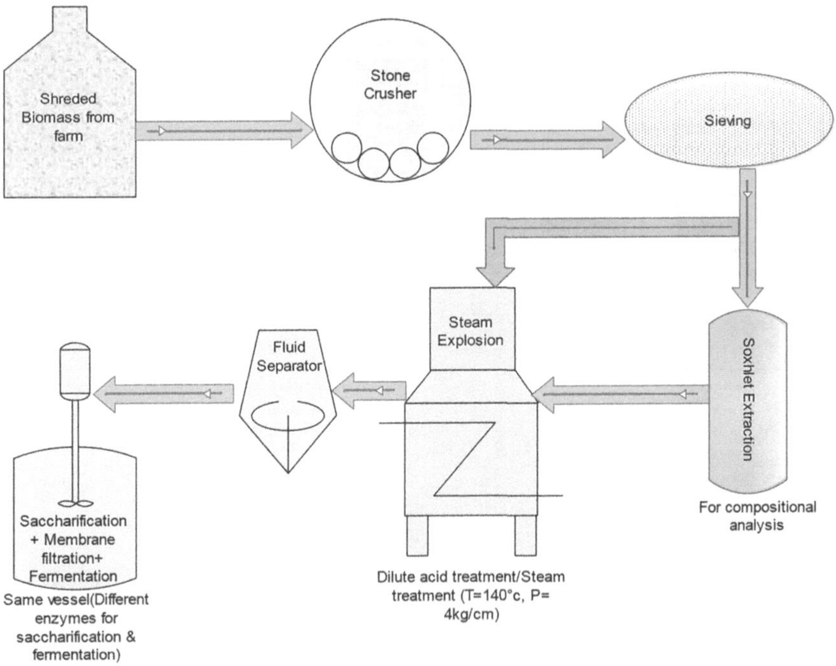

FIGURE 25.2 Mechanical unit operations for biomass pretreatment.

25.2 ROLE OF MEMBRANE FILTRATION TECHNOLOGY

The use of membrane technologies, such as microfiltration, ultrafiltration (UF), nanofiltration (NF), reverse osmosis (RO), electrodialysis (ED), pervaporation (PV), and membrane bioreactor (MBR), could be effective in achieving high bioethanol yields at low cost. The critical role of membrane processes in converting biomass to bioethanol is to reduce capex/opex, enhance process safety, reduce footprint, and increase recovery of valuable products. Table 25.1 presents the scope for applying membrane processes in bioethanol production. Mandalika et al. (2025) have detailed the scope of membrane separations in biomass processing. Mansy, El Desouky, Saleh (2024) used bacterial cellulose membranes for bioethanol separation and, in the same year, reported another study on bioethanol purification from the processing of office paper waste.

Membrane filtration is a proven, promising method primarily used in industrial processes, with increasing adoption in biofuel production and biorefineries. Membranes are physical barriers used in various processes for separating liquid-liquid and liquid-solid mixtures. Membranes allow the preferential passage of particles depending on their specific size and shape. Membrane filtration is widely used across various industrial sectors, including water purification, wastewater treatment, food processing, pharmaceuticals, biotechnology, and medicine (Rafik et al., 2015).

Figure 25.3(a) depicts an example of membrane intervention in biorefinery through a schematic of an electrodialysis process for the recovery of acid, alkali, or alkaline peroxide, along with isolation of lignin from the spent aqueous stream.

TABLE 25.1
Application of Membrane Processes in Various Steps of Bioethanol Production

Membrane Process	Application in Biorefinery
ED/NF (Elecrodialysis/Nano filtration)	Recovery of spent acid/alkali
UF (Ultrafiltration)	Retention of enzymes and substrates in a continuous enzyme reactor, permitting the removal of reaction-inhibiting components, enzyme concentration, concentration of lignin macromolecules with permeation of separation of hemi cellulose and cellulose and salts
MF (Microfiltration)	Isolation of the enzyme from a microorganism to obtain a clear enzymatic broth. MF for pretreatment to UF, NF, or RO
NF (Nanofiltration)	Concentration of dissolved solids and sugars in biomass
PV (Pervaporation)	Dehydration of rectified spirit (92%) to absolute alcohol (99.5%)
MBR (Membrane bioreactor)	Continuous extraction of ethanol from the fermenter to enhance yield
RO (Reverse osmosis)	Biomass effluent treatment for water reclamation

Alkaline peroxide is preferred because it separates both C5 and C6 sugars, whereas acid pretreatment separates hemicellulose only, and plain alkali pretreatment separates only cellulose, with the other sugar retained with lignin. Cation- and anion-transfer membranes are arranged alternately between the anode and the cathode, to which a DC power supply of 10 to 50 V is applied. The pretreatment step uses 2–4% alkaline peroxide to break down lignin in the biomass, after which the spent liquor contains alkali, along with water, lignin, cellulose, and hemicellulose. This solution can be introduced into an ED system that separates ionizable species, such as alkali, into concentrate chambers. At the same time, lignin and water will exit in a separate stream for further processing to separate lignin. As peroxide decomposes during pretreatment, the alkali-rich stream is collected in deionized water flowing through the parallel concentrate compartments. It can be reclaimed at 80–90% for the next pretreatment cycle of a fresh biomass batch (Figure. 25.3(b)).

Similarly, ED can be employed to recover 2–4% of the alkali used in other pretreatment steps that involve only alkali or alkaline peroxide. However, H_2O_2 does not ionize in water and cannot be separated by ED. Another process with potential for acid/alkali recovery from the spent pretreatment solution is nanofiltration using acid/alkali-resistant membranes, such as HF-NF AR with a 300 MWCO, which allows water and acid/alkali to pass through while retaining other impurities and mass residue. While previous sections presented novel but theoretical concepts for utilizing membranes in biorefineries, this section presents

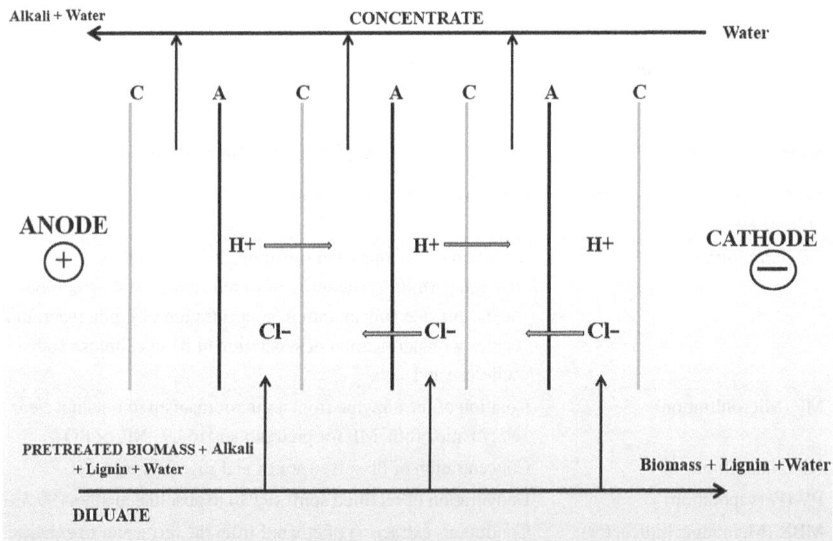

FIGURE 25.3A Principle of electrodialysis process for recovery of spent acid from biomass pretreatment step

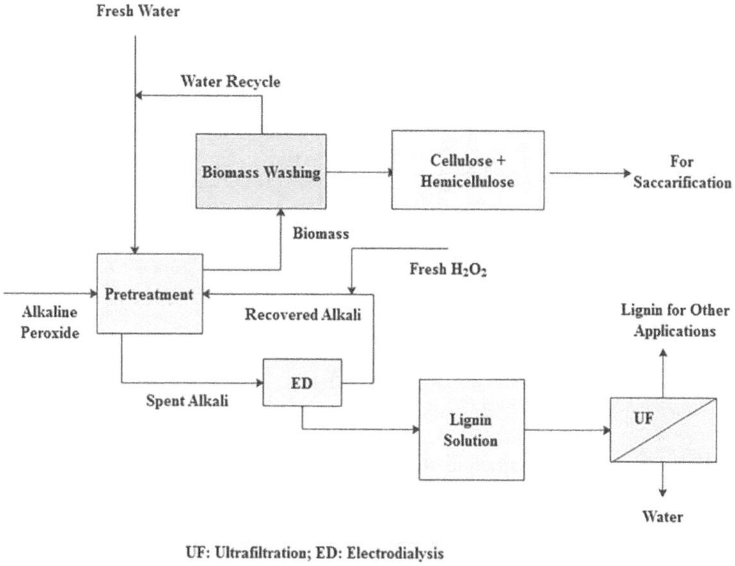

FIGURE 25.3B Alkaline peroxide-based biomass fractionation with alkali and water recycling.

authentic results from real-time experiments on sugar concentration, continuous ethanol separation during fermentation to enhance bioethanol yield, and, finally, biorefinery effluent treatment.

Membranes can be deployed in modular configurations for higher-capacity biorefineries. Membrane technology is used in biodiesel production by enabling the reuse of water and the dehydration of bioethanol (Ang et al., 2025). Li et al. (2025) recovered a concentrated saccharide solution from microalgal residue by combining hot-compressed water treatment with membrane separation. Wandscher Busanello et al. (2024) have investigated the role of membranes in biodiesel and bioethanol production.

25.3 RESULTS AND DISCUSSIONS

25.3.1 Sugar Concentration

The MWCO of the nanofiltration process lies between that of RO and microfiltration. The pore diameter size of these membranes ranges from 2 to 5 nm, with the applied pressure gradient across the membrane is being 100–400 psi (Figure 25.4). Commercially, nanofiltration is primarily used for the separation of monovalent ions from bivalent salts, treatment of industrial effluents to reclaim water, solvent recovery in pharma industry, etc. (Wyman and Dale, 2005). In biorefinery, Diaz-Arenas et al. (2025) have recovered xylooligosaccharides from steam-exploded hydrolysates using nanofiltration. Concentrated sugar can give

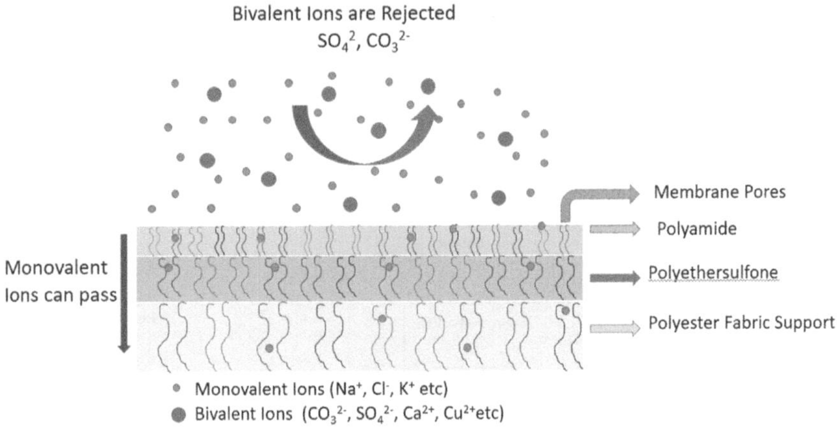

FIGURE 25.4 Working principle of the nanofiltration process.

higher fermentation yields, as investigated by Jiang H. et al. (2024), who used a pervaporation membrane bioreactor to isolate bioethanol from a cassava-fed fermentation unit. In the present study, tightly porous nanofiltration membranes, such as HFT 150, HPA 150, and HPA 100, were evaluated at both bench and pilot scales for the concentration of a glucose solution. NF is also used for the concentration of dairy, food products, sugar, starch, wine, and enzymes (Bowen et al., 2005). In the saccharification step, enzymes catalyze reactions that convert cellulose and hemicellulose into monomeric sugars. One limitation to improving alcohol yield is the formation of inhibitory products, such as monomeric sugars, during the saccharification step, which can reach specific concentrations over time. In the present work, attempts have been made to concentrate the C5 sugar from 2–5% to 12–20% post-saccharification by using NF. The concentrated sugar is then fed to the fermentation reactor for conversion to alcohol, while the lean sugar is returned to the saccharification reactor. This enables an increase in ethanol yield, typically 50% of the weight of the sugar fermented, meaning that every kg of sugar fermented yields 500 g of bioethanol.

A low-concentration sugar solution was used as the feed solution, which was passed through the membrane at high pressure. The retentate (concentrate) was collected from the feed tank, as shown in Figure 25.5. The feed solution was 25 L for the pilot scale and 2 L for the bench scale, with sugar feed concentrations ranging from 2% to 5%. The pressures applied were 7, 14, and 21 kg/cm^2 in each case study, until a specific permeate recovery was achieved. NF results were evaluated on the basis of operating parameters, including % water recovery, flux, and % sugar concentration, as shown in Table 25.3, with a % recovery of 71.33%.

The concentrated sugar solution from the retentate line was collected in the feed tank and recirculated to the NF membrane module, yielding a highly concentrated solution. After the experiment was completed, the highly concentrated

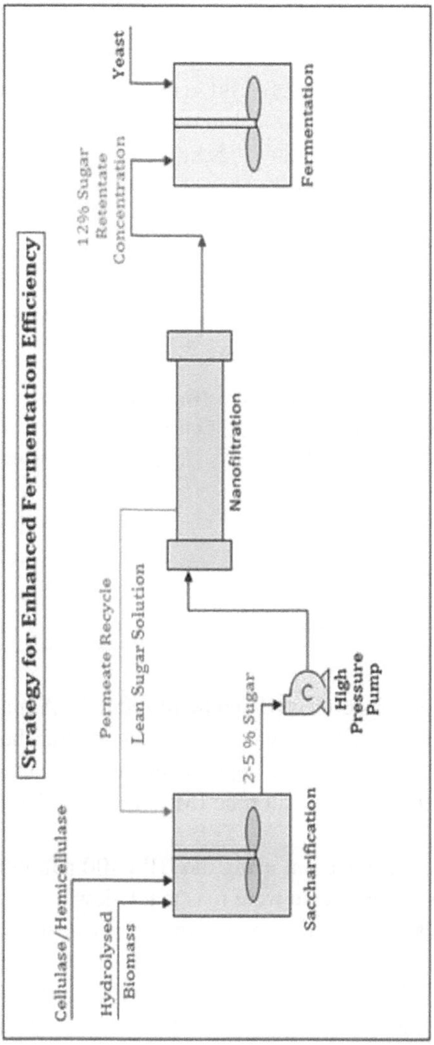

FIGURE 25.5 Sugar concentration by nanofiltration for enhanced productivity.

TABLE 25.2
Nanofiltration-Based Sugar Concentration Using Three Different Membranes

Membrane Type	Pressure (kg/cm^2)	Permeate Flux ($L/m^2/hr$)	% Water Recovery	Sugar Concentration (g/L) (%) Feed	Permeate	Conc.
HFT-150	7	1.26	83.5	91.94 (9.19%)	65.92 (6.59%)	228.4 (22.84%)
HPA-150	15	13.86	86.6	49.75 (4.97%)	30.15(3.01%)	177.1 (17.71%)
HPA-100	21	1.26	71.3	29.8 (2.98%)	0.6 (0.06%)	119.1 (11.91%)

TABLE 25.3
Nanofiltration Results for Sugar Concentration for HPA 100 at Pressures of 7, 14, 21 kg/cm²

Pressure (kg/cm^2)	Flux ($L/m^2/hr$)	Initial Sugar Concentration (g/lt)	Final Sugar Concentration (g/lt)	% Sugar rejection	% Permeate Water Recovery
7	15.5	1.7	5.6	50.82	88
14	30.3	1.61	5.55	69.4	90.8
21	54.5	1.4	4.3	65.57	90.8
21	6.58	3.0	11.91	89.79	71.33

retentate sugar solution was collected and analyzed (J.E. Almazan). For a particular membrane, the higher the applied pressure, the greater the pore compaction, leading to increasing retention of the sugar solute and greater water flux through the hydrophilic polyamide NF membrane [Moulik et al., 2015] as illustrated by Figure 25.6.

Further studies were carried out using the HPA-100 nanofiltration membrane, as the sugar losses in the permeate were reasonably low.

Figure 25.6 shows the effect of feed pressure on permeate flux and retention of sugar in the concentrate stream through the HPA-100 nanofiltration membrane. As pressure was varied from 7 to 21 kg/cm^2, flux ranged from 15.5 to 54.5 $L/m^2/hr$, while sugar retention ranged from 50.8% to 69.4%. The initial concentration was maintained constant at 1.5 g/L, and the final retentate concentrate was 5.5 g/L. Higher pressure allowed lower losses of sugar in the permeate due to the solution-diffusion mechanism [Sridhar, 2002], which states that the solvent (water) flux increases because of the preferential affinity of the hydrophilic membrane, containing —CONH— groups, with polar H_2O molecules. As described earlier, pore compaction theory predicts that, with increased sugar concentration

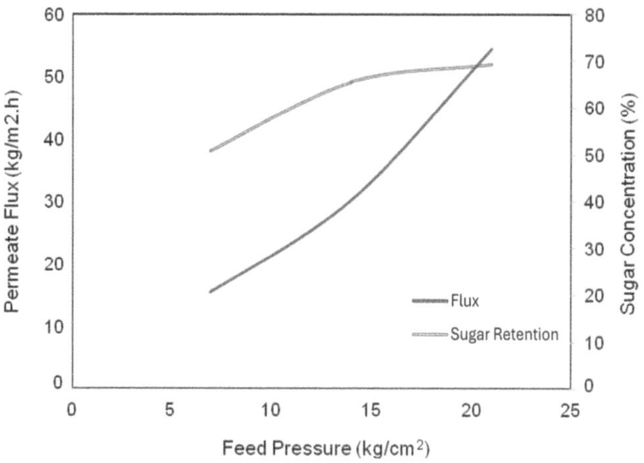

FIGURE 25.6 Effect of feed pressure on permeate flux and sugar retention in concentrates stream for HPA-100 nanofiltration membrane.

in the retentate, the solute flux remains more or less the same; however, in the present case, sugar molecules have some polarity, which limits their permeation to a lesser extent. HPA-100 was also subjected to a trial where the feed concentration was changed to 3% while the pressure was maintained at 21 kg/cm^2. However, it was possible to concentrate the sugar to 11.91%, which is nearly four times the initial content, but at a water recovery of 71.3% and a water flux of 6.58 L/m^2/hr, due to the high osmotic pressure. However, the losses in the permeate were negligible at only 0.06%, indicating great commercial potential for the NF process in biorefineries.

25.3.2 Fermentation Aided by Pervaporation

The production of bioethanol from lignocellulosic biomass is mainly classified into three series of steps: (a) to produce fermentable sugars, (b) conversion of fermented sugars into bioethanol, and (c) separation and concentration of bioethanol through the process of distillation (Demirbas, 2005; Asgher et al., 2014). Jiang et al. (2025) used a pervaporation-aided MBR to produce bioethanol from cassava feedstock in a batch fermenter, while Liu et al. (2025) designed a pilot plant to analyze the performance of a pervaporation membrane bioreactor with mechanical vapor compression for bioethanol production. Enzymatic hydrolysis breaks down polysaccharides into simple sugars, such as hexoses and pentoses, for fermentation by microorganisms. However, bioethanol formation itself inhibits microbial activity, limiting the maximum yield to only 4–6%.

Mokaram and Esfahanian successfully used polydimethyl siloxane (PDMS) membrane for bioethanol separation. To overcome this limitation, hydrophobic PV using a dense polyvinyl chloride (PVC) membrane can be coupled to the

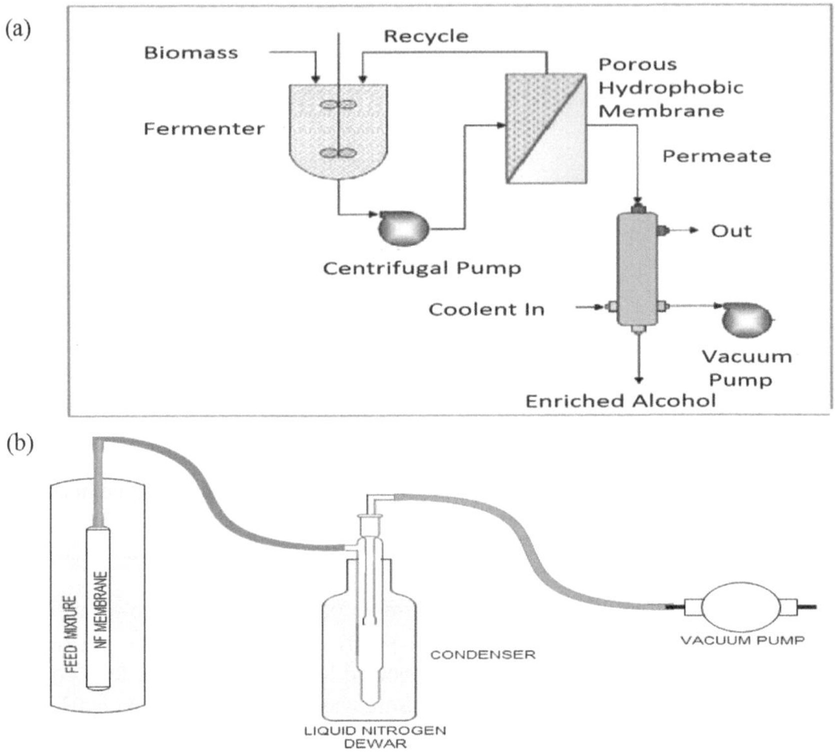

FIGURE 25.7 Selective separations of ethanol from aqueous fermentation medium by hydrophobic and hydrophilic pervaporation.

fermenter for the continuous, selective removal of ethanol, thereby enhancing ethanol yield by retaining yeast activity (Figure 25.7(a)). Synthetic ethanol-water mixtures were subjected to pervaporation as shown in Figure 25.7(a). Even hydrophilic pervaporation using a nanoporous hydrophilized polyamide membrane yielded promising results for ethanol extraction from water owing to ethanol's greater volatility [Figure 25.7(b)].

Table 25.4 shows high selectivity for the extraction of ethanol from aqueous solutions using the hydrophobic PVC membrane due to preferential sorption, diffusion, and desorption of ethanol through the organophilic PVC membrane. On the other hand, reasonable selectivity was observed with the nanoporous membrane, as water molecules would experience lower resistance to mass transfer through the nanopores. The lower flux through the nanoporous membrane is attributed to the lesser vacuum (higher permeate pressure during these experiments (Figure 25.7 (b)).

From Figure 25.8, it can be seen that an increase in feed ethanol concentration from 0.3% wt. to 7.55% wt. resulted in an increase in alcohol content in the permeate from 2.27% wt. to 50.24% wt. On the other hand, the ethanol flux increased from 0.004 to 0.50 kg/m²/hr. The hydrophobic PVC membrane preferentially sorbs more ethanol due to its organophilic nature.

TABLE 25.4
Performance of Various Membranes for Pervaporation-Based Extraction of Ethanol from Aqueous Synthetic Glucose Solutions

Membrane Type	Feed Ethanol Concentration (wt%)	Permeate Ethanol Concentration (wt%)	Ethanol Flux (kg/m²/hr)
Hydrophobic flatsheet PVC membrane	7.55	50.24	0.50
Hydrophobic flatsheet PVC membrane	3.30	19.21	0.19
Hydrophilic spiral wound PA membrane	2.68	9.47	0.002
Hydrophobic flatsheet PVC membrane	0.43	2.34	0.01
Hydrophobic flatsheet PVDF membrane	0.12	0.72	0.22

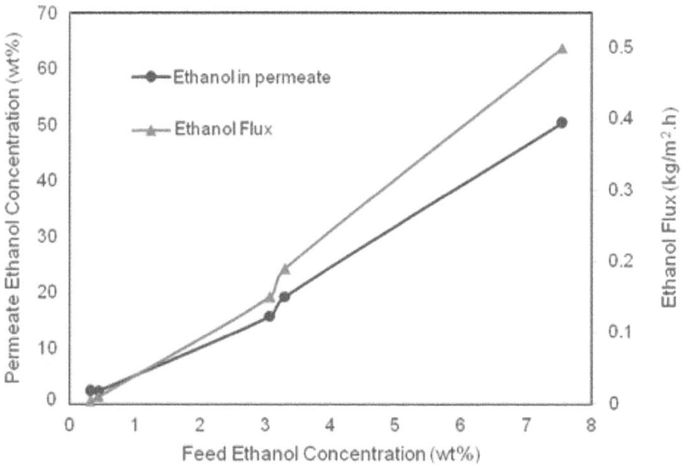

FIGURE 25.8 Effect of feed ethanol concentration on permeate ethanol content and flux through hydrophobic PVC membrane.

Hydrophilic PV membranes, such as polyvinyl alcohol (PVA), can also be used to dehydrate rectified spirit from 92% to absolute alcohol (99.5%) [Huang, 1991]. This would enable the exclusion of azeotropic distillation, which employs hazardous entrainers and is energy-intensive due to the high ethanol vaporization rate (92.1%) compared to the water (8%) separation by pervaporation.

25.3.3 MBR+RO Hybrid Process to Recover Spent Water from the Pretreatment Step

25.3.3.1 Reverse Osmosis

Reverse osmosis (RO) is aimed at the separation of ionic solutes, metals, and macromolecules from aqueous streams such as industrial wastewater and mining water (Sourirajan, 1970). Water is, in principle (Figure 25.9), the only material that passes through the membrane, while essentially all dissolved and suspended materials, both organic and inorganic, are rejected by RO membranes. The operating pressure of an RO system depends on the osmotic pressure of the solution and typically ranges from 15 to 60 bar (Wang et al., 2010). Separation of species is a function of the shape and size of the permeating species, their ionic charge, the membrane material properties and composition, and the interaction between the permeating species and the membrane. The most common applications of RO are desalination of seawater and brackish water and treatment of groundwater containing pollutants such as fluoride, arsenic, iron, nitrate, and heavy metals such as Hg and Pb. The ultimate goal of RO application is to retain feed components as product, to produce pure filtrate, or to reduce wastewater volume for disposal.

As shown in Figure 25.10, the hybrid process of MBR + RO achieved a high reduction in COD, from 2,850 mg/L to 120 mg/L, indicating potential for low-cost treatment of biomass wastewater on an industrial scale. A mixed microbial

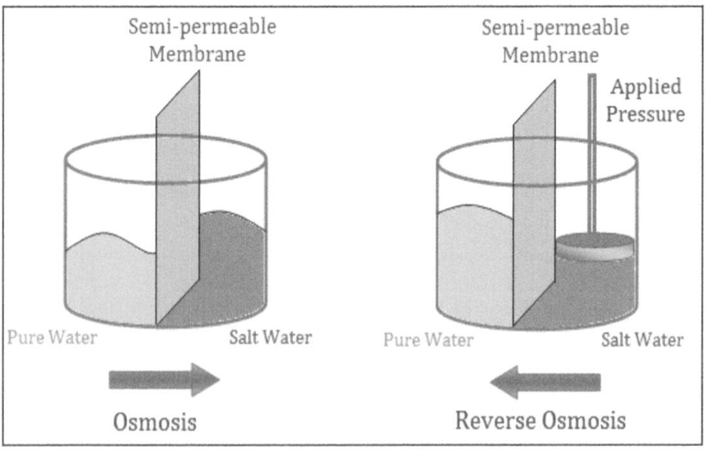

FIGURE 25.9 Schematic diagram of the reverse osmosis process.

The effluent from a biorefinery contains wash water from all pretreatment, hydrolysis, and fermentation steps. It therefore contains TSS, TDS, COD, BOD, and turbidity as impurities that should be removed to reclaim the water. TDS, comprising mostly inorganic salts and some organic impurities, was removed by more than 95%. However, COD comprises organics that can interact with the membrane and pass through. The presence of VSS, TSS, and COD in the effluent (Table 25.5) can easily form on the RO membrane and also reduce flux and rejection. However, their larger molecular sizes, as compared to water, which is also more polar, resulted in a reduction in COD by the RO step. Hence, a membrane bioreactor (MBR) was employed to reduce these contaminants by aeration followed by submerged UF to clarify the water. The UF-treated permeate is then sent to RO for further purification, reducing COD, inorganic salts, and other impurities to make the water fit for reuse in the biorefinery for washing.

TABLE 25.5
Reduction of COD (Chemical Oxygen Demand), TSS (Total Suspended Solids), and VSS (Volatile Suspended Solids) by MBR (Membrane Bioreactor)-RO (Reverse Osmosis) Integrated Process

Parameters	Feed	MBR+RO
COD (mg/L)	2850	120
Total suspended solids (mg/L)	7256	600
Volatile suspended solids (mg/L)	4354	823

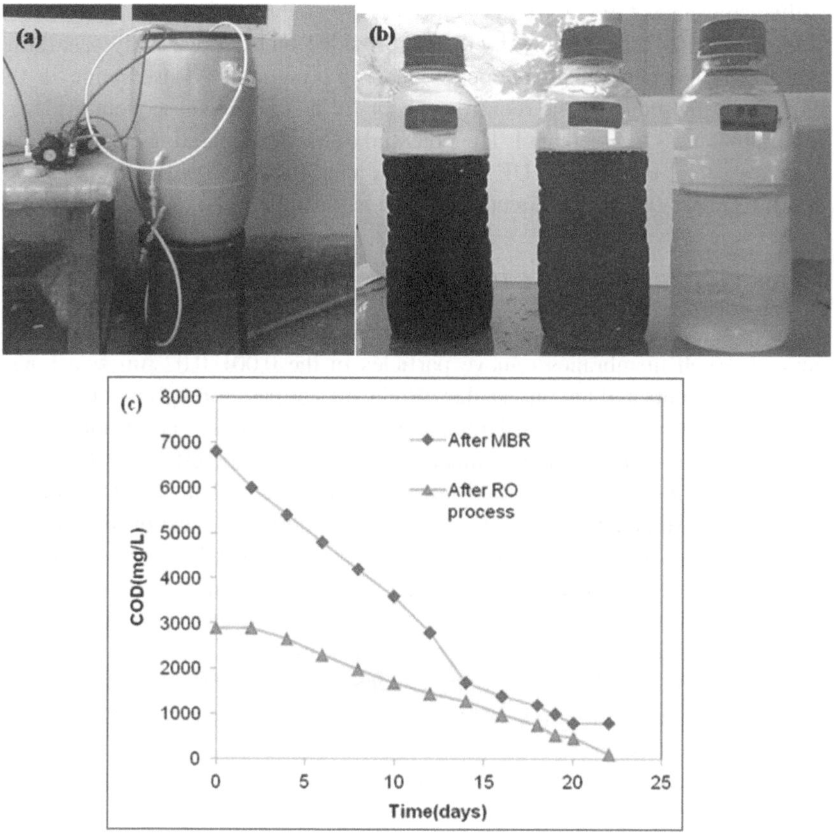

FIGURE 25.10 COD reduction with time.

culture was used in the aerobic process to break down COD and VSS. The anaerobic is to be tried. The acclimatization period was 7 days, with a sludge retention time of 22 days and a hydraulic retention time of 2 days. The sludge can undergo anaerobic digestion to produce biomanure and biogas. SRT (sludge retention time) was 22 days, while HRT (hydraulic retention time) was 2 days.

25.4 CONCLUSIONS

This study presents both hypothetical concepts and practical experimental results of membrane application at various steps of biorefinery. NF proves to be a promising technology for sugar concentration, with the HPA-100 spiral wound nanofiltration module capable of concentrating glucose from 3% to 11.91% (w/v) with minimal losses in permeate, thereby enhancing the feed sugar concentration for yeast fermentation and, thereby, bioethanol yield. Selective separation of bioethanol from synthetic aqueous solutions containing water and nutrients by pervaporation using dense PVC membranes enables increased bioethanol yield by preventing the product ethanol from inhibiting fermentation. PV produced a permeate with a high ethanol concentration, which would be easily and economically achievable at high purity (>99%).

Anaerobic MBR combined with RO provided reusable water by separating inorganics and degrading organic COD, promoting water conservation in the biorefinery by reducing the requirement for fresh water in subsequent cycles of refining biomass to bioethanol. The potential of MF for separating enzymes from their microbial cultures, of UF for enzyme concentration, and of ED for acid/alkali recovery from the pretreatment stage is illustrated.

25.5 FUTURE PROSPECTS

Ultrafiltration: Ultrafiltration (UF) is another pressure-driven membrane process in which membranes remove particles in the 0.001–0.02 μm size range, allowing solvents and low-molecular-weight salts to pass through while simultaneously rejecting or retaining larger molecules. The primary application of the UF process is the separation of macromolecules. Osmotic effects in UF membranes are minor, and an applied operating pressure of 1–10 bar is primarily required to overcome the viscous resistance of liquid permeation through the membrane matrix's pore network. On the other hand, the MF separation process involves membranes with pore diameters of 0.1 to 10 μm. It can be designed for two operating configurations: dead-end filtration and cross-flow filtration, as shown in Figure 25.11, wherein operating pressure varies over a smaller range of 0–2 kg/cm^2. Dead-end filtration, as demonstrated in Figure 25.11(a), is the most basic form of filtration, where the feed flow is forced through the membrane, and the filtered matter accumulates on its surface. Dead-end filtration is a batch process because the accumulation of matter on the filter reduces its filtration capacity due to clogging. This process requires another step to remove the accumulated matter. This filtration technique can be beneficial for concentrating enzymes used in the saccharification step or yeast in the fermentation process. During indigenous enzyme production, UF can facilitate the retention of enzymes and substrates in a continuous enzyme reactor, permitting the removal of reaction-inhibiting components.

In cross-flow filtration, a constant flow is maintained along the membrane surface, which prevents accumulation of solutes and suspended solids. The feed flowing through the membrane has an elevated pressure as a driving force for

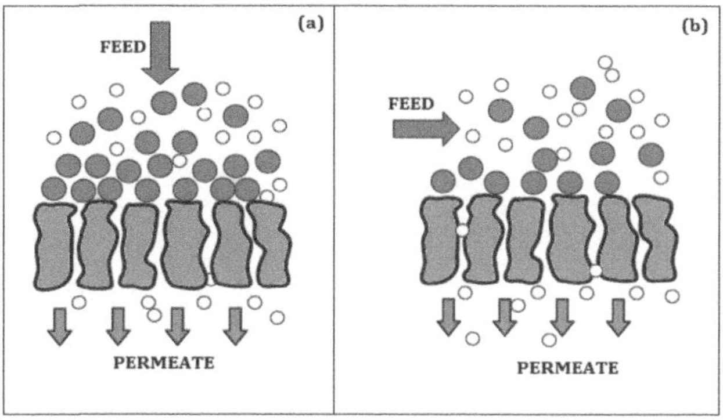

FIGURE 25.11 Schematic comparing (a) dead-end microfiltration with (b) cross-flow microfiltration.

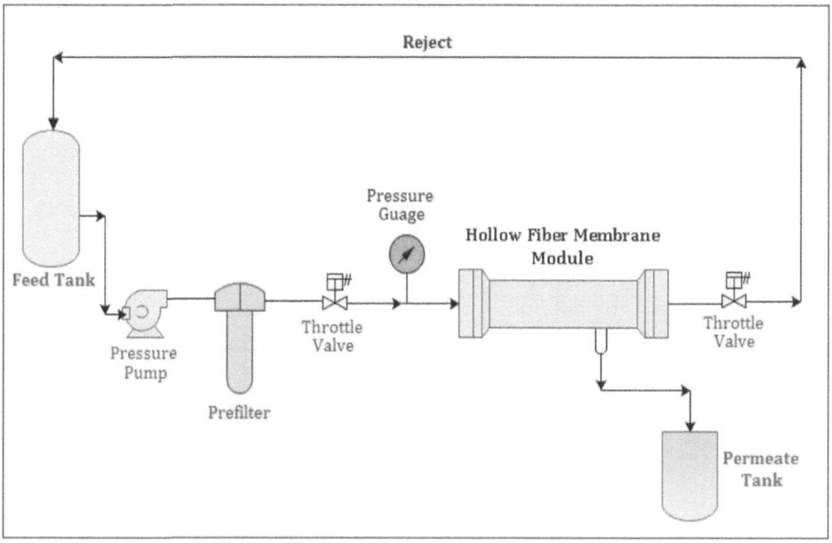

FIGURE 25.12 Schematic drawing of MF/UF experimental manifold.

the filtration process and a high flow speed to create turbulence. This process is referred to as "cross-flow," as the feed flow and filtration flow directions make a 90° angle. Cross-flow filtration is an excellent way to filter liquids having a high concentration of filterable matter as shown in Figure 25.12, which is applicable to both MF and UF processes though the methods for synthesis of MF and UF membranes are different.

MF can be used to isolate the enzyme from the microorganism that produces it, obtaining a clear enzymatic broth that can be further concentrated by UF, as shown in Figure 25.13. Figure 25.14 shows the schematic of a biorefinery facilitated by membrane processes.

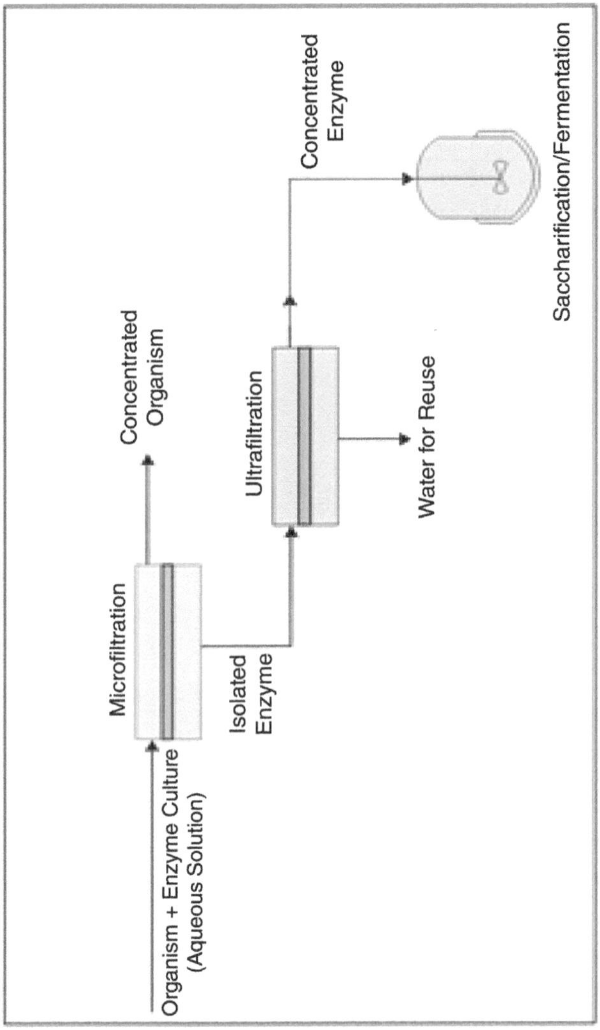

FIGURE 25.13 Indigenous enzyme clarification by MF and concentration by UF.

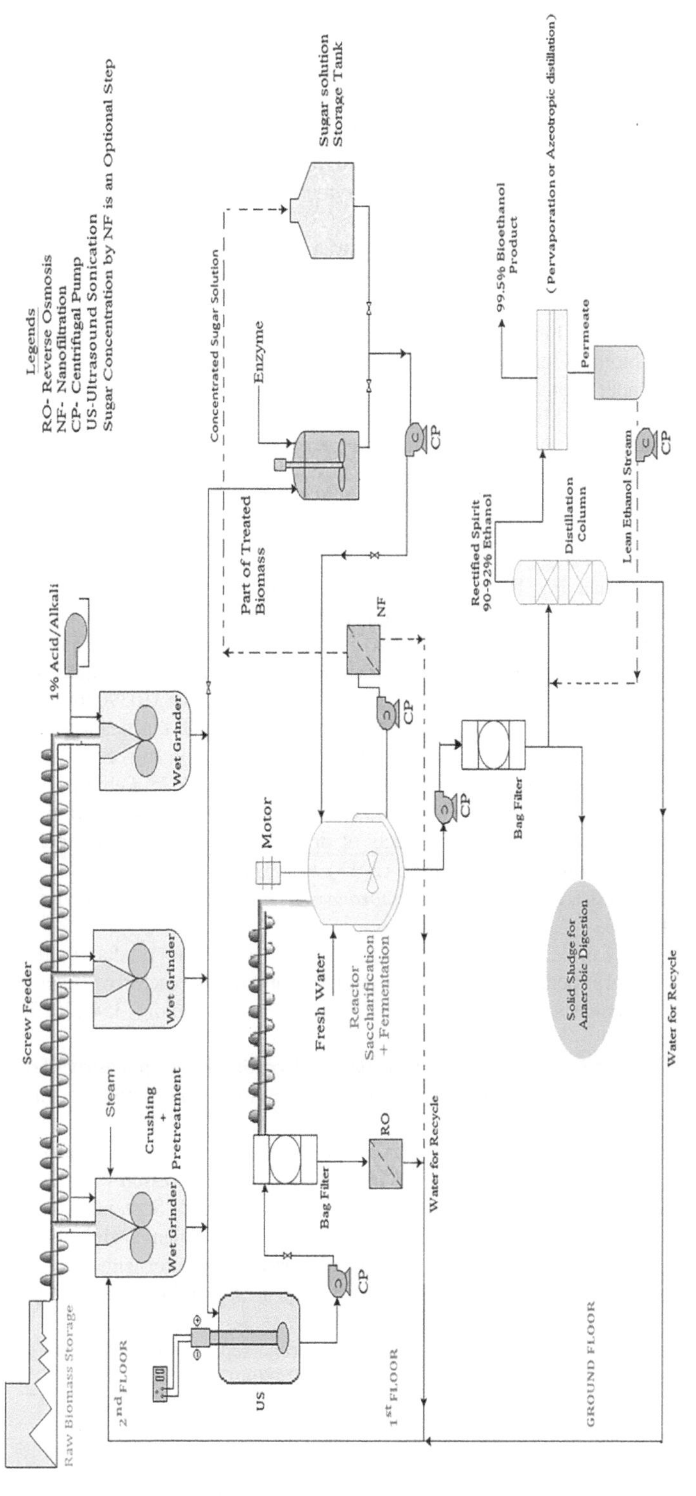

FIGURE 25.14 Biorefinery facilitated by membrane intervention.

REFERENCES

Almazan JE, Romero-Dondiz EM, Rajal VB, Castro-Vidaurre EF. Nanofiltration of glucose: Analysis of parameters and membrane characterization. *Chemical Engineering Research and Design* 94 (2015) 485–493.

Ang MB, Chou HY, Millare JC, Huang SH. High-performance polyurea thin-film composite membranes: Tailored interfacial polymerization for efficient bioethanol dehydration. *Journal of Membrane Science* 725 (2025, May 1) 123985.

Anwar Z, Gulfraz M, Irshad M. Agro-industrial lignocellulosic biomass a key to unlock the future bioenergy: A brief review. *Journal of Radiation Research and Applied Sciences* 7 (2014) 163–173.

Asgher M, Ahmad Z, Iqbal HM. Recent developments in enzymatic hydrolysis of lignocellulosic biomass for ethanol production. *Abbreviated Science* (also cited in some databases under related journals like Advances in Life Sciences) 2(2) (2013) 106–128.

Asgher M, Bashir F, Muhammad Nasir Iqbal H. A comprehensive ligninolytic pre-treatment approach from lignocellulose green biotechnology to produce bio-ethanol. *Chemical Engineering Research and Design* 92(8) (2014) 1571–1578.

Bowen T, Namboodiri V, Vane LM. *Emerging technologies for bioethanol recovery using membrane processes*. Presented at EPA Science forum, oral face-to-face post doc meeting, Washington, DC, 2005.

Chandel AK, Chan ES, Rudravaram R, Narasu ML, Venkateswa Rao L, Ravindra P. Economics and environmental impact of bioethanol production technologies: An appraisal. *Biotechnology and Molecular Biology Review* 2(1) (2007) 14–32.

Demirbas, A. Bioethanol from cellulosic materials: A renewable motor fuel from biomass. *Energy Sources* 27(4) (2005) 327–337. doi:10.1080/00908310390266643.

Diaz-Arenas GL, Stocker CW, Sadiq MM, Garnier G, Tanner J. Purification of Eucalyptus globulus steam explosion hydrolysates via nanofiltration to recover xylooligosaccharides. *Separation and Purification Technology* 354 (2025, February 19) 128898.

Hamzeha Y, Ashori A, Khorasani Z, Abdulkhani A, Abyaz A. Pre-extraction of hemicelluloses from bagasse fibers: Effects of dry-strength additives on paper properties. *Industrial Crops and Products* 43 (2013) 365–371.

R.Y.M. Huang (Ed.), *Pervaporation Membrane Separation Processes*, Elsevier, New York, 1991.

Jiang H, Han L, Liu W, Zhang Y, Liu J, Xiao Z, Fan S. Bioethanol production from cassava fed-batch fermentation in pervaporation membrane bioreactor with permeate fractional condensation. *Separation and Purification Technology* 354 (2025, February 19) 128807.

Jiang H, Liu J, Liu W, Xiao Z, Fan S. Bioethanol production from cassava fermentation in pervaporation membrane bioreactor fed with high concentration sugar. *Fuel* 362 (2024, April 15) 130744.

Li F, Kawajiri S, Al-Duri B, Oshima Y, Akizuki M. Recovery of concentrated saccharide solution from microalgal residue via combined hot compressed water treatment and membrane separation. *Biomass and Bioenergy* 200 (2025, September 1) 107975.

Liu J, Zhang Y, Liu W, Jiang H, Han L, Xiao Z, Fan S. Pilot plant design and technology performance analysis of pervaporation membrane bioreactor with mechanical vapor compression for bioethanol production. *Chinese Journal of Chemical Engineering* 82 (2025) 57–66.

Mandalika AS, Runge TM, Ragauskas AJ. Membrane separations in biomass processing. *ChemPlusChem* 90(2) (2025, February) e202400497.

Mansy AE, El Desouky EA, Saleh AK, Abu-Saied MA, Taha TH, El-Zawawy WK, Abdel-Fattah YR. Separation of bioethanol using in situ composite membrane of bacterial cellulose/poly (2-acrylamido-2-methylpropane sulfonic acid) (AMPS) and their characterization. *Biomass Conversion and Biorefinery* 14(16) (2024 August) 18697–18706.

Mansy AE, El Desouky EA, Taha TH, Abu-Saied MA, El-Gendi H, Amer RA, Tian ZY. Sustainable production of bioethanol from office paper waste and its purification via blended polymeric membrane. *Energy Conversion and Management* 299 (2024, January 1) 117855.

Moiser N, Wyman C, Dale B, Elander R, Lee YY, Holtzapple M, Ladisch M. Features of promising technologies for pretreatment of lignocellulosic biomass. *Bio. Res. Technol.* 96 (2005) 673–686.

Mokaram MM, Esfahanian M. Bioethanol fermentation integrated with PDMS membrane modified by carbon nanotube and graphene oxide from sugarcane bagasse. *Biomass Conversion and Biorefinery* (2024, August 14) 1–5.

S. Moulik, Pavani Vadthya, K. Yamuna Rani, C. Sumana, and S. Sridhar, Production of fructose sugar from aqueous solutions: nanofiltration performance and hydrodynamic analysis, *Journal of Cleaner Production*, Vol. 92 (2015) 44–53.

Rafik M, Qabli H, Belhamidi S, Elhannouni F, Elkhedmaoui A, Elmidaoui A. Membrane separation in the sugar industry. *Journal of Chemical and Pharmaceutical Research* 7(9) (2015) 653–658.

Sourirajan S. Reverse osmosis. Loeb-Sourirajan process. "The Seminal Book: Reverse Osmosis", Logos Press, London/Academic Press, New York, 1970.

S. Sridhar, Aniket Kale and A. A. Khan, "Reverse Osmosis of Edible Vegetable Oil Industry Effluent", *Journal of Membrane Science*, Vol. 205 (2002) pp 83–90.

Wandscher Busanello F, Sérgi Gomes MC, Paschoal SM, Rodrigues da Silva Baumgärtner T, Barp G, Fiorentin-Ferrari LD. The influence of membrane separation technique in the biodiesel and bioethanol production process: A review. *Biofuels* 15(7) (2024, August 8) 903–928.

Wang LK, Paul Chen J, Hung Y-T, Shammas NK. Membrane and desalination technologies, Humana Press (imprint of Springer Science & Business Media), 2010.

Wyman CE. Ethanol from lignocellulosic biomass: Technology, economics, and opportunities. *Bio. Res. Technol.* 50 (1994) 3–16.

Wyman CE, Dale BE. *Energy consumption analysis of integrated flow sheets for production of fuel ethanol from lignocellulosic biomass*, Dartmouth College, Hanover, NH, United States, 2005.

Wyman CE, Hinman ND. Ethanol: Fundamentals of production from renewable feed stocks and use as a transportation fuel. *Appl. Biochem. Biotech.* 24–25 (1990) 735.

Yang B, Wyman CE. Characterization of the degree of polymerization of xylooligomers produced by flow through hydrolysis of pure xylan and corn stover with water. *Bioresource Technology* 99(13), 5756–5762. DOI: 10.1016/j.biortech.2007.10.054.

Index

B

C

D

E

F

G

H

I

J

K

L

N

O

P

Q

R

T

U

V

Y

Z